PRESCHOOL ASSESSMENT

Preschool ASSESSMENT

Principles and Practices

MARLA R. BRASSARD
ANN E. BOEHM

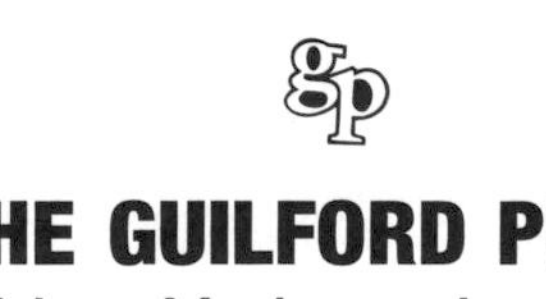

THE GUILFORD PRESS
New York London

A Division of Guilford Publications, Inc.
72 Spring Street, New York, NY 10012
www.guilford.com

Printed in the United States of America

This book is printed on acid-free paper.

Last digit is print number: 9 8 7 6 5 4 3 2 1

Library of Congress Cataloging-in-Publication Data

Brassard, Marla R.
Preschool assessment : principles and practices / Marla R. Brassard, Ann E. Boehm.
p. cm.
Includes bibliographical references and index.
ISBN-13: 978-1-59385-333-4 (hardcover : alk. paper)
ISBN-10: 1-59385-333-5 (hardcover : alk. paper)
1. Child development—Evaluation. 2. Ability—Testing. 3. Education, Preschool.
I. Boehm, Ann E., 1938– II. Title.
LB1131.B623 2007
372.126—dc22

2006039103

To our beloved husbands,
George Litchford and Neville Kaplan

To our fellow early childhood assessors,
committed to improving the lives of young children

In memory of the late Mary Alice White,
who trained us as scientist-practitioners

About the Authors

Marla R. Brassard, PhD, Associate Professor in the School Psychology Program at Teachers College, Columbia University, has been assessing preschool children and their families in research settings, public schools, and university clinics for over 25 years. Her research focuses on psychological maltreatment of children—its assessment, the emotional/behavioral injuries that result, and contextual factors that moderate the effect of maltreatment (particularly the role of schools, teachers, and peer relationships). Dr. Brassard has published two books on this topic—*Psychological Maltreatment of Children and Youth* (coedited with Robert Germain and Stuart N. Hart, 1987) and *Psychological Maltreatment of Children* (coauthored with Nelson J. Binggeli and Stuart N. Hart, 2001)—and many articles, chapters, special issues of journals, and pamphlets for parents and educators. In addition, she cochaired the task force that wrote the *Guidelines for the Psychosocial Evaluation of Suspected Psychological Maltreatment* (American Professional Society on the Abuse of Children, 1995). Instrument development in the area of psychological aggression/maltreatment has been another area of focus (Psychological Maltreatment Rating Scales, Teacher Psychological Aggression Scale). Dr. Brassard also investigates psychological aggression in teacher–student and peer relationships, and its impact on children's functioning, in a longitudinal study of secondary school children. She has worked in prisons, preschools, schools, and clinics with disabled, maltreated, and other troubled children and youth, and has taught courses and supervised practica in the university clinic in this area for over 25 years.

Ann E. Boehm, PhD, Professor Emerita in the School Psychology Program at Teachers College, Columbia University, is well known for her groundbreaking work in identifying the importance of young children's knowledge of basic relational concepts (e.g., *next to,* *after, first*) to their understanding of teacher and text directions. She has developed two widely used early childhood tests to assess this knowledge—the Boehm Test of Basic Concepts, Third Edition, for grades K–2 (2000), and the Boehm Test of Basic Concepts, Third Edition: Preschool (2001)—and is working on editions of both tests for children with visual impairments. She is the author (with Richard Weinberg) of *The Classroom Observer* (third edition) and has written extensively on assessment issues at the early childhood level. Dr. Boehm also cosponsors an annual conference and teaches a graduate course entitled "Observing and Assessing the Preschool Child." Her research interests include cross-cultural development of relational concepts used in different direction formats, the role of comprehension in direction following, and intergenerational literacy. She has been a preschool psychologist, a teacher, and a consultant for Head Start. Most of her teaching has been focused on the psychoeducational assessment of young children, practica on cognitive functioning, and issues regarding the practice of school psychology.

Preface

This book presents an integrated analysis of the issues and practices of preschool assessment, from our perspective as practicing clinicians-researchers. The book is written both for graduate students and for practicing assessors, including school and child clinical psychologists, early childhood and special educators, learning disability specialists, and speech–language specialists. Designed to be a primary text in courses on preschool/early childhood assessment and a manual for clinical practice, the book focuses on how to think about assessment issues, select appropriate measures and procedures (extensive test reviews are presented), and integrate diverse information for use in decision making; there is less emphasis on how to administer tests. The book offers a synopsis of current research, federal laws, and practice relevant to preschool assessment, illustrated with actual case examples. It describes our thinking as we (1) share a comprehensive developmental model of preschool assessment; (2) describe how to establish and evaluate screening programs for instructional and child-finding purposes; (3) present suggestions for establishing good working relationships with families of children ages 3–6 from diverse backgrounds; (4) collect information relevant to understanding developmental problems and making diagnoses; and (5) link assessment findings to intervention and program planning.

With the passage of the No Child Left Behind (NCLB) Act of 2001, promoting children's early language and cognitive development has become federal policy. The requirements of the NCLB legislation have further prodded state policymakers into defining the goals of formal schooling and articulating early learning standards for their preschool populations. States are increasingly funding universal programs as legislators take note of the research supporting the efficacy of these programs in preparing young children to learn when they start formal schooling, especially children from low-income and minority populations.

The need for preschool programs to promote *all* areas of children's development is only gradually being acknowledged. When Scott-Little, Kagan, and Frelow (2006) reviewed 46 early learning standards documents developed by state-level organizations and compared them with the five domains of school readiness identified by the National Education Goals Panel (NEGP, 1997), they found an almost universal emphasis on the domains of language and communication development and of cognition and general knowledge. There was a relative lack of attention to the domains of physical well-being, social and emotional development, and approaches to learning (e.g., task persistence)—all of which research shows to be important for school success. We hope that states' early learning standards will evolve into comprehensive multidomain standards that target the whole child, as emphasized in this text.

These government initiatives expand the role of early childhood assessors—hitherto focused primarily on assessment and placement of preschool children with disabilities—into consultation around what to assess, what measures to use, and what curricula to select in order to achieve these early learning standards. This book covers assessment of all of the NEGP domains of school readiness except physical well-being. Moreover, it goes beyond these domains by covering assessment of the strengths and needs of preschool/kindergarten children within the contexts of the home, childcare center, school, and other learning environments, and the integration of this information in planning interventions that address the whole child. The focus on children 3 through 6 years of age includes the traditional transition points from early intervention to preschool, from preschool to kindergarten, and from kindergarten to the formal learning demands of first grade.

The two of us have been preschool psychologists and have taught and supervised practica in this area for over 20 years. We contributed equally to the conceptualization and writing of this book and flipped a coin to determine the order of authorship. The two chapters on cognitive assessment and assessment of children with mental retardation were written by Susan Vig, PhD, and Michelle Sanders, PsyD. We are grateful that our readers can benefit, as have we, from their extensive experience and scholarship in these areas.

ORIENTATION TO THE BOOK

Chapter 1 surveys the contexts (legal, demographic, social) in which preschool assessors do their work, as well as the protective and risk factors that affect children's functioning. Chapter 2 presents our theoretical model of preschool assessment, describes the assessment process, and notes the characteristics of preschool children that are relevant to assessment. In Chapter 3, we review the technical characteristics of assessment measures administered to preschool children, in order to help assessors select tests and interpret results. Chapter 4 presents what we consider the key technique for assessment of preschoolers: observation of the child. Chapter 5 describes observation of the childcare/preschool environment. In Chapter 6, developmental screening practices and assessment are covered in detail, so that readers can select appropriate measures for their population and implement a program in their district or agency. Chapter 7 critiques traditional approaches to readiness assessment and details the importance of instructional screening for emergent literacy. Curriculum-based assessment, portfolio assessment, strategy assessment, and testing modifications are also presented. Chapter 8 reviews the major models of family assessment and intervention; discusses how to develop a productive working relationship with families; and presents a model of family assessment as a collaborative approach to identifying critical aspects of family functioning for support and/or change. Chapter 9, on the assessment of culturally and linguistically diverse children and their families, examines a great deal of information on becoming culturally sensitive and self-aware; it also discusses bilingualism, bilingual education, and culturally sensitive assessment practices.

Chapter 10 covers the major areas that early childhood assessors, who are not speech–language specialists, need to know about language development and assessment, in order to promote development in this area. In Chapters 11 and 12, Susan Vig and Michelle Sanders describe critical aspects of cognitive development during the preschool period, and then review current measures in terms of how validly they capture the cognitive functioning of preschool children—especially those most likely to be referred for a cognitive evaluation, children with mental retardation. Chapter 13 discusses the screening, diagnosis, and treatment of children with autism spectrum disorders. Chapter 14 is based on the research-supported premise that emotional development leads directly to social development, and socioemotional competence is as important as cognitive skills in determining school success. It presents emotional milestones and the factors that influence them; a model for assessing emotional skills, as well as curricula that promote such skills; diagnostic models for children with emotional and behavioral problems; and an assessment approach for these children, along with useful measures. Case studies are used throughout the book to illustrate assessment strategies and measures, as well as possible interventions.

ACKNOWLEDGMENTS

Many people have encouraged us and have contributed to the development of this book; we are very grateful to them all. Many years ago we were motivated by Sharon Panulla, who then worked at The Guilford Press, to write the book. After Sharon's departure, we were encouraged by Chris Jennison, who had confidence in us through the years of research and writing the chapters. Craig Thomas has helped us greatly to pull everything together with high-quality suggestions. Finally, we deeply appreciate the marvelous editing by our copy editor, Marie Sprayberry, and production editor, Anna Nelson.

We would also like to thank the many graduate assistants who have been of great help in finding and reviewing tests and materials, including Pooja Vekaria, Anna Ward, Kera Miller, Natascha Crandall, Arjan Graybill, Chris Mullen, Melania Puza Pearl, and Lindsay Reddington; the secretaries who have worked with us throughout this project, Colleen Wood and Laura Stellato; our students, anonymous reviewers, and colleagues (Lois Dreyer, Richard Weinberg, Virginia Stolarski, Denise Green, Maria Hartman) who have critiqued chapters, offering many helpful recommendations; and the family members who co-read chapters (including our husbands and Lydia and Shaina Brassard). Most importantly, we would like to thank our husbands, George Litchford and Neville Kaplan, for their unending patience, encouragement, and pressure to finish "THE BOOK" that has consumed our lives for these many years.

Contents

Chapter 1

A Framework for Preschool Assessment

The impact of a child's early years on later development is widely recognized by early childhood educators and researchers. Economic, social, and legislative forces are all focusing attention on the importance of these years for the child's physical, emotional, language, cognitive, and social development. The topic of this book is assessing the strengths and needs of children ages 3–6 years within the context of the home, childcare, school, or other learning environments. The focus on children in this age group includes the traditional transition points from preschool to kindergarten and from kindergarten to the formal learning demands of first grade, as well as the less traditional transition from early intervention to preschool. (Note that although we sometimes use the term *preschool* as we have done just now—that is, to refer to educational experiences prior to kindergarten—we also use the term *preschool assessment* throughout this book in a broader sense, to refer to assessment of all children from age 3 from until the traditional first-grade entry age of 6. The book does not, however, cover assessment of preschool children who have sensory or motor impairments. Assessment of the gifted is covered briefly in Chapter 11.)

The purpose of this chapter is to develop a framework for considering important risk and protective environmental factors in relationship to a given child. This framework provides assessors with a foundation for interpreting assessment outcomes and developing intervention. In the sections that follow, legislation that affects assessment practices is reviewed, followed by a summary of key interacting influences on child development: (1) poverty; (2) effects of parental substance abuse; (3) work constraints, childcare, and caregiving; (4) early intervention; (5) multiple risk factors; (6) violence and maltreatment; (7) protective factors; (8) resilience in children; (9) environmental forces in childcare and educational settings; (10) sociocultural considerations; and (11) the nature of child development itself. First, however, we define preschool assessment and consider its functions.

DEFINITION AND FUNCTIONS OF PRESCHOOL ASSESSMENT

The term *preschool assessment* covers a broad range of procedures used to gather information relevant to understanding the functioning of young children. It includes standardized testing; observation; parent and teacher interviews and ratings; and evaluation of work samples, records, and environmental factors. There is widespread agreement on the part of educators and other early childhood specialists (e.g., school psychologists, early childhood special educators, social workers, speech pathologists, pediatric nurses, physicians, occupational and physical therapists) that the ultimate goal of preschool assessment needs to be the improvement of learning experiences for all young children. In a position statement regarding standardized testing, the National Association for the Education of Young Children (NAEYC, 1988) succinctly states the issue: "The purpose of testing must be to improve services for children and ensure that children benefit from their educational experiences" (p. 14). This purpose can best be served when assessment is an *ongoing* and *dynamic* process that:

- Is multifaceted (i.e., it uses a variety of measures and approaches).
- Focuses not only on an individual child, but also on his or her learning environments of home, school, and community.
- Is used to discover children's learning strengths, emerging areas of development, problem-solving strategies, and personal styles, as well as their weaknesses and needs.
- Informs the development of appropriate instructional and behavioral strategies and interventions.
- Is tied to teaching goals, which in turn need to be evaluated and refined over time.
- Is carried out with the expectation that children will change, and that the earlier an intervention occurs, the greater its prospects for producing beneficial outcomes.
- Respects the diversity of children's backgrounds and experiences.

Assessment serves another essential function—that of progress evaluation. In the United States, this function has become an area of central concern with the passage of the No Child Left Behind (NCLB) Act of 2001 (see below). This act mandates accountability for student performance, even as early as the preschool years.

Therefore, it can be expected that preschool assessment in its varying forms will play a major role in making decisions and in developing learning experiences/curricula tailored to meet child and family needs. Assessment needs to incorporate research evidence and needs to focus on both learners and their learning environments, including the contributions of parents, family members, members of the community, teachers, all other relevant school personnel, and specialists. Integrating assessment outcomes into successful intervention in school settings can take place through initiatives funded under the Early Reading First Program (an aspect of the NCLB legislation). Such initiatives should use curriculum-relevant measures and the real-life tasks of play, ongoing consultation, and intensive workshops with teachers and parents to illustrate the meaning of assessment results and their implications for learning and intervention activities with children. This process requires participants to focus not only on scores (if formal testing procedures are used), but on the pattern of children's errors, successes, strategies used to arrive at responses, and environmental supports and teaching strategies that facilitate learning both at school and at home. To achieve these goals, it is important that assessors and early childhood specialists work collaboratively with classroom teachers, childcare staff, and parents—not only discussing individual children, but also modeling behaviors, facilitating home–school partnerships, obtaining culturally relevant data on effective strategies, and learning themselves from parents and teachers/caregivers. When this model is followed, the results of assessment can help teachers and parents alike enhance their understanding of children, achieve their goals and objectives, and realize their own importance in affecting the quality of instruction.

Translating assessment into successful intervention in clinical settings also involves ongoing consultation with parents and other important adults in a child's life (e.g., grandmothers, nannies, teachers, childcare personnel). However, clinical intervention may include a variety of more intensive approaches than are typically used in school settings, such as a support group for parents of children with autism or other disabilities, behavioral family treatment for a family with a highly disruptive child, or psychotherapy with a child suffering from posttraumatic stress disorder.

Parents need to be involved in the assessment process in many ways—not only to provide information about their child's development and particular needs, but also to gain an increased awareness of their own importance in their child's early development and of the need for their participation in the child's schooling. Within this context, assessment takes on a new dimension; it becomes an ongoing process integral to teaching, intervention, and adjusting learning experiences to meet child and family needs. Using the research literatures in developmental and cognitive psychology, education, and early childhood disabilities, as well as on the effects of different instructional and educational procedures, assessors can play a major role in improving services for children and in assisting teachers, parents, and important others in helping them benefit from their educational experiences.

Attention to the role of preschool assessment and intervention has become an area of national interest. The importance of the preschool years in providing the basic foundations for children's later learning was documented by researchers in the early 1960s (Bloom, 1964; Bruner, 1960; Hunt, 1961) and continues to be an area of research concern in our increasingly diverse society. In the United States, the importance of the preschool years was also recognized in the passage of Public Law 99-457 (the Education of the Handicapped Act Amendments of 1986), the downward extension of Public Law 94-142 (the Education for All Handicapped Children Act of 1975). Both of these laws were incorporated into Public Law 101-476 (the Individuals with Disabilities Act [IDEA] of 1990), then Public Law 105-17 (the IDEA Amendments of 1997), and finally Public Law 108-446 (the IDEA Improvement Act of 2004, which is generally known as IDEA 2004). Public Law 99-457 mandated a free and appropriate public education for all disabled children 3–5 years of age, and early intervention services to disabled children (0–2 years of age and their families. Passage of Public Law 107-110 (the NCLB Act of 2001), mandating accountability, has again highlighted the importance of the preschool years. Details of this legislation follow.

U.S. FEDERAL AND STATE LEGISLATION

Over the past 30 years, increased federal and state involvement has focused on improving the development of preschool children. At first, most of the major programs that were introduced focused on specific target groups of children with special needs, such as children from low-income backgrounds and those with particular disabilities (Gallagher, 1989). This changed with passage of the Education of the Handicapped Act Amendments of 1986 (Public Law 99-457). The broad purposes of this legislation were to (1) enhance the development of infants and toddlers with disabilities and to minimize their potential for developmental delay; (2) reduce the educational costs to society by minimizing the need for special education and related services after infants and toddlers with disabilities reach school age; (3) minimize the likelihood of institutionalization of individuals with disabilities and maximize the potential for their independent living in society; and (4) enhance the capacity of families to meet the special needs of their infants and toddlers with disabilities. Part H of the legislation established for the first time a national policy to serve infants and toddlers through age 2 with disabilities and their families. Part B of this legislation focused on children ages 3–5 and allowed states to serve children within this age group without labeling them. Since the legislative provisions of the IDEA Amendments of 1997, subsequently reaffirmed in IDEA 2004, do not require states to classify 3- to 9-year-old children into disability categories and have added the eligibility designation of "developmental delay," how such delay (or the risk for such delay) is determined is a critical issue. The definition of delay or risk in turn, determines how many children need to be provided with services. The outcome of this decision will also affect the funds states will need to contribute, in addition to those funds provided by the federal government and the amount districts spend on each child. However, there are no uniform criteria across states regarding developmental delay.

IDEA 2004 for children ages 3–9 designates a "disability," at the discretion of the state and local educational agency, as the experience of developmental delays in one or more of several areas (physical, cognitive, communicative, social or emotional, or adaptive development), and the resulting need for special education and related services. Some states use the 13 disability categories specified by 34 C.F.R. 300; plus general descriptors "at risk" or "developmentally delayed." These 13 categories include hearing impairments (including deafness), deaf-blindness, mental retardation, autism, orthopedic impairments, emotional disturbance, traumatic brain injury, multiple disabilities, other health impairments, serious emotional disturbances, specific learning disabilities (LD), speech or language impairments, and visual impairments. The flexibility in definitions given to states sometimes results in children's qualifying for services in one district but being denied services in another. Such a varying yardstick in turn may affect a family's mobility. On the other hand, local criteria allow greater sensitivity to community and cultural perspectives regarding how development unfolds and how developmental delay is perceived by families. Great caution, however, needs to be exercised in labeling children to be served. Barnett and Escobar (1987) point to a sobering conclusion that still holds true today: The vast majority of the children identified as having disabilities at school age are not thus identified as preschoolers, and many of them are disadvantaged.

Although multiple child and environmental factors are associated with developmental disorders and are of concern for assessors, they generally are not accounted for in any systematic way when assessors are determining delay and planning intervention. Furthermore, as noted earlier, projecting the number of children eligible for services varies according to how risk is determined. Simeonsson (1991) indicates that with children ages 0–3, this number can range from 33% of the population if a single risk factor is used to 25% if multiple risk factors are used, and to 16% if a particular combination of multiple risk factors is used. Thus, while Public Law 101-476 made a major advance in not requiring states to classify 3- to 5-year-old children into disability categories, many states or districts still *do* categorize children based on their performance on tests and do not focus on the interplay of child and environmental factors. And although the designations "developmentally delayed" or "at risk" do not refer to specific disabilities, they are still labels that are of great concern to parents and many early childhood specialists.

IDEA 2004 reaffirms the federal government's commitment to providing services to all children with disabilities, and in particular providing a "free and appropriate education" (FAPE) to all children with disabilities ages 3–21. In IDEA 2004, the U.S. Congress took note of the fact that although prior legislation (Public Law 94-142, IDEA, IDEA Amendments of 1997) had succeeded in providing children with disabilities and their families access to FAPE, nonetheless a number of factors had impeded full implementation of these laws—specifically, low expectations and an insufficient focus on applying research-supported methods for teaching children with disabilities. Among the effective practices supported in research, the law takes note of the following:

- The importance of having high expectations for children with disabilities and having these children participate in the regular curriculum as much as possible, with the goal of productive, independent living as adults.
- Strengthening the ability of parents to participate meaningfully in the education of their children at home and at school.
- Coordinating improvement efforts from the local to the federal level, such that special education becomes a service rather than a place where children are sent.
- Providing appropriate special education services and regular classroom supports to children with disabilities wherever and whenever appropriate.
- Supporting high-quality preservice and professional development, such that all personnel are trained to be effective in using scientifically supported practices to improve the academic performance and functional behavior of children with disabilities.
- Providing incentives to use whole-school approaches, such as research-supported early reading programs, positive behavior interventions/supports, and early intervention to reduce the number of children labeled as having disabilities.
- Focusing efforts on teaching and learning while reducing nonessential paperwork.
- Supporting the development and use of adaptive technology.

Other provisions of IDEA 2004 of relevance to preschool assessors include the following:

- Parents of a child receiving early intervention services for a toddler may request to continue to have an individualized family service plan (IFSP) rather than an individualized education plan (IEP) when their child turns 3 and would otherwise move to an IEP, as long as the IFSP includes services that will promote school readiness, including preliteracy, language, and numeracy.
- States and local educational agencies cannot require a child to take medication (a controlled substance) as a requirement for attending school.
- School districts must screen for disabilities in populations that have long been neglected: children attending private schools, living in shelters for homeless persons, or from migrant families.
- Assessment tools and strategies must not only be valid for deciding that a child has a disability; they must directly assist the IEP team in determining the educational needs of the child by comprehensively assessing all areas related to the disability as appropriate (e.g., vision, health, social and emotional functioning, intelligence, hearing, communication, motor and academic achievement), even if such areas are not commonly linked to the child's disability category.
- Children with limited English proficiency (LEP) must be assessed in the language they use and know best, if at all feasible.

- Children cannot be found to have a disability if the basis of the determination is either LEP or a lack of appropriate instruction in the essential components of reading and math.
- In developing the IEP, the team must take into consideration the child's strengths; the concerns of the parents; the results of the most recent evaluation; and the academic, functional and developmental needs of the child.

Another landmark piece of legislation that affects educational practice with preschool children is the NCLB legislation of 2001. The NCLB Act emphasizes four key points: accountability for results; greater flexibility for states, districts, and schools in the use of federal funds; more choices for parents of disadvantaged backgrounds; and the use of empirically supported methods of teaching (U.S. Department of Education, n.d.). Also stressed are reading for young children, improving the quality of teachers, and ensuring that all students master English prior to graduation.

In terms of accountability, annual assessments are mandated for reading and math in grades 3–8. This affects preschool and kindergarten children directly: In order to do well by third grade, children need to get off to a strong start. The NCLB legislation supports scientifically based reading instruction in the early grades under the Reading First Program and in preschool under the Early Reading First Program; it also calls for discretionary grants to the states for curriculum development, professional development, implementation, and evaluation. With NCLB's heavy emphasis on mastery of literacy and numeracy in English, much of the first-grade curriculum is being moved to kindergarten and the kindergarten curriculum to preschool.

The ramifications and specific aspects of IDEA 2004 and the NCLB Act are discussed throughout the book as they relate to information in each of the chapters.

KEY INTERACTING INFLUENCES ON DEVELOPMENT

There is little question that the family and the home are the most critical influences on the development of young children. And parenting is probably the most difficult job facing most adults. The family provides the physical means for the child's physical and psychological well-being and development. It is through the family, home, and community environments that the child gains concepts of the world and of interpersonal relationships, and develops cognitive, language, communication, and social skills. Interacting parental and contextual factors that have an impact on the family, and therefore on the child, include prenatal and postnatal care, substance abuse, illness, poverty, homelessness, divorce and single-parent status, teenage mothers, inconsistent childcare, maternal and paternal adjustment, English as a second language, cultural diversity, immigration, and maltreatment. Although space does not allow us to detail the contribution of each of these forces here, we raise a number of important concerns.

Poverty

Poverty (and the associated incidence of low birth weight and premature births) relates more often to vulnerability in young children than any other identifiable factor (Thurman & Widerstrom, 1985). Such vulnerability lasts throughout the preschool period, due to factors such as malnutrition, negative mother–child interaction patterns, and language experiences. The data suggest that children who live in poverty are much more likely to suffer from one or more disabilities. Natriello, McDill, and Pallas (1990) projected that by the year 2020 there will be a 33% increase in children reared in poverty—a trend already apparent with evidence that the economic plight of young families is increasing. Data from 2005 indicate that of 24 million children under age 6 in the United States, 42% live in low-income families that are just above the poverty line, and 20% in poor families. The federal poverty level in 2006 is about $20,000 for a family of four. (It varies by location.) Poor families have an income level that is below the poverty level, while low-income families are those that are above it but have less than the amount research suggests is needed to meet their most basic needs. In 2006 this would include families of four who have an income of less than $40,000 in Chicago or $36,000 in Houston. After a decade of decline, the proportion of children under 6 living in low-income families is rising (National Center for Children in Poverty, 2005). Not only is child poverty widespread geographically, but children of all racial and ethnic groups and family types are affected. Contrary to stereotypes, there are more poor European American than poor African American or Hispanic children (National Center for Children in Poverty, 2005), although the percentage of European American children who are poor is lower than the percentage of African American and Hispanic children who are poor. Sixty percent of children under age 6 from immigrant parents live in low-income families. The percentage of children from low-income families also varies by the region of the country where children live and by urban, suburban, or rural area (National Center for Children in Poverty, 2005).

A Children's Defense Fund (CDF, 1993b) special report on child poverty summarizes the following consequences of poverty for a child's overall well-being: lower measured intelligence, stunted growth, high lead blood levels (which place children at risk for impaired mental and physical development), difficulty in keeping up at school, and a three times greater likelihood of death during childhood. These issues are described in detail by McLoyd (1998) and the National Institute of Child Health and Human Development (NICHD) Early Child Care Research Network (2005). A number of other conditions are often related to poverty, such as late or no prenatal health care. Lack of prenatal care in turn greatly increases the probability of low birth weight and later health problems.

Brooks-Gunn and Duncan (1997) focused on national longitudinal data sets to estimate the effects of family income on children's lives. These researchers found that family income is more strongly related to children's ability and achievement than to their emotional outcomes (although these are also affected), and that the worst outcomes are for children who live in extreme poverty or below the poverty line for multiple years. They also point out that the associations between income and child outcomes are complex and varying. These authors document that low income during a child's preschool and early school years has a stronger relationship to school completion than during the childhood and adolescent years—an outcome which can be exacerbated by poor schooling and neighborhood poverty. These points are underscored by McLoyd (1998), who also highlights the importance of the neighborhood. Families residing in neighborhoods characterized by poverty frequently experience multiple stressors: less access to jobs, high-quality public or private services, and informal social supports, while at the same time greater exposure to street violence, homelessness, and negative role models.

The NICHD Early Child Care Research Network (2005) longitudinal study found that while any experience of poverty was associated with less favorable family situations and child outcomes, being poor later (from ages 4 to third grade) was more detrimental than being poor only early in life (birth–age 3). Persistent poverty was the most detrimental. Children from persistently poor families had the lowest performance on tests of language and school readiness. These children, along with those from families who were poor later, were also rated by mothers and teachers as having more externalizing and internalizing behavior problems.

The outcomes of poverty early in life are thus multifaceted and have important implications for learning. Based on an extensive synthesis of the outcomes of more than 3,000 studies, Walberg (1984) identified four major aptitude, instruction, and environmental factors that consistently affect learning. These include (1) the educationally stimulating psychological climate of the home; (2) the classroom social group; (3) the peer group outside the school; and (4) the use of out-of-school time (specifically, the amount of leisure-time television viewing). Important instructional variables cited by Walberg included the amount of time students engaged in learning and the quality of their instructional experience. No single factor was predominant; all factors were important. However, out-of-school factors, particularly the home environment, were powerful influences on learning. Supportive characteristics of the "alterable curriculum of the home" that were found to have strong influences on learning included

> informed parent–child conversations about school and everyday events; encouragement and discussion of leisure reading, monitoring and joint critical analysis of television viewing and peer activities; deferral of immediate gratification to accomplish long term human capital goals; expressions of affection and interest in the child's academic and other progress as a person; and perhaps, among such unremitting efforts, smiles, laughter, caprice, and serendipity. (Walberg, 1984, p. 25)

Although these factors play a critical role with school-age children, most are important as well with preschool children. Promotion of these activities can be built into parenting programs and home focused interventions, with a particular focus on those activities that promote literacy (such as joint storybook reading).

Effects of Parental Substance Abuse

Throughout the 1990s and into the 2000s, the use of psychoactive substances has increased dramatically, accompanied by the rapid spread of AIDS and the virus that causes AIDS (HIV). Parental substance abuse in particular is on a sharp rise, and this has important effects on childcare. In a survey of 915 professionals working in the field of child welfare, and in a review of the literature, the National Center on Addiction and Substance Abuse at Columbia University (CASA, 1999) found that the number of abused and neglected children in America jumped from 1.4 to 3 million in the period from 1986 to 1997. Alcohol and drug abuse are fueling this explosion. The use of alcohol in combination with other drugs is the most frequent problem. Children whose parents abuse drugs and alcohol, according to the CASA reports, are almost three times likelier to be physically or sexually assaulted and almost four times likelier to be neglected than children whose parents do not abuse substances. The costs are "incalculable" in terms of broken families and of children who are malnourished, neglected, and beaten. Today most cases of abuse and neglect by substance-abusing parents involve children under 5, and approximately 10% of all American children in this age range live with at least one parent who abuses substances (National Household Survey on Drug Abuse, 2003). Among the significant findings of the CASA reports are that substance abuse and addiction severely compromise or destroy the ability of parents to provide a safe and nurturing home for children (see also Accornero, Morrow, Bandstra, Johnson, & Anthony, 2002;

Messinger et al., 2004). Some of the relationship between parental substance abuse and poor child well-being is likely due to the co-occurrence of other risk factors in parents who abuse substances, such as limited education, poverty, and conflictual and unstable home environments (Clark, Cornelius, Wood, & Vanyukov, 2004). Many children of substance-abusing parents thus live in unstable, often dangerous environments (Howard, Beckwith, Rodning, & Kropenske, 1989), and the risks are considerably higher when both parents have substance abuse problems (Osborne & Berger, 2006).

Although there is great variation in the effects of substance abuse on children, these children often are cared for inconsistently by parents whose primary commitment is to chemicals, not to their children. The thoughts, attention, memory, and perceptions of such parents may be so impaired or distorted that they cannot function as protectors and advocates for their children. Based on their earlier research, Howard et al. (1989) found that toddlers who were raised in substance-abusing families scored within the low-average range on developmental tests. However, they showed striking deficits in free-play situations that required self-organization, self-initiation, and follow-through. Their play tended to be sparse and disorganized. Using data from the Fragile Families and Child Well-Being Study that included over 3,000 three-year-olds in families with at least one substance-abusing parent, Osborne and Berger (2006) found significant health and behavior problems in these children, including much higher rates of aggressive, anxious-depressed, attention-deficit/hyperactivity disorder, and oppositional defiant disorder behavior. Prenatal/birth characteristics, such as low birth weight and maternal cigarette and substance use during pregnancy, accounted for limited variance in the relationship between current parental substance use and poor child outcomes. This indicates that it is ongoing parental substance use that place children at risk, rather than prenatal substance exposure and/or problems at the time of birth.

Preventing parental substance abuse needs to be a top priority. The neglect or maltreatment that often results can have serious consequences for a child's physical, social, and cognitive development. Moreover, according to the CASA (1999) children exposed to substances during pregnancy tend to be medically fragile because of prematurity and/or low birth weight. These children may have health problems that place greater care demands on their parents, which in turn often lead to repeated abuse and neglect. Such youngsters tend to be angry, antisocial, and aggressive; frequently perform poorly in school; and may have low self-esteem or be depressed. Early intervention for these children and their parents is critical. The CASA reports also indicate that the number one barrier is the lack of motivation on the part of parents to seek treatment. Even when parents are thus motivated, the lack of funding for appropriate substance abuse treatment often sabotages the efforts of child welfare intervention. The extensive literature in this area is beyond the scope of this chapter to cover (see, e.g., Luthar, Burack, Cicchetti, & Weiss, 1997).

Work Constraints and Childcare

Increasing numbers of mothers are in the workforce and are using a variety of childcare arrangements. According to 2003 data (National Center for Children in Poverty, 2005), 52% of children under age 6 in low-income families have at least one parent who works full-time year round. Another 18% have at least one parent who works part-time year round, or full-time part of the year. Such families therefore need to arrange for childcare. In a longitudinal study of children in childcare, Howes (1988) found that the quality and stability of childcare, not enrollment in childcare per se, were the important factors in predicting school adjustment for both boys and girls. In fact, maternal education was more closely associated with children's school adjustment than was maternal employment or marital status. These conclusions are consistent with those of other investigators, such as Belsky (1984), Espinosa (2002), McCartney (1984), Pianta and Walsh (1996), and the NICHD Early Child Care Research Network (2003). Other studies of nonparental child care report more negative outcomes, such as problem behaviors (Belsky, 1999; NICHD, 2003; Vandell, Burchinal, Friedman, & Brownell, 2001) or deleterious effects on cognitive development (Russell, 1999). Shpancer (2006) presents a review of factors that affect these inconsistent findings. For example, because the political and social climate changes over time, findings "valid five, 10, or 20 years ago may no longer be valid in the present" (p. 228). In addition, many factors interact when childcare arrangements are studied, and the correlational outcomes reported do not allow causal inferences. High-quality childcare programs are not widespread. Hirsh-Pasek, Kochanoff, Newcombe, and de Villiers (2005), citing the work of the Cost, Quality, and Outcomes Study Team (1995), indicate that the overall quality of 70% of childcare programs has been rated as "fair" and 13% as "poor" on the Early Childhood Environment Rating Scale (Harms & Clifford, 1983; see Chapter 5). Espinosa (2002) reports a series of other studies using this scale with similar outcomes. The term "quality" is problematic. As Shpancer (2006) points out, although group size, staff–child ratio, and training correlate with quality, they do not account for how quality of care is produced in daycare centers. Furthermore, detrimental effects can occur even when quality of care is controlled (Vandell, 2004).

Increasingly, fathers are playing an important role in providing child care. In some families, mothers find employment more readily, placing fathers in the childcare role. Young African American men have particularly suffered from lack of security at work (Hernandez, 1993). In other cases, mothers may be working the day shift and fathers at night. For many fathers who do provide childcare, this is a new role for which they have had little previous preparation. For some such fathers, this role may influence their perceived status in their cultural group. In a study of 50 low-income African American fathers participating in fatherhood programs, Gadsden, Brooks, and Jackson (1997) found that many fathers felt challenged by their fathering roles. Some of these fathers had low literacy skills but had the desire to help their children—a desire that may be common in fathers of preschool children (Turbiville & Marquis, 2001). The impact of fathers' involvement in day-to-day caregiving interactions with their young children (play, storybook reading, basic care activities) has been an area of considerable recent research. Some of the extensive findings are as follows: (1) Fathers with lower levels of education are less likely to be involved than fathers with higher levels (Nord, Brimhall, & West, 1997); (2) fathers who had or have a romantic relationship with the mother are more involved than those with no relationship with the mother (Cabrera et al., 2004); (3) Head Start outreach programs to involve fathers resulted in greater participation and improved child readiness scores in mathematics (Fagan & Iglesias, 1999), more complex father–toddler social toy play, and better social and cognitive child outcomes (Roggman, Boyce, Cook, Christiansen, & Jones, 2004), increased confidence in teaching their children, and parenting satisfaction (Fagan & Stevenson, 2002); and (4) fathers can play an important role through engaging in early literacy activities (Gadsden & Bowman, 1999; Gadsden & Ray, 2003). Programs therefore need to reach out to fathers and encourage their participation (e.g., through fathers' nights, play groups, support groups).

An expanding literature on fathers' involvement in child care is now exploring their role in the daily care of children during their early development. The nature of this role in turn is linked to cultural, family, and child characteristics (see, e.g., Cabrera, Tamis-LeMonda, Bradley, Hofferth, & Lamb, 2000; Lamb, 2004).

Early Intervention

The importance of adequate environmental stimulation for a child's development was stressed by Hunt (1961), and increasing such stimulation was a critical reason for the introduction of the Head Start program in 1965. Much research has examined the effects of high-quality childcare programs and preschool programs such as the High Scope Program, Head Start, and state prekindergarten programs on children of low socioeconomic status (SES) (Barnett, Lamey, & Jung, 2005; Belsky & Steinberg, 1978; Berrueta-Clement, Schweinhart, Epstein & Weikert, 1984; Guralnick, 1997; Lazar & Darlington, 1982; White & Boyce, 1993; Zigler & Muenchow, 1992, among many others). These studies have demonstrated short-term gains in intellectual performance (a benefit that does not occur with children from average-SES backgrounds), as well as an increased orientation toward peers. Although preschool intervention has resulted in substantial gains in IQ scores and other cognitive measures during prekindergarten and kindergarten, the evidence also reflects a progressive decline in differences between experimental and control groups during the primary grades (Zigler & Muenchow, 1992). However, both Lazar and Darlington (1982) and Weikert and his colleagues have demonstrated various long-term benefits of early intervention, including fewer retentions and fewer assignments to special education, lower dropout, lower delinquency, lower adult crime, less welfare among those who participated in preschool intervention versus controls (Berrueta-Clement et al., 1984; Schweinhart & Weikart, 1998). A key feature of these positive outcomes is the quality of programs. These findings are confirmed by other research with preschool programs, such as the Family and Child Experiences Survey (FACES) study of Head Start programs (Commissioner's Office of Research and Evaluation & Head Start Bureau, 2001b) and research on state preschool programs. Access to and enrollment in high-quality preschool programs is highly uneven across states, and many children who qualify—40% of 3- and 4-year-olds below the poverty line, according to the National Institute for Early Education Research (NIEER, 2003)—are not enrolled.

In a comprehensive review of the literature, Ramey and Ramey (1998) focused on studies of Head Start programs with rigorous research designs. They cite characteristics of programs that result in greater benefits to participants. These programs:

1. Begin intervention early in children's development.
2. Are more intensive.
3. Provide services directly to children, in contrast to focusing mainly on caregivers.
4. Provide a broad range of comprehensive services (such as health, social services, transportation, and parent training and counseling), in addition to strong educational programs for children.
5. Attend to individual differences; not all programs benefit all children. Programs need to be related to both child and family characteristics.
6. Lead to ongoing environmental support (home, school, community), which is necessary for children to maintain the effects of early intervention.

Children's prekindergarten experience not only can affect their early school success; it also may enhance the amount of parental involvement in their children's later schooling and direct children toward later school success (Reynolds, 1991; Reynolds, Ou, & Topitzes, 2004). Research has consistently found that parental involvement contributes importantly to school success (Alexander & Entwisle, 1988; Burchinal, Peisner-Feinberg, Pianta, & Howes, 2002; Connell & Prinz, 2002; Dearing, Taylor, & McCartney, 2004;

NICHD Early Child Care Research Network, 2000; Reynolds, 1991; Snow, Barnes, Chandler, Goodman, & Hemphill, 1991). For example, Dearing et al. (2004) studied the effects of parent involvement in kindergarten on children's literacy performance and the children's feelings about literacy at grades three and five. The sample included children from 91 schools serving low-income families. The results indicated that (1) children with more educated mothers who were highly involved reported the most positive feelings about literacy, (2) children with less educated mothers who were highly involved reported less positive feelings about literacy at kindergarten but demonstrated a dramatic increase in positive feelings between kindergarten and fifth grade, and (3) higher levels of involvement were significantly related to literacy performance at grade five, especially for children whose mothers were less educated. These researchers concluded that for children living in low-income families, family involvement matters most for children whose mothers are least educated, as they note in the following: "although children of less educated mothers displayed lower than average literacy performance than children of more educated mothers when involvement was low, this gap was non-existent when involvement was high" (p. 467).

Multiple Risk Factors

All of the factors that have a negative impact on a family—health problems, marital and economic strain, neglect, abuse—are likely to increase a child's vulnerabilities for later problems in school. Many children are born into families where several of these factors are operating. Researchers are increasingly pointing to the importance of considering the cumulative effects of multiple child and environmental risk factors during the assessment process, in order to avoid high rates of error and misclassification (Furstenberg, Brooks-Gunn, & Morgan, 1987; Kochanek, Kabacoff, & Lipsitt, 1987, 1990; Luster & McAdoo, 1991; Sameroff, Seifer, Barocas, Zax, & Greenspan, 1987; Shonkoff & Meisels, 1991). However, research is needed to determine the contribution and interplay of specific factors. One of a series of studies by Sameroff (Sameroff et al., 1987) examined the impact of 10 risk factors (maternal anxiety; other aspects of maternal mental health; stressed life events; family social support; occupation; education levels; parent perspectives regarding child development; mother–child interaction behaviors; nonwhite status; and family size) on Verbal IQ scores when children were 4 years of age. As the number of risk factors increased, intellectual performance decreased. Sameroff (1993) also indicated that multiple risk factors are persistent over long periods of time: The same risk factors as those found at age 4 are still having an effect when children reach age 13. Unfortunately, this indicates that these families do not change very much. Therefore, assessment of such families is critical, and financial support of programs for families is a critical component of the process.

The contribution of multiple risk factors (collected before 12 months of age) to the prediction of disabilities reported between 14 and 20 years of age was studied by Kochanek et al. (1987, 1990). In their 1987 study, maternal factors such as level of educational attainment were more accurate predictors of adolescent status than the child data gathered at 4, 8, and 12 months of age. In their 1990 study, these researchers detailed the contributions of child-centered data (birth to age 7) collected serially over time and familial factors to the prediction of disabilities in adolescence. Using a sample of 268 disabled adolescents and 268 nondisabled adolescents matched on sex, age, and race, Kochanek et al. concluded: (1) There was no significant difference between groups with regard to prenatal and perinatal data; (2) parental traits, specifically maternal education, were more accurate predictors of adolescent disability status than a child's own behavior from birth to age 3; and (3) child-centered skills at ages 4 and 7 were better indicators of disabling conditions than was maternal educational level. Of interest is the fact that the relative weight of specific factors changed over time. No one child factor or isolated environmental factor could accurately predict outcome. This indicates that attention needs to be addressed to the interplay of child and environmental factors.

Luster and McAdoo (1991) examined factors related to cognitive and behavioral success among young African American students. Subjects included female respondents from the National Longitudinal Survey of Youth data set who had been interviewed annually since 1979 and their children. This study focused on 364 children between the ages of 6 and 9 and their families. Outcomes indicated that children who did well on achievement tests tended to have mothers who were relatively intelligent and well educated, and to come from more financially secure, smaller, and more supportive families. Factors not predictive of cognitive competence included father absence, age of mother at first birth, and maternal education (when maternal intelligence was controlled for). Children's behavioral adjustment was related to mothers' self-esteem, the number of children in the family, and low income. More recently, Rauh, Parker, Garfinkel, Perry, and Andrews (2003) examined the relative contribution of individual and community levels of risk on a 3,600+ population of African American and Hispanic children born in New York City who attended Head Start and then public school. Poor reading scores were related to the individual risk factors of low maternal education, low birth weight, being male, having an unmarried mother, and close spacing between births of siblings. After controlling for individual risk, lower reading scores were related to the community concentration of poverty and higher reading scores to a high percentage of immigrants in the community. These researchers, like others (Rutter, 1987; Sameroff et al., 1987; Sameroff, Gutman, & Peck, 2003; Werner, 1988), recommended considering a cumulative advantage–risk index to predict outcomes. Such predictions need to take into account not only the cumulative impact of multiple and diverse risk factors, but also the age of the child when these factors came into play and the outcome variables that are the focus of concern.

Violence and Maltreatment

Violence within both families and neighborhoods is another major stressor that must be considered in early childhood assessment. The increased numbers of young children living in violent environments are particularly troublesome (Crockett, 2003). In their article "Parenting in Violent Environments," Osofsky and Jackson (1993–1994) point to the psychological effects on parents of living with violence—in particular, their own feelings of frustration, helplessness, stress, and fears of being victims of violence. These feelings and fears can interfere with parents' attending to their children's needs, such as signs of distress, fears, and behavioral outbursts. Some families, however, are resilient despite these adverse circumstances. Citing the work of Hill (1972) and Hill and Billingsley (1993), Osofsky and Jackson (1993–1994) cite five factors that contribute to resilience: (1) strong kinship bonds, (2) flexibility of family roles, (3) strong spiritual/religious orientation, (4) strong work orientation, and (5) high achievement orientation. We discuss protective factors and resilience in more detail below.

Within the home, child maltreatment clearly impairs children's functioning. Psychological and physical abuse are both manifestations of harsh, hostile parenting. Across the developmental period, maltreatment's effects are seen in poor interpersonal relationships and resultant problems in emotional and behavioral regulation. In some maltreated children, learning is also affected—either because security issues are foremost in children's focus, interfering with their readiness to learn; because emotional undercontrol interferes with focus, discipline, and/or motivation; or because of head injuries resulting from physical abuse (Brassard & Rivelis, 2006).

Interparental conflict/violence (both verbal and physical) witnessed by young children can also have a serious impact. Fantuzzo, De Paola, Lambert, Anderson, and Sutton (1991), for example, studied 84 children and their mothers enrolled in Head Start centers, and 23 mothers temporarily residing in shelters for battered women and their young children. The Head Start mothers and children were divided into a group experiencing verbal conflict within the home and a group experiencing both verbal conflict and physical violence at home. All participants were from low-income backgrounds (59% were white, and 41% were from minority groups). Children from the shelter group exhibited higher levels of internalized problems than did children from either of the Head Start groups. The shelter groups also exhibited the lowest levels of social competence and maternal acceptance. There were no gender differences. Overall child outcomes indicated that (1) witnessing verbal conflict only was associated with a moderate level of conduct problems; (2) witnessing both verbal and physical conflict was associated with a clinical level of conduct problems plus a moderate level of emotional problems; and (3) witnessing both types of conflict *and* residing in temporary shelter situations were associated with clinical levels of conduct problems, higher levels of emotional problems, and lower levels of social functioning and perceived maternal acceptance. These findings, according to Fantuzzo et al. (1991), are supportive of Rutter's (1980, 1981) cumulative risk hypothesis. These authors also hypothesized that the shelter situation separated children from important mechanisms that helped them cope in their natural home settings, such as toys, peers, and neighbors or family members. Research in the past decade has substantiated their findings about children's reactions to interparental violence and coping. Twin studies have shown that young children exposed to a high level of domestic violence have IQs that are on average 8 points lower than those who are not exposed, consistent with animal models showing the harmful effects of extreme stress on brain development (Koenen, Moffitt, Caspi, Taylor, & Purcell, 2003). Increasingly research has moved to a focus on prevention and intervention (e.g., Jaffe, Baker, & Cunningham, 2004). We are hopeful that the next decade will show a marked improvement in societal responses to this major threat to children's well-being.

In addition to within-family violence, children are increasingly exposed to violence in their communities, particularly urban communities. Children living in urban communities frequently witness both intentional and random violent behaviors, often involving guns or knives (Gorman-Smith & Tolan, 2003; Osofsky, 1995). Mascolo (1998) cites a growing body of research indicating that exposure to such violence can have emotional and social effects (behavioral difficulty, fear, and aggression), as well as academic consequences. Early childhood is a particularly vulnerable time for exposure to violence. Perry and colleagues (Perry, 1997; Perry, Pollard, Blakely, Baker, & Vigilante, 1995) have shown that substantial, and possibly permanent, changes in the brain can occur as the result of trauma, altering children's ability to cope with stress and increasing overall arousal. This is reflected in elevated startle response, sleep disturbance, and cardiovascular regulatory abnormalities (Perry & Pate, 1994). Regressive behavior in traumatized preschool children is also seen in terms of loss of verbal skills, bed wetting, and dependent behavior (Gorman-Smith & Tolan, 2003). The causes of such problems are often not identified by professionals working in schools; instead, the problems are attributed to the children (Mascolo, 1998). Because of the centrality of the caregiver–child relationship in the early years, the response of the caregiver to the traumatic event is particularly important in influencing children's adaptation. When caregivers are calm and effective, but realistic in their response to the dangerousness of the situation, children do better (Gorman-Smith & Tolan, 2003). A family environment that is safe and cohesive and a community that provides connectedness and support from neighbors are other protective factors. Unfortunately, children exposed to community violence are those most likely to be exposed to multiple stressors, such as poverty, unstable environments, and lack of social supports. Moreover, as Sameroff (1993; Sameroff et al., 2003) caution when considering how to intervene in the face of these many difficulties, all children are different, and early intervention programs are only one facet of their life experiences. A program may be on target for some children, but may not provide enough support for others if other facets of the children's lives do not provide support. Within this context, it is important to consider as well those factors that are related to such support and to resilience in children during the preschool years.

Protective Factors

As important as the studies of risk factors are, they do not capture the wide variability among interacting circumstances or the degree to which families can cope with adversity. In their classic book *Overcoming the Odds: High Risk Children from Birth to Adulthood*, Werner and Smith (1992) highlight possible buffers of relevance to preschool assessors, interventionists, and caregivers. Based on their own longitudinal study (see below) and the work of other investigators, these authors stress that when such buffers are present, they "make a more profound impact [than do risk factors] on the life course of children who grow up under stressful life events. They appear to transcend ethnic, social class, geographical, and historical boundaries" (Werner & Smith, 1992, p. 202). Therefore, taking protective factors into account can provide a more optimistic outlook than focusing largely on risk factors; they can provide a "corrective lens" as we consider those factors "that move children toward normal adult development." The interacting effects of home environments and other caregiving environments are critical. According to Werner and Smith, factors contributing to the supportiveness of these environments include having options, having adequate financial resources, expecting that children will remain in school 10–12 years, expecting that children will become literate, recognizing that children will be socialized by a series of teachers and important others, preparing children to enter into a competitive society, and valuing human control over circumstances.

Werner and Smith go on to summarize Rutter's (1987) work, which focuses on factors that might change children's life trajectories. These include factors that (1) reduce risk impact, (2) reduce the likelihood of negative chain reactions of events, (3) promote self-esteem and self-efficacy, and (4) open up opportunities in people's lives. Stressing that some of the most critical determinants of adult outcomes are present in the first decade of life, Werner and Smith detail a number of general protective factors:

1. Structure and rules in the household.
2. Time with caring adults, which may occur outside the household.
3. Promotion of self-esteem and self-efficacy.
4. Academic competence and effective reading skills by grade 4.
5. Supportive relationships, including a close bond early in children's lives.

6. Opportunities and events that open up during the path to adulthood.
7. Confidence in their ability to cope and to combat the odds.

Resilience in Children

Since there is wide variation in how individuals respond to both risk and protective factors, some children will need more assistance than others. Therefore, assessors need to focus continually on children's responses to protective as well as risk factors, in addition to the children's own personalities. The longitudinal study reported by Werner (1988) and Werner and Smith (1992, 2001) explored the roots of resilience in young children. This ongoing study is based on a multiracial cohort of 698 infants born in 1955 in a rural Hawaiian island. Beginning with the prenatal period, the study has monitored a variety of biological and psychosocial risk factors, stressful life events, and protective factors at ages 1, 2, 10, 18, 30, 32, and the early 40s (Werner & Smith, 2001).

The majority of Werner and Smith's subjects were born without complications and lived in supportive home environments. One-third, however, were considered "at risk" due to a variety of factors. Three-quarters of this vulnerable group (those who encountered four or more risk factors before the age of 2) did subsequently develop serious learning and/or behavioral problems by age 10, or had delinquency records, mental health problems, or pregnancies before age 18. However, one-quarter of the vulnerable group developed into "competent, confident, and caring young adults" (Werner & Smith, 1992, p. 2). Personal qualities that existed among this resilient group included temperamental and behavioral characteristics that were exhibited during the first years of life. As infants, these children were active, cuddly, good-natured, and easy to deal with; they also elicited positive attention from others. As toddlers, they were robust, alert, and responsive. They had advanced communication and self-help skills, and they displayed significantly more signs of autonomy and independence than high-risk toddlers who later developed problems, as well as a more positive social orientation in response to others. A number of family factors were also important: (1) the presence of four or fewer offspring, with a space of 2 years between offspring; (2) consistent caregiving without prolonged separations from the primary caregiver during the first year of life; and (3) opportunity to establish a close bond with one caregiver. These factors continued to play an important role in the 30-year follow-up of subjects, which was initiated in 1985.

In addition to establishing a close bond with a caregiver, resilient young children gain increasing control in directing their attention and in regulating their emotions and behavior, according to Masten and Coatsworth (1998). These skills are important for academic and social success in school. These authors also caution that children "have different vulnerabilities and protective systems at different points in development" (p. 213)—a point of particular importance for assessors. Therefore, the family and neighborhood, as well as the child (including his or her areas of individual resilience), all need to be considered in assessment and intervention planning.

Benard (1995) views the characteristics of resilience as including social competence (e.g., the ability to elicit a positive response from others), problem-solving skills (e.g., the ability to plan and seek help from others), a critical consciousness of strategies to use in the face of adverse events, autonomy, and a sense of purpose and hopefulness. These characteristics are fostered by a caring other who provides a positive model and respects the child (parent, grandparent, teacher). The child, in turn, develops a sense of trust and the desire to work for and please these individuals. Caring others can set high expectations for children and give them the support necessary to succeed and believe in themselves. Such an outcome was demonstrated in the work of Burchinal et al. (2002) in the school setting.

Environmental Forces in Childcare and Educational Settings

Assessment of all the different environments experienced by children is absolutely essential for understanding child behavior and developing effective intervention. Environments that need to be focused on include not only the home and community (as suggested in the previous sections), but school and childcare settings. Taking account of these environments is fundamental to ecologically valid assessment, as emphasized by most current experts focusing on the early childhood years (e.g., Adelman, 1982; Barnett, 1984; Lidz, 2003; Paget, 1985, 1990; Paget & Nagle, 1986; Paget & Barnett, 1990; Reynolds, Gutkin, Elliot, & Witt, 1984; Thurman & Widerstrom, 1985, 1990). Central to an ecological model of assessment is an approach in which "behavioral and learning difficulties are not viewed as deficits residing in the child or his or her parents; rather such deficits are viewed as variations resulting from ecological forces that affect parent, child, and family behavior" (Paget & Barnett, 1990, p. 461). Key features of an ecological model, according to Paget and Barnett (1990), include (1) analyzing children's interactions with and reactions to people, objects, and events; (2) observation and consultation with significant adults across major settings; and (3) matching strategies and techniques to the unique qualities of each child and family. We advocate an ecocultural approach to assessment (see Chapter 2). That is, as assessors, we need to take account of the pervasive images and messages that all environments communicate to a young child, along with the cultural and linguistic heritage of the child.

Instructional environments are of critical importance. Based on a summary of a report to the National Research Council (Heller, Holtzman, & Messick, 1982), Messick (1984) urges assessors to appraise student performance in relation to instructional quality. Although this summary is focused on school-age children, it addresses our concerns in this book and is instructive for preschool assessors. For example, Messick indicates that assessment procedures for special education need to entail two successive phases or steps: first, ruling out deficiencies in children's learning environment by systematically examining the nature and quality of instruction received; and, second, administrating a comprehensive assessment battery covering intellectual/cognitive functioning and adaptive behavior (including social and emotional functioning), as well as screening for biomedical disorders.

Features of assessment during the first phase should include (1) documentation by schools of their use of programs and curricula that are effective across the ethnic, SES, and linguistic groups served by the school; (2) evidence (including observational data) that children are being adequately exposed to these programs and curricula, through both regular school attendance and through effective curriculum implementation (including flexible instructional strategies, appropriate directions, feedback, and reinforcement); (3) objective evidence (such as criterion-referenced tests) that children have or have not learned what has been taught; and (4) evidence of past efforts to identify and correct learning difficulties through using alternative procedures in the regular classroom. In addition to standardized achievement tests and criterion-referenced tests geared to curriculum objectives, systematic classroom observation is viewed as critical to sustain the first-phase process. Messick's (1984) recommendation for research on the assessment of learning environments, along with the development of measurement procedures to identify dimensions of curriculum effectiveness and alternative instructional strategies with reference to low-achieving pupils, is particularly relevant. But at the preschool level, children may or may not have been exposed to systematic preschool teaching in Head Start, nursery schools, or high-quality childcare programs. Our hope is that with the accountability demands of NCLB, this will change.

Sociocultural Considerations

Along with acknowledging the rich body of evidence regarding the value of early education programs in preventing or ameliorating many disabilities among preschool children, Bowman (1992) raises important sociocultural concerns about determining "at riskness" among preschool children. Possible dangers include the following:

1. Confusing what particular cultures value and teach with mainstream values when judging the development of children's knowledge and skills. It is important to understand children's daily lives before interpreting their behavior. Therefore, "We must frame evaluation strategies which do not consciously or unconsciously lead us to devalue differences that are developmentally equivalent. This means that we must develop instruments and clinical practices which assess a range of learned behavior that represent similar developmental steps" (Bowman, 1992, p. 103).
2. Blaming the victim and assuming "that risks to development inherent in unequal social conditions can be 'cured' by services to individuals, when for many children and families failure resides with the social system and disruptions to development with too few resources (particularly with respect to pre- and postnatal services, nutrition, hopelessness and despair, non-responsive parenting, disorganization, depression) all of which make children more vulnerable" (Bowman, 1992, p. 104).
3. Segregating young children with special needs from other children, which occurs in many programs. Bowman stresses that while some children have profound physical or mental disabilities, most special needs are "tied to the social context in which children live" (p. 106), and many special-needs children function well within the normal limits necessary to function in society. Bowman recommends environments that are consistent and provide opportunities to explore, together with teachers who scaffold skills and knowledge, who accept what children can and want to do, who guide them toward skills needed for school success, and who recognize the importance of and support parents. Early childhood teachers and special education teachers would work together in programs, which would last until children reach 6 or 7 years of age, to foster such outcomes.

Bowman's recommendations are consistent with the NAEYC and NAECS/SDE (2003) policy statement on early childhood curriculum, assessment, and program evaluation.

In our pluralistic society, assessors will work with children from many cultural backgrounds. Their sensitivity to these backgrounds is essential to planning for children and to addressing the concerns raised by Bowman, especially the first one. Assessors must gain cultural insight into community stressors (such as violence) contributing to children's learning or emotional difficulties, and must also become aware of the feelings and reactions they themselves might have when working with diverse populations. As Hilliard (1989) points out, "Culture provides group members with a deep sense of belonging and often with a strong preference for behaving in certain ways" (p. 66). Hilliard believes that "children, no matter what their style, are failing primarily because of systematic inequities in the delivery of whatever pedagogical approach the teachers claim to master—not because students cannot learn from teachers whose styles do not match their own" (p. 68). Understanding differences in behavioral style has important consequences for assessors, who must strive to reduced erroneous estimates of children's intellectual potential, mislabeling, misplacement, and inappropriate teaching; to increase their sensitivity to different structures for expressing ideas, such as storytelling styles; and to increase their openness to language expression that is not standard English. Predominant questions relevant to assessment include these:

1. What child cognitive, social, and behavioral abilities does a child's culture value and teach?
2. How does this culture teach children to behave with adults and strangers?
3. How does this culture view disabilities?
4. What extra steps are required to gain an understanding that daily pressures place on families?
5. How does one deal with cultural and language barriers and frequent family mobility?

These are complex issues that need systematic study and direction. Nonetheless, many school systems are faced with extraordinary challenges. In large urban school districts, children come from many cultures and speak many languages or dialects—a trend that is likely to increase. This challenge is not limited to urban areas. Large numbers of immigrant families are finding their way to counties across the country (Perry & Schachter, 2003). An assessor/translator/teacher fluent in one language (e.g., Cantonese) may not be fluent even in a related one (e.g., Mandarin). Families from some cultures are often highly mobile because of poverty, joblessness, and homelessness, so that children are placed in and out of programs. Some children enter school without prior kindergarten or first-grade experience. Many families have had little schooling or unsuccessful schooling themselves. Other families are unfamiliar with the North American school system. Since sensitivity to issues of cultural and language diversity is essential for preschool assessors, these issues are referred to repeatedly throughout this text and are explored in depth in Chapter 9.

The Nature of Child Development Itself

Understanding young children's developmental progression within physical, motor, speech–language, cognitive, and socioemotional domains of growth is vital for assessors who focus on these children. Research points to the need to be familiar with the normal range of behavior across areas, to be alert to signals of possible problems, and to understand the progression of emerging skills. These emerging skills often follow developmental paths in which errors are systematic across groups of children and not random. Such errors, then, generally make sense and need to be explored for planning learning experiences. Since young children's development is so rapid, their strengths and needs often change across brief periods of time. Accordingly, assessment of preschool children needs to be frequent and ongoing, and needs to encompass a "feedback loop" (Boehm & Sandberg, 1982) that takes into account development, instruction, and intervention. A rich developmental research literature exists to help us understand how children think, reason, and behave. It is essential to keep up to date with this literature and imbed it into assessment practices, to support their "empirical validity" (Hirsh-Pasek et al., 2005).

Although assessors clearly recognize the importance of understanding the nature of child development, it often is difficult to sift through the huge developmental literature in order to understand the specific details of normal and abnormal growth. In part, what assessors need are developmental maps across areas for the ages of 3–6 years, tailored to the child population of interest, a point raised by Lichtenstein and Ireton (1984). Professionals working with preschool populations with sensory deficits (visual, hearing, or motor impairments), and those working with children from diverse cultural backgrounds, emphasize the need for assessors to consider developmental progressions that are "normal" for these populations.

SUMMARY

The importance of a child's early years for his or her later physical, cognitive, language, social, and emotional development has been well documented in the research literature. In the United States, nationwide attention is currently being focused on developing home and school conditions that foster such development. Early childhood programs for children living in poverty, children with disabilities, and children at risk, such as Head Start and those available under IDEA 2004 and the NCLB legislation of 2001, are available to address these concerns. Assessment of child and family strengths and needs plays an important role in improving such services for children and in ensuring that children benefit from their learning experiences. The outcomes of the various forms of assessment used at the preschool level must in turn be linked to learning activities and parent programs. In order to achieve these goals, assessment needs to focus not only on children, but also on their learning environments. Using the research literatures relating to development and disability conditions during the early childhood years, assessors can play a major role in improving services for children; in facilitating the role of teachers, parents, and important others; and in documenting children's progress.

Important environmental risk factors—poverty, parental substance abuse, violence seen and experienced, and many more—can have an impact upon children in the course of their early development. These can be countered by critical protective factors, such as maternal education, a caring adult, consistent routines, and a child's own resilience. Based on the overview presented in this chapter, Table 1.1 summarizes the numerous interacting factors that need to be considered in the assessment process. This table can serve as a checklist for assessors as they consider the interplay of the multiple forces that influence children's lives and behaviors.

The likelihood of variation among states and districts in their definition of what constitutes "developmental delay," along with the use of different standards and procedures for assessment and diagnosis, continues to influence the possibility that children and families will gain or lose services on the basis of where they live as much as their actual need for services—an issue raised by Short, Simeonsson, and Huntington (1990). Moreover, sometimes it is difficult to know what causes a child's problem in learning or behavior—

TABLE 1.1. Summary of Risk and Protective Factors: A Checklist

Buffers/protective factors	Risk factors
	Child
• Prenatal care, beginning in first trimester • Proper nutrition	• Low birth weight/prematurity • Poor prenatal care • Known disabilities • Malnutrition
• Resilient behaviors	
• Good-natured temperament	• Difficult temperament
• Ability to elicit positive attention from others	• Poor peer relationships
• Good communication and self-help skills	• Low intellectual status
• Independent behavior	• Low mental health status
• Early success with literacy activities and social relationships	• Need for remedial education

(continued)

TABLE 1.1. *(continued)*

Family	
• Time with caring and interested adults	• Child maltreatment
• Higher maternal educational level (high school graduate or above)	• Lower maternal educational level
• Expressions of caring and affection/strong bonds	• Maternal mental health problems (anxiety, depression)
• Support from family members	• Sibling with a developmental disability
• Financial security/average to high SES	• Extreme poverty/economic strain
• Four or fewer offspring	• Large families (more than four offspring)
• Children born more than 2 years apart	• Birth spacing less than 2 years
• Strong work orientation	• Restricted environments
• Regular, consistent routines and caregiving	• Disorganized routines
	• Excessive sensory stimulation
• Monitored TV watching	• Unlimited TV watching
• Frequent storybook reading and discussion	• Minority status/discrimination
• Stable school experience through Grade 1	• High degree of family mobility
• Expectation that child will remain in school 10–12 years and become literate	
• Involvement with child's school and parent programs	
• Sense of control over circumstances	• Low self-efficacy
School/child care	
• High-quality programs tied to child strengths and needs	• Rigid or exclusively skill-focused curriculum
• Adults who provide rich language models	• Few language exchanges with children
• Discouragement of retention	• Retention during early years
	• Belief that difficulties lie within the child
Community	
• Support from friends/religious groups	• Social isolation
• Childcare and educational opportunities available	• Violence frequently observed
• Community programs (literacy, job training, parenting)	• Few community supports for families

Research supports that . . .
- Buffers are more powerful than risks.
- The more risks a child faces, the more buffers are needed.
- The impact of both risk factors and buffers differs in relation to the age of the child.
- Further research is needed to determine the contribution and interplay of risk factors and buffers in identifying child strengths and needs.

the child's own biological and neurological makeup, trauma, abuse, persistent poverty, inadequate childcare or preschool experiences, inadequate early intervention, or some combination of these. Given the variability among assessment settings and the potential complexity of an individual child's difficulties, the assessment process must be thorough and must be informed by ongoing research.

Chapter 2

A Multifactor Ecocultural Model of Assessment and the Assessment Process

Improving learning, social, and emotional experiences and enhancing competence for all young children—the ultimate goals of preschool assessment as presented in this text—are grounded on six fundamental assumptions:

1. Assessment is a dynamic and complex process that addresses various purposes. Moreover, it needs to be ongoing, to reevaluate the changing needs of the child at home and at school.
2. Children develop embedded in a culture(s) consisting of home, school, and community. They, in turn, change their environment by their presence and their behavior. These sociocultural influences must be accounted for in the assessment process, and assessors must be knowledgeable about local community influences. Family functioning needs to be a central area of concern.
3. Whenever possible, assessment needs to include observation of the young child in a familiar environment and to include meaningful structured and unstructured tasks.
4. Assessment and intervention planning centered on instruction and/or behavior change need to be considered as reciprocal processes, in which assessment guides and evaluates the effectiveness of instruction and intervention strategies.
5. Assessment is a collaborative process involving multiple individuals—classroom teachers, caregivers, and early childhood specialists (such as school psychologists, speech therapists, special educators, social workers, occupational and physical therapists, and pediatric physicians/nurses). Family members need to be involved as full partners throughout assessment and intervention.
6. The focus of assessment can be on consultation with the parent and/or teacher, rather than directly on the child.

These assumptions are addressed throughout this book.

As noted in Chapter 1, preschool assessment serves multiple functions. Specifically, it enables assessors to (1) describe children's strengths and needs across developmental areas, in order to plan instruction and other forms of early intervention; (2) predict possible developmental delay and academic preparedness for school; (3) determine eligibility for special education, including the possible causes of behavior and specific recommendations for intervention; (4) consult with teachers in order to adjust teaching activities, monitor progress, and set goals; (5) plan and monitor family intervention activities; (6) evaluate the effectiveness of teaching and intervention programs; (7) inform administrative planning related to service and staffing needs; and (8) evaluate programs for purposes of accountability. Different types of assessment are needed to address these multiple purposes (see Figure 2.1). Assessment for purposes of accountability has taken on a major role in the NCLB legislation of 2001 in the United States, with tests used to evaluate the progress of Head Start children twice a year in language, literacy, and pre-math skills. The narrow focus of this law on cognitive development as the critical factor in evaluating children's school readiness, without consideration of children's physical development, health, social competence, and emotional development, is controversial for a number of reasons (Meisels & Atkins-Burnett, 2004; Raver & Zigler, 2004). We discuss this issue in this chapter and throughout this text.

There are numerous, often interrelated approaches to preschool assessment; these can be used individually or in combination, depending on the assessment purpose. They

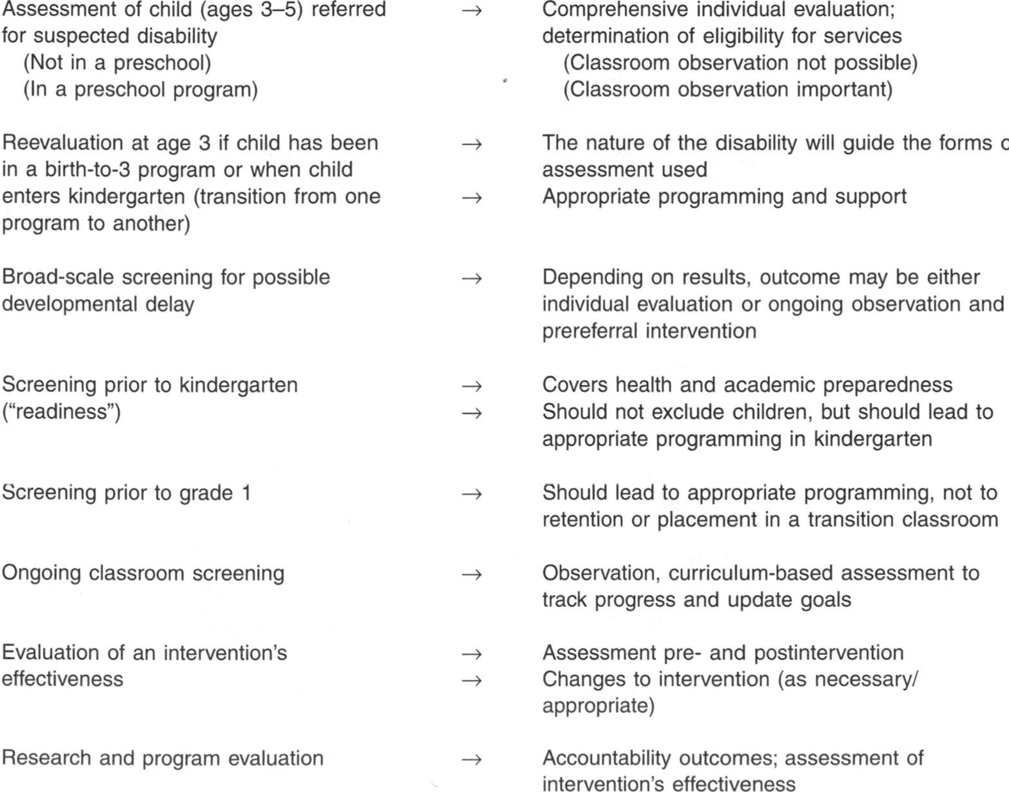

Assessment of child (ages 3–5) referred for suspected disability (Not in a preschool) (In a preschool program)	→	Comprehensive individual evaluation; determination of eligibility for services (Classroom observation not possible) (Classroom observation important)
Reevaluation at age 3 if child has been in a birth-to-3 program or when child enters kindergarten (transition from one program to another)	→ →	The nature of the disability will guide the forms of assessment used Appropriate programming and support
Broad-scale screening for possible developmental delay	→	Depending on results, outcome may be either individual evaluation or ongoing observation and prereferral intervention
Screening prior to kindergarten ("readiness")	→ →	Covers health and academic preparedness Should not exclude children, but should lead to appropriate programming in kindergarten
Screening prior to grade 1	→	Should lead to appropriate programming, not to retention or placement in a transition classroom
Ongoing classroom screening	→	Observation, curriculum-based assessment to track progress and update goals
Evaluation of an intervention's effectiveness	→ →	Assessment pre- and postintervention Changes to intervention (as necessary/appropriate)
Research and program evaluation	→	Accountability outcomes; assessment of intervention's effectiveness

FIGURE 2.1. Types and outcomes of assessment.

include interviews, informal and formal methods of observation, norm-referenced testing, criterion-referenced testing, performance-based or curriculum-based assessment, play assessment, dynamic and strategy-based approaches, work sampling, parent and teacher consultation, and family-based procedures. Examples of each of these approaches are described throughout this text, and they need to be viewed in relation to what each approach can contribute to understanding children and their learning environments. There is no reason to hope or imagine that one assessment approach will answer all questions. Rather, multiple methods need to be used to explore questions of interest. As Abbott and Crane (1977) pointed out many years ago, "the method of assessment used with young children is not as important as the accuracy and appropriateness of the technique in relation to what is being assessed" (p. 118).

In addition to the purpose(s) for which assessment is carried out and the approach(es) that are employed, a number of critical factors will affect all types of assessment. These include the sheer number of children needing to be served; cultural and language diversity among children, and the assessor's cultural sensitivity, knowledge, and insight; availability of specialized personnel trained to assess and serve preschool populations, including those at risk, those with low-incidence disabilities, and those coming from backgrounds different from the mainstream culture; the range of program and intervention options available; state and local mandates; the adequacy of financial support; and other pragmatic factors. The interplay of these factors will affect the nature and outcomes of even the best-planned assessment programs. The purposes of this chapter are (1) to consider essential features of a multifactor ecocultural model of assessment, and (2) to provide an overview of issues and procedures involved in the assessment process.

A MULTIFACTOR ECOCULTURAL MODEL OF PRESCHOOL ASSESSMENT

In our multifactor ecocultural model of preschool assessment, assessment is viewed as an ongoing problem-solving task with the goals of understanding the child within his or her daily environments and planning appropriate instruction or other forms of intervention. The work of researchers such as Bandura (1978, 1986), Hobbs (1975), and Sameroff and MacKenzie (2003) has been key to our understanding of the reciprocal interactions among adult and child characteristics and behavior, within the context of diverse environments and situations. This interplay of adult, child, environmental, and situational factors sets the stage for children's skill development and behavior. An ecological model of assessment is therefore endorsed by most authors in this field (e.g., Bailey & Rouse, 1989; Bagnato, 1992; Bracken, 2000; Barnett & Carey, 1992; Boehm & Sandberg, 1982; Boehm & Weinberg, 1997; Lichtenstein & Ireton, 1984; Lidz, 1983a, 1991, 2003; Nagle, 2000; Paget, 1985, 1990; Paget & Nagle, 1986; Thurman & Widerstrom, 1990). That is, assessors need to collect information from and about all of the persons and settings relevant to a child. We refer to our model as *ecocultural* rather than simply *ecological*, because of our emphasis on how children's ethnic, cultural, and linguistic backgrounds affect their development and their interactions with assessors. While children from different backgrounds achieve many developmental milestones at roughly the same time, cultures value behaviors differently. Paget (1990) succinctly states the issues: "Whether assessing social, cognitive, language, or motor functioning, we must remain open to the possibility that the questions and tasks we present to a young child may not be making contact with the child's understanding of the world" (p. 107).

Roles of Preschool Assessors

Constructs that guide assessment roles include obtaining and organizing information regarding children's strengths, limitations, and learning styles; supports needed from others; and the nature of family systems and learning environments (Barnett, 1984). Comprehensive assessment of preschool children therefore requires consideration of behavior in the classroom, at home, and during interaction with peers (Boehm & Sandburg, 1982; Bracken, 2004; Lidz, 2003; Nuttall, Romero, & Kalesnik, 1999). Moreover, assessors need to look beyond individual child factors and take into account (1) instructional practices, including adults' providing a stimulating and caring environment, using reinforcement to encourage learning and appropriate behavior, serving as language models, providing bridges to learning, and being sensitive to stress and other behavioral and emotional signals; (2) the belief systems and goals of parents, caregivers, and teachers; and (3) the characteristics of a child's environments (including both stressors and buffers, as described in Chapter 1). Parent and teacher consultation is an essential aspect of this process and provides a "foundation for assessment because it is based on problem solving and a collaborative relationship between participants" (Bagnato, 1992, p. 6). Finally, current literature (see, for example, Boehm, 1990, 2001; Ginsburg, 1997a; Peverly & Kitzen, 1998; and Lidz, 1991, 2003) points to the importance of understanding the cognitive processes that underlie learning goals, along with the problem-solving strategies used by young children and the adult supports needed for successful functioning.

Focusing on assessment for early intervention with infants and toddlers, Bagnato (1992) recommends a collaborative approach by a team consisting of family members and professionals in decision making. The comprehensive multidimensional model for assessment and research detailed by Bagnato and Neisworth (1991), and Bagnato, Neisworth, and Munson (1997) includes the use of (1) multiple measures of different types (including curriculum-based and other alternative assessment procedures to gather converging information about children); (2) information gathered from multiple sources and across multiple environmental contexts; (3) information collected across multiple developmental areas and across time; and (4) multiple assessment functions, including description, placement, prediction, and prescription. Linking assessment to curriculum and intervention planning is a key outcome gained through integrating the information gathered and through collaborative problem solving. Parents need to be involved and enabled throughout the process to support the child's development and experiences at home and at school. The work of Paget and Barnett (1990) and Barnett and Carey (1991), and the model proposed by Bagnato and Neisworth (1991), serve as the foundation for the multifactor ecocultural model employed throughout this book. Building on this basic model, we emphasize understanding the interplay of children's multiple environments, along with their cultural and linguistic diversity. The interrelated components of comprehensive preschool assessment need to be carefully planned and systematically carried out. The sections that follow describe some of the key considerations assessors need to keep in mind as they address different assessment purposes. Figure 2.2 is a graphic summary of such considerations.

Adults (general)

Knowledge and experience in working with preschool children
Knowledge of assessment approaches
Ability to break down tasks and provide needed supports
Ability to develop a caring relationship with a child
Sensitivity to child cues and emerging behaviors

The assessor

Personal belief systems and sensitivity to cultural and linguistic diversity
Training and experience
Familiarity with wide range of traditional and alternative assessment approaches
Familiarity with intervention possibilities
Willingness to confront dilemmas and advocate for children

School

Teachers' belief systems
Teachers' qualifications and in-service activities
Approaches to diversity and bilingualism
Nature of curriculum
Availability of alternative programs
Flexibility for movement within and across programs
Teacher–child ratio

Child characteristics

Cognitive
Mental health
Physical
Interpersonal
Communicative
Memory
Strategies/styles
Risk and protective factors

Daycare

Quality of programs available
Coordination with preschool

Family

Length of time in country
Language(s) spoken
Child-rearing beliefs and practices
Beliefs about disability and intervention
Family stress and areas of strength
Support systems available
Parental mental illness
Parent–child conversations and shared book reading
Involvement with school

Community

Safe/reasonable housing available
Financial resources available
Violence
Support services available (daycare, health, jobs)
Political climate and local issues
Attitudes toward diversity

FIGURE 2.2. Key considerations in early childhood assessment.

Language and Cultural Diversity of Local Student Populations

As noted in Chapter 1, the face of North American education is undergoing radical change, with increasing numbers of children from minority and linguistically diverse backgrounds. In particular, the number of Hispanic children has increased dramatically in the United States. In 2000, Hispanics of any race constituted 16.24% of the U.S. population under 5 years of age, as opposed to 9.31% of the 40- to 44-year-old population (U.S. Census Bureau 2002). Some cities (Miami, Los Angeles, New York, Chicago) and states (California, Colorado, Florida, Illinois, New York, and Texas) already have very large numbers of Hispanic children for whom English is their second language. As of October 2003, 20.1% of all nursery and kindergarten children in the United States had at least one foreign-born parent, but this was true of 62.2% of all Hispanic children in this age group (U.S. Census Bureau, 2003). Many of these children come from immigrant families that tend to be living in poverty. Preschool-age children from these families attend preschool at slightly less than half the rate of their non-Hispanic white counterparts (55% vs. 39%), and they tend to do poorly in U.S. schools in reading and all other academic areas as early as grade 1, "demonstrating low performance even when they are taught and tested in Spanish" (Goldenberg, 1996, p. 10). Gersten and Woodward (1994) cite research indicating that larger numbers of Hispanic children than the national average (1) are retained, (2) drop out of school, and (3) have parents who have had little formal education. Their parents, however, have high expectations for their children's education as a road to success in life.

Moreover, as Goldenberg (1996) points out, the Hispanic population is extremely diverse, with large numbers from families from Mexico, South America, Puerto Rico, Cuba, and other parts of the Caribbean. And, of course, many, many other immigrant groups are now also represented in U.S. schools—numerous Asian groups, as well as increasing numbers of children from Eastern Europe and Africa. Although these population changes are almost staggering in their complexity, they must be reflected in assessment practice and in assessors' knowledge base and sensitivities, such as considering which children are referred and for what reasons. IDEA 2004, major professional organizations, and the current literature all call for assessment to be carried out in an unbiased manner and in a child's predominant language.

The importance of cultural and background factors in assessment models has consistently been emphasized in the research literature. A number of examples are the social learning theory model of Bandura (1978) and the ecological model proposed by Paget and Nagle (1986), although Keogh and Becker drew attention to these same issues as early as 1973. Paget and Nagle (1986) urge that preschool assessors assume a perspective in which both child variables and environmental influences are viewed as reciprocally influencing each other and mutually determining assessment results. This view requires assessors to spend considerable time developing their understanding of the populations they are to serve and assuring the use of appropriate practices (see Chapter 9).

A major, ongoing issue with critical implications is the disproportionate representation of several language and ethnic minorities in special education classes. Gersten and Woodward (1994) cite evidence indicating that many teachers, when faced with children who do not speak English, are uncertain and stressed about how to proceed. As a result, they often turn to special education for assistance when these students are experiencing difficulties. Frequent outcomes include misidentification, misuse of tests, and misplacement of language minority children into special education. The same problems relate to some ethnic minorities, including African Americans and Native Americans. Gersten and Woodward (1994) go on to identify a widespread paradoxical condition that consists of both overreferral and underreferral. In some districts, Hispanic students are often erroneously diagnosed as having LD or mental retardation; in other districts, teachers are reluctant to refer language minority children for special education services, fearing charges of discrimination. Furthermore, few support services are available in many locations for students speaking languages other than English until they are reasonably proficient in English. Continuing problems with school success in Hispanic and other language minority populations, and state and district accountability for addressing them, are a major emphasis of the NCLB legislation in the United States.

The Critical Importance of Assessing Environments

Environments are complex and multifaceted in their influence on child functioning (see Chapter 5). Assessing home, school, and community environments is indeed difficult (teachers, parents, or others often feel judged, and the process takes time); as a result, unfortunately, it is not a systematic part of many screening approaches or in-depth assessment. Therefore, most screening and diagnostic assessment outcomes need to be viewed cautiously, and the following question should be raised: "To what extent does the assessment process consider the features of each environment's physical settings, instructional practices (both direct and indirect or inadvertent), and interactions among key individuals and agencies, all in relationship to families' cultural beliefs and child-rearing practices?" Unfortunately, it is often impossible for individuals conducting outside evaluations, school "roundup" screening, and large-scale developmental screening to take this question into account. However, direct observation and reported information concerning daily environments are key to the ecocultural assessment of children determined to be at risk, in order to understand the reciprocal interactions of the child, home, school, and community. These are critical to the development of IEPs, recommendations, and instructional or other forms of intervention.

In addition to understanding the developmental status of children, along with child and family risk and protective factors, it is particularly important to consider educational expectations and teacher beliefs as they guide curricular practices at each of the preschool levels (age 3 through kindergarten) and the scope of programs available. More specifically, it is important for assessors in educational/caregiving environments to obtain information about how the child interacts with family members (when present), teachers, other adults, and peers; routines, materials available, and instructional approaches and curricula used; and the caring relationships and supports that are present in each setting. For example, within classroom environments it is important to observe instructional activities, physical arrangements, access to educational materials and toys, the use of feedback, and specific adaptations used by teachers to meet children's needs and support learning (see Chapter 5, for a discussion of these issues). The assessor who is not able to conduct observations in relevant settings over time needs to construct the assessment situation to include not only tests or curriculum-based materials, but culture- and age-appropriate play activities to capture important child behaviors in a familiar context. The assessor must also work with parents, obtaining their past observations and checking out whether or not assessment outcomes are consistent with their observations; teachers need to be contacted for their observations as well, where appropriate.

Using a Developmental Perspective to Guide Practice

The preschool years are years of rapid development for all children. This development is likely to be an uneven process, with spurts of growth across areas such as comprehension, language, motor functioning, and play interactions. Children also present individual differences in how they learn and in what they have learned in the past. As noted in Chapter 1, it is therefore necessary for assessors to be familiar with both typical and atypical developmental milestones that are culturally appropriate and take into account the past learning experiences of each child. A multifaceted approach, in which assessors use a variety of methods to collect information from many sources, provides a comprehensive picture of children's development across domains.

Integrating Assessment with Intervention

From the beginning, assessment and intervention need to be viewed as reciprocal activities and as ongoing processes. Assessment supports intervention in many ways: through

(1) monitoring children's progress; (2) guiding the choice and sequencing of teaching objectives; (3) providing a basis for communication with parents; (4) facilitating the diagnosis and treatment of children with special needs; (5) monitoring the effectiveness of intervention activities and programs; (6) contributing to teachers' and schools' accountability for students' learning; and (7) furthering public understanding of young children's development. Dangers include (1) a narrow focus for purposes of accountability on paper-and-pencil tests, as well as on cognitive and preacademic results rather than a comprehensive approach across developmental domains; (2) inadequate consideration of cultural issues, such as proficiency with the English language; and (3) basing high-stakes accountability judgments on the results of a single test. The Goal 1 Early Childhood Assessment Resource Group (Shepard, Kagan, & Wurtz, 1998) formulated the following safeguards: Assessment must consider all domains of development, be carried out in natural learning contexts with familiar tasks, be linguistically appropriate, be carried out by multiple observers, be addressed to the specific purposes and ages of children for whom it is intended, and "bring about positive benefits for children and increased understanding for parents and teachers" (p. 11). These safeguards are consistent with the model developed in this book. However, they require appropriate funding, which is often not available in financially stressed schools (Schemo, 2004).

Since assessment serves multiple purposes, it is natural that its outcomes be used for multiple forms of intervention, including prevention; enrichment; psychotherapeutic and behavioral treatment; curriculum-based remedial activities; and other special education services, such as speech therapy and appropriate schooling for children with physical disabilities or developmental disorders. Although some assessment specialists (e.g., Braden & Plunge, 1994) have indicated that psychologists have long linked traditional assessment to planning intervention, others (e.g., Meisels, 1999; Reschly, 1988) dispute their views and criticize traditional assessment as requiring high levels of inference, as not directly linked to outcomes or performance measures, and as promoting a focus on child pathology in problem identification. Braden and Plunge (1994) have countered that valuable criticisms such as these are often used to polarize the issues, to justify the elimination of traditional assessment methods, and to present alternative approaches to assessment as incompatible with traditional approaches. We believe that a balanced view is appropriate—a position consistent with the "flexible assessment" position endorsed by the School Psychology Educators Council of New York State and the New York Association of School Psychologists (Lidz et al., 1999), which allows professionals to use "considered" choice in decision making.

Because intervention is an integral component of assessment, a number of goals and opportunities for intervention are indicated below. These can and should be considered in the development of assessment procedures.

1. *Intervene early, before persistent educational and/or emotional problems develop.* Early intervention can take a number of forms, one of which is prereferral intervention. In this case, observation and consultation with parents and/or teachers are used to develop a short-term prereferral plan, to recommend modifications in instruction or responses to behavior, or to alter aspects of the physical environment. The outcomes of these activities are then evaluated and modified. Only if the problem persists is a referral made for formal evaluation. This approach is particularly important for children who perform at borderline levels based on developmental or readiness screening, or who are demonstrating behavioral problems.

2. *Offer enrichment programs.* Enriched instructional opportunities can be provided for children whose environments may place them at risk. Such enrichment can take place at home, during preschool, during the early years of schooling, or through parent programs, and it is often essential for developing emergent literacy skills. Examples of parent programs that can take place in the home or in workshops at school are those helping parents to provide activities that foster child development, to manage behavior, to engage in intergenerational literacy activities, or to learn about nutrition and healthcare. Another form of enrichment can take place within the context of the school program. Goldenberg and Gallimore (1991), for example, demonstrated a successful change process when specialists met regularly with teachers of Hispanic children to discuss child development, to enrich their curriculum and track small steps, and to involve parents. Webster-Stratton and her colleagues have developed and validated teacher-, parent-, and child-focused interventions that increase children's social skills and understanding of feelings, academic engagement, school readiness, and cooperation with teachers, in addition to decreasing behavior problems at home and in school (Webster-Stratton, Reid, & Hammond, 2004).

3. *Focus on teachers' beliefs and instructional interactions.* The nature of instruction and of teachers' beliefs makes a significant contribution to children's development. Where teachers hold high but realistic and developmentally appropriate expectations, children perform better (Goldenberg & Gallimore, 1991; Ysseldyke & Christenson, 1988)—and teachers are judged by observers to have higher quality classrooms than those who endorse developmentally inappropriate beliefs (McCarty, Abbott-Shin, & Lambert, 2001). Questions such as the following are important: Do teachers believe there is one correct way of delivering material, and that it is up to children to understand it? Or do teachers continually create new ways of presenting material if it is not understood? To what extent do teachers establish a supportive learning environment and use positive motivational strategies? Thus assessors (often as members of a screening team) must become familiar with local instructional practices used at the preschool and kindergarten levels, and with what is expected once children enter first grade. Often teachers need a support system that includes ongoing training and consultation. The Success for All program (Slavin et al., 1994), for example, is based on the belief that reading failure in the primary grades is preventable. The program focuses on prevention and immediate intensive intervention in the context of the classroom. The program involves three components: (a) curriculum revision to foster excellent instruction in prekindergarten, kindergarten, and the primary grades, with regular periods for reading and writing; (b) one-to-one in-class tutoring support if problems begin to surface; (c) parent support, with a team at school available to make families feel comfortable in the school and involve parents in providing support for their children; and (d) regular reassessment of child performance and consultation with teachers. The naturalistic intervention design detailed by Barnett and Carey (1992) and Barnett, Bell, and Carey (1999) is another excellent example of ecobehavioral analysis of interacting environmental systems. Here the focus is on identifying important behaviors needed for children to be successful and on developing interventions that easily can be incorporated into the routines of caregivers. This approach seeks to capitalize on everyday incidental activities (shopping, play, and mealtime) as opportunities for practice and learning at home and in the classroom. Examples of effective instructional interventions based on these principles are recent studies conducted in Head Start Programs that (1) significantly increased rhyme detection over control groups by embedding it in introductory and closing singing during circle time (Majsterek, Shorr, & Erion, 2000), (2) significantly increased children's vocabularly at the end of the year over control classrooms by training teachers in specific storybook reading and conversa-

tional strategies that promoted language development (Wasik, Bond, & Hindman, 2006), and (3) significantly increased math ability and enjoyment over control classrooms by training teachers in how to promote emergent math skills and interest during daily routines (Arnold, Fisher, Doctoroff, & Dobbs, 2002). The positive behavior supports model is similar in its ecological systemic approach to intervention with children with severe disabilities (Lucyshyn, Dunlap, & Albin, 2002).

4. *Promote emotional and social competence.* Emotional development is as important as cognitive development in the later academic success of young children (Raver, 2003). Emotional skills and regulation play a key role in the development of children's interpersonal relationships, problem-solving behaviors, and readiness to learn. From longitudinal and early intervention studies, it is clear that emotional and behavioral problems appear very early in life and can quickly become entrenched and difficult to remediate if professional help is delayed until children start formal schooling (U.S. Department of Health and Human Services [DHHS], 1999). Thus social and emotional competence should be routinely assessed in early childhood programs, and curricula should be implemented as necessary to promote such competence (see Chapter 14).

5. *Develop strong parent–professional partnerships to support child development.* Families have a powerful role in shaping early child development, and yet they need the support of culture and of cultural institutions to perform this role successfully. The quality of parent–professional partnerships influences the ability of parents and professionals to work together for children's benefit, the parents' receptiveness to intervention, the professionals' willingness to learn from parents, and the quality of later such partnerships. Some professional practices that can promote these partnerships include a welcoming environment; respect for cultural diversity; positive and nonjudgmental interest in the whole family; maintaining confidentiality and keeping agreements; sharing information and resources; and focusing on parents' hopes, concerns, and needs (see Esler, Godber, & Christenson, 2002; Fish, 2002).

6. *Ensure the psychological and physical safety of children at home and in schools or daycare centers.* Early childhood professionals should be attuned to the quality of parent–child relationships and family life, and sensitive to negative changes in children's well-being. If abuse or neglect is suspected, it should be reported, and supports should be put in place to enhance the functioning of the child and the family. Although it may be difficult for school or center personnel to ensure that children are treated properly outside of the school or center building, abuse or neglect by staff or peers should be not be tolerated. Staff training in conflict resolution, appropriate discipline techniques, behavior management, and stress and anger management will provide teachers and caregivers with the support and resources to address problematic interactions as they arise (see Brassard & Rivelis, 2006). Abused children often inaccurately identify their own and others' emotional states, and are inclined to attribute negative intent to the neutral behavior of others (Crittenden, 1989). They often suffer from poor self-control and low levels of self-esteem and self-confidence (Fantuzzo, 1990). Teaching children to control, regulate, and modulate their emotions, and to cooperate with adults and peers, can significantly reduce aggressive and impulsive behavior (Webster-Stratton et al., 2004) that elicits negative responses from others.

Possible Barriers to Assessment and Intervention

Four sets of possible barriers to assessment and intervention are discussed below: family issues, system issues, professional issues, and measurement issues.

Family Issues

The work of numerous researchers highlights key issues that may impinge on the assessor–family relationship (Bailey & Wolery, 1992; Hanson & Lynch, 2004; Nihira, Weisner, & Bernheimer, 1994; Sameroff & MacKenzie, 2003). These include (1) assessors' lack of openness to families' culture or to parental input and style, along with parental skepticism or unwillingness to participate in assessment/intervention; (2) lack of available support to help families cope with stress and interact effectively with their children; and (3) lack of cooperation between home and school or other intervention settings, including lack of outreach to families or of assistance in interaction with other social service agencies.

System Issues

Considerable confusion and inequity may exist regarding the implementation of desired programs, policies, regulations, or procedures for children to qualify for services. It is essential, therefore, to consider policy issues that can hinder assessment or impede intervention. For example, although compensatory education programs such as Early Head Start, Head Start, and Title I represent the promise of equal educational opportunity regardless of SES or family income, these promises are often not kept. Only a small percentage of eligible children receive services, and these programs are particularly underutilized by children who have or are at high risk for disabilities, especially by those whose parents are in a minority group or are non-English speaking (Beauchesne, Barnes, & Patsdaughter, 2004; Peterson et al., 2004). Many poor or linguistically diverse children are placed in early childhood special education programs, with beginning reading often the basis of an LD designation (McGill-Franzen & Allington, 1991). Many states require the administration of developmental tests prior to entrance into Head Start and kindergarten, and children who are not able to perform these tasks may be referred for special education. Furthermore, Head Start programs need to serve a percentage of children with disabilities, and the children of poor families are those most likely to be labeled as having disabilities (McGill-Franzen, 1994). Researchers also point out that the focus of these programs is largely on child deficits, not school practices. And school districts widely engage in practices of retention or extra-year placements for low-achieving kindergarten children (Shepard & Smith, 1989). McGill-Franzen (1994) summarizes these issues well: "Many low-achieving children who formerly would have been called poor or educationally disadvantaged become handicapped instead" (p. 26), and these practices shape teachers' beliefs. Other system issues that may constitute barriers include (1) strict or confusing state or local administrative policies, regulations, or procedures for children to qualify for services, as well as rigid bureaucracies; (2) lack of trained staff, limited or no time for training, and shortage of personnel from diverse backgrounds; and (3) lack of funding (Bryant & Graham, 1993; Peterson et al., 2004).

Professional Barriers

The knowledge, skill, attitudes, experience, and training of individuals who work with preschool children are all critical to appropriate assessment practices and to integrating outcomes into meaningful intervention. Many assessors have not been trained to work with preschool children and their families, are unfamiliar with the range of measures available, and are not familiar with the strengths and drawbacks of instructional practices used prior to grade 1. In addition, assessors need to have a comprehensive command of the research literature across developmental areas. This literature provides evidence on how children develop physically, learn, acquire language and their concepts of the world, and develop social-interactional behaviors. For example, the research literature on how young children acquire concepts and the errors they make on the path to mastery can be used to probe responses, provide the needed adult supports, and develop learning experiences.

Measurement Issues

A number of important measurement issues can constitute barriers to assessment and intervention at the preschool level. Among these are (1) the small number of reliable and valid measures for determining developmental delay; (2) the lack of instruments available in languages other than English (although the number of measures available in Spanish has been increasing); (3) the lack of understanding of how developmental norms and expectations may differ from culture to culture; and (4) practical difficulties related to professional training and cost. These issues are detailed throughout this book.

THE ASSESSMENT PROCESS: CHALLENGES AND CONSIDERATIONS IN PLANNING

Many educators and early interventionists are openly skeptical about the use of standardized testing for preschool children, citing the nature of such tests' demands for information-processing skills that young children do not possess, the negative influence of the tests' results on parents and teachers' perceptions about children, and many other objections. Of particular concern are screening practices that exclude children from entering kindergarten, and readiness screening prior to first grade that results in extra-year kindergarten or "transition" year placements. The arguments are well articulated by Genishi (1992), Kim and Kagan (1999), Martin (1988), Meisels (1989b, 1999), and Shepard et al. (1998), who point out the problems created by categorizing young children in this way. These include the following: Few allowances are made for differences in learning styles and developmental patterns; decisions are based on minimal samples of behavior, and often based on the use of unfamiliar tasks; children are labeled to receive services, usually on the basis of deficits alone; and the outcomes of many standardized tests used are not directly translatable into instruction or intervention. Martin (1988) is particularly concerned with the expression "at risk," noting that it is a "prediction of danger" and can become a self-fulfilling prophecy. Her concern that labeling children who encounter difficulty as being "at risk" often deflects attention from how the teacher and the classroom could adapt to the child's difficulties is well founded. Particularly problematic issues include (1) inappropriate labeling of children as "disabled" who are not disabled, in order for them to receive otherwise unavailable services; (2) use of labels that are irrelevant to instructional needs; (3) use of arbitrarily defined deficit categories, rather than a focus on the individual child's psychoeducational needs; (4) use of limited funds to determine eligibility rather than to develop effective educational programs; and (5) reluctance to take responsibility for modifying curricula and programs to meet diverse child needs (Dawson & Knoff, 1990). These issues present ongoing challenges to assessors and early childhood educators who are faced with federal and state mandates under the NCLB Act and IDEA 2004.

Professional organizations such as the NAEYC (2003) and the National Association of School Psychologists (NASP; Bracken, Bagnato, & Barnett, 1990; Dawson & Knoff, 1990) spell out essential principles for assessors at the early childhood levels. Assessment is simply "a means for answering questions about young children's knowledge, behavior, skill, or personality" (Meisels & Atkins-Burnett, 2005). As such, it needs to be conducted in relationship to specific purposes. We believe that all preschool assessors should engage in developmentally appropriate practices; that standardized tests should be used only when they are appropriate for improving services for children and making sure they benefit from their educational experiences (NAEYC, 2003); and that such tests must be reliable and valid for their purposes. Their contribution depends on what information they yield, how this information is used to guide instruction or behavioral intervention, and how it is used to document progress.

The principles described thus far, however, are often compromised. The bottom line involves the financial resources of communities, schools, and other agencies, as well as current pressures for accountability. In other words, in addition to getting assessment done according to state timelines, there is often pressure to use the least expensive procedures. Once children enter kindergarten, this sometimes involves using outside assessors at the lowest acceptable level of training—who often lack familiarity with the school's structure, curriculum, student population, programs available, and local issues, and who often bypass such appropriate practices as observation in the classroom or the home.

Challenges to the Assessment Process

In order to achieve the multiple goals of assessment, a number of major challenges need to be taken into account, including the effects of labeling; child characteristics and differing responses to variable learning demands; and characteristics of the testing situation. (Technical issues related to assessment approaches are covered in Chapter 3.) Each of these concerns is addressed briefly in the sections that follow and throughout this text.

Effects of Labeling

Some specialists raise important questions about the potential negative effects of labeling and the overall poor predictability of early childhood measures to later school achievement (Adelman, 1982; Genishi, 1992; Hobbs, 1975; Keogh & Becker, 1973; Lichtenstein & Ireton, 1984; Lidz, 1983b; Linder, 1996; Meisels, 1985, 1989b). An early NAEYC (1988) policy statement on standardized testing also raised cautions about "the possible effects of failure on the admission test on the child's self-esteem, the parents' perceptions, or the educational impact of labeling or mislabeling the child as being behind the peer group" (p. 44). This concern continues to be voiced by many teachers and early childhood specialists.

There are two major reasons why a label is assigned: (1) to determine eligibility for preschool special education services provided for by IDEA 2004; and (2) to identify children's preparedness for kindergarten or first grade in order to place children into transitional classes or to hold them back or place them in classes for the gifted. A number of problems related to assigning labels for purposes of eligibility are addressed in a NASP (2003a) position statement, "Advocacy for Appropriate Educational Services for All Children." Such problems include (1) mislabeling of some children as "disabled" because assessors lack knowledge regarding racial, cultural, and linguistic diversity, which would permit them to recognize developmental milestones in varying forms and design instruction to address diverse learning styles; (2) the irrelevance of labels to many children's instructional needs; (3) reduced expectations for children placed in special education; and (4) limited modifications of instructional programs to meet the diverse needs of children. Some specialists (Smith & Shakel, 1986) have advocated many years for broad, noncategorical labeling of children (e.g., "developmentally delayed"), rather than the use of existing special education categories in order to determine eligibility for special services. Such noncategorical definition has been possible for children ages 3–5 under Public Law 99-457, and has been extended through age 9 under IDEA 2004. Smith and Shakel (1986) have also suggested that "deferred diagnosis" may be a useful category for children who show defined developmental delays with unclear etiology. This category could be assigned a limited time (allowing assessment to take place over time) until either the delay is remedied or more accurate diagnosis can be made. The NASP Division of Early Childhood recommended that eligibility criteria include the noncategorical option of "developmental delay" and that intervention take place where possible in regular classrooms (NASP, 2003b). Issues related to labeling children as "immature" or as "not ready" for kindergarten or first grade are covered in Chapter 7. Issues related to determining giftedness are reviewed briefly in Chapter 11.

Child Characteristics

Preschool children's day-to-day behavior is highly variable (Boehm & Sandberg, 1982; Lidz, 1983b; Nagle, 2000; Ulrey, 1982), so that responses available one day or in one context may not be accessible the next day or in another context. There will be significant fluctuations in their day-to-day behavior, sudden growth spurts, and vulnerability to such events as the birth of a new sibling. Moreover, while early childhood specialists point out general stages and sequences of development, they also recognize that broad variation occurs in the "normal" patterns and time of development (NAEYC, 1988). Therefore, except in extreme cases such as developmental disorders and severe emotional problems where behavior is quite stable, the results of much preschool assessment need to be viewed as tentative. Test or observation results need to be confirmed through periodic observation and rescreening, and to be corroborated by other sources of information. Furthermore, development is highly interconnected across areas, so that outcomes of screening or in-depth evaluation in one domain (e.g., communication) must also be interpreted in relationship to other areas (e.g., the physical/motor, cognitive and socio-emotional domains) and to the environmental context.

In any review of assessment procedures and goals, it is also important to bear in mind some age-related characteristics of preschoolers that are highlighted in the literature (Boehm & Sandberg, 1982; Bracken, 2000; Greenspan & Meisels, 1996; Lidz, 2003; Nagle, 2000; Paget, 1990, 1991; Shepard et al., 1998; Ulrey, 1982), and that can make these children a challenge to assess:

1. Many preschoolers may be unfamiliar with the procedures required by the testing situation, such as test-taking skills, the materials presented, comprehension of the instructions (which might contain multiple steps or concepts they have not yet learned), and task demands.
2. Some children lack well-developed verbal skills, particularly when responding to unfamiliar adults, particularly if children have cognitive or language difficulties.
3. Young children's developing perceptual–motor skills may not match task demands.

4. Some preschoolers may have difficulty in separating from adults, which may result in distress, negativism, or oppositional behavior when the children are entering the assessment situation.
5. Limited ability to pay attention, as well as possible anxiety and other response tendencies, must be considered. Young children typically do not sit for long periods of time with focused attention; they move around a lot and are sensitive to distractions. Some preschoolers are shy, and their discomfort may result in task refusals.
6. Young children's tolerance for frustration is often poor, and they may not necessarily try to please the assessor and comply with task demands. They may become particularly frustrated with tasks they do not like or with repeated failure. Since they may not have the language skills to express their frustration verbally, they are more likely to express their distress behaviorally. Children from diverse cultures may have styles of expressing themselves that are different from those of the assessor.
7. Adults may need to demonstrate what is expected to a child in order for him or her to understand the task.
8. Children who have had preschool experience may relate more readily to a new adult—in this case, to the assessor.
9. Physical well-being, including health, hunger, or fatigue, may affect young children's performance more than that of older children.
10. Disability conditions, particularly those relating to vision, hearing, speech, language, and motor ability, may impede performance (see Bagnato & Neisworth, 1991, Paget, 1991, and Sattler, 2001, for guidelines for assessing children with low-incidence disabilities).

Other characteristics of young children help to offset these challenges, including the facts that they generally respond positively to adult attention, are spontaneous, are eager, and are interested in preschool assessment materials. Many are also delighted to have an enthusiastic adult focus all of his or her attention on them. Moreover, little children like to play, and the more play-like the assessment situation is, the more likely assessors are to obtain needed information. However, the session, while fun, should not be too play-like, in that the child should know that he or she is expected to comply with assessor requests and directives. We like Susan Vig's term "special work" to describe the assessment activities to the child (see Chapter 11). A child's response to assessment can vary greatly, depending on how the assessment situation is set up: (1) at one point of time in a strange room, with strange tasks and a strange tester; (2) within the context of play situations, with several observers watching the child engage in play with familiar objects; or (3) in the everyday context of home or classroom, allowing multiple observations in a familiar setting.

A major challenge comes when a child is referred by a parent or medical professional for developmental testing and is brought to a clinic where the opportunity for observation in a natural setting over time is not present. Under these circumstances, it is important for the assessor to spend time with the child in a play situation prior to testing, or to have the parent engage in a play activity with the child. Many assessors allow a parent to be present during the assessment or observe through a two-way mirror—not only to help the child feel more at ease, but to confirm whether or not the child's performance is typical, and to contribute other observations.

Finally, children's needs change over time. A verbal child who complies easily with the demands of nursery school may encounter difficulty in kindergarten when learning letter–sound associations. A child with poor attention at age 3 may have settled down by age 4 or 5. Given these issues, the reliability and validity of preschool assessment measures and procedures present special challenges; we will return to this topic in later chapters.

The Assessment Setting/Situation

As suggested above, the characteristics of the testing situation itself and the procedures used can pose challenges to the assessment process. In most large-scale developmental screening programs, for example, a child may be brought to an unfamiliar environment and be seen by a team of strangers. Rarely does the screening take place in the classroom or home, or under conditions that simulate classroom or home learning situations (Adelman, 1982). However, a child may be highly distracted by the materials typically present in a home or classroom. An early childhood assessor therefore needs to be aware of alternative ways to put a child at ease and elicit the child's best responses, interest, attention, and cooperation. Effective strategies include being enthusiastic, using humor, playing with the child on the floor to establish rapport prior to formal assessment, and so forth (see, e.g., Paget, 1990, 1991). It is important to set up the room so that it is appealing and so that distracters (such as mirrors or other materials) are not easily visible or are removed. Toys, furniture, and other materials should be age-appropriate and should be adapted as necessary for a child with a particular disabling condition. Assessors need to provide the necessary physical and verbal supports for children to be successful (including modification of tasks and the pace of presentation to meet the needs of children with behavioral difficulties, sensory disabilities, or poor language skills), as well as praise for children's efforts. Other strategies we have found to be effective in engaging children's cooperation include the following: giving 3–5 minutes of play time after so many tasks; turning away from a child and not responding for a minute if a child is not cooperating, followed by warm praise for appropriate behavior as a child settles into the task; posting a pictorial schedule of the testing session on a Velcro strip (e.g., special work, snack, special work, play time, special work, a small reward) that a child can remove as each activity is completed; and use of a more elaborate token system or other reinforcement schedule. Strategies used should be described in the report. As emphasized throughout this chapter, assessors also need to be sensitive to cultural variation (i.e., to respond appropriately to behaviors that may be culturally appropriate but different from expected responses), and to engage in nonbiased administration and accurate scoring of assessment measures. A successful early childhood assessor needs to have had training and experience with a wide range of very young children, including those with various disabling conditions as well as with those who are gifted, and to know how to adapt tasks appropriately. Finally, an assessor needs to be alert to and observe the competencies a child demonstrates in an area not being assessed (i.e., spontaneous use of language, or fine and gross motor skills).

Considerations in Planning Assessment

A common set of questions applies to planning any assessment. The answers to these questions will shape the assessment plan.

1. *What is your assessment question? How will the results be used?* Most assessment questions can be answered in a variety of ways, depending on how the results will be

used. For example, consider the following question: How competent is a child socially and emotionally? If the purpose is to assess emotional skills in 3-year-olds to plan a curriculum, an informal teacher test of knowledge and use of emotional skills may suffice. If the purpose is to screen an early childhood population for potential emotional or behavioral problems, then a parent or teacher/caregiver screening measure designed for that purpose should be used. If a significant problem in emotional or behavioral functioning has been reported and the purpose of assessment is to rule in or out a diagnosis, then multiple measures with demonstrated validity for this purpose from multiple sources should be used to address the assessment question.

2. *From what sources will information be obtained?* The purpose of the assessment, the ease of obtaining information, and the quality of information that is likely to be obtained will all guide the sources of information to be used. For example, if a child is having great difficulty learning at school, an assessor might solicit informal observations by parents, teachers, and others; conduct parent and/or teacher interviews; administer a questionnaire or rating scales to multiple informants; observe the child in one or more settings; administer tests to the child; engage the child in play activities; and collect ongoing work samples. All are likely to provide useful information about how the child learns and when and why there are difficulties.

3. *How comprehensive will the assessment be?* The purpose of the assessment, the skills of the assessor, and the resources of the agency or school for whom the assessor works will all determine how comprehensive the assessment will be. In general, the more severe the problem that a child is having (or that those in a particular setting are having with a child), the more comprehensive the assessment will be. Diagnostic assessments are more comprehensive than developmental screenings or measures for planning instruction. They generally involve multiple sources of information and measures, and often professionals from multiple disciplines.

4. *How will children's strengths as well as difficulties be assessed, and what variables will be considered?* How will children's learning strategies be assessed across development areas? Given the problem-driven nature of many assessments, and the frustration often experienced by parents and/or teachers before referring a child, it may take a concerted effort on the part of assessors to identify areas of strength. Assessment across developmental areas (e.g., communication, interpersonal relationships), strategic interviewing to identify areas of emerging knowledge (see Chapter 7), and asking parents and teachers/caregivers about the child's strengths are ways of ensuring that a more complete picture of the child is obtained.

5. *In what ways will assessors review the technical adequacy of approaches used and become familiar with (and use) new and alternative approaches?* The technical adequacy of early childhood measures is highly variable. It is the ethical responsibility of all assessors to ensure that the measures they administer have demonstrated validity for the purposes for which they are used. Using unvalidated measures to make major life decisions for young children is unconscionable. Chapter 3 offers a guide to evaluating measures for this age group.

6. *How will families be involved in the process?* Preschool children are highly dependent on their families in every area; families are the most important context for children this age. Assessments that focus both on the child and on the family surround (including needs, strengths, and environmental supports, as well as stressors) are those most likely to lead to interventions that will be accepted by and useful for both the family and the child. Relationships forged as part of the assessment can lead to ongoing home–school–agency collaboration.

7. *How will home and school learning environments be assessed? What variables will be reviewed?* The development of environmental measures, and their use in home and educational settings (particularly the latter), have lagged behind the development of measures of the child. Parents and educational personnel are often sensitive about being evaluated and possibly implicated in a child's learning or behavior problem. Nonetheless, the quality of disciplinary and instructional approaches, the beliefs of parents and teachers, and the use of reinforcement and consequences are all casually related to competent child functioning. Assessment of such variables is an essential component of evaluating children in context (see Chapters 5 and 8).

8. *How will adaptations to cultural, language, or disability conditions be made?* The diversity of languages and cultural backgrounds in some North American school districts is so great that no school can have the personnel or expertise to provide culturally appropriate assessments for all children. However, various practices can be followed to minimize the bias inherent in evaluating children from cultural and linguistic backgrounds for which no appropriate normed tests exist, and from backgrounds not represented on the assessment team (see Chapter 9 for a review of these practices).

9. *What will intervention involve?* Intervention needs to be broadly conceived in order to promote child competence to the greatest extent. It may include activities and strategies directed toward child behavior and learning; changes in teaching content; modified instructional approaches; teacher in-service activities; special placements or intervention services; parent involvement outreach programs; family therapy; greater use of informal social support by families; family planning and health; and interaction with community organizations, agencies, or other services.

SUMMARY

In the multifactor ecocultural model of assessment presented in this chapter (and visually displayed in Figure 2.3), assessment is viewed as an ongoing problem-solving process that informs intervention. This process needs to take account of the child's interactions within his or her home, school, and community environmental contexts, including risk factors and buffers. Assessors need to be sensitive to diversity, to define their assessment question(s) clearly, and to use approaches that address this question and improve services for children and families. Information needs to be gathered from multiple sources and across contexts and time, using multiple approaches (especially observation). It is important as well to consider children's learning strategies and the supports needed from others to foster emerging behaviors and skills. Our idea of a consummate preschool assessor is someone who knows child development across all domains, and who is familiar with the full range from highly deviant to exceptional functioning. Assessors need to know what different cultures value and expect on the part of their children, as well as the range of early childhood environments children experience. They need to be aware of the major childhood disorders, and to seek information and consultation as necessary when they encounter less common disorders. They also need a sound understanding of psychometrics and must keep up with the research literature and identify areas they do not understand. Nothing can replace a combination of experience, training, and seeking knowledge. Assessment is a product of the professional and what he or she brings to the situation, including keen observational skills, knowledge of diagnostic procedures, the ability to develop plans drawing on a variety of intervention approaches, and an ability to work with others.

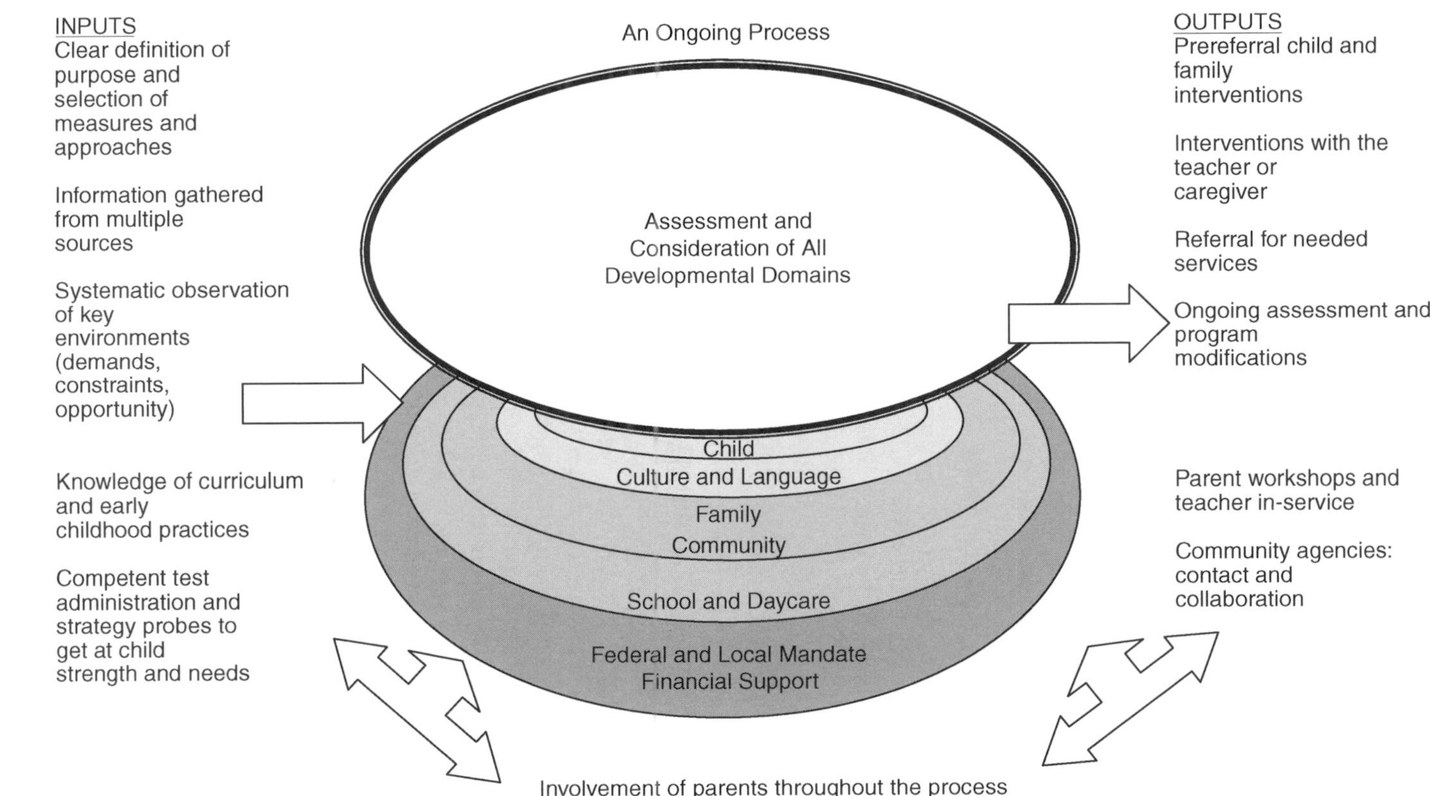

FIGURE 2.3. Multifactor ecocultural model of assessment: assessment ↔ intervention.

Chapter 3

Technical Concerns

Although early childhood researchers and educators agree the early identification of potential problem areas and early intervention are worthy goals, they also generally agree that the procedures used to achieve these goals often fail to meet minimal technical standards in the areas of validity, reliability, and standardization (Adelman, 1982; Boehm & Sandberg, 1982; Bracken, 1988, 2000; Lichtenstein & Ireton, 1984; Meisels, 1989a, 1999; Paget & Nagle, 1986; Salvia & Ysseldyke, 2004; Sattler, 1988, 2001; Thurlow, O'Sullivan & Ysseldyke, 1986). For example, assessors screening large numbers of preschool children as the first stage in the identification process must consider possible problems with predictive validity, due to either identifying children as having problems who in fact do not (*false positives*) or by missing children who turn out to have problems (*false negatives*). Good screening instruments must have a low percentage of both false positives and false negatives. The technical adequacy of a measure depends on documentation of validity, reliability, and (for norm-referenced tests) normative data. Of particular concern is the extent to which decision errors are likely to occur with the use of a specific measure or approach. These errors may result from child behaviors on the day of assessment, assessor errors, and/or test content. Detailed standards for judging the quality of educational and psychological tests are spelled out in the *Standards for Educational and Psychological Testing* (American Educational Research Association [AERA], American Psychological Association, & National Council for Measurement in Education, 1999). The application of these standards to preschool assessment is the purpose of this chapter.

Along with the technical characteristics of assessment procedures, it is also important to consider the (1) extent to which the items represent the construct assessed; (2) clarity and cultural appropriateness of the items and illustrations; (3) complexity of directions (both syntax and the inclusion of basic concepts unfamiliar to many children); (4) complexity of administrative and scoring procedures; (5) training required on the part of the assessor; (6) length of the procedure; (7) modifications suggested to meet the special needs of children with disabling conditions; and (8) the attractiveness of test stimuli to young children.

RELIABILITY AND RELATED ISSUES

Reliability, an essential requirement of all assessment measures, tells assessors how confident they can be in the scores obtained or in the observations collected. An assessment procedure must be reliable in order for it to be valid. When selecting measures, assessors need to consider how high the reliability coefficient (r) is as well as the nature of the reliability data presented and sources of possible error (e.g., if the reliability data are based on a small sample the chances of error are greater). Reliability addresses a number of questions, which are covered briefly in the sections that follow.

Consistency/Stability

The consistency of a child's test performance (or behaviors within and across observations) is of major concern in determining whether an assessor has obtained a representative picture of the child's performance. When the concept of consistency stability is applied to test reliability, it takes the form of this question: "If we could give a child many opportunities to take a test in a short period of time without the effects of practice, how consistent would the child be in responding to the same items?" Of course, it is not really possible to achieve this ideal situation in real life, and so methods of estimating reliability can provide only approximate answers to this question. Moreover, several characteristics of preschool children pose challenges to the consistency/stability concept.

First, as parents and early childhood educators will attest, young children's growth is rapid across developmental areas. It is exciting to watch the unfolding of competence with each day, week, and month. This time of rapid development presents a dilemma: Little children are often not reliable. Their skills and abilities are emerging—available or expressed on some occasions but not on others, or elicited by some examples and not others. Young children are also likely to be highly sensitive to the testing situation, including the personality of the tester, format of the test, particular examples used, and constraints of the situation (which is often new and unfamiliar). An assessor thus needs to gain and maintain a child's attention and make the situation an enjoyable experience. Furthermore, young children frequently have limited expressive skills, which may preclude them from accurately communicating what they know. Assessors therefore need to be attuned to children's styles, use multiple assessment procedures so that convergent or disconfirming data are collected over time, and interpret findings in view of all this information.

In addition, assessors need to look for an adequate sample of a child's behavior or knowledge. Developmental screening tests, for example, are by definition brief and include only a few items per area or sample very few areas (e.g., copying shapes and hopping, skipping, and jumping for the visual–motor and gross motor areas, respectively). Thus an assessor using such a test may or may not gain a representative picture of a child's functioning. The child who performs poorly will either be rescreened at a later point or referred and assessed in depth. The child who performs at a borderline level may be passed by. In general, longer tests covering each area in detail will provide a more representative picture of a child's performance and result in greater reliability. The assessor can also confer with parents and teachers regarding the accuracy of test findings.

Measures of reliability typically reported in test manuals take the following forms (see texts such as Anastasi & Urbina, 1997, and Taylor, 2005, for more details).

Internal Approaches to Reliability

The first question of interest is how consistently items on the same test measure the area(s) of concern. The focus is on performance on a single test. Two major approaches to this question are split-half reliability and the use of coefficient alpha or related statistical procedures. *Split-half reliability* is obtained by dividing the test into two halves (alternate items, first half vs. second half, or other combinations of items), with the child's performance correlated between halves. Statistical procedures generally used include the (1) *Spearman–Brown prophecy formula*, to account for the underestimates of reliability that may result from shortened tests; (2) *Küder–Richardson formula*, which is a measure of the relationship of all possible splits; or (3) *coefficient alpha* (Cronbach, 1951), which represents the correlation of every item with each other and the total score. The greater the correlation between items within a subtest or across the test, the greater the confidence assessors can have that the test or subtest measures the same construct.

Measures of Stability across Time

Two approaches to measuring stability across time are used: test–retest reliability and alternate-form reliability. *Test–retest reliability* is determined by administering the same test to the same child or group of children on two occasions separated by a brief period of time (usually 2–3 weeks) to assess consistency of responding. Children's performance at the first administration is then correlated with their performance at the second administration. Test–retest reliability brings with it a number of challenges that can inflate or deflate reliability estimates. In many areas, growth can be expected if the retest occurs several weeks later. Or some direct teaching may intervene, particularly with performance-type items (e.g., skipping). And the preschool child encountering a testing situation for the first time may have learned something about taking the test by the time of the retest. Other issues include familiarity or unfamiliarity with the material covered (e.g., vocabulary used in items), which may put the child at an advantage or disadvantage, and the transient effects of attention or physical well-being. Accounting for this form of reliability is essential in test manuals.

To obtain *alternate-form (parallel-form) reliability*, two equivalent forms of the test are administered to the same children within a 2- to 3-week interval. The scores from the first form are then correlated with scores from the second form. While avoiding some of the problems of practice, and therefore providing the best measure of consistency over time, parallel forms are not available for most preschool tests. It is difficult to devise parallel examples of such items as copying a circle, jumping, or counting to 10. Moreover, as with test–retest approaches to reliability, intervening practice and familiarity with the format can inflate or deflate outcomes. Nevertheless, alternate forms of tests are particularly valuable when assessing student progress and are more prevalent beginning at the kindergarten level. Interobserver agreement scores can be considered a type of alternate-form reliability, in which two observers are analogous to two parallel forms of a testing instrument (Page & Iwata, 1986).

Factors Affecting Reliability

Although an accepted rule of thumb is to use the most reliable test available for a particular purpose, a number of critical factors that need to be considered in any review of reliability data have been detailed by Bailey and Brochin (1989). These include procedural reliability and scoring reliability. *Procedural reliability* reflects the extent to which assessors adhere to the procedural requirements of administering a particular test or observational approach and responding to children's answers. *Scoring reliability* involves (1) the extent to which scoring follows the procedures detailed in assessment manuals; (2) the objectivity of scoring and the extent to which scorers agree with each other (e.g., when scoring a practice protocol or coding an observational example); and (3) the extent to which the forms of bias that apply to observers also apply to assessors (see Chapter 4). These reliability concerns can be addressed in large part through adequate training of assessors. Training should include witnessing test administration or observational approaches (either directly or through the use of training videotapes), obtaining practice in test administration and scoring, cross-checking scoring, and reaching a criterion level of procedural and scoring reliability before evaluating child clients.

In addition to the issues raised above, several other factors affect reliability data:

1. *The variability of the group tested.* The larger the spread of scores, the greater the reliability. Groups of children that represent diverse abilities allow for more variability, which in turn leads to higher reliability coefficients than do groups in which children are more similar. However, if most children get most items correct on a test (which is appropriate when a test reflects mastery of specific instructional objectives or areas of knowledge desired on the part of all children), the reliability is likely to be lower. The more diverse the group in terms of age, ability, and SES, the higher the reliabilities are likely to be. High reliabilities need to be viewed with great caution. Some preschool test manuals, for example, report reliabilities based on only 30–40 children covering a large age span (e.g., 4–6 years of age). Such variability in age results in higher reliabilities and masks the extent of the variability that occurs at each age.

2. *The number of items on a test.* Longer tests allow for more variability in student performance than brief measures, and thus are likely to report higher reliability coefficients. Many tests used with young children, however, cover broad content areas with only a few items per area; the result is that these tests have lower reliability coefficients than tests with many items in one or two more narrow content areas.

3. *The difficulty of test items.* Difficult tests also allow for more variability than tests that measure areas most children have mastered. During the development of many standardized tests, those items that most children pass may be deleted from final forms. At the preschool level, however, it is important for tests to have a sufficient number of easy items (referred to as the test *floor*) to assess children who have low ability (i.e., children should be able to answer some questions correctly). Adequate floor and *ceiling* (the inclusion of more difficult items) are essential for tests used at multiple age levels and are major concerns at the preschool level. The Wechsler Preschool and Primary Scale of Intelligence—Third Edition (WPPSI-III; Wechsler, 2002), for example, has insufficient floor levels at age 3 for testing children for possible mental retardation.

Additional reasons for the lower reliability of preschool assessment measures than of those for school-age children (which need to be accounted for in the interpretation of results) may include poorly defined constructs, standardization samples that do not include atypical children, and factors related to assessors' training and experience with young children (Bracken, 1987, 1991b; Harrison, 1992). Bracken (1991b) urges that short-term reliability should be emphasized when assessors are selecting preschool screening measures.

Deciding Whether a Test Is Reliable Enough for a Particular Purpose

It is well known that reliability will be the highest for total test scores, followed by subtest scores; item scores are the least reliable. Issues related to reliability, documented many years ago, still pertain today. For example, Guilford (1956) provided the following guidelines for interpreting *Pearson product–moment coefficients* of correlation:

<.20: Slight, almost negligible.
.20–.40: Low; definite, but small, relationship.
.40–.70: Moderate; substantial relationship.
.70–.90: High; marked relationship.
.90–1.00: Very high; dependable relationship.

Many reviewers of preschool tests tend to use the same yardstick in judging the adequacy of all tests, regardless of the type/purpose of each test (e.g., screening, curriculum planning, or diagnosis). Generally these judgments focus on the internal consistency of the test and test–retest coefficients. Often test–retest coefficients have been determined with small samples and samples that do not include children with special needs. A better approach is to consider reliability data in relationship to the purpose and comprehensiveness of the assessment measure. Here are several recommendations made by testing experts:

- For important (high-stake) decisions, such as whether children qualify for special services, high reliability is needed:
  - .90 minimum, .95 desirable (Nunnally, 1978).
  - .90 minimum standard for individually administered diagnostic tests; .80 for group-administered tests (Salvia & Ysseldyke, 1988).
  - .80 minimum, .90 desirable for tests with a small standard error of measurement (see below) (Bailey & Brochin, 1989).
  - .90 for total test scores, .80 for subtest scores (Bracken, 1987).
- For purposes of screening that will lead to further assessment, a *slightly* lower level is acceptable:
  - .80 (Salvia & Ysseldyke, 1988).
- Lower levels of reliability are acceptable for screening that informs instruction but does not result in a referral.

On observational measures, a number of other factors related to reliability take on particular importance; these include observer agreement, the form of observation used (such as a rating scale or observational schedule), and the consistency of the observed behaviors over time and across settings or activities. These concerns are detailed by McCloskey (1990) and are covered in Chapter 4.

Standard Error of Measurement

Reliability is closely related to the standard error of measurement (*SEM*) of a test. This statistic estimates how consistently a child would score if tested repeatedly on the same test, without the effects of practice and with the child's random errors canceling each other out. Because (as noted earlier) this ideal situation is not possible, it is estimated statistically, based on the standard deviation of the sample taking the test as reported in test manuals. Since assessors want low error rates, test developers seek to report studies with a low *SEM*—as close to 0 as possible. The lower the *SEM*, the greater the confidence assessors can have in the accuracy of the score, and the greater the reliability of the test. The greater the *SEM*, the lower the confidence assessors can have regarding the score, since more of this estimate of a child's functioning is based on errors in the test itself or in procedures for administering, scoring, and interpreting the test outcomes. For example, a child who receives a score of 90 on a test that has an *SEM* of 3 can be expected to score:

Between 87 and 93, or within ±1 *SEM* (68% of the time).
Between 84 and 96, or within ±2 *SEM* (95% of the time).
Between 81 and 99, or within ±3 *SEM* (99% of the time).

The *SEM* will differ at different age and grade levels, as well as for students from different backgrounds. This information needs to be reported in test manuals. Concerns related to the *SEM* are essential for labeling and classifying children, such as those falling at the low end of the IQ range. For this reason, it is a growing practice for assessors to present scores as falling into *SEM* bands such as those suggested above. This step helps us understand the amount of error surrounding a score, and reminds us that scores are not fixed points. Assessors at the early childhood level have been slow to adopt this procedure, except in the area of cognitive functioning.

VALIDITY AND RELATED ISSUES

Validity is "the most fundamental consideration in developing and evaluating tests" (AERA et al., 1999, p. 9). The most important question one can raise about observation, norm-referenced, and performance-based assessment procedures is whether they are valid. *Validity* concerns the meaningfulness of what a test (or other assessment procedure) measures, in addition to how well it does so (Anastasi & Urbina, 1997). That is, does the test provide a true picture of what assessors are trying to assess? With young children, validity estimates are typically dependent on the use of concurrent measures of the same construct (i.e., basic concepts), of which standardized tests represent only one type of sampling; systematic observation and behavioral measures need to be part of the process as well. Validity also needs to be documented for each purpose stated in test manuals, and needs to be evaluated in relationship to an assessor's particular purpose. Sources of validity, detailed in the *Standards for Educational and Psychological Testing* (AERA et al., 1999), of concern to assessors are summarized in the sections that follow.

Evidence Based on Test Content

Content-related validity reflects the extent to which the content (items and tasks) of a test or observational measure samples the domain being assessed. Content validity is determined by carefully analyzing each skill area included, reviewing relevant developmental research, and drawing on the knowledge of experts. When selecting an assessment measure and evaluating its content, users need to evaluate the measure's content in relationship to (1) their assessment purpose (e.g., screening, instruction); (2) the research documentation provided in the manual related to the domain covered; and (3) the extent to which a measure reflects local objectives and curricular expectations (Bailey & Brochin, 1989). In addition, professionals need to consider whether the content of the assessment procedures selected is sufficiently detailed to meet their assessment purpose, review the appropriateness of the items for children from culturally and linguistically diverse backgrounds, and consider the utility of the measure for instructional planning.

Evidence Based on the Relationship to Other Variables

The relationship of test scores with other variables is obtained to "assess the degree to which these relationships are consistent with the constructs underlying the proposed test interpretations" (AERA et al., 1999, p. 13). Two forms of evidence (usually presented in the form of correlation coefficients) regarding the confidence one can have in the outcomes generally used at the preschool level include (1) providing congruent (concurrent) evidence and (2) providing predictive evidence. *Congruent* evidence refers to the extent to which a child's scores on one measure match the child's scores on other related measures (i.e., other tests of language competence or teacher observations) administered at approximately the same time. The more independent evidence collected to support inferences, the greater the confidence in the outcomes can be.

Predictive evidence refers to the criterion against which an assessment measure is evaluated, which is fixed at a future point in time. For example, to what extent does a score on a test of early academic learning obtained at the beginning of the kindergarten year (or a teacher judgment or observational measure) accurately predict later performance, such as achievement in reading at the end of grade 1? Another example is the extent to which a preschool developmental test correctly identifies as "at risk" or not those children who demonstrate learning problems and those who do not at the end of grade 2. Predictive evidence is essential for preschool assessors who need to identify developmental delay, and according to Meisels and Atkins-Burnett (2005) and Lichtenstein and Ireton (1984), it is among the major criteria for considering use of a particular preschool developmental screening measure. Developmental screening tests that miss many children who later encounter difficulty have little utility. Assessors want to see positive correlations between two measures—the closer to 1.0, the better. However, perfect agreement is not likely to happen, since different tests or observational approaches are likely to tap somewhat different content (even with subtests that have the same name). When determining the desired extent of the correlation, assessors also need to consider the criterion measure used. Typical criterion measures include achievement tests and teacher ratings. Many years ago, Thorndike and Hagen (1955) identified the following qualities desired of criterion measures, in order of importance: (1) relevant behaviors, (2) freedom from bias, (3) reliability, and (4) practicality.

Evidence Based on an Accumulated Database

The assessment purposes detailed by diverse assessment procedures and the constructs they represent (the set of behaviors they are developed to sample) need to be supported through the accumulation of research results. Evidence of validity needs to be demonstrated across multiple sources, including development of ability or skill with age; factor analysis; correlation with other measures of the same construct; and evidence from content and criterion-related studies showing that the constructs are correlated with one another, not with different constructs. As part of this process, it is important to gather evidence based on an analysis of children's individual responses. Such evidence can be gained through questioning children about their responses or strategies to particular items; maintaining records of response development on a given task; obtaining raters' evaluations; or examining other aspects of performance, such as response time (AERA et al., 1999, p. 12).

Hirsh-Pasek et al. (2005) present a case for what they call "empirical validity." Specifically, tests need to reflect "state-of-the-art research that charts developmental process that best predict later outcomes in reading, language, mathematics, social skill, to name a few" (p. 3). Assessment activities need to measure aspects of learning central to developmental milestones in each of these areas as children develop over time. Researchers and developers of assessment tools need to collaborate, so that the most recent findings regarding developmental processes are incorporated into assessment. Hirsh-Pasek et al. underscore the point that predictive validity needs to capture the full range of constructs detailed in early childhood developmental research and to consider the interactions among domains using examples of situations familiar to children (such as a birthday party). The focus needs to be on *how* children learn, in contrast to *what* they learn. In particular, the focus needs to be on the strategies children use to solve problems (see also Chapter 5).

Messick (1995a) urges that validity be viewed as a unified concept—one reflecting an overall evaluative judgment of the degree to which the empirical evidence and theoretical rationales support the adequacy, appropriateness of interpretation, and actions based on test scores or other modes of assessment. According to Messick, validity is not a property of a test or assessment as such, but rather the meaning of the test scores. *Meaning* refers to the interpretation of scores, as well as to their implications for action and the possible social consequences that might result (Messick, 1995a, p. 5). An integrated view of validity is reflected in the AERA et al. (1999) *Standards* document, referred to throughout this section.

Additional Validity Issues

A number of other issues affect validity, including the following:

1. *What is the timeline of prediction?* Except for individuals performing at the extremes, the farther away in time the criterion behavior is, the greater the probability of error. Making long-term predictions in reference to preschool children is inherently difficult, for a number of reasons. First, as Keogh and Becker (1973) pointed out, "it is not possible to sample the broad spectrum of skills needed for successful school performance years later" (p. 8). In other words, preschoolers cannot be tested on reading skills they have not yet been taught. Second, school and home environmental factors are rarely accounted for in the long-term prediction matrix. Third, the quality and form of instruction, as well as the nature and extent of intervention, are rarely detailed. Therefore, preschool assessors need to look for predictive studies carried out over brief intervals (e.g., the beginning to the end of a school year), where the nature of the instruction/intervention and teacher support can be documented.

2. *What criterion measures are used?* Assessors need to consider the relevance and reliability of the criterion measure used, as well as its sensitivity to the form of intervention used, when evaluating the magnitude of validity coefficients. Is there, for example, a match between the preschool problems identified (such as speech–language problems or motor problems) and the content of criterion measures, which generally are achievement

measures and sometimes involve teacher judgment? Or a child may perform poorly during screening, due to attention or behavioral problems; if the criterion measure is an achievement test, the outcomes may not reflect improvement in behavior.

3. *To what extent have intervening variables been accounted for?* If preschool intervention has beneficial effects—the hoped-for outcome of early intervention—one would expect the power of predictive validity to decrease with time, except at the extremes. Keogh and Becker (1973) called attention to this methodological paradox:

> If early identification and diagnosis were insightful and remedial implementation successful, the preschool or kindergarten high risk child would receive the kind of attention and help which results in successful school performance. In essence, he would no longer be high risk and instead would be a successful achiever. Predictive validity of the identification instruments would, therefore, be low. In such a case, success of the child would negate accuracy of prediction. (p. 7)

The effects of intervening variables on outcome measures have received little systematic attention. However, assessors clearly need to consider intervention when trying to evaluate the effectiveness of readiness screening measures for the prediction of risk. Furthermore, the prediction of risk must also be related to changes in learning expectations from a developmental perspective. For example, a well-functioning 3- or 4-year-old child with good language skills may later encounter difficulty with other tasks related to early reading, and at this later point may be at risk for later academic difficulties.

4. *What are the consequences of flexible definitions of risk?* Definition problems are also an issue relating to validity, because definitions of risk vary by school district. There is no consistent standard for what constitutes a potential (or actual) problem. In the case of developmental screening, definitional issues, along with local economic constraints, result in districts' using different criteria for labeling children's performance as problematic; such differences can result in missing children who later demonstrate problems (false negatives), along with false identifications. In addition, the tolerance for child behavior varies by teacher/educator/assessor, as does the objectivity of the rater. Adelman (1982) and Keogh and Becker (1973) noted other problems that are still relevant today, such as (a) the limited behavior samples obtained, due to restrictions in time or instrument availability; (b) the limited range of competencies tapped, as well as greater concern about conditions of deficit or disturbance within a child than about strengths; and (c) a lack of clarity regarding outcome goals—long- or short-term, and socioemotional as well as academic. Adelman (1982) clearly states the issue: "Varying standards may be applied in indicating cut-off points for labeling a child as a problem. As a result, children with the same behaviors and level of skills could be seen as problems in one situation (e.g., one school) and not in another" (p. 259). (See also Chapter 6.)

5. *Are validity data presented for various assessment purposes?* The authors of assessment measures often cite more than one purpose for which a measure can be used. Although Shepard and Graue (1993) underscore the importance of presenting validity data for each intended use, this practice is not widely followed. Citing Messick (1989), these authors also indicate that the validity of tests for the purpose of identifying student needs must be separate from validation for the purpose of intervention decisions. Therefore, "tests cannot be used to assign children to different educational treatments unless it can be shown that those treatments are differentially effective" (1993, p. 295). In addition, Shepard and Graue point out that the correlation coefficients often presented in test manuals in support of validity do not document their relevance for intervention.

TECHNICAL ISSUES ASSOCIATED WITH NORM-REFERENCED TESTS

Norm-referenced tests (NRTs) are used to compare individual children's performance with that of other typical children of the same age, gender, race, and SES represented in the standardization sample. These tests are important when the assessment purpose is identification of developmental problems. The standardization data reported in a test manual provide important information regarding the samples of children used to establish the basis for interpreting the meaning of test scores. When assessors are reviewing the information provided in a test manual, it is important to raise questions such as the following:

1. For what purpose(s) was the test developed, and to what extent are the domains covered measured?

2. How was the test developed, including the selection and field testing of items, as well as procedures for scoring and interpretation of outcomes?

3. When was the test developed, and what is the date of the most recent data collection (norming)? Some currently used tests and assessment procedures were developed and normed more than 15–20 years ago, the generally accepted "age" of educational tests. Thus, the interpretations that result may be misleading (Bailey & Brochin, 1989). Periodic review and renorming are important, therefore, to support the ongoing utility of tests. However, a few tests with old norms (e.g., McCarthy Scales of Children's Abilities [McCarthy, 1972]; Griffiths Mental Development Scales [Griffiths, 1970]; see Chapter 11) may appropriately measure areas of concern. Some assessors may choose the McCarthy because they believe it provides a better sample of children's abilities in the 4–6 age range than other measures do. In this case, local norms can be collected (this is discussed in a later section), or the assessor can make general statements ("average range," "low range") rather than provide an IQ score or level of mental retardation.

4. What are the characteristics of the normative sample, including age, sex, SES, geographic region of the country, ethnic and language background, urban–rural residence, and disabling conditions? In particular, it is important to compare the characteristics of the test's reported sample with the characteristics of the local group with which the test will be used. If there is a mismatch, this does not necessarily mean that the test is poor or that assessors need to develop their own. If the test is well constructed and addresses the assessment purpose, assessors need to take this into account when interpreting outcomes and may wish to collect local norms.

5. What types of scores are provided to assist interpretation? Typically, the scores provided based on norms include the percentage of the normative sample passing each item; the mean and standard deviation (*SD*) for the total score and each subtest score; and other statistical procedures (standard scores, stanines, etc.) that give meaning to raw scores (the number of items correctly answered). A fuller discussion of these scores and procedures is provided in Appendix 3.1. In each case, scores are related to what is referred to as the normal curve or *normal distribution*, a mathematical construct used to describe behaviors that are distributed normally; that is, most cluster near the middle of a distribution (the average range). Fewer individuals perform very well or very poorly—that is, at either extreme. The normal curve represents this distribution in relation to the *SD*. There is an exact mathematical relationship between the *SD* and the proportion of cases. The same proportion of cases will always be found within the same standard devia-

tion limits. Thus if we know the mean and *SD* of a given test, we know a great deal of information, such as the following:

- The distribution of scores for the normative group as a whole, and the position of an individual score in relation to the group.
- The fact that approximately 68%, 95%, and 99.9% of all children taking the test fall within ±1, ±2, and ±3 *SD* of the mean, respectively.

Based on the normal distribution, the cumulative percentage of children falling below each *SD* value can be determined. This information is particularly important with reference to developmental screening. Often children who score 2.0 *SD* below the mean in one developmental area, or 1.5 *SD* below the mean in more than one developmental area, are referred for comprehensive assessment. If –2.0 *SD* is the cutoff, we are referring to the lowest 2.3% of children, versus 6.7% if the cutoff is –1.5 *SD*—a huge difference. Assessors also need to review how many additional items children need to miss or answer correctly to fall at a lower or higher *SD* unit (sometimes only one or two items on brief screening instruments).

NRT information is widely employed across states to provide the cutoff points used to establish children's risk for later learning problems, readiness for entrance into kindergarten or first grade (areas of great debate), and qualification for special services. To meet these policy and administrative needs, NRTs will continue to have an important place in the assessment process (Fewell, 1984), including screening and diagnosis. What NRTs cannot tell us is why an individual scored in a particular way or how we might plan appropriate intervention. Many early childhood specialists take a negative view of NRTs or standardized tests, because they measure isolated skills and their scores do not inform intervention. NRTs, however, can present more information than simply comparing an individual's score with that of the normative group can do—an area often overlooked by critics. They can present area scores that can be used to create a profile of the child's performance. These scores can help identify areas in need of observation, instruction, or additional assessment, as well as areas of relative strength. Some NRTs also provide criterion-referenced information that is useful to review for intervention planning (e.g., the Boehm Test of Basic Concepts–3: Preschool; Boehm, 2001), or they have been well researched in relation to identifying severe emotional and behavioral problems (e.g., the Child Behavior Checklist for Ages 1½–5; Achenbach & Rescorla, 2000b). Although it is possible to review items on some NRTs to identify instructional or behavioral objectives, the features of other NRTs limit criterion-referenced interpretations (see the next section). First, some NRTs cover multiple domains with a limited number of items in any one area, or items are not sufficiently specific to guide instruction. Second, items that all children either miss or answer correctly may be excluded during the construction of an NRT, in order to shorten the length of the test and increase the reliability. Thus items testing important instructional objectives may be eliminated on NRTs, particularly at the floor or ceiling level, but may be included on criterion-referenced measures in the same domain. Nevertheless, assessment measures can provide both norm-referenced and criterion-referenced information and scores. The use of NRTs does not need to be limited to comparisons of scores to the norm group—a criticism voiced by many early childhood assessors. From our perspective, the use made of score outcomes is the real issue. When used appropriately, the outcomes of NRTs can provide useful information—as, for example, when children's profiles are reviewed in order to determine areas mastered and those needing development. In addition, an error analysis can be made of the content of items missed by individual children or groups of children. These outcomes can be refined through ongoing assessment and the observations of teachers, therapists, and parents.

TECHNICAL ISSUES ASSOCIATED WITH CRITERION-REFERENCED TESTS AND OTHER PERFORMANCE-BASED ASSESSMENT PROCEDURES

The use of criterion-referenced tests (CRTs) and other performance-based assessment procedures has become increasingly widespread among preschool assessors. Each of these forms of testing focuses on determining whether or not a child has attained a specified standard of performance related to academic functioning or daily living. Objectives may be chosen from any well-defined domain: cognitive, language, sensory, motor, social, or emotional. An advantage of both CRTs and other types of performance-based assessment is that they focus on the child's mastery of an instructional or behavioral objective or of specified tasks, not on comparing a child's performance to that of others in the standardization group. A second advantage is that the results can be directly translated into targets for instruction, instructional objectives, or IEPs. Whereas most CRTs focus on mastery to a criterion level of specified behaviors/skills deemed important across developmental and achievement areas, curriculum-based assessment (CBA), a particular form of CRT, focuses on mastery of those behaviors/skills that are specified in a particular curricular sequence (see Chapter 7 for additional details on these two forms of assessment).

Although criterion-referenced measurement provides a conceptual framework for thinking about the various types of performance-based assessment, the fundamental concept of criterion-referenced measurement has been imprecisely defined and often results in confusion (Linn, 1994). Areas of confusion include

> a) the view that norm-referenced and criterion-referenced interpretations cannot coexist for a single measure, b) the interpretation that criterion-referenced measurement necessarily involves the use of a cut score to determine mastery, c) the equating of criterion-referenced measurement and domain-referenced measurement, and d) the limitation of criterion-referenced measurement to a narrowly behaviorist conception of many discrete and typically hierarchical skills and behaviors. (Linn, 1994, pp. 12–13)

Developing CRTs requires multiple steps, including (1) specification of objectives in terms of specific behaviors; (2) task analysis of the objectives in terms of both the subskills and cognitive processes needed for successful performance; (3) specified standards for both successful performance and the nature of the testing conditions; (4) adequate sampling of the skill area; (5) scoring and reporting of results so that they clearly describe a child's performance; and (6) consultation with others to determine which objectives are important (e.g., knowledge of letter names and sounds). Setting criterion levels, while guided by understanding the degree of mastery that is necessary in order to move on to the next level of instruction, is often subjective and not determined by research. For instance, the frequently used criterion level of "80% correct" is seldom supported by any particular evidence or rationale. The questions that need to be addressed are "Does this standard of performance make sense?" and "What is the rationale for setting this level of performance?" CRTs often provide raw scores, domain scores, or sets of behavioral observations; these may be interpreted in a number of ways, such as the percentage of total items correct, the percentage of objectives mastered, or the degree to which performance standards set by the program or school are met. Bailey and Brochin (1989, p. 37), citing Berk (1986), note that these standards are frequently set unsystematically and thus are often controversial. In addition, the thinking processes that underlie successful performance are often not defined as objectives. Finally, when possible, evidence from other sources needs to be collected to support interpretation. Useful resources for developing CRTs include publications by AERA et al. (1999), Berk (1984), Gronlund (1973), Popham (1984), Stiggins (1994), and Taylor (2005).

Content validity is fundamental for CRT and CBA procedures. Content validity is determined through (1) documentation of the exhaustiveness with which a learning area is covered, (2) judgments by specialists regarding the relevance of items, and (3) meaningful sampling of content areas. In addition, other forms of validity need to be addressed, including (1) predicting future performance (e.g., success at the end of an instructional unit) and (2) relating a child's CRT or CBA performance to other measures of children who have or have not achieved the objectives specified. Finally, it is expected that children who have received instruction relative to a particular objective should perform better than those who have not received this instruction.

Most measurement specialists point out that neither CBA nor other types of CRTs answer all questions, and they may not address complex learning outcomes. Both types of measures, however, need to provide documentation of technical adequacy. Technical data for forms of CBA are often not reported. In particular, issues of reliability and validity, other than content validity, are usually not addressed (Shinn, 1989a), but this has begun to change (Shinn, 1998). As stated by Messick (1995a), the principles of validity apply to all forms of assessment and are critical for performance-based assessment. At the preschool level, performance-based measures are used for a variety of purposes (e.g., attention to tasks, behavior across instructional activities). It is essential for documentation to include justification that the domain of concern is covered through a representative set of tasks (items). Such justification is required in terms of both content validity and sampling of the domain.

Reliability procedures that need to be considered include (1) test–retest procedures, which look at the consistency with which a CRT measures mastery or nonmastery of an objective; (2) use of alternate-form procedures, to avoid the effects of practice and forgetting that occur when the same test items are readministered (Martuzza, 1977); and (3) when observers are used, issues related to interrater and intrarater agreement. Again, the consistency with which raters judge the mastery or nonmastery of an objective is at issue. The common practice of simply providing data to support content validity is not sufficient if the test results contribute to important decisions.

Issues related to validity are particularly important when the outcomes of the performance assessment are used to determine eligibility for special services or readiness for moving into first grade. When outcome data are used to make decisions about eligibility or retention, the extent to which performance can be generalized across tasks needs to be addressed, as well as the reliability of observers (Brennen & Johnson, 1995). Furthermore, since the nature of the task presented to a child will affect performance, objectives need to be measured through multiple tasks. Brennen and Johnson (1995) raise key questions about both task quality and rater quality: What is the criterion and is it used consistently across students, across tasks, and across classes? What observational and scoring procedures are used? And are these clearly understood and adhered to among raters? When performance-based assessments are used to compare student progress from year to year, they must mean the same thing from one year to the next and from one assessor to another.

The use of CRTs, however, often does not address the issues of how a child solves a problem (i.e., the cognitive strategies used to arrive at a response); what accounts for a child's failures; or what assistance a teacher or other interventionist needs to provide to foster successful task performance, such as breaking down tasks or providing concrete materials (Lidz, 1981, 2001, 2003). The basis of the objectives included on CRTs is another issue. Although CRTs are composed of items selected because of their importance to school performance or daily living, and although such items typically become teaching targets when missed, curriculum objectives need to be established by early childhood specialists prior to the use of any test (Bailey & Brochin, 1989). A potential danger exists when users allow a CRT, such as the Brigance Inventory of Early Development-II (Brigance, 2004), to set the curriculum.

THE TECHNICAL ADEQUACY OF PRESCHOOL ASSESSMENT APPROACHES

Evaluating instruments based on statistical outcomes, referred to as determining their *predictive utility*, is problematic from a number of perspectives. In particular, users need to be aware of the criteria used to make decisions. Mercer, Algozzine, and Triffletti (1979b) over 25 years ago demonstrated that use of the traditional prediction matrix can result in a number of different interpretations:

Performance on the prediction measure (time 1)	Performance on the criterion measure (time 2)	
	Learning difficulty	No learning difficulty
Poor (at risk)	+ Correct identification (true positive) A	– False positive B
Good (not at risk)	– False negative C	+ Correct identification (true negative) D

Note. A, needs services; B, receives services not needed (overidentification); C, services were needed but not received (underreferral); D, services were not needed or received.

- If the overall hit rate (percentage of correct identifications—quadrants A and D) is of concern, the percentage of children correctly identified as being at risk and not at risk is (A + D)/(A + B + C + D).
- If the percentage of children who actually need services is of concern (as is the case during screening, since these children need to be referred) the children of quadrant A will be considered. The percentage of children correctly flagged for further assessment is A/(A + C).
- If the proportion of children identified at time 1 as needing further assessment (quadrants A and B) is of is a concern, this percentage is (A + B)/(A + B + C + D).

- If the accuracy of the instrument in identifying those children who later encounter problems is of concern, we need to look across quadrants A and C: A/(A + D) and C/(C + D).
- The proportion of overreferrals is B/(A + B + C + D), and the proportion of underreferrals is C/(A + B + C + D).

Looking only at A/(A + C) or A/(A + B) can lead to inaccurate conclusions. According to Mercer et al. (1979b), looking across all quadrants to determine overall accuracy is the desired procedure. These researchers describe how different outcomes were found for 15 studies, based on how the results of these studies were reviewed. Thus assessors need to consider the completeness with which outcomes are presented when reviewing the technical data presented in manuals and when determining cutoff scores. A change in cutoff scores, moreover, will affect the predictive validity of a measure (Mercer et al., 1979b; Sicoly, 1992). For example:

- Wider cutoff point → More sensitive to possible areas of risk
  (–1.5 *SD* vs. –2.0 *SD* below mean) → More false positives (overidentification)
- Narrower cutoff → More false negatives (misses)
  (–2.0 *SD* vs. –1.5 *SD* below mean) → More utility in terms of cost

Therefore, the predictive validity of a screening instrument must be considered in light of both its *sensitivity* to risk conditions and its accuracy in identifying children without difficulty (*specificity*). Sicoly (1992) presents expectancy tables for converting a validity or test–retest reliability coefficient into measures of classification accuracy for different cutoff scores on a test or criterion measure. He points to the importance of reporting the degree of classification accuracy for various cutoff scores. Screening tests are widely criticized for their lack of validity data or their low rates of predictive validity data (Gallerani, O'Regan, & Reinherz, 1982; Lindeman, Goodstein, Sacks, & Young, 1984; Meisels, 1985, 1987, 1989a, 1999; Shepard & Smith, 1986). Thus children's progress needs to be monitored frequently, so that "false positives will progress rapidly, meet exit criteria, and be placed in an appropriate program. False negatives, on the other hand, will progress slowly, meet entrance criteria, and be placed in the special intervention program" (Mercer, Algozzine, & Triffiletti, 1979a, p. 22). When tests are designed to predict mild risks, increased decision errors should be expected (Fletcher & Satz, 1982).

Although many preschool assessment instruments lack technical adequacy in relation to the *Standards for Educational and Psychological Testing* (AERA et al., 1999), these standards are general, and their application varies from study to study. However, increasingly authors (e.g., Alfonso & Flanagan, 1999, and Flanagan & McGrew, 1997) are applying the same adequacy criteria across studies when measures are used for a specific assessment purpose, such as screening to identify individuals who are possibly at risk. In addition, few researchers have specifically addressed issues of particular relevance to preschool assessment. Bracken (1987) set out to address this issue and reviewed a total of 10 commonly used school instruments (5 used for diagnosis of specific skills and 5 for placement purposes). The adequacy of each instrument was reviewed according to the following criteria. (Note that these recommendations did not extend to tests used primarily to make curriculum-based decisions.)

1. Median subtest reliabilities of .80 or greater.
2. Total test internal consistencies of .90 or greater.

3. Total test stability coefficients of .90 or greater over an average period of 2–4 weeks.
4. Subtest floors 2 *SD* below the normative mean subtest score, to allow differentiation at that degree of disability.
5. Total test floor 2 *SD* below the normative total test mean score (score of 70 or below).
6. Subtest *item gradients* of no fewer than three raw score items per standard score deviation unit. "Item gradient refers to how rapidly standard scores increase as a function of a child's success of failure on a single test item" (Bracken, 1987, p. 322).
7. Evidence of validity data present or absent and based on the projected use of the instrument.

Bracken's recommendations have been broadly applied in the field.

Bracken also suggested that some standards need to be considered with flexibility, depending on the intended use of the test. For example, the floor of the test is not the critical issue in the assessment of gifted children. Nevertheless, Bracken concluded that many instruments used for preschool assessment are severely limited in floor, item gradient, and reliability at lower age levels, or do not report validity data. The lack of a test floor to assist assessors in establishing the point of intervention is often a characteristic of the lowest age levels of preschool tests. This point has been underscored by the work of Bradley-Johnson and Durmusoglu (2005) in their review of floor and item gradients for reading and math tests for young children. These authors document that ignoring test floors can have serious consequences, such as underestimating the performance of children with serious academic delays, and thus the need for intervention. Such problems are most likely with the lowest-performing children and those at the youngest age levels covered by a measure. Shepard and Smith's (1986) point is essential here: "The more crucial the decision for an individual child, the greater are the demands for test validity evidence and due process" (p. 83).

INTEGRATING AND INTERPRETING ASSESSMENT OUTCOMES

A critical component of the assessment process is integrating the outcomes from different assessment procedures in order to make recommendations and design interventions. Profiles are often used to summarize outcomes. Hills (1993) cautions assessors not to plot scores from tests by different publishers on the same profile, since they are based on different normative groups. He also recommends the following:

- When scores from different subtests of a measure are plotted, it is important to plot each score as a band to allow for error of measurement. "Bands that touch or overlap are usually not interpreted as representing different levels of score" (Hills, 1993, p. 32).
- Attention should be paid to the fact that scores from subtests from different tests with the same name may measure different facets of skills within the same domain.
- With low scores, it is important to be aware of possible floor effects. As noted earlier in this chapter, floor effects occur when a test is so difficult for the individual that the assessor does not get a good picture of what the individual can and cannot do—that is, what the poor performance really represents. For example, getting a scale score of 0 on

three out of five subtests on the Verbal scale of the WPPSI-III means that no inferences about the child's verbal ability can be made, other than that his or her verbal ability is below the floor of the test.

• Attention is also needed to scores at the middle of the distribution, where only a few items more that are correct or incorrect may result in a large change in percentiles. For example, on the WPPSI-III a child might earn a standard score of 90 on the Verbal scale, which is at the 24th percentile and earn a standard score of 100 on the Performance scale which is at the 50th percentile. If one focuses on the percentile scores, it looks as if one score is twice as high as the other, yet both scores are within the average range and indicate similar levels of functioning. Therefore, assessors need to review manuals carefully to see what changes in percentiles may result from one or two more correct or incorrect responses, particularly on screening tests at the end of the age range.

STEPS IN COLLECTING LOCAL NORMS

Local norms may be developed for a number of reasons, such as to compare the performance of local groups to school or local objectives, or to that of groups included in the normative sample when standardized tests are used. Such data collection in relation to standardized tests is important when a test's reported norms have been based on a sample representing a restricted geographic area, SES composition, and range of diversity, or have been collected more than 20 years earlier. Such norms may not represent the groups to be assessed in a particular community (e.g., a Native American population). This concern applies in particular to language and ethnic diversity, as well as diversity based on disabling conditions. Although increasing numbers of children come from homes where a language other than English is spoken, few tests are translated and normed in languages other than English and Spanish. Since each language group may speak a unique form of its particular language—for example, Panjabi—there may be no appropriate norms available, even if there is a Panjabi version of the test. A group may have immigrated from a particular part of India that speaks a particular dialect of Panjabi. Moreover, the version of Panjabi spoken in the local group may well have, through its interaction with the local form of English being spoken, become a unique form or dialect of Panjabi that makes it difficult to use anything other than local norms to gauge a child's developing language competence. Issues such as this can only be assessed by doing some research in the language in question and the geographic origin of local speakers (Stokes & Duncan, 1989). One cannot assume that a translation of a test into a child's primary language "produces a version of the test that is equivalent in content, difficulty level, reliability, and validity to the original untranslated version" (AERA et al., 1999, p. 92).

Local norms can also be important to determine the utility of the local results when standardized NRTs are used or when standardized curriculum-based measurement (CBM), one form of CBA, is used. As detailed by Cantor (1995), Shinn (1989), and Stewart and Kaminiski (2002), collecting local norms can decrease potential bias in decision making. Such information is important when test outcomes are used to make decisions about prereferral intervention or other problem-solving prevention efforts, about referral for in-depth assessment, or about placement. In particular, local norms can be used in prevention efforts to avoid such practices as placing kindergarten children in transition classrooms prior to first grade when they might have performed as well in the regular first-grade classroom with appropriate adaptive instruction.

When CBM is used, the performance of students from the local group can be analyzed to determine the extent to which the students have achieved important instructional goals in areas such as early literacy, and can be compared to the benchmarks established by the community (Stewart & Kaminski, 2002). To achieve this outcome, it is essential to detail the behaviors that are included in goals and to establish clear criterion levels. As Stewart and Kaminski (2002) point out, this is a process that needs to be updated regularly. The local database can be used to document progress; to identify students who are not keeping up with an established standard; and to report results to teachers, parents, or other agencies. Stewart and Kaminski (2002) provide excellent guidelines for developing, collecting, and interpreting local norms related to curricular expectations across instructional areas. Data can be organized to facilitate various levels of interpretation of scores at the individual, classroom, school, and district levels (e.g., rank ordering, means, percentile ranks, cutoff scores). The development of local norms can help community schools engage in problem solving, communicate what is expected of students, and base decisions on tasks related to curricular content. However, Stewart and Kaminski also caution that local norms collected on small samples (fewer than 100 children per grade) can be unstable; such norms should be used cautiously and not as the basis for eligibility decisions.

When NRTs are used, the scores of the local group can be compared to that of the normative group to determine whether the local group exhibits differences in performance on any items, and whether these differences occur by cultural or language group, by gender, or by disabling condition. Item bias may exist if there are significant differences between the norm group and the local reference group. The reasons for these differences need to be determined, and the items possibly replaced with more appropriate representations if bias is indeed detected. Furthermore, if a translated test is used, vocabulary items may have a different level of difficulty across language groups and the local dialect of the language in question. Local data need to be collected over a number of years to determine whether patterns develop and updated as student populations change. It is important as well to maintain records regarding the relationship of assessment results with other data collected about each child (i.e., teacher observation, prereferral interventions used, and later achievement or student behavior). For example, to what extent do scores relate to teacher judgments collected at the same time?

Empirical support for the efficacy of restandardization is presented by Stokes and Duncan (1989). These researchers provide a very helpful description of the modification and restandardization of an English receptive language test into Panjabi. Their model can be used to guide local districts in developing their own measures. To develop local norms, the following general steps are important:

1. Convene a good team for the task (i.e., speech pathologist, school psychologist, bilingual education teacher, artist, and four fluent speakers of the target language in its local dialect).
2. Choose the best available English measure to modify.
3. Have three fluent speakers translate the measure, resolve their differences, and then have it back-translated by the fourth fluent speaker. (It should be noted, however, that back-translation is no longer recommended by the AERA et al. *Standards*, since this procedure may possibly provide an "artificial similarity of meaning across languages"; 1999, p. 92).
4. Eliminate items that *do not* translate meaningfully or *cannot* be depicted in the second language.

5. Pilot-test the measure on 10–25 children at each age level and modify items that are missed by many students.
6. Draw test pictures for new items if needed to multiculturalize the whole test.
7. Standardize and norm the test on the local monolingual English population and second-language bilingual population, using as large numbers as possible, but at least 100 per age or grade.
8. Collect related demographic data on the normative sample; these data should include SES, language dialect, and length of residence in the United States or Canada.
9. Analyze data by chronological age, calculating means and *SD* such that any child falling 1.5 *SD* below the mean would be referred for further assessment.
10. Maintain records regarding the relationship between the test results and other data collected about the children. These records should take into account the nature of programs or other interventions recommended, how these children performed, and the extent to which children who were not identified by the test as having a problem needed services, were retained, and were referred for other services.
11. Maintain data that contribute to documentation of the effectiveness of interventions.

SUMMARY

The technical characteristics of NRTs, as well as of CRTs and other performance-based procedures, have been reviewed in this chapter. Our review has reflected the *Standards for Educational and Psychological Testing* (AERA et al., 1999) and research in the field. Early childhood specialists have criticized the technical adequacy of many preschool measures for many years. Preschool assessors therefore need to be particularly attentive to the technical adequacy of the procedures they use in relationship to their assessment purpose, including reliability, validity, and normative or field data. Procedures for collecting local norms have also been summarized. A format for reviewing tests is presented in Table 3.1.

TABLE 3.1. Points to Consider in Reviewing a Test

1. Title, author(s), publisher, and date of publication
2. Description
   - Purpose: Briefly state the purpose(s) for which the test was designed, age group(s) it is intended for.
   - Content: Describe the content areas/subtests included and the types of responses expected from children.
   - Format: Describe the overall format (individual vs. group, norm-referenced vs. criterion-referenced), organization (e.g., rating scale, pass–fail, no opportunity to observe vs. observation of specific behaviors), availability of parent and/or teacher questionnaires, materials required, and availability of alternate forms.
   - Time needed for administration and cost.
   - Scores: Describe how scores are expressed (standard scores, percentiles, etc.).
3. Technical data
   - Norms: How many individuals were sampled?
   - How representative is the sample (age, gender, race/ethnicity, language, SES, geographic location, urban vs. rural)?
   - Are individuals with disabling conditions included?
   - Reliability: State briefly how reliability was determined, including the procedure (test–retest [over what time span], interrater, etc.) and the size of the sample.
   - Validity:
     - Evidence based on test content.
     - Evidence based on the relationship to other variables, including concurrent (the extent to which individuals' scores on this measure match their scores on other related measures) and predictive (the extent to which scores on this measure predict later performance, such as achievement).
     - Evidence accumulated from diverse sources (development with age, factor analysis, other sources).
     - Issues of sensitivity and specificity addressed where needed (e.g., for a developmental screening test).
     - Evidence provided for each of the stated purposes of the test.
4. Comments
   - Ease of administration, scoring, and interpretation.
   - Appeal of materials and space on response forms to record observations.
   - Adequate range of easy items.
   - Availability in other languages besides English (if so, which?).
   - Provisions for individuals with disabling conditions.
   - Training required and activities recommended in the manual or with supplementary materials.
   - Your opinions regarding desirable and undesirable features.
   - The opinions of outside reviews of the test (e.g., those included in the *Mental Measurement Yearbooks*); include references.
   - Your overall evaluation.
   - If the test is a recent revision that has not yet been reviewed, the ways the authors took into account the criticisms of past reviews.

APPENDIX 3.1. Norm-Referenced Scores and Statistical Terms

Scores on NRTs take a number of forms, which serve as the basis for describing the normal distribution of scores, as well as for interpreting a child's performance on both subtests and the entire test. These include the following:

- *Median*—The middle score of a group of scores; that is, 50% of scores fall above and 50% below this point.
- *Mean*—The average of all scores (= 50th percentile) for a particular group. Mean scores generally increase with age.
- *Standard deviation* (*SD*)—A measure that represents the average variability (scatter) of the group. A large *SD* means that there is a lot of variation, whereas a small *SD* indicates little variation between children in the normative sample.
- *Quartile*—One of four groups into which a standardization sample is divided, so that 25% of the scores fall into each group. The performance of individuals scoring in the first (bottom) quartile is often of concern to assessors.
- *Decile*—One of 10 groups into which a standardization sample is divided, so that 10% of scores fall into each group. The top 10% of children (those scoring at or above the 90th percentile) might be considered for an enrichment program in some settings, whereas those scoring in the lowest decile in a particular developmental area may be considered for intervention.
- *Stanine*—One of nine groups into which a standardization sample is divided, with the fifth stanine serving as the middle group. Stanines are infrequently used with preschool assessment procedures.
- *Percentile rank*—A commonly used means of interpreting scores, based on comparison of a particular score with those of the sample on which the test was normed. A particular percentile indicates the percentage of individuals in the normative sample who scored at or below a certain score. A percentile rank of 25 means that 25% of those in the group have the same or lower scores. The mean of a test always represents the 50th percentile. One of the problems with percentiles is that they do not have equal meaning throughout score distribution. In the middle of the distribution, where most children perform, a small change in score (children's answering more or fewer questions) results in a much higher (or lower) percentile. In contrast, at the low end or high end of the distribution, a large change in score will result in a small change in percentile. This issue is of particular relevance for brief screening tests, which contain few items.

Sometimes we want to compare a child's performances on different tests. The meaning of a child's score varies in relationship to the mean of each test taken. If the mean and *SD* are different for each test used, it is difficult to compare the meaning of scores from different tests. The use of standard scores addresses this issue.

- *Standard scores*—A means of translating raw scores into equal units. Standard scores, based on the normal curve, are statistically derived so that the mean and *SD* stay the same across age groups. On the Wechsler scales, for example, the mean is 100 and the *SD* is 15 across age groups. For the McCarthy Scales of Children's Abilities, the mean is 100 and the *SD* is 16. When *z*-scores are presented, the mean is 0 and the *SD* is 1. The meaning of these scores is comparable across tests. Standard scores are developed by use of the following procedure:

$$\text{Standard score} = \frac{(\text{Child's raw score}) - (\text{Mean of test})}{(SD \text{ of test})}$$

- *Developmental age scores*—Scores indicating the average age at which 50% of the normative group answered the item correctly, achieved a particular raw score, or manifested a skill. Developmental age scores involve a number of problems, the major one being that a year of growth does not represent the same thing at different points in a child's life. This is of particular concern for young children—let's say, 3, 4, and 5 years of age, for whom 1 year represents one-third, one-fourth, and one-fifth of their lives, respectively (Bailey & Brochin, 1989). Sattler (2001) raises a number of other problems related to developmental age scores:

1. The same raw score in an area may reflect a different pattern of items missed and passed.
2. Many age scores are extrapolated scores—that is, estimated for children of certain ages who may not actually have been tested, such as children with extremely high or low scores or children who fall outside of the age range and norms of the test.
3. Differences between developmental ages (a) are not necessarily equal and (b) do not indicate what portion of improvement is due to maturation.

Many kinds of developmental quotients are reported in test manuals (including reading age scores, social age quotients, IQ, etc.). The basic meaning is the same. While developmental quotients are appropriate for use with very young children, since they are relatively stable at this level (Bailey & Brochin, 1989), their use becomes inappropriate as children get older (with higher chronological ages), and as the content of the test includes fewer and fewer harder items or as growth increases no longer occur (a child scores at the ceiling of the test, having mastered the skill area tested).

- T *score*—Standard scores with a mean of 50 and a standard deviation of 10.
- *Normal curve equivalents (NCEs)*—Standard scores with a mean of 100 and a standard deviation of 21.06.
- *Grade scores*—Similar to developmental age scores, but organized by grade units. Grade scores are easily misinterpreted. A 6-year-old child who attains a grade score of 3.0 does not read or perform like an average third grader. The score simply reflects that the child is performing considerably above average.
- *Correlation coefficient*—A statistic for expressing the relationship between scores of children on two tests or assessment procedures. This statistic is important to understand how similarly (consistently) children perform on two forms of a test or on the same test given at two points in time (see the text discussion of reliability); how children's performance on one test relates to performance on other tests or rating scales administrated at the same time (see the text discussion of concurrent validity); and how scores on one test predict (relate to) scores on measures given at a later date (see the text discussion of predictive validity). A readiness test must provide such information.

If two test forms were perfectly consistent (so that children scored the same way on both), we would have a perfect positive correlation of +1.0. If children who scored the highest on one test scored randomly on the second administration of that test, there would be little relationship between the scores on the two tests, and the correlation would be near 0. If children who scored highest on one test scored lowest on the next test after a 6-week intervention, we would have a perfect negative correlation of –1.0. Correlations can thus range from –1.0 to +1.0, although they generally range from 0 to +1.0 when used with tests. The closer to +1.0, the better the relationship of two tests given at the same time, and the better the prediction of behavior at a later point of time. High accuracy is the goal with testing measures.

When assessors are reviewing correlational data presented in test manuals and research reports, it is important to be mindful of several factors that affect the size of correlations:

1. *The number of cases reported.* The size of the sample on which the study was conducted is likely to influence the degree of the resulting relationships. Correlations are likely to be lower in small samples than in large samples of children, because in small groups there is less opportunity for behavior to vary, whereas in large samples variation is likely.
2. *Restriction of range.* Correlations are likely to be lower in more homogeneous than in more heterogeneous groups. For example, if a language screening test was only used with

children exhibiting language difficulties, it would result in lower correlations than it would if administered to the full range of children.

3. *Correlations versus causes*. Correlations do not indicate causes. For example, the finding that poor vocabulary relates to poor comprehension does not indicate that poor vocabulary causes poor comprehension, or vice versa.

• *Extrapolated scores*—Estimates that are used to provide meaning to extreme scores. Bailey and Brochin (1989, p. 32) point out that extrapolated scores are often necessary in the testing of disabled children, particularly those with severe disabilities. They recommend that these scores should only be used when a minimal level or score is obtained, and that their use should always be indicated in a report.

Chapter 4

Observation of the Child

Observation has consistently been cited as the major tool for assessing the behavioral, socioemotional, and learning needs of young children (e.g., Alessi & Kaye, 1983; Almy & Genishi, 1983; Bagnato & Neisworth, 1991; Boehm & Sandberg, 1982; Boehm & Weinberg, 1997; Bracken, 1991a; Cohen, Stern, & Balaban, 1997; Genishi, 1992; Lichtenstein & Ireton, 1984; Lidz, 1983b, 1991, 2003; Meisels & Atkins-Burnett, 2005; Meisels, 1999; Shepard et al., 1998; Volpe & McConaughy, 2005), and it is mandated by IDEA 2004 when a child is referred for a suspected learning disability. Specifically, IDEA 2004 requires that either information from observation during routine classroom instruction and monitoring of the child's performance prior to referral occur or that observation of the child and his or her learning environment, subsequent to referral and parental consent, be conducted by one member of a school's or school district's committee on students with disabilities. This is to document academic performance and behavior relevant to the area of difficulty. In the case of preschool children, observation should also take place in nonschool environments that are appropriate for this age group. Observational approaches are fundamental to monitoring progress toward instructional goals, conducting behavioral assessment, planning intervention, and conducting developmental assessment to identify children for special services. Observation is the most common assessment method used by school psychologists (Wilson & Reschly, 1996).

Observation across time allows observers to gain a comprehensive understanding of a child's behavior as it occurs across natural contexts. Accordingly, observations by parents, teachers, caregivers, and early childhood specialists of children engaged in a variety of activities, ranging from play to daily routines, are essential to ongoing assessment. In contrast to formal testing techniques, which present children with a set of tasks to be completed or questions to be responded to, observation has the major advantage of focusing on children's behaviors during naturally occurring events. This approach is particularly important with young children, who often have difficulty expressing themselves verbally or who may find it threatening to respond to questions posed by an unfamiliar examiner or in an unfamiliar format. Observation is essential for assessing a wide range of children's behaviors, such as interactions with peers, self-help skills, motor behaviors, emergent literacy, emotional states, and attention. It is also essential for identifying children's problem-solving strategies and current methods of coping with day-to-day situations, as well as the influence of environmental settings and adult interactions on children's behaviors. Finally, observation serves as a means of validating information collected with other assessment tools and is critical for identifying appropriate intervention strategies. The observations of the assessor are important in answering questions such as these:

- "What factors might be influencing a child's performance—cultural or linguistic differences, hearing, vision, health, outside distractions (such as noise or missing a favorite activity), anxiety, fatigue, and so forth?"
- "What language or other communicative activities, such as pointing, does the child use during assessment?"
- "What kinds of adult supports or contingencies help the child to succeed?"
- "To what extent does the child sustain attention and persist with tasks?"
- "Does the child display unusual behaviors?"

Two reciprocal systems need to be assessed via observational techniques: the child and the child's daily environments, including the home, school, and community. An ecological approach to assessment must include observational data on both these systems. The purposes of the present chapter are to (1) review the strengths and limitations of the major forms of child observation; (2) detail critical features of systematic observation; (3) present an overview of two observational approaches widely used at the preschool level (behavioral observation and observation of children at play); and (4) consider issues related to observation during formal testing. Observation of environments and the role of observation in family assessment are covered in Chapters 5 and 8, respectively.

Observation can be used in a number of ways during ongoing assessment, screening, and comprehensive developmental assessment (diagnosis). For example, when a school-age child is assessed for special services under IDEA 2004, the child's performance in the regular classroom needs to be observed. When a preschool child is being evaluated, observation needs to occur in environments appropriate for a child of that age, as noted earlier. If the child is not enrolled in a preschool, these environments may include a childcare setting or the home. Not only do teachers and childcare workers play an essential role in referral; they are in a key position to track developmental changes in behavior over time, evaluate the effects of instruction or behavioral intervention, and contrast the behavior of an individual child with that of other children of the same age and background. And the observations of parents and other caregivers are of course critical for understanding the child, as well as his or her pace of achieving important developmental milestones (e.g., walking and talking) and the daily environment that the child experiences. Their ongoing observations ("slow to talk," "doesn't get along with others," "engages in unusual behaviors") may be the basis of a referral and are essential to developing effective intervention.

MAJOR FORMS OF OBSERVATION: THEIR STRENGTHS AND LIMITATIONS

The major forms of observation used in early childhood assessment include direct measures (diary accounts, anecdotal records/logs, running records, and observation schedules) and indirect measures (checklists, questionnaires, and rating scales). A number of the latter may be used during ongoing direct observation as well. Interviews, while qualitatively different from other observational procedures, constitute an essential prelude or follow-up to these other procedures and allow the assessor to explore with parents important areas of child development, family life, and family concerns. Interviews are described in later chapters.

Direct Obsesrvation

Various forms of direct observation are used to record ongoing behavior. These include narrative systems (diary accounts, anecdotal records, running records) and detailed observation schedules.

Diary Accounts

Diary accounts can range from brief entries to comprehensive accounts; they are generally used to document developmental milestones or target behaviors of interest. Written diary entries, whether made regularly or sporadically, are usually retrospective; written accounts may be accompanied by photographs or work samples. Increasingly, however, videotape may be the preferred format for keeping a diary. Teachers, parents, or other caregivers may maintain diaries about children in order to document the unfolding of development over time and progress once an intervention has been initiated. These accounts can provide important assessment information if they include specific factual details. Many of the points made below about anecdotal records also apply to diary accounts. The "informal diaries" (baby books, photograph albums, or videos) often maintained by parents may be very useful when in-depth evaluation is called for. The review of materials such as these during parent interviews can be used to gain an understanding of the child's growth and important others in the child's life.

Anecdotal Records/Logs/Descriptive Notes

Anecdotal records, logs, or descriptive notes are brief narrative accounts written by teachers or other childcare workers and may include important developmental milestones or events that are a source of concern (e.g., persistent fights or particularly difficult separations from a caregiver). Anecdotal records or logs are useful to help teachers or workers chart development, test their hypotheses, identify possible problem areas, or review the effects of instruction or other forms of intervention. Such accounts are essential when teachers use alternative assessment procedures to document skill development in such areas as language, emergent literacy, and independence. Descriptive notes may be regularly collected on all children to monitor skill development and are an important component of portfolio assessment.

Several problems are associated with anecdotal information, however. These include (1) vulnerability to observer bias/subjectivity; (2) dependence on memory, since records, log entries, or notes are usually written after the event; and (3) difficulty related to their analysis and quantification. In order to address these problems, observers should follow these guidelines (based on Boehm & Weinberg, 1997; Brandt, 1972; Everston & Green, 1986; Thurman & Widerstrom, 1990):

- Record an event soon after it occurs.
- Separate the observation from the inferences based on that observation.
- Include objective descriptions about the context of the event (setting, activity, time); key persons involved; and what happened (its sequence, who was involved, what was said, and how others responded).

When these cautions are heeded, anecdotes and other field data can be entered as specific examples of a child's performance in a portfolio.

Running Records (Specimen Descriptions)

Running records are complete narrative records of what a child does and says in sequence during a given period of time, as well as of related contextual events. The goal is to determine how a child's behaviors unfold in natural contexts and why these behaviors occur. The collection of running records is labor-intensive and not feasible in most assessment situations. Today, video recording of an individual child (or small groups of children) can be an aid to the detailed understanding of child–environment interactions. However, when videotape (or audiotape) is used, accompanying information is still needed, such as setting, time, and the context of the events recorded. An advantage of a running record is that it allows assessors to gain an in-depth understanding of activity sequences that lead up to and follow behaviors of interest, and to learn about features of the environment that influence behavior. Collecting samples of children's talk to determine mean length of utterances and which language forms are used is a form of this procedure (see Chapter 10 for greater detail). Another advantage of running records is that assessors can subject them to in-depth analysis, using a coding system with predetermined categories. The data reported by Hart and Risley (1999) regarding the interplay of adult and child variables in language development were based on such a procedure.

Observation Schedules

Observation schedules are systematic recording systems that allow assessors to focus on predetermined and carefully defined aspects of development for referred children, based on problem identification and consultation with parents and teachers. They are developed to collect detailed information about an area of interest so that it is representative of a child over time. It is important for observation schedules to include all behaviors of concern, but for categories not to overlap. Using observation schedules, assessors can determine the frequency (or duration, accuracy, latency, etc.) of these target behaviors during specified observation periods across natural settings.

Hoge (1985) recommends that whenever possible, assessors use existing observation schedules rather than creating their own—not only to save time, but to take into account supportive reliability and validity evidence. Increasingly observation schedules focus on target behaviors that are operationally defined with standardized coding procedures. They, therefore, "can be tested for reliability and validity across different observers, time periods, and settings" (Volpe & McConaughly, 2005, p. 452).

The consistency of observations over time can be determined by repeated observations with the same schedule. Sufficient data need to be collected for decision-making purposes and should lead to intervention planning (Barnett et al., 1999). However, if no observation schedules exist for particular behaviors of interest, assessors will have to create their own. For example, an assessor who is interested in how a preschool child persists with tasks might develop a procedure such as the one illustrated below.

Purpose: Determine how often and for what reasons a child leaves a task, and how the child responds to teacher redirection.

Child *Jared* Date *3/7/06*

Setting (describe): Time Observation Starts:

Ends:

People present (describe):

Time	Activity	Nature of task behavior	Nature of teacher redirection	Child response to teacher redirection
1. 10:01	Block play	Pulls block from another child	Asks child to look for similar block on shelf	Goes to shelf
2. 10:02		Selects blocks		
3. 10:03		Builds a tower		
4. 10:04		Kicks down blocks of boy next to him	Tells Jared he may not do that	Starts to cry
5. 10:05		Pushes boy	Moves Jared from block area	Crying continues
6. 10:06		Crying continues	Yells at Jared	Crying and kicking
7. 10:07		Crying and kicking	Sends aide to intervene	Crying continues
8. 10:08		Yells at aide	Aide redirects Jared to blocks	Crying ceases
9. 10:09		Starts to build		

Again, use of a procedure such as this should lead to decision making and intervention planning. Assessors need to consider what kinds of observational data best address their assessment question, represent what is observed, and provide appropriate information about the setting. Different sampling techniques yield different information about behavior, such as rates of responding, percentage of time on task, or average length of time to respond. The use of different techniques often makes it difficult to compare findings across studies and can affect assessment outcomes (Mann, ten Have, Plunkett, & Meisels, 1991). However, the ability to tailor a technique to a specific observational purpose is a major advantage.

Challenges to Direct Observation

Challenges to the use of many direct observation procedures include the interpretation of outcomes, and often the lack of norms or standards with which to compare the data collected on a child of concern. In order to address this issue, Nelson and Bowles (1975) recommended collecting normative data across children to facilitate the assessment of a particular problem or the evaluation of an intervention program. For example, in order to identify withdrawn children in four schools, Nelson and Bowles asked two randomly selected teachers at each grade level (1–6), to select one boy and one girl from their class they considered to be typical. These 24 children were then observed for 15 minutes in each of four class situations on 12 target behaviors, using a time-sampling procedure consisting of 20-second intervals. Thus, when assessors were judging the extent of withdrawn behavior on the part of a child of concern, rough normative data were available. Fortunately, many recent observation approaches include data on large numbers of children.

Judgment-Based, Indirect Observation

The various forms of indirect observation are widely referred to as *judgment-based assessment* (JBA)—a term introduced by Neisworth and Bagnato (1988). These researchers indicate that JBA "collects, structures, and usually quantifies the impressions of professionals and caregivers about child/environment characteristics" (Neisworth & Bagnato, 1988, p. 36). JBA is generally used to record past observations during an assessment session or in the classroom. Forms of JBA/indirect observation include checklists, rating scales, questionnaires, and interviews. Since interviews allow assessors to probe areas of interest and thus are qualitatively different from checklists and rating scales, their use is described in Chapter 8. Indirect observation forms can be completed by several members of the assessment team, as well as by parents and teachers; they thus provide information regarding convergent/contrasting observations, an important check on reliability.

Checklists

Completing a checklist requires the assessor to make judgments about the presence or absence of the specific behaviors or skills listed. Checklists therefore are a dichotomous form of rating, and many of the issues covered in the next section on rating scales apply here as well. Only infrequently is descriptive information provided about the quality of behavior. Checklists are widely used in early childhood assessment and need to be carefully prepared to be specific, objective, and representative of child behavior. Although they are easy to use and are appealing to assessors, caution needs to be exercised, since many checklists are brief and superficial.

Most assessment instruments of emotional and social behavior are checklists or rating scales, such as the Autism Behavior Checklist (Krug, Arick, & Almond, 1993), a parent rating scale, and the Checklist for Autism in Toddlers (Baron-Cohen, Allen, & Gillberg, 1992), a yes–no checklist based on caregiver interview and direct observation. Other examples include the Hawaii Early Learning Profile (Vort Corporation, 1994), which displays the child's progression on 650 sequenced skills in six domains: Cognitive, Language, Fine Motor, Gross Motor, Social, and Self-Help. This criterion-referenced checklist spans the ages 0–3 years and is widely used to establish intervention activities and goals. The Work Sampling System, Fourth Edition (Meisels, Jablon, Marsden, Dichtelmiller, & Dorfman, 2001), widely used in portfolio assessment, includes a developmental checklist of the child's learning behaviors and teaching guidelines as one of its three components (see Chapter 7 for a detailed description).

Rating Scales

Completing a rating scale involves making qualitative judgments about specific behaviors. These judgments can take a number of forms, involving what McCloskey (1990) refers to as *anchors*, which "can be thought of as scoring [guides]" (p. 46). Depending on their wording, anchors can call for simple subjective ratings about the presence or quality of behavior, as "Always" and "Rarely" do in this example:

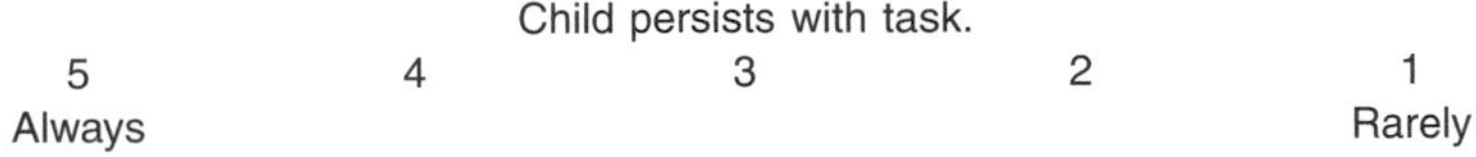

Or they can call for broad descriptive judgments, in this example:

Cuts with scissors.

4	3	2	1
Superior	Satisfactory	Needs improvement	Unsatisfactory

Or they can refer to specific defined points along an evaluation continuum, as in this example about a child's ability to follow teacher two-step directions:

4	3	2	1
Follows two-step directions	Follows two-step directions when these are broken into successive steps	Follows one-step directions only	Unable to follow one-step directions

McCloskey (1990) indicates that the use of two or more anchors facilitates the understanding of score differences.

Rating scales and checklists are widely used as part of "the screening and identification process for children who have been referred for special education services" (Elliott, Busse, & Gresham, 1993, p. 313). In addition, ratings completed by parents prior to meeting with assessors are important to a consultation approach to service delivery (Elliott et al., 1993). Teacher-completed ratings can provide useful information about aspects (activities, expectations, etc.) of the environment for a referred child. Many preschool tests are rating scales, particularly in areas such as adaptive behavior, socioemotional development, attention, and physical/motor behavior; a well-known example is the Social Skills Rating System (SSRS; Gresham & Elliott, 1990).

Although rating scales appear easy to construct and to use, Kerlinger (1973) long ago cautioned that this ease carries a heavy price related to lack of validity, due to three sources of bias: (1) errors of severity, which result in rating individuals in the deviant direction on all characteristics; (2) errors of leniency, which result in giving all individuals the benefit of the doubt; and (3) errors of a central tendency, or avoiding all extreme judgments. Since rating scales are so widely used in assessment, some attention needs to be directed to improving their use. A number of other challenges to obtaining valid and reliable ratings have been pointed out by Boehm and Weinberg (1997), Elliott et al. (1993), Everston and Green (1986), Hintze (2005), Kerlinger (1973), McCloskey (1990), and others, many of which draw attention to the central role of the rater:

- The objectivity–subjectivity of raters' impressions. Personal biases, beliefs, and previous experiences will all influence ratings.
- Raters' willingness to take the necessary time to respond thoughtfully and analytically.

- The tendency to base ratings on overall impressions or superficial knowledge of a child. Ratings are often derived from a limited number of observation opportunities. This concern is particularly relevant during screening, where only the briefest of behavior samples are obtained.
- Ambiguity in the meaning of the dimension to be rated (e.g., "attention" or "cooperation").
- The ease with which behaviors or traits can be observed. Many rating scales focus on abstract traits, which are not easily observable.
- Raters' knowledge of normal developmental variations. This concern is particularly relevant when minimally trained individuals are involved in the assessment process.
- Raters' knowledge of cultural expectations with regard to the behaviors of concern. Such variability is not taken into account on most rating scales, which generally reflect a mainstream value system.
- Raters' sensitivity as to where to follow up, probe, or ask for clarification, particularly when ratings are based on interview. For example, a teacher might endorse the item "Child talks to self." Probing might indicate that when the child is solving problems, like puzzles, he or she thinks aloud.
- Raters' appreciation of the effects of the setting, activities, standards of behavior, and individual characteristics (such as gender) on the behaviors rated.

Although different raters are likely to vary in their judgments, training and the layout of the scale can help reduce this variability. Since children's behaviors are often situation-specific, ratings also need to be reported in relationship to a specific context or to be carried out over time. Moreover, it is important to review whether data regarding test–retest reliability, interrater reliability, and the internal consistency of the scale have been reported (test–retest reliability is the most important form of reliability for rating scales) (McCloskey, 1990). McCloskey (1990, p. 51) presents an excellent table detailing factors that affect reliability, including (1) the nature of the trait being rated, (2) personal characteristics of the rater, (3) characteristics of the rating scale, and (4) the amount of time between ratings.

Documentation of the validity of the scale is also essential. For example, are studies reported in the scale's manual that document the utility of the rating outcomes for specific decision-making purposes, program planning, or intervention activities? Does the scale represent current knowledge regarding the traits measured? Is the number of items included per trait sufficient for screening or diagnostic decisions or for planning intervention? McCloskey (1990) urges users to pay careful attention to content validity in relationship to their purpose in using the scale, and further notes that for purposes of planning intervention and evaluation, the "scale should attempt to accurately represent all key behaviors related to [each] trait" consistent with "current knowledge about how that trait develops over time, or changes with new learning" (p. 59). For example, are data presented that relate the scale to other scales measuring similar traits? In addition, the use of decision grids, such as those used for determining the prediction accuracy of preschool screening tests, is a helpful procedure (McCloskey, 1990). Such a grid (like the one in Chapter 3, p. 54) includes four quadrants representing the relationship of children identified by a screening test to their performance on a criterion measure (true positive, false positive, false negative, and true negative). The Modified Checklist for Autism in Toddlers (Robbins, Fein, Barton, & Green, 2001) and the SSRS (Gresham & Elliott, 1990), for example, present excellent technical characteristics.

Among the advantages of rating scales is that they can contain many items covering multiple domains (McConaughy, 1993), involve brief time demands to administer and score, and can be completed by multiple observers. In reviewing and selecting scales, potential users need to bear in mind how the results will be used, who will do the rating, and what the setting will be (McCloskey, 1990). In addition to reviewing critiques of rating scales, McCloskey (1990) suggests a number of useful questions for reviewing, evaluating, and selecting among available rating scales:

- Are the directions for using the scale clearly stated, avoiding technical jargon?
- Are the items worded clearly?
- Is the readability level appropriate for those who will be doing the rating (an important issue for parent rating scales)?
- Does the scale measure behaviors that raters will view as meaningful (the *face validity* of the scale)?
- How much training will be required to use the scale?
- How are the items presented and scored? What types of anchors are provided (i.e., adjectives vs. fuller behavioral descriptors, numbers vs. percentages) and how well are these defined? What types of scores are yielded by the rating scale—scores referenced to norms, to mastery levels, or to developmental skill objectives?

McCloskey, in this comprehensive article, also provides useful information about the desired technical qualities of rating scales in relationship to different assessment purposes.

Although judgment-based observations yielded through checklists and rating scales are very useful in the assessment process, users need to be mindful that they do not provide information regarding the causes of behavior, or suggest the nature of teaching or other forms of intervention (McConaughy, 1993). If rating scales are to be used to make important decisions, they must be well defined and confirmed by other forms of assessment, such as direct observation or clinical interviews. Elliott et al. (1993) suggest five issues that need to be considered in using and interpretating of behavior rating scales:

1. Practical utility in terms of item clarity, scale format, training required, and interpretation for the situation.
2. Test–retest reliability of .80 or better (.70 or better over time periods of 6 months or more); internal consistency; and interrater agreement on scale items at acceptable levels, depending on the situation.
3. Diverse forms of validity, including content representative of the domain of interest; social validity in relationship to the usefulness of the information provided; internal validity determined through item review by experts, references to research, and user surveys; and criterion-related information, including other measures, both similar and dissimilar.
4. Recognition that raters will view behaviors differently across settings.
5. Recognition that child characteristics, such as appearance and gender, are likely to influence ratings.

Questionnaires/History Forms

Both questionnaires and history forms consist of sets of structured questions responded to by caregivers or others, often prior to assessment. Across settings there is great variation in questionnaire and history formats, although most cover questions about family composition and background, medical/health history, developmental history, preschool educational experience, sources of concern about the child, and the nature of past assessment or intervention. In general, relatively little information is gathered with regard to child or family strengths, although this situation is changing. Many widely used questionnaires are covered in detail in Chapters 8, 13, and 14. Considerable information sought on these forms is based on the recollection of past observations. When such forms are sent to the home and filled in prior to the time of assessment, their readability and complexity are important considerations, as well as family members' concern that a child's difficulties will reflect poorly on the family. Related to these concerns is the availability of forms in a family's primary language. If family members are recent immigrants, the language and format of a questionnaire or history form may be completely unfamiliar, and therefore may yield incomplete or inaccurate information. The recommended practice under these circumstances is to complete the form(s) in the context of an interview where areas of difficulty can be clarified.

A useful series of questionnaires for the preschool level is the second edition of the Ages and Stages Questionnaires (ASQ; Bricker & Squires, 1999), a parent-completed system for screening infants and young children (ages 4–60 months) for possible developmental delays. Nineteen age-specific questionnaires cover five developmental areas: Communication, Gross Motor, Fine Motor, Problem Solving, and Personal–Social. Parents check "Yes," "Sometimes," or "Not yet" for each of the 30 items included on each questionnaire. Additional information is gathered regarding hearing, vision, health, and general concerns. Each questionnaire takes 10–15 minutes to complete and is written at a grade 4–6 reading level, with assistance provided where needed. The questionnaires are also available in Spanish, French, Korean, and a number of other languages, and they may also be used as interview tools. The *ASQ User's Guide* (Squires, Potter, & Bricker, 1999) is clearly written, with many examples provided to help users administer the questionnaires and interpret the results. Ratings are converted into point values, which are totaled and can be compared to screening cutoff points. Validity data, collected since 1981, on 1,763 assessments using age-appropriate developmental measures are presented. Overidentification ranged from 7% to 16%, sensitivity from 38% to 90%, and specificity from 81% to 91%. Test–retest reliability over a 2-week span was .94. Interrater agreement between 112 parents and 3 trained observers was reported as greater than 90%. The questionnaires can be used as part of screening prior to kindergarten, during evaluation of eligibility for special services, or by parents prior to an appointment with primary healthcare providers, so that the parents' concerns can provide a focus for the exam. Activity sheets are also included in the system. Reproducible Ages and Stages learning activities (Twombly & Fink, 2004) linked to the ASQ are provided in both book and CD-ROM formats. (We urge that questionnaires such as these be used as part of the developmental screening process described in Chapter 6.)

Also available are the Ages and Stages Questionnaires: Social–Emotional (ASQ:SE; Squires, Bricker, & Twombly, 2002), which cover ages 6–60 months in the areas of Self-Regulation, Compliance, Communication, Adaptive Functioning, Autonomy, Affect, and Interaction with People (see Chapter 14).

CRITICAL FEATURES OF SYSTEMATIC OBSERVATION

Although it serves essential assessment purposes and is mandated by IDEA 2004, observation (especially direct observation) involves a number of challenges, including the major time commitment and training required of observers. The benefits of collecting data about children in their natural environments while engaged in everyday tasks, however, far outweigh the costs in terms of their value for intervention planning. As noted earlier, another set of concerns relates to the difficulties encountered in analyzing the outcomes of observation, determining their reliability, and evaluating issues related to their validity. These issues, however, should not be viewed as limitations, but rather as challenges to good practice. Most of the same challenges apply to all approaches to assessment during the preschool years. To yield dependable information about children, observation must be focused, organized, and systematic.

The Observer

The outcomes of observation are only as good as the observer. Being a good observer requires self-awareness, sensitivity, knowledge about young children and their development, knowledge about cultural differences and environmental expectations, and the ability to integrate observational information with other assessment results and to translate these results into meaningful instruction or intervention strategies. Although these topics are covered throughout this book, a number of points are stressed here.

As human beings, we all have our personal biases, beliefs, and approaches to situations. Some of us are critical; others are inclined to give the benefit of the doubt. Recognition of these tendencies is critical to obtaining dependable observational data. Thus, as observers, we need to become aware of our own biases, beliefs, and tolerance levels—which may be based on past experiences with a particular child, family, or instructional approach. What behaviors do we, for example, select to observe? How objectively do we record observations? How accurate are our memories? How sensitive are we with regard to diversity? Have we collected enough information to arrive at an appropriate conclusion and to facilitate intervention planning?

It takes considerable training to be an accurate and systematic observer who collects reliable and dependable information. Steps that lead to this end, along with practice, are provided by Boehm and Weinberg (1997). These include (1) posing clear questions that can be answered through observation (see the next section); (2) separating objective from subjective observations; (3) supporting inferences with specific observational data; (4) recognizing sources of personal bias; and (5) employing procedures that are specific, systematic, and that cover the question at hand. Some rules of thumb for observers include the following:

- Sample and record behaviors that provide insight about a child and are useful for guiding teaching or intervention, such as important developmental and behavioral areas (e.g., a child's response to particular teacher reinforcers). It is important for early childhood assessors and interventionists to focus on and clearly define behaviors for modification that are "truly useful" (Hintze & Shapiro, 1995). High priority should be given to skills that are prerequisites for other skills to develop and to "keystone" variables that have "widespread positive consequences" (Barnett et al., 1999, p. 77).
- Record important aspects of the environment, including environmental arrangements, activities, and adult–child interaction styles. Barnett, Ehrhardt, Stollar, and Bauer (1994) suggest group instructional time, transitions, and free play as important focal points.
- Provide accurate and factual accounts, with enough information about the setting, event, and child or caregiver behaviors and interactions to make the accounts meaningful.
- Avoid generalities; instead, provide specific, concrete details.

- Provide information that is typical of a child (e.g., "José participates frequently during circle time by contributing to discussions and responding to questions").
- Hold off on making judgments about the meaning of observations while recording.

Questions Posed by the Observer

The questions we pose as observers will, in large part, determine the type and procedures of observation we use. For example, how finely tuned do we want observations to be? Do we need only a rough measure (typical of developmental screening), such as the general range of physical agility of children on the playground, where brief descriptions of each child's large motor behaviors would suffice? Or do we need finely tuned information that leads to differential diagnosis or to developing intervention targets, as would be appropriate if a particular child appeared poorly coordinated in contrast to other children of the same age on the playground? In the latter case, we would need specific data about the quality of the child's large motor behaviors (running, skipping, hopping, climbing, etc., as well as the environmental circumstances under which these are best demonstrated) and would need to carry out such observations over several days during playground sessions. In addition, we would want to support these observations by conducting interviews with the child's teachers and parents, and by comparing the child's playground motor activities with performance on a series of structured tasks to understand the extent of the difficulty and the form of intervention needed.

Another question regards clear specification of our exact concerns. Are we interested in assessing a specific child, evaluating a group of children, capturing the flow of events in the classroom setting, or detailing behaviors of concern? If, for example, we are interested in assessing the nature of play interactions among 4-year-olds in a preschool setting, we would first need to define the types of play behaviors that are likely to be observed at this age level (solitary, parallel, or cooperative); the settings in which play is observed (classroom, playground); with whom the play activity occurs (no one, a single other child, a subgroup, the whole group); the type of play activity (block building, imaginative play in housekeeping corner, game, etc.); the tone (behaviorally described) of the interaction with others during play (aggressive, creative, cooperative, directive, destructive, etc.); and so forth. We would then build these behaviors into an observation schedule and record the play behaviors of a representative sample of children over time, or use an existing schedule such as the Penn Interactive Peer Play Scale (PIPPS; Fantuzzo, Coolahan, & Manz, 1996), described later in this chapter.

Training Required

Observation, like other assessment procedures, requires training. If structured observation schedules are to be used, the amount of training needed varies in relationship to the complexity of the system, with more complex systems requiring greater practice to make accurate and reliable observations. Most systems require practice until observers reach a criterion level, such as agreement 80% or more of the time. Training can involve (1) discussion of the categories; (2) memorization of category definitions; (3) quizzes on these definitions; (4) practice using written descriptors of behavior or videotape examples, with trainers discussing agreements and disagreements and encouraging high levels of agreement; (5) practice with a criterion videotape protocol; and (6) practice in the field with a co-observer. A useful example is provided by Bramlett and Barnett (1993) in the development of the Preschool Observation Code, a measure that focuses on problematic behaviors of children in relation to classroom events. The frequencies of a child's "state" behaviors and "event" behaviors are recorded over 20- to 30-second intervals, using momentary time sampling (see Table 4.1). States are recorded first at the moment of the interval prompt when the observer looks at the target child. The rest of the interval is used to record event behaviors. According to Bramlett and Barnett, the initial training of observers included memorization of category definitions, quizzes on these definitions, coding five practice tapes, and repeated viewings of a criterion tape until full agreement was reached compared with a criterion protocol. Evidence is provided regarding the technical adequacy of the procedure.

Extensive training is usually required when observation schedules are used in research. One example is presented in the book *The Social World of Children Learning to Talk* Hart and Risley (1999). These researchers collected 60 minutes of data every month from 42 children for 2½ years. Audio recordings were made in the home of these sessions and transcribed by the observer. Observers were trained for 9 months until they achieved 90% levels of interobserver agreement on both the videotaped interactions and audio-

TABLE 4.1. Categories and Brief Descriptions of the Preschool Observation Code

Category	Brief description
States	
Play engagement	Oriented toward play materials, games, and/or activities
Preacademic engagement	Activities designed to teach specific skills (e.g., numbers, concepts, etc.)
Nonpurposeful play	Play with no apparent goal or purpose
Unoccupied/transitional behaviors	Not engaged in, or in between, activities
Disruptive behaviors	Yelling, throwing objects
Self-stimulating behaviors	Mouthing objects, twirling hair
Other behaviors	Behavior not otherwise specified
Social interaction—peer	Verbally interacting or playing with a peer
Teacher monitoring—interacting	Teacher is monitoring activities
Events	
Activity changes	Moves from one activity to another
Disruptive behaviors	Yelling, throwing objects
Negative verbal interactions	Negative statements toward others
Positive motor interactions	Sharing, hugging, positive events
Child approach teacher	Asking for permission
Teacher commands—alpha	Clear and direct commands
Teacher commands—beta	Ambiguous commands
Child compliance	Child complies with request
Teacher approval	Verbal or physical approval
Teacher disapproval	Nonacceptance of child's behavior

Note. From Bramlett and Barnett (1993). Copyright 1993 by the National Association of School Psychologists, Bethesda, MD. Reprinted with permission of the publisher.

recordings of two actual families. Among the checks included to document reliability was independent transcription of 56% of the audiorecordings.

Training in using all other forms of observation, including checklists, ratings, and interviews, is essential as well. For example, if codes are used, the steps suggested by Bramlett and Barnett (1993) are particularly useful. Other approaches included reviewing videotapes or audiotapes of language interactions or of an interview. Observations that take place during screening are of particular concern. During large-scale screening, many individuals need to be involved, such as aides, volunteers, and teachers who often have worked mainly with older children. A morning training session in observation may heighten awareness, but cannot build in the necessary sensitivity to developmental variation of children, cultural difference, bias, observer drift, and reliability. Practice with supervision is required as these individuals work with children who come from different backgrounds and who demonstrate different styles, strengths, and limitations.

Features Specific to Direct Observation

Features specific to systematic direct observation have been detailed by a number of authors (i.e., Alessi & Kaye, 1983; Barker & Tyne, 1980; Boehm & Weinberg, 1997; Cohen et al., 1997; Good & Brophy, 1991; Hintze, 2005; Hintze & Shapiro, 1995; Hintze, Volpe, & Shapiro, 2002; Sattler, 1988, 1998, 2001; Wolery, 1989). These include the following.

Clear, Objective Operational Definitions

As noted earlier, the observer needs to delimit the problem area, detail specific examples of child behavior (or of parent or teacher behavior) to be changed or documented, and to record contextual information. Systematic observation schedules are coded in relation to predetermined categories that have been field tested and refined. An excellent example is provided by McGill-Franzen, Lanford, and Adams (2002), who provide a framework for coding teacher talk during storybook reading.

A Systematic Plan for Collecting Observational Information

The plan for collecting observational information needs to involve repeated observations over time and across settings, in order to obtain a representative picture of the child (this may not be possible when a child is referred outside of the school for developmental assessment). Whenever possible, the plan needs to include eliciting corroborative observations of others, including teachers, parents, early childhood specialists, medical personnel, and so forth.

Reducing Reactivity

Observers need to consider how children may react to them, and to change their behavior accordingly. To reduce problems of reactivity, the following steps are suggested (Alessi & Kaye, 1983; Boehm & Weinberg, 1997; Shapiro & Skinner, 1990): (1) Spend time in the setting (i.e., school, childcare, or home) before collecting observational data; (2) videotape observations where possible, so that you can focus on children rather than on recording responses; (3) situate yourself in the room to be as unobtrusive as possible; (4) sample as many situations as needed to gain a representative picture of child behavior across times of day and activities; and (5) take into account the physical, social, and cognitive demands of the setting.

Recording Formats

Recording formats need to be developed for direct observation that capture what has taken place. Not only must observers consider the frequency of a behavior or whether or not it occurred (as in many observation schedules and checklists); they must also provide brief behavioral descriptions of what happened or what justifies a rating, as well as descriptions of the context. Time needs to be spent developing formats that facilitate recording and summarizing these observations.

Approaches to Sampling Behavior

Numerous approaches are used to sample behavior. Here are some examples:

- Focusing on counting the frequency with which specific behaviors occur, such as "How frequently does a child use questions during play in the dramatic play or housekeeping area?" This is the use of a *sign system* or *event sampling*—every time the child asks a question (the event or sign), this is recorded. Event sampling can be used with behaviors that occur frequently, but is most useful with behaviors that occur infrequently (e.g., a tantrum or a very quiet child's contributing to a discussion) and is most successful with behaviors that have a defined beginning and ending (Hintze & Shapiro, 1995). Event sampling captures events as they naturally occur and is important as children acquire skills or control of their behavior. The observer may wish to account for what triggers and/or follows an event.
- Developing a list of all categories of language used (nonoverlapping and operationally defined) in the dramatic play or housekeeping area ahead of time, and simply tallying the frequency with which each language form is used during the observation period. This is the use of a *category system*. A video or audio recording of this activity would allow review and a reliability check. A teacher or aide can step back and record on a sheet attached to a clipboard or wall when a limited number of behaviors are of interest for one or two target children in a class. The use of a more detailed system would require an outside observer.
- Making tallies every minute during a given activity or period of time, such as recording the language forms that are used every minute. This is the use of *time sampling*. Time-sampling procedures are appropriate only for behaviors that occur fairly frequently and are frequently used in systematic observation (Hintze & Shapiro, 1995). The briefer the interval (10 seconds, 20 seconds), the more training required for accurate recording. The nature of the behaviors of interest will help users determine the length of the interval.
- Breaking up observation time into units or intervals (1 minute, 5 minutes, etc.). The observer then records whether or not the behaviors targeted for observation occur during the interval. Later, the number of intervals in which the behaviors of interest were observed to occur can be divided by the total number of intervals to yield the rate of the target behaviors. A sample format is presented in the top portion of Figure 4.1.
- Using observation cycles in which there is a period of observation followed by a period of recording. The Classroom Assessment Scoring System (CLASS) (Pianta, La Paro, & Hamré, 2007), for example, uses 30-minute cycles, during which 20 minutes are used to observe classroom interactions and 10 minutes to record three detailed aspects of classroom quality: Emotional Support, Classroom Organization, and Instructional Support in relation to student outcomes (see Chapter 5).

Observer 1			
		On-task[a]	Off-task[b]
Task	10:01	×	
	10:02	×	
	10:03	×	
	10:04		×
	10:05	×	
	10:06		×
	10:07		×
	10:08	×	
	10:09	×	
	10:10	×	
Totals		7	3

Observer 2			
		On-task[a]	Off-task[b]
Task	10:01	×	
	10:02	×	
	10:03		×
	10:04		×
	10:05	×	
	10:06		×
	10:07		×
	10:08		×
	10:09	×	
	10:10	×	
		5	5

Agreements:	On-task—5	Off-task—3
Disagreements:	2	
Total agreements:	10/10 × 100	= 100%
Interval total agreements:	8/10 × 100	= 80%
On-task agreements:	5/10 × 100	= 50%
Off-task agreements:	3/10 × 100	= 30%

[a]On-task: looking at work, playing with materials, sharing idea with another child.
[b]Off-task: looking around, wandering from play area.

FIGURE 4.1. Estimating agreement about a target child's on-task behavior.

The data that result from approaches such as these include (1) frequency; (2) percentage of occurrence (number of occurrences divided by total time or number of opportunities; (3) rate (occurrences divided by number of time units); and (4) duration (length of each event across intervals). Depending of the question of interest, observers may be interested in whether the behavior persists over the whole interval (such as with task engagement) or only part of it. In this case, a simple form can be developed in which a plus or minus is recorded in each interval (specify the interval's length).

Child: Target behavior:

Date:

Activity:

Time observation begins:

1_____	2_____	3_____	4_____	5_____	6_____
7_____	8_____	9_____	10_____	11_____	12_____
13_____	14_____	15_____	16_____	17_____	18_____
19_____	20_____	21_____	22_____	23_____	24_____
25_____	26_____	27_____	28_____	29_____	30_____
31_____	32_____	33_____	34_____	35_____	36_____
37_____	38_____	39_____	40_____	41_____	42_____
43_____	44_____	45_____	46_____	47_____	48_____
49_____	50_____	51_____	52_____	53_____	54_____
55_____	56_____	57_____	58_____	59_____	60_____

Other observation systems focus on (1) *latency*, which addresses the question of how long it takes for the child to respond after the presentation of a particular stimulus, such as complying with a teacher's request; (2) *intensity*, which addresses the question of how extreme or extensive a behavior is, such as a seizure; and (3) *accuracy*, which addresses the degree to which a given behavior is related to a stated criterion.

Sampling child behavior during representative times of day (e.g., opening activities, shared book reading, snack time) and across activities is essential to determine the generality of target behaviors across settings. Ensuring representativeness is a key step in the PASSkey (Planned Activity, Systematic Sampling, and Keystone behavior) model detailed by Barnett et al. (1994), in which the time for each activity is recorded. These observations can yield information about the frequency and duration of events (such as learning and/or behavioral problems), the sequencing of events, and the child's interactions with others. Such observation can lead to the selection of target ("keystone") behaviors for intervention, which is carried out in consultation with teachers or parents and is described in step-by-step intervention guidelines. Teachers and/or parents work collaboratively with consultants to collect baseline data prior to intervention, and then track the trend of behaviors during intervention. (Behavioral assessment is discussed later in this chapter.) Alessi and Kaye (1983) suggest that assessors consider sampling behavior (1) in both structured and unstructured settings; (2) in the child's strongest and weakest school activities; and (3) in both group and one-to-one activities. Suggestions that have been offered to guide observers in making decisions when using time-sampling procedures include basing the percentage of occurrence on a minimum of 20 opportunities to respond (Wolery, 1989) and using time sampling with behaviors that occur fairly frequently—at least once every 15 minutes (Irwin & Bushnell, 1980), or at a moderate but steady rate (Alessi & Kaye, 1983).

In addition to these general forms of recording, Wolery (1989) also recommends *levels-of-assistance recording*. This form of recording is used when the child is presented with an opportunity to comply with a behavior request independently and then at various levels of assistance or support (e.g., a verbal cue if a response is not forthcoming) until child performs the behavior. Wolery also recommends *task-analytic recording*, which is particularly important with *chained* skills (those involving a number of behaviors that need to be performed in sequence, such as dressing, eating, or riding a tricycle). For some children, failure to do one step may preclude the performance of the others, and an adult may need to help a child complete this step. Excellent examples of this approach are presented by Barnett et al. (1999).

Technical Concerns for Observers

A number of technical concerns regarding observation have been suggested throughout this chapter, and some solutions to these are presented in this section. (For a more detailed discussion, see Boehm & Weinberg, 1997 and Hintze, 2005).

Subjectivity and Bias

In order to reduce errors due to subjectivity or bias, it is essential to (1) differentiate objective from subjective observations, (2) separate observations from inferences, (3) train assessors in observation techniques, and (4) follow through with an interview and possibly a home visit when parents provide observations.

Memory Lapses

Memory problems can be addressed by recording observed behaviors as soon as possible after an event or by using systematic observation schedules (after practice to a criterion level).

Representativeness of the Behavior Sample

The extent to which the sampling of behavior is genuinely representative of the problem at hand is improved by (1) collecting observations over time; (2) conducting observations in relation to a comparison child; (3) collecting behavior samples from converging sources; and (4) using systematic data collection procedures, with clear, nonoverlapping categories that are exhaustive descriptions of the problem. The purpose of the observation guides the amount of observation required. Wolery (1989) makes a number of recommendations: (1) If the purpose is instructional planning, at least two to three observations are needed (if the data from these are quite different, then additional observations are needed); (2) if recommendations are to be monitored and modified on an ongoing basis, fewer data may be needed; and (3) if the purpose is to monitor the effectiveness of a behavioral (or other) intervention, then frequent observation is needed.

Reliability of Observation

Reliability is critical to the use of observational techniques and is increased by training and spot checks. Kent and Foster (1977) remind us that while training can enhance agreement between observers, spot checks need to be carried out in actual observation situations to keep observers' reliability finely tuned; knowing that supervisors will co-observe results in greater reliability than if there are no such checks (a point underscored by Volpe, DiPerna, Hintze, and Shapiro [2005]). Kent and Foster (1977) also call attention to the fact that not all behaviors, individuals, and situations can be viewed with equal reliability. Some situations are easier to observe than others, and observers are more familiar with some situations than others.

The reliability of two users of a rating scale will be determined through correlation procedures. These may focus on observers' making the same point judgment along the rating scale, but more frequently on whether they are within ±1 scale point of each other. Reliability is enhanced when points along the scale are behaviorally defined and when systems that are not overly complex are used (Alessi & Kaye, 1983; Hintze, 2005). Observer agreement regarding the occurrence of target behaviors over time also needs to be considered. Assessors with limited time may not have the opportunity to make repeated visits to a classroom, but they can check their observations against those of a parent or teacher. The most frequently used procedure is for two individuals to observe, using the same system, and then to divide the number of agreements between observers regarding whether the behavior did or did not occur (within each time interval) by the total number of observations made by both observers:

$$\frac{\text{Number of agreements}}{(\text{Agreements} + \text{disagreements}) \times \text{Number of observers}}$$

This statistic can be inflated when behaviors are very frequent or infrequent. Computing the kappa statistic (Cohen, 1960) will address this issue. Additional interobserver indices are detailed by Suen, Ary, and Ary (1986).

Observers may also want to know more than the overall rate of agreement. They may be interested in whether observers agreed that the same behavior occurred in each interval, that the same frequency of a target behavior occurred within each interval, or that a behavior did not occur in some intervals. Each of these is a more rigorous form of agreement. Page and Iwata (1986) indicate that the calculation of occurrence agreement is a more conservative measure for low-rate behaviors than interval agreement. In contrast, nonoccurrence agreement is a more conservative measure for high-rate behaviors. An example of using these procedures is presented in the bottom portion of Figure 4.1.

Refinements of these procedures are detailed by Barker and Tyne (1980), Hartmann (1982), Hintze (2005), Kratochwill and Wetzel (1977), Kent and Foster (1977), and Page and Iwata (1986), among others. According to Kent and Foster (1977), "the method of computing reliability is an important determiner of the magnitude of the reliability coefficient and, therefore, of the conclusions reached about the quality of one's data" (p. 308).

The relative instability of children's behavior requires observation over time and during multiple activities. Such reliability data are needed to determine whether a skill (e.g., turn taking during conversations) has been acquired and can be applied across activities.

Validity of Observation

Validity depends on (1) comprehensive coverage of behaviors that make up the area of concern (e.g., fighting); (2) sampling each behavior a sufficient number of times and ways to obtain a representative picture of that behavior; and (3) the degree of interpretation required on the part of the observer (e.g., the behaviors that will constitute "fighting"). First of all, attention needs to be directed to the content validity of the observational procedure. Rating scales, checklists, and formal observation schemes need to include clear behavioral descriptions of the categories of behaviors that make up the area of concern/interest. Developers of assessment procedures that rely on observation need to describe in detail how they have accounted for comprehensive coverage through task analysis, review of the literature, and discussion with other developmental specialists.

Attention next needs to be addressed to adequate sampling of behaviors for assessment to be predictive or representative (see "Representativeness of the Behavior Sample," above). If observations are based on one brief session with a child, as in the typical screening program, the observer can have only limited confidence that an accurate picture of the child has been obtained, particularly if the child is encountering moderate difficulty. Assessment procedures that build in systematic observation checks over 1 or 2 weeks begin to address this problem, as well as to provide information that will guide instruction. Certainly, ongoing observation checks are likely to have the highest assessment validity. Barker and Tyne (1980) specify that the responses targeted should be quantifiable and occur with sufficient frequency to serve as a basis for making decisions (e.g., forms of language use, engagement with tasks, disruptive behavior, etc.). Furthermore, sampling needs to take place at a time when observers can see behaviors of concern. If, for example, observers are interested in social interactions with peers, they need to watch children interacting with peers. Although an observation of children at play might be built into screening, follow-up observations would be necessary to verify any problematic behavior before referral decisions are made. Finally, information from other measures collected at the same time, in the form of interviews, questionnaires, or rating scales, provide concurrent information about target behaviors of concern, as do children's work or behavior samples and performance on tests. At issue is whether or not a consistent picture is presented about the child across measures and across contexts. According to

Hintze (2005), moderate to high correlations are needed to support adequate concurrent validity. Depending on the purpose of the system, predictive validity evidence may also need to be presented in relationship to future performance on criterion measures of specified outcomes.

Finally, the construct validity of observation systems used for assessment purposes can be determined by seeing whether observation data discriminate between children who are identified as having problems and those who are not, and by checking these data against later performance in school. The relationship between the observational outcomes and the concepts predicted by theories or in response to intervention also needs to be investigated (Hintze, 2005). Hintze (2005) presents a useful table of quality indicators of direct observation methods.

The interpretation of outcomes based on systematic observation procedures depends on the complexity of the system used, training of observers, and the psychometric properties detailed. But, as McConaughy (2005) cautions, even direct observations of children's behavior are based on perceptions of the observer of a particular situation. Thus, outcomes need to be used to generate hypotheses to be followed up by targeted observation and integrated with other test data.

Volpe et al. (2005) present a review of seven coding systems school psychologists might find useful for observing students in classroom settings who present problem behaviors. One of these scales, the Direct Observation Form (DOF; Achenbach, 1986), is appropriate for use below grade 1. The DOF was developed to be used as part of the Achenbach System of Empirically Based Assessment (ASEBA; Achenbach & Rescorla, 2000a). This system is detailed in Chapter 14. Volpe et al. (2005) indicate that the seven systems reviewed require considerable training and multiple observation occasions to achieve a reliable estimate of student behavior. These researchers also point out that although most systems provide documentation of interobserver agreement, predictive validity, and treatment sensitivity, the evidence is based on single studies with small to moderate size samples. Thus, the collection of local normative data is recommended. These factors make the use of the systems difficult for professionals with limited time to work with individual students.

Technical concerns such as the ones covered in this section are addressed in two observational approaches widely used at the preschool level: behavioral assessment and observation of children at play.

TWO OBSERVATIONAL APPROACHES WIDELY USED AT THE PRESCHOOL LEVEL

Behavioral Assessment

A fundamental technique in addressing such behaviors as inattention, hyperactivity, fighting, lack of engagement with tasks, and social interaction skills is observation—a central component of behavioral assessment. This type of observation needs to include what sets off a behavior (the antecedents), the behavior itself, and the responses to that behavior (the consequences)—in other words, the ABCs of behavior management or applied behavior analysis. The teacher or specialist needs to determine how the child's interaction with the environment influences desired or undesired behavior. Systematic observation is central to tracking and documenting changes in behavior that occur as a result of intervention focused on both the child and the environment (see Chapter 5). Quantitative methods are used, including documenting data on both behavior prior to intervention and the behavioral patterns that result from intervention. Behavioral intervention is the major type of intervention for hyperactivity and autism spectrum disorders (ASD) in preschool children, as well as most behaviors of concern in regular preschool settings. A simple example in a preschool setting follows:

> Jack has been observed to move around the room starting, but rarely finishing, various activities during free play. Not only does he make a mess; he is not following through on his work. Before the teacher tried to modify this behavior, the parents are notified and asked for their input and support at home. The goals are to help Jack complete the activities he starts and put away the materials he has used. In order to encourage him to reach these goals, the teacher allows him to play in one area only during free play, and develops a checklist of behaviors with him that he must successfully complete for a reward (a sticker on a badge). He will be told whether he is successful, and what he needs to do if he is not. As he becomes more successful, he will be allowed to move around during free play. The teacher will check what he has done and he can check off the behaviors listed (in picture format) on the checklist. If he reverts to his previous behaviors, he will go back to the structured checklist and single activity area. Every day when his mother comes to pick him up, she will be told what Jack has done and shown the checklist.
>
> Antecedent (free play) → Behavior (includes not moving around room, completing tasks, and putting away materials) → Consequence (checklist, sticker, and report to mother)

Many researchers interested in the preschool population focus on applied behavior analysis (Barnett & Carey, 1992; Barnett et al., 1994, 1999; Mash & Terdal, 1997). Detailed discussion of this topic is beyond the scope of this chapter, however. An excellent resource is *Designing Preschool Interventions: A Practitioner's Guide* (Barnett et al., 1999).

Observation of Children at Play

Early childhood assessors consistently point to the need to observe children at play as an essential component of the assessment process (see, e.g., Coolahan, Fantuzzo, Mendez, & McDermott, 2000; Leff & Larkin, 2005; Linder, 1996; Paget, 1990; Pellegrini, 1998). Play affords assessors the opportunity to observe children engaging in familiar activities, in order to learn how they interact with a variety of materials, with other children, or with caregivers, and to understand their skill development. In addition, assessors may (1) study target areas of interest, such as language/communication development, socio-emotional development, separation from caregivers, emergent literacy in reading and writing, and the ability to follow directions; (2) monitor the achievement of instructional objectives, many of which can be measured only by using an observational technique (e.g., self-help skills and peer interactions); (3) evaluate the effectiveness of a particular intervention (e.g., time out as a consequence of aggressive behavior); or (4) provide empirical support for other identification procedures.

According to Piaget (1951), play progresses in the following sequence: (1) exploratory; (2) relational (objects are used for the purpose they were intended for, such as a brush for hair); (3) constructive (objects are used for creating something with an end goal in mind); (4) dramatic; and (5) games with rules. Children may engage in one or more of these types of play, depending on their developmental level and interests. Unusual play behaviors described by parents and other caregivers are also important, such as obsessively opening and closing doors, banging, and lining things up in rows; these are often observed among children with ASD (see Chapter 13).

Play is instrumental to developing all aspects of language (Vygotsky, 1962), such as phonology, semantics, syntax, and the pragmatics of interacting in everyday situations. Children play with fantasy and nonsense words, speech acts, and discourse conventions. Morrow (1992) cites evidence that links play to literacy development, including story comprehension, story retelling, and vocabulary development. Diverse cognitive abilities can also be observed while children are at play, such as memory, reasoning, abstraction, problem solving, and attention span. Children's play will be affected by the physical environment, the toys available, and the number of children at play, as well as by each child's personality, physical condition, gender, and culture. Furthermore, the nature of children's preschool program affects the nature of their play activities (Johnson, Ershler, & Bell, 1980).

In addition to children's individual play activity, observing their play interaction with peers provides critical insight into their social and emotional development. Social play has been the focus of considerable research in determining how children develop the skills to get along with one another since Mildred Parten first looked at preschoolers' social participation in the late 1920s. Based on her observations of free play among 42 children ages 2–5 years, Parten (1932) developed a scale of social participation skills that defined six broad sequential behavior categories of social participation: unoccupied behavior, onlooker behavior, solitary independent play, parallel activity, associative play, and cooperative play. This scale provides a broad view of the social and cognitive levels of play. However, a careful observation of a child's play over a day in a preschool setting can provide many insights for targets of intervention.

In more recent years, a number of observational rating scales have been developed to focus on different aspects of play. Leff and Lakin (2005), for example, view the playground as an important natural context in which to study social competence and social conflicts as children progress through school. These researchers reviewed six playground observation scales with manuals based on Hintze et al. (2002) criteria, including "(a) the goal of the system is to measure specific, targeted behaviors; (b) the behaviors being observed are operationally defined a priori; (c) observations are conducted using standardized procedures and are highly objective in nature; (d) the times and places are carefully selected; and (e) the scoring and summation of data are standardized" (p. 993). Of these six scales, two are appropriate at levels prior to first grade: the Child-Peer Observation Code (Synder et al., 1998) that codes play activity and the presence or absence of aggressive acts and the Ostrov Early Childhood Play Project Observation System (Ostrov, 2005) that focuses on antisocial and prosocial behaviors. Leff and Lakin (2005) indicate that both of these scales are recently developed and have limited research with diverse populations. These researchers also stress the importance of observation of targeted behaviors across multiple settings. Although such observation across settings can be time-consuming, it helps identify the context of problem behaviors and the effect of intervention on target behaviors.

Numerous other scales that have been developed to focus on aspects of play as part of the diagnosis-intervention process are detailed by Gitlin-Weiner, Sandgrund, and Schaefer (2000). Others, such as the Howes Peer Play Observation Scale (Howes, 1980; Howes & Stewart, 1987), are used to document play interactions in studies of childcare and Head Start settings, such as in the Head Start FACES study (Commissioner's Office of Research and Evaluation & Head Start Bureau, 2001a).

Two scales are described in the sections that follow. Others are included in Appendix 4.1. The first scale focuses on play behaviors that can be readily observed in preschool classrooms. The second focuses on systematic use of play during in-depth evaluation.

The Penn Interactive Peer Play Scale

The Penn Interactive Peer Play Scale (PIPPS; Fantuzzo et al., 1995, 1996; Fantuzzo, Mendez, & Tighe, 1998) is a 4-point rating scale ("never," "seldom," "often," "always") of both positive and negative play behaviors completed by parents and teachers. The revised version of this scale consists of 32 interactive free play behaviors. The purposes of the scale are to (1) differentiate the behaviors of children who are more versus less successful in sustaining interactive play, (2) identify the play strengths of resilient preschool children living in high-risk urban environments, and (3) inform early childhood classroom-based intervention. The Teacher Report version of the PIPPS is shown in Figure 4.2. Content was based on the descriptions of 38 Head Start teachers of children's typical play behaviors and upon Parten's (1932) basic categories of social interaction, revised for use in Head Start. These revised categories include the following (Fantuzzo et al., 1996):

Nonplay—unoccupied behavior (standing or sitting without playing) or watching without playing.

Negative—child hits, pinches, or otherwise attempts to physically injure other child, or grabs an object from other child; child maliciously insults, teases, curses, screams at, or threatens other child.

Solitary—child plays independently without looking or talking to other children.

Social Attention—child plays independently but shows awareness of what another child is doing (i.e., looks at other child); child does not speak to other child.

Associate—child talks to, smiles at, and/or exchanges toys with the other child, but does not adjust own behavior to what the other is doing.

Collaborative—child collaborates with other child in play activity in a mutual, complementary way; child may take on a reciprocal role that is distinctively different than that of the other child and adjust his or her behavior according to the actions of the other child.

The play behaviors of 800 children were videotaped, with observers determining the highest and the lowest levels of interactive play. Fantuzzo et al. (1995) performed an exploratory factor analysis that revealed three reliable underlying dimensions: Play Interaction, Play Disruption, and Play Disconnection. Concurrent validity with the SSRS (Gresham & Elliott, 1990) demonstrated a similarity in the factor structure between the two scales. In a later study with 1,186 ethnically diverse urban Head Start children (Fantuzzo et al., 1996) the same three factors were supported by a common factor analysis. Concurrent validity was reported in this study with three criterion measures: the Conners' Teacher Rating Scale (Conners, 1989), a sociometric measure developed by Howes (1987), and the Interactive Peer Play Observational Coding System (Fantuzzo & Sutton-Smith, 1994). These dimensions have been supported in subsequent studies (Coolahan, Fantuzzo, Mendez, & McDermott, 1998; Fantuzzo, Coolahan, Mendez, McDermott, & Sutton-Smith, 1998; Gagnon & Nagle, 2004).

PENN INTERACTIVE PEER PLAY SCALE

Teacher Report

Child name ______________________ School/Classroom ______________________

In the past two months, indicate how much you have observed the following behaviors in this child during free play by circling Never, Seldom, Often, or Always observed.

1.	Helps other children	Never	Seldom	Often	Always
2.	Starts fights & arguments	Never	Seldom	Often	Always
3.	Is rejected by others	Never	Seldom	Often	Always
4.	Does not take turns	Never	Seldom	Often	Always
5.	Hovers outside play group	Never	Seldom	Often	Always
6.	Shares toys with other children	Never	Seldom	Often	Always
7.	Withdraws	Never	Seldom	Often	Always
8.	Wanders aimlessly	Never	Seldom	Often	Always
9.	Rejects the play ideas of others	Never	Seldom	Often	Always
10.	Is ignored by others	Never	Seldom	Often	Always
11.	Tattles	Never	Seldom	Often	Always
12.	Helps settle peer conflicts	Never	Seldom	Often	Always
13.	Destroys others' things	Never	Seldom	Often	Always
14.	Disagrees without fighting	Never	Seldom	Often	Always
15.	Refuses to play when invited	Never	Seldom	Often	Always
16.	Needs help to start playing	Never	Seldom	Often	Always
17.	Verbally assaults others	Never	Seldom	Often	Always
18.	Directs others' action politely	Never	Seldom	Often	Always
19.	Cries, whines, shows temper	Never	Seldom	Often	Always
20.	Encourages others to join play	Never	Seldom	Often	Always
21.	Grabs others' things	Never	Seldom	Often	Always
22.	Comforts others who are hurt or sad	Never	Seldom	Often	Always
23.	Confused in play	Never	Seldom	Often	Always
24.	Verbalizes stories during play	Never	Seldom	Often	Always
25.	Needs teacher's direction	Never	Seldom	Often	Always
26.	Disrupts the play of others	Never	Seldom	Often	Always
27.	Seems unhappy	Never	Seldom	Often	Always
28.	Shows positive emotions during play (e.g., smiles, laughs)	Never	Seldom	Often	Always
29.	Is physically aggressive	Never	Seldom	Often	Always
30.	Shows creativity in making up play stories and activities	Never	Seldom	Often	Always

FIGURE 4.2. Penn Interactive Peer Play Scale (PIPPS)—Teacher Report. From Fantuzzo et al. (1995). Copyright 1995 by Elsevier. Reprinted by permission. *Note.* The two additional items on the current version of the PIPPS (2002) are "Demands to be in charge" and "Is disruptive during transitions."

The construct and concurrent validity of the revised 32-item teacher version of the PIPPS was supported by Fantuzzo, Coolahan, et al. (1998) based on a study of 523 African American children enrolled in a large central-city Head Start program. Outcomes were based on teacher report of social skills using the SSRS, peer report based on a pictorial sociometric measure, and direct play observation data. The same three constructs of interactive play were again confirmed. Outcomes indicates that children who demonstrated interactive play behaviors, received high teacher ratings for more general social skills and were well-liked by their peers, as indicated by sociometric data. In contrast, children who received high observer ratings of disruptive peer play also received teacher ratings indicating a lack of self-control. In addition, these children were not well accepted by their peers. Children who received high ratings for disconnected peer play were observed to be attending to but not participating in play with other children.

The construct validity of the parent version of the PIPPS was supported by Fantuzzo, Coolahan, et al. (1998) with data collected on 297 predominantly African American urban Head Start children. Support was demonstrated for the same three constructs of interactive peer play: play interaction, play disruption, and play disconnection, obtained from prior studies with the teacher version. The parent version of the PIPPS was also validated in this study with the teacher version. Results indicated that there is a significant, but relatively low, degree of similarity between parent and teacher reports of play at home and at school.

Coolahan et al. (2000) found a significant relationship between high ratings on Play Interaction and engagement in classroom learning activities, motivation, and attention. Using the parent version of the PIPPS, Fantuzzo and McWayne (2002) found that play competencies exhibited in the home environment were significantly associated with behavior in the classroom and motivation to learn. Finally, in this unfolding body of research, Gagnon and Nagle (2004) conducted a study with a sample very different from the Head Start samples reported above. The sample consisted of 85 largely Caucasian 4-year-old children who attended an early intervention program in a rural area in the southeast. A significant relationship was found between the Parent PIPPS and the Vineland Social-Emotional Early Childhood scales (SEEC; Sparrow et al., 1998). This outcome suggests that children who are competent players also display strong social-emotional skills, while children who are negative and aggressive during play interactions tend to display lower levels of social-emotional development. Significant correlations were also found between the teacher PIPPS and each of the SEEC scales. Positive correlations emerged between the Play Interaction scale and negative correlations between the Play Disruption and Play Disconnection scales and each of the SEEC scales and the Composite. Positive correlations were also revealed between the Play Interaction factor and the social skills factors on the SSRS. In contrast, negative correlations were found between the Play Disruption and Play Disconnection factors and the social skills factors on the SSRS.

Gagnon and Nagle (2004) indicate that these findings have important implications for early childhood assessors and suggest that the evaluation of play using a brief measure such as the PIPPS become standard practice, particularly in the area of social-emotional functioning.

In sum, this scale can be useful for assessors, parents, and teachers to understand aspects of the environment that constrain or facilitate development, and to guide them in devising intervention activities. A Spanish version of the PIPPS is documented in a study of Hispanic children in a southeast region of the United States (Castro, Mendes, & Fantuzzo, 2002).

Transdisciplinary Play-Based Assessment

The most comprehensive play-based assessment system to date for a referred child at the preschool level is the revised version of Transdisciplinary Play-Based Assessment (TPBA), developed by Toni Linder (1996). TPBA is a team process used for identifying individual intervention objectives, including those related to specific skill deficits, and for tracking a child's progress related to these objectives. It involves structured and unstructured play situations in which the child can be observed interacting alone with toys, another child, parent(s), and a facilitating adult. TPBA is a comprehensive method that can be used with children between infancy and 6 years of age to observe development in four domains: Cognitive Abilities, Social-Emotional Functioning, Communication and Language Skills, and Sensory–Motor Development. Detailed developmental charts are provided to guide observation. Linder claims that this model is developmental, transdisciplinary, holistic, and dynamic. The transdisciplinary aspect of assessment integrates the observations of team members and reflects an understanding that each domain of development is not distinct, but is associated with other domains. All members of the team observe the child's behaviors at the same time, leading to an integrated view of the child's functioning. TPBA is designed to supplement, or in some cases to replace, traditional, structured individual assessments. Unlike traditional assessment that uses a particular set of activities, TPBA is a flexible approach. Different materials can be used, and the content, sequence, and language used can be changed, depending on the needs of the child and his or her native language. Parents are actively involved in the process as both information providers and participants.

TPBA usually takes 1–1½ hours to complete and is usually videotaped for more careful analysis. Before the session, members of the professional team learn as much as they can about the child to be assessed, so they can appropriately structure the room and the tasks to be presented. The assessment process is divided into six phases:

Unstructured Facilitation. The child is given 20–25 minutes to explore the testing room and become more comfortable, with the facilitator following the child's lead.

Structured Facilitation (10–15 minutes). The facilitator directs the child to engage in specific activities that need to be evaluated and were not observed in the first phase. The facilitator attempts to promote problem solving through scaffolding. At times a team member may interact directly with the child (e.g., a physical therapist may want to "feel" the child's muscle tone).

Child–Child Interaction (10 minutes). Another child (one with whom the index child may be familiar, but who has slightly higher-level play skills) is brought into the room to play with the subject, in order to assess the subject's interactive play skills.

Parent–Child Interaction (10 minutes). One or both parents are brought in to engage in structured and unstructured play activities with the child, in order to assess the parent–child interaction style. The parent or parents leave the room and then return during this phase, in order to observe the child's reactions to separation and reunion.

Motor Play (10–15 minutes). Motor play is elicited in order to assess the child's physical abilities.

Snack (5–10 minutes). The child is given a snack to determine his or her level of self-help skills, social interaction, language, and motor functioning.

After the play session, the following take place: a postsession meeting with parents to address immediate concerns; videotape analysis and guideline review; assessment of strengths, rating of abilities, and justifications on summary sheets; development of preliminary recommendations; a meeting of the full team, including parents; and the writing of a formal report. The detailed results can be used to develop home and school interventions, and a companion guide, *Transdisciplinary Play-Based Intervention* (Linder, 1993), provides many useful suggestions for intervention by developmental domain.

TPBA can provide the assessment team with rich information. It is conducted in a nonthreatening play environment that is conducive to eliciting a child's natural behaviors. It is particularly useful for children presenting special needs or at risk for developmental delay. The multidisciplinary team observes the interaction of skills across developmental areas, providing an integrated view of the child's developmental levels. The involvement of parents not only allows the child to "check in" when necessary, but enables the parents to offer additional insight into the child's particular behaviors as members of the assessment team. The information obtained is easily translated into functional, skill-based interventions. Multiple observations are made of the strategies the child uses across tasks and the time the child is engaged with materials or activities as the child interacts with the facilitator, a parent, and a peer. The manual provides guidelines and worksheets for observing play, sample timetables, and specific suggestions for ensuring children's optimal performance.

However, there are drawbacks to this type of assessment. It is labor-intensive (significant team members all need to be present at one time) and requires much preparation. The assessment procedure is complex and requires practice (although the videotapes that are available help address this issue). The team members must work closely together to assure accurate observation and interpretation of behaviors. Results are qualitative and rely on clinical observations and professional judgment, and there is an overall lack of validity and reliability data. There are also no norms, which may present a problem when state guidelines require standardized testing for eligibility for special services. Still, early childhood experts support the content validity of the TPBA approach, and Linder indicates that the procedure can be as accurate as norm-referenced tests in identifying children who need special services. Test–retest and interrater reliabilities are reported as good, although no specific ratios are given. Little available published research exists that analyzes the use of TPBA in determining development. Some important behaviors may not be observed and evaluated adequately, such as receptive language. However, the use of TPBA provides detailed information for intervention planning.

In most time-limited assessment situations, it would be hard to conduct TPBA in full. However, assessors may use aspects of this system in developmental areas of concern. The guidelines provide an excellent framework from which to observe children in any type of assessment situation and to develop intervention strategies.

ISSUES RELATED TO OBSERVATION DURING TESTING

Observation during testing, while widely advocated as an essential clinical skill to interpret the reliability and validity of the child's behavior in the testing situation and to generalize the results to similar situations outside of testing, has received little empirical research attention. The few studies to date suggest that this practice needs to be engaged in with great caution. Glutting, Oakland, and McDermott (1989), for example, studied the validity of test session observations as they related to test session performance on the

Wechsler Intelligence Scale for Children—Revised (WISC-R) administered by school psychologists, and to performance on the Adaptive Behavior Inventory for Children (Mercer & Lewis, 1982) obtained outside the testing situation. The WISC-R was administered to a sample of 311 children, ages 7 years, 6 months (7-6) to 14-4 years, drawn randomly from a south central U.S. school district which included children from a representative sample of black, white, and Mexican American middle- and lower-SES backgrounds. Intrasession observations were recorded with 15 of 19 items from the Test Behavior Observation Guide (TBOG; Caldwell, 1951). These included performance rate, orientation to examination, initial adjustment, interest, cooperation, expressive ability, attention, self-confidence, motivation, effort, persistence, ability to shift, reaction to praise and encouragement, reaction to failure, and self-criticism. Each item was rated on a scale from 1 ("optimum behavior") to 5 ("least satisfactory") with points along the scale, in general, behaviorally defined. The findings of this study revealed three major factors on the TBOG, which the authors labeled Task Attentiveness, Task Confidence, and Cooperative Disposition. The moderately strong correlation of the TBOG with the WISC-R demonstrated a fairly strong relationship between test session observations and test performance (r = .48), supporting the validity of the clinical observations made during testing. However, there was only a marginal relationship between the test session observations and out-of-session performance (r = .17). Glutting and McDermott (1988) demonstrated a similar lack of generality of findings with kindergarten children when classroom behaviors were rated. Thus generalizing from observations obtained during testing to everyday functioning in the school and community is problematic. Clearly, the brief observations obtained during testing need to be supplemented by observation of the child's routine activities and interviews with parents and teachers.

More recently McConaughy (2005) reviewed the characteristics and psychometric properties of three standardized instruments for test session or interview observations. One of these, the Test Observation Form (TOF; McConaughy & Achenbach, 2004) is appropriate for children under age 6. This form was developed for children ages 2 to 18 and was designed to be used with other instruments from the Achenbach System of Empirically Based Assessment (ASEBA) (Achenbach & Rescorla, 2000; Achenbach & Rescorla, 2001). The TOF consists of 125 items rated on a 4-point scale and focuses on largely maladaptive behaviors (e.g., apathetic or unmotivated; argues). Extensive information is provided for scoring. The TOF is completed after testing and takes 5 to 10 minutes to complete by trained observers and another 10 to 15 minutes to score. Factor analyses were used to derive the five TOF syndrome scores. Test–retest reliabilities range from .53 to .87. Interrater reliabilities ranged from .42 to .78. The validity studies reported were not based on preschool children. While reasonable technical data are presented, McConaughy underscores that issue of situational variability and cautions against overgeneralizing from test session observations to other settings. Rather, outcomes should be used to develop hypotheses about problems that can be targeted through more specific observation in everyday settings.

Focusing specifically on preschool children, Kaplan (1993) presented data supporting the lack of generality of test session behaviors to less structured nontest situations, such as the classroom. He raised the question of reliability with which assessors observed examinees' behavior within the testing situation during administration of the WPPSI-R. A 42-item, 4-point rating scale was developed and used to rate the test session behavior of preschool children (covering comments, facial expressions, gestures, and other verbal and nonverbal behaviors). Twenty-six children were videotaped while tested by an experienced tester. Ratings were completed after the session, using notes gathered during testing. Observer agreement data (collected by the researcher and a second trained observer, using the rating scale with five tapes) revealed that the two observers often disagreed on their test session ratings, in regard to both occurrence–nonoccurrence of behaviors and the level of ratings. Item correlation ranged from –.26 (disagreement) to .89, with a mean of .52. Fewer than 20% of the items had interrater coefficients of .80 or better. Kaplan urged that assessors consider observations collected during testing as hunches only, to be followed up by systematic observation over time of children engaged in everyday tasks.

In summary, behavioral observations during formal assessment cannot be generalized directly to nontest situations and need to be considered only as hunches (based on the assessor's perceptions). Bracken (1985) has noted that within the testing situation itself, both test and nontest behaviors need to be described, and diagnosticians need to be cautioned to describe and evaluate a child's behavior as enhancing or impeding performance without feeling the need to label that behavior as "normal" or "abnormal." These hunches can be followed up by observation in the classroom or other naturalistic settings. Although the use of standardized observation measures greatly increases the reliability and validity of test session observations based on anecdotal reports (McConaughy, 2005), the time required to complete and score these observations may be problematic for many assessors.

SUMMARY

Observation is central to all forms of early childhood assessment. It allows assessors to gain a comprehensive understanding of children's behavior as it occurs in the natural context of familiar tasks. Observation of children's behavior across settings and across time is fundamental to instructional planning, behavioral assessment, and intervention, and is a major component of screening and in-depth evaluation.

The strengths and limitations of various forms of observation have been detailed, including diary accounts, anecdotal records, running records, observation schedules, checklists, rating scales, and questionnaires. These can all play an integral part in assessing the child's cognitive, physical/motor, language, social, and emotional strengths and limitations. Observation also serves as a means for validating information collected with other assessment tools and is critical for identifying appropriate intervention strategies.

The major features of systematic observation have been detailed, including the roles of the observer, task, setting, and the observational procedure used. Essential technical characteristics of reliability and validity have been reviewed.

An overview of two widely used observation approaches—behavioral assessment and play assessment—is presented. Finally, issues related to the lack of generalizability of observations made during formal testing to nontest situations are raised.

APPENDIX 4.1. Review of Measures

Measure	**Ages and Stages Questionnaires (ASQ) (2nd ed.). Bricker and Squires (1999).**
Purpose	A parent completed system for screening infants and young children for possible developmental delays.
Areas	There are nineteen age-interval questionnaires that cover five developmental areas: Communication, Gross Motor, Fine Motor, Problem Solving, and Personal–Social. Additional questions are asked regarding the child's health history.
Format	Parents check "yes," "sometimes," or "not yet" for each of the 30 items per questionnaire; may be completed through interview.
Scores	The three response options are then converted to point values, and a summary score (consisting of items belonging to each area) is calculated for each of the five areas. The scores are then compared to empirically derived cutoff scores for each area.
Age group	4–60 months.
Time	10–15 minutes to complete.
Users	Parent or caregiver with at least a fourth- to sixth-grade reading level.
Norms	Norms were derived from 1,763 assessments using age-appropriate developmental questionnaires.
Reliability	The test–retest reliability (2-week interval) was .94 and the interrater reliability was also high, with agreement between 112 parents and 3 trained observers being greater than 90%.
Validity	Overidentification ranged from 7–16%, sensitivity from 38–90% (median .75), and specificity from 81–91% (median .86) across age groups.
Comments	The questionnaires can be used as part of screening prior to kindergarten, during child find, or by primary healthcare providers with parents prior to an appointment so that parent concerns can provide a focus for the exam. The questionnaires are also available in Spanish, French, Korean and a number of other languages, and may also be used as an interview tool. Other materials and questionnaires that are associated with the ASQ are the ASQ User's Guide, Ages and Stages Learning Activities, and Ages and Stages Questionnaires: Social-Emotional. All available on CD-ROM for training purposes and to facilitate scoring. A database program manager is also available. These questionnaires can be quickly completed by parents and can be used over time to track growth across developmental areas.
References consulted	Boehm in text; Boyce (2005); Meisels and Atkins-Burnett (2005); Poteat (2005). See book's References list.

Measure	**Child–Peer Observation Code. Snyder et al. (1998).**
Purpose	Observing playground behaviors of young children to identify the presence or absence of seven different child behaviors.
Areas	Negative Interaction, Rough Play, Positive Interaction, Parallel Play, Solitary Focused Play, Solitary Unfocused Play and Other.
Format	Paper-and-pencil coding system. Coding is performed across consecutive 10-second intervals for 5-minute periods. System includes coding flow chart.
Scores	Coder records behaviors as either absent or present.

Age group	Preschool and kindergarten children.
Time	Not reported.
Users	Trained observers.
Norms	Not reported.
Reliability	Interrater reliability ranged from .65 to .80; intraclass correlations ranged from .79 to .84.
Validity	Promising convergent and predictive/discriminant validity.
Comments	The strengths of the Child-Peer Observation Code include well-defined behaviors, coding flow chart sheets, and promising initial reliability and validity studies. A limitation is that the system has only been used with European American kindergartners from one school.
References consulted	Snyder et al. (1998); Leff and Lakin (2005). See book's References list.

Measure	**Howes Peer Play Scale (Revised). Howes and Matheson (1992).**
Purpose	Assessing the developmental sequences in children's social play with peers.
Areas	From the original Howes Peer Play Scale, four of the five scale points were used (Parallel Play, Parallel Aware Play, Simple Social Play, and Complementary and Reciprocal Play). The fifth scale point that was created is Complex Social Pretend Play. Measures children's interactions with other children, teachers, and other adults during free play.
Format	Paper-and-pencil coding system. Coding is performed across consecutive 20-second intervals for 5-minute periods, for a total of 20 minutes.
Scores	Behaviors are coded as absent or present.
Age group	Toddler through 59 months.
Time	Approximately 20 minutes.
Users	Trained practitioners.
Norms	Age norms.
Reliability	Not reported for revised version.
Validity	A series of studies by Howes and Matheson (1992) with children 10 to 59 months old document the validity of the scale. While play forms emerged in the predicted sequence, only 80% of children engaged in the highest form of peer play. Play forms also varied as a function of the children's childcare setting with less complex play demonstrated in lower-quality settings.
Comments	The revised version of the Howes Peer Play Scale seems to capture a developmental sequence in children's interactive behaviors. Children appear to display continuity over developmental periods in their use of play forms, and individual differences in play forms seem to be connected to more general indexes of social competence with peers. Initial studies, however, were completed on small samples of infants and children, with greater than half of the sample being of European American descent. These scales have been used in studies of children in childcare and Head Start settings, and they were among the measures used to document play interactions in the Head Start FACES study. These scales can be useful for evaluating the effects of intervention directed at an entire class, rather than a referred child.
References consulted	Boehm review; Commissioner's Office of Research and Evaluation and Head Start Bureau (2001a); Howes (1980); Howes and Stewart (1987); Howes and Matheson (1992). See book's References list.

Measure	Ostrov Early Childhood Play Project Observation System. Ostrov (2005).
Purpose	An observation system that records child behaviors using six codes.
Areas	The six behavior codes are divided into two groups: aggressive behavior and play behaviors. The aggressive behavior codes are as follows: Relational, Verbal, and Physical. The play behavior codes are Cooperative, Parallel Play, and Solitary Play.
Format	Paper-and-pencil coding using a continuous event recording system. A target child's behavior is coded any time he/she exhibits target behaviors during the observation period, which can last anywhere from 3 to 10 minutes.
Scores	Behavioral counts are summed to derive scores per code.
Age group	3 to 6 years.
Time	Not reported.
Users	Trained professionals.
Norms	Not reported.
Reliability	Interrater agreement was adequate with intraclass correlations ranging from .74 to .95 per code.
Validity	There is initial evidence for the convergent validity.
Comments	The manual is very clear, and the codes are well defined. The system addresses behaviors in very young children. It can be used across different contexts, such as playground, classroom, or play lab. Unfortunately there is limited research with diverse populations.
References consulted	Leff and Lakin (2005); Ostrov and Keating (2004). See book's References list.

Measure	Penn Interactive Peer Play Scale (PIPPS). Fantuzzo et al. (1995; Fantuzzo et al., 1998).
Purpose	(1) Differentiating the behaviors of children who are more versus less successful in sustaining interactive play; (2) identifying play strengths of resilient preschool children living in high-risk urban environments; and (3) informing early childhood classroom-based intervention
Areas	Play Interaction, Play Disruption, and Play Disconnection.
Format	4-point rating scale per item; parallel parent and teacher versions.
Scores	Scores for the three domains (Play Interaction, Play Disruption, and Play Disconnection); frequency data provided.
Age group	Preschool children.
Time	Not specified.
Users	Professionals, teacher assistants, and parents.
Norms	Developed on a sample of 800 preschool children and then on a sample of 1,186 ethnically diverse urban Head Start children. Revised teacher version based on 523 African American children. Parent version based on 297 Head Start children.
Reliability	Internal consistency for teacher version, .92 for Play Interaction, .91 for Play Disruption, and .89 for Play Disconnection; for parent version, .84 for Play Interaction, .81 for Play Disruption, and .74 for Play Disconnection.
Validity	Content, based on descriptions of 38 Head Start teachers' descriptions of children's typical behavior and Parten's (1932) categories of social interaction.

	Concurrent (for teacher version), established through canonical correlation analyses, indicating that the PIPPS measures components of social competence. Convergent and divergent, demonstrated across studies with correlation with the Social Skills Rating Scale, Conners' Teacher Rating Scale, and Communication subscale of the Vineland Adaptive Behavior Scales—Classroom Edition. Bivariate and multivariate correlation analyses demonstrated that the PIPPS predicts first-grade academic performance. Explorations of the relationships between the teacher and parent versions found that the two versions measure congruent constructs. Concurrent validity for the parent PIPPS was supported by correlations with the Vineland Social-Emotional Early Childhood Scales.
Comments	Useful for understanding aspects of the environment that constrain or facilitate development and designing intervention activities. Spanish translation available. The PIPPS has much strength, including strong validity data. In addition to obtaining measures of peer interactions, the PIPPS can be used to facilitate home–school relationships. A manual recently has become available.
References consulted	Fantuzzo et al. (1995); Fantuzzo, Mendez, and Tighe (1998); Fantuzzo, Coolahan, Mendez, McDermott, and Sutton-Smith (1998); Gagnon and Nagle (2004); Hampton and Fantuzzo (2003). See book's References list.

Measure	**Preschool Child Observation Record (COR) (2nd ed.). HighScope (2003).**
Purpose	An observational assessment tool designed to measure children's progress in all early childhood programs.
Areas	Focuses on 32 dimensions of learning in six broad categories critical for school success: Initiative, Social Relations, Creative Representation, Movement and Music, Language and Literacy, and Mathematics and Science. For statistical purposes, some of the categories were combined resulting in four: Initiative, Social Relations; Creative Representation, Movement and Music; Language and Literacy; and Mathematics and Science.
Format	Teacher or caregiver rates child's behaviors on a 5-point scale. Assesses the ways in which young children initiate their own activities, as well as how they respond to questions and demands.
Scores	Subscale scores are averaged for each of the six developmental categories. Mean scores and standard deviations are provided for each item.
Age group	2½ to 6 years.
Time	N/A; charts child's progress three times over the course of the school year.
Users	Teachers or caregivers with training.
Norms	There were two studies: one conducted in spring 2002 with 160 children and the other in fall 2002 with 233 children, with ages ranging from 3-0 to 5-5 years from Head Start centers in one location in Michigan.
Reliability	Overall internal consistency ranges from .91 to .94; interrated reliability was .73 for total COR; and the categories range from .69 to .79.
Validity	Internal validity was affirmed using confirmatory factor analysis, which identified four factors that fit with the four categories; external validity was supported by correlations between Total COR and the Cognitive Skills Assessment Battery, ranging from .46 to .62. Sekino and Fantuzzo (2005) documented the concurrent and predictive validity with three dimensions (Cognitive Skills, Social Engagement, and Coordinated Movement). High ratings on the Cognitive dimension were associated with rater reading skills as well as with engagement on the PIPPS.

Comments	Easy to use. Available in Spanish. For the 1992 version, there were no directions as to what to do with the scores, or how best to interpret them. The second edition seems to have addressed this problem and includes additional information in the manual. Although the COR has potential, results need to be interpreted with caution. Limited information is provided about the sample other than it is likely to have a low SES. Mean score and SDs are not broken down by age groups, which limits the comparisons that might be made. Validity data provided by the author are limited but a study by Sekino and Fantuzzo (2005) provides some validity data. A teaching guide and parent guide (in Spanish and English) are available.
References consulted	Aylward (2001); Chittooran (2001); Sekino and Fantuzzo (2005). See book's References list.

Measure	**Symbolic Play Scale. Westby (1980, 1988, 1991).**
Purpose	Observing the play and language skills of young children and older children with learning problems.
Areas	Decontextualization, Thematic Content, Organization, Self–Other Relations, and Language.
Format	Completion of an observation form, and selection of the specific developmental stage most suitable. The practitioner provides toys (doll figures, utensils, and furniture). There is no specific arrangement or order for presentation. The child plays freely, and the assessor completes a checklist to determine developmental levels suggested by toy combinations, sequences, decontextualization, and planning. It is useful to make a written record of everything the child does.
Scores	Behaviors checked off if present; scale is broken down into Play and Language behaviors. The 1980 original play checklist provides age ranges for symbolic play and developmentally comparable language abilities.
Age group	8 months to 5 years (and older children with learning problems).
Time	5–10 minutes
Users	Professionals with knowledge of child development and language.
Norms	Technical data are not provided.
Reliability	Technical data are not provided.
Validity	Content, supported; ratings based on research-supported developmentally sequenced observations of play. Other technical data not provided.
Comments	Some experienced clinicians find 1980 version more useful for diagnosis than 1988 version. Useful for diagnosis in young children who function cognitively at very low levels.
References consulted	Parker (1996); Westby (1980, 1991). See book's References list.

Measure	**Symbolic Play Test (2nd ed.). Lowe and Costello (1988).**
Purpose	Assessing young children's cognitive functioning through unscaffolded play.
Areas	Cognitive and expressive language.
Format	Presentation of four sets of toys in standardized arrays; scoring is based on the child's spontaneous toy combinations.
Scores	Age equivalents, standard scores (*z*-scores).
Age group	12–36 months.

Time	Untimed; usually 10–15 minutes.
Users	Professionals with extensive training.
Norms	Normed on a small sample of 241 (sometimes described as 137) British children (representative for SES but lacks data about race and ethnicity). Children with disabilities were excluded.
Reliability	Split-half, .81 for the whole test; test–retest, ranging from .64 for a 3-month interval to .81 for a 9-month interval.
Validity	Content, supported; ratings based on research-supported developmentally sequenced observations of play. Scores increase with age, with significant floor and ceiling effects. Correlations with the Reynell Developmental Language scales and sentence length vary significantly across age levels. Power and Radcliffe (1989) found significant, but low correlations with the Bayley Scales of Infant Development and the Stanford Binet: Form L-M. The test appears to be most sensitive between the age of 15 and 24 months.
Comments	Useful as a way to structure observations for older preschoolers who function at earlier developmental levels. Scoring very clear. A drawback of the test is that it was normed on a sample of British children. Influence of British culture evident in the use of item sets (e.g., a doll with blonde hair and a traditional brush and comb; a tablecloth as well as chair, table, knife, and fork). Due to issues of cultural fairness, the test may not be appropriate for children representing diverse ethnic groups. Validity data are weak. The test is easy to administer and score, with the exception of a vague "stop" rule. Materials may not be appropriate for children from culturally diverse backgrounds. The norms and technical data are inadequate and were not updated for the second edition of the test. While purporting to measure symbolic play, the test may more accurately measure functional play or the appropriate use of play objects. The test, however, is used in many languages and has provided some useful data. A revision with updated toys and norms would be useful.
References consulted	Lyytinen, Poikkeus, and Laakso (1997); Paolito (1995); Power and Radcliffe (1989, 2000); Switzky (1995). See book's References list.

Measure	**Test Observation Form (TOF). McConaughy and Achenbach (2004).**
Purpose	A standardized instrument for rating test session observation.
Areas	The empirically based scales include: Withdrawn/Depressed, Language/Thought Problems, Anxious, Oppositional, Attention Problems, Internalizing, Externalizing, and Total Problems. The DSM-oriented scales include: Attention Deficit/Hyperactivity (ADHD) Problems, Inattention and Hyperactivity/ Impulsivity.
Format	125 items rated on a 4-point scale; 0 = no occurrence, 1 = slight or ambiguous occurrence, 2 = definite occurrence with mild to moderate intensity and less than 3 minutes duration, and 3 = definite occurrence with severe intensity or 3 or more minutes duration.
Scores	*T* scores and percentiles for separate samples of boys and girls at each age range.
Age group	2–18 years.
Time	Rating takes approximately 5–10 minutes; scoring takes an additional 10–15 minutes.
Users	Trained professional.
Norms	Normative sample consisted of 3.943 children ages 2–5, 6–11, and 12–18.

Reliability	Test–retest reliability ranges from .53 to .87 for 10 scales and Total Problems; average *r* across scales = .80; average interval = 10 days. Interrater reliability ranges from .42 to .73 for 10 scales and Total Problems; average *r* across scales = .62.
Validity	Construct validity was supported by correlations of .60 to .76 between scores on comparable TOF and Guide to Assessment of Test Session Behavior scales; criterion validity was established by comparing clinically referred children to nonreferred children—the clinically referred children scored significantly higher on all TOF scales than nonreferred. Discriminant validity was established by differentiating children with ADHD from clinically referred children without ADHD and controls.
Comments	The TOF was designed to be used with other instruments from the Achenbach System of Empirically Based Assessment including: the Child Behavior Checklist (CBCL); Teacher's Report Form (TRF); and Youth Self-Report (YSR). Computer scoring is available.
References consulted	McConaughy (2005). See book's References list.

Measure	**Transdisciplinary Play-Based Assessment (TPBA) (revised edition). Linder (1996).**
Purpose	A multidimensional approach to identifying service needs, to developing intervention plans, and to evaluating progress in children.
Areas	Cognitive Abilities, Social-Emotional Functioning, Communication and Language Skills, and Sensory–Motor Development.
Format	Observation of structured and unstructured play situations in which the child can be observed interacting alone with toys, another child, parents, and a facilitating adult. The manual provides guidelines and worksheets for observing play. All activities are videotaped by a team member.
Scores	Results are qualitative. Summary worksheets are provided.
Age group	Infancy–6 years of age.
Time	60–90 minutes.
User	Team of professionals. Parents are involved both as information providers and participants.
Norms	Not normed.
Reliability	Minimal detail provided in the manual.
Validity	Content supported; ratings based on research-supported developmentally sequenced observations of behavior in different domains (e.g., cognitive, socio-emotional, motor). Other technical data not provided.
Comments	Can provide the assessment team with rich information, but is labor-intensive. Assessors, however, can incorporate many aspects of the approach. A training video is available as well as a volume on intervention activities. The lack of reliability and validity data is a limitation of the TPBA. Use of the system requires extensive training of team members. The TPBA, however, can be very valuable for evaluating children who are difficult to assess or in a setting that serves children with low cognitive or motor functioning, or severe behavioral or mental disorders. Worksheets and guides are useful as a tool for developing IEPs and charting acquisitions of skills across developmental areas or in an area of concern.
References consulted	Boehm review (see text). Overton (1992); Stainback (1992). See book's References list.

Chapter 5

Observation of Environments

The influence of environments—childcare, preschool, community, healthcare, religious setting, and particularly the family—on the development of young children has been well documented (e.g., Barker, 1968; Bronfenbrenner, 1977, 1979; Burchinal et al., 2000; Gump, 1975; Harms & Clifford, 1993; Hobbs, 1966, 1978; Moos, 1976; NICHD Early Child Care Research Network, 2005; Smith & Connolly, 1980). Up until the early 1980s, psychological and psychoeducational assessment focused almost exclusively on the child. Increasingly, however, attention is being addressed to understanding the interplay of the characteristics of environments in which children develop and learn with child behaviors. According to Ysseldyke and Christenson (1987, p. 22), "No student assessment can be considered complete without an assessment of the nature of the student's instructional environment." Heller et al. (1982) state the issue even more strongly: "valid assessment of the learning environment is as critical as valid assessment of the individual" (p. 1). IDEA (2004) supports this position through its requirement that a member of the IEP team observe both the child and the learning environment, to document academic performance and behavior in the area(s) in which the child is having problems, unless there is observational data from routine classroom monitoring of a child's performance available prior to referral for a suspected learning disability.

Some forms of assessment take this concern about environmental effects on children's learning into account. For example, behavioral assessment of a student's academic behaviors must include evaluation of natural aspects of the classroom environment that have an impact upon academic performance (Shapiro, 2004a). As detailed by Shapiro, whose focus is on grades 1 and above, these include opportunities to respond, procedures for facilitating on-task behavior, instructional procedures, and procedures for monitoring student behavior. This information is obtained through student and teacher interviews, review of student work products, and direct observation. Another example is the extensive work in applied behavior analysis, which uses behavioral observation to understand the effects of different types of environmental input on social and emotional behavior problems (see Mash & Terdal, 1997, for examples).

In order to explain the influence of contextual variables on behavior, Bandura (1978) has developed a model of reciprocal determinism. This model reflects the belief that the environment influences behavior, also that people's actions, physical characteristics, and socially conferred attributes (e.g., roles and status) also influence the environment. Although most early childhood experts call for ecologically sound practices that incorporate this model and include assessment of the environment as an integral component of the assessment process, environmental assessment is not yet a widespread practice when a preschool child has been referred. Assessors need to play a major role in collecting relevant data through observation and interview, despite the fact that time pressures may make this difficult. For a child with a possible disability, Thurman and Widerstrom (1985) urge assessors to describe as many aspects of the child's functioning as possible (physical, intellectual, social), in as many settings as possible (home, school, community), when planning a comprehensive intervention program.

The first goal of this chapter is to review important physical, interpersonal, interactional, and instructional features of environments identified in the research literature that play an important role in preschoolers' functioning. Some components of environments can be changed—an essential concern for early childhood specialists and teachers. Features are reviewed first in relation to a referred child and then in relation to general concerns for preschool environments. A second goal is to review the relatively few instruments currently available that are appropriate for observing preschool environments, and to generate a checklist of environmental concerns for assessors.

Four objectives of environmental assessment are detailed by Bailey (1989): (1) determining the extent to which given environments are likely to facilitate children's development; (2) evaluating whether they are safe, warm, and generally comfortable places for the care of children; (3) establishing the degree to which they are "normalized" or least restrictive, in order to meet the mandates of IDEA and its successors; and (4) determining the extent to which certain skills are required for children to function successfully in a given environment. To this list, we would add understanding teacher and parent behaviors related to engaging children, motivating them, reinforcing their attempts, providing language and behavioral models, and providing the foundations for literacy and social competence.

THEORETICAL FOUNDATIONS FOR ASSESSING ENVIRONMENTS

The work of Bronfenbrenner (1977, 1979) has been particularly influential in the development of environmental assessment. Bronfenbrenner (1979), in his acclaimed text *The Ecology of Human Development*, details his theoretical perspective on the interaction between the developing child and the environment. Bronfenbrenner conceives the ecological environment "as a set of nested structures, each inside the next, like a set of Russian dolls. At the innermost level is the immediate setting containing the developing person" (p. 3). Bronfenbrenner then describes four spheres of environmental influence on children's behavior: (1) the *microsystem*, or all of the immediate settings that contain the child, including physical arrangements, other people present, and instructional procedures; (2) the *mesosystem*, or factors outside these immediate settings that directly influence the child (e.g., the teaching practices of a school program); (3) the *exosystem*, or events outside the immediate settings that indirectly influence the child (e.g., teacher in-service training and parents' work situation); and (4) the *macrosystem*, which includes belief systems and other factors common to a particular culture or subculture (e.g., government funding) that influence parents, teachers, and children. Bronfenbrenner argues that the interconnections between settings (i.e., home, school, and community) can be as decisive for development as events taking place within a given setting. But, as Harms and Clifford (1993) point out, the mesosystem and exosystem are generally not addressed directly in assessment procedures.

Bronfenbrenner (1979) also indicates out that "much of developmental psychology as it now exists is *the science of the strange behavior of children in strange situations with strange adults for the briefest periods of time*" (p. 19; emphasis in original). The same comment could be made about frequently used screening practices when children are brought into new and strange settings for testing. Furthermore, Bronfenbrenner cautions that carrying out an investigation in natural settings with objects and activities from everyday life does not necessarily make it ecologically valid. Rather, we must be concerned as assessors not only with how environmental factors influence a child, but also with how the child experiences these factors, and how in turn the child influences the environment. Although we may never fully understand how the child experiences his or her world, we can use diverse strategies to approximate this understanding—including observation of behavior as it occurs spontaneously within a familiar context, interviewing participants to gain their retrospective view of the situation, and viewing the same activity (i.e., the child's use of language) in different settings in order to identify any systematic effects of context.

However, it is not sufficient to understand the interactions of the spheres of environmental influence. It is also important to know how environmental characteristics (such as how families use space, time, and language) affect specific kinds of development, and to avoid the types of discontinuities between home and school expectations that might interfere with classroom interactions (Silvern, 1988). Assessors need to be knowledgeable about diverse home cultural and child-rearing practices, so as "to provide continuities that allow children to make sense of the world and discontinuities that afford children important experiences they do not obtain at home" (Silvern, 1988, p. 149). For example, to what extent (1) are home expectations in line with teacher expectations; (2) do styles and forms of communication between home and school match; and (3) are the extent to which opportunities to learn at home continuous with school expectations and experiences? These are points of possible intervention with parents or teachers, such as consultation, parent workshops, or teacher in-service programs.

Harms and Clifford (1993) apply Bronfenbrenner's model to early childhood educational settings and detail the multiple levels of external influence on the child in his or her immediate setting. At the center of their model is the educational setting in which a child is placed. What happens in the classroom is influenced by the personnel involved and by program characteristics. The classroom program in turn is influenced by local, state, and professional organizations' regulations; funding; local efforts to improve quality; guidelines of sponsoring agencies; teacher training; the economic climate and other characteristics of the community; and the child's family. For example, programs for income-eligible children (e.g., Head Start and school-based prekindergarten) are highly regulated, resulting in important differences in program philosophy and content. These issues are clearly illustrated in McGill-Franzen et al.'s (2002) extensive observational study of literacy support (materials and activities) available to children in five types of early childhood programs. Book-reading activities were extensive in some classrooms, but peripheral in others; in one setting, story reading was limited to 15 minutes at the end of the day, with a very limited selection of books chosen for the teacher by the central office. Similarly, in some programs children learned to identify and write letters; in other programs children did not experience activities with letters or writing. In the income-eligible programs observed (Head Start, public school prekindergarten, and child development daycare), children had less access to books and print and less experience with literacy activities than children in either a university-run daycare center or a religion-affiliated nursery school. Thus it often will be necessary for assessors to build such activities into their recommendations, and for preschool specialists to focus on these essential activities.

Harms and Clifford (1993) also present a useful framework for assessing early childhood educational settings. *Structure components* include the people present, the organization of space and availability of materials, and the nature of recurring patterns or routines. *Interaction components* include interactions between caregivers and other adults in the immediate setting with children. These two components, along with what we refer to as *instructional activities*, are used as the framework for considering the environmental assessment activities presented in this chapter. (Assessment of home environments is covered in Chapters 8 and 14.)

APPROACHES TO ASSESSING ENVIRONMENTS

Environmental Issues in Relation to a Referred Child

Because the interactions of people within and across environments are complex, isolating the factors that interact with and predict child behavior and inform intervention is a major challenge. As the child develops through the early childhood years, and as instructional variables become more diverse, no one easily used procedure can be expected to address all concerns. One's assessment question needs to drive the selection of specific observation procedures.

Major interactions to consider as a child develops over time are presented in Figure 5.1. Assessment of each of these interactions, as well as of the interconnections between settings, is needed to understand the effect of the environment on all children (particularly children with special needs). However, as Shapiro and Skinner (1990) point out, it is difficult and often impractical to observe all environments that influence child functioning. These researchers recommend the use of problem-solving interviews to determine relevant issues regarding the influence of the environment, along with observation.

Hobbs (1978) presents a schematic approach to viewing a child within what he refers to as the *ecosystem* of families and communities. He not only focuses on these interacting systems, but stresses the importance of considering the developmental changes in child–environment interactions that occur over time. Describing or diagramming the child's ecosystem, including the valence (positive or negative) of interactions between individuals within and across settings, will help assessors to understand where areas of discord occur and points of possible intervention. An example of such a description is presented in Figure 5.2.

This recommendation is developed by Cantrell and Cantrell (1985), who detail a sequence for systematic ecological problem solving that includes assessment and analysis of the problem, planning intervention, implementation, and evaluation (pp. 279–280). Here is a brief synopsis of the steps involved for a child of concern:

Major Players	Key Issues
Home • Parents • Extended family • Siblings • Hired caregivers	• Safety vs. violence/abuse • Child-rearing practices • Adult talk and child–adult conversations • Availability of toys and literacy-related materials
	↕
Child	• Sensitivity to environmental stimuli • Adaptability and interpersonal skills • Interests • Attention and engagement with tasks • Cognitive skills • Physical and sensory abilities • Speech and language abilities
	↕
Community • Immediate neighborhood • Religious groups • Healthcare services • Community agencies • Daycare services • Shopkeepers • Other children	• Community size and density • Safety vs. exposure to violence • Availability of playground and library • Availability of services and services already engaged in by the family • Opportunity to explore and solve problems
	↕
Media	• Supervised TV watching • Availability of VCR/DVD, computer • Violence portrayed on TV or in video games

Cultural and linguistic background (child/family's and community's)

↕

Changes in the interactions above with child's development from birth to school age

FIGURE 5.1. Environmental interactions and key issues to be considered over time.

1. Identify critical settings where and persons with whom the child spends time (e.g., home, school, peer groups, other settings), along with the relative impact of each of these on the child and on each other.
2. Identify areas of discord between the child and his or her environments (e.g., child becomes highly hyperactive when younger brother is in the room), along with possible sources of intervention.
3. Determine areas of possible stress or deficiency, as well as strength, between the child and his or her environments (including economic, childcare, medical, and legal areas).
4. Identify characteristics of settings and behaviors of persons relevant to the areas of discord.
5. Determine expectations of individuals across settings, based on their values and behavioral norms.
6. Determine critical agents to be involved in change and their approaches to problem solving.
7. Identify the resources required to solve problems and the steps needed to interface with other agencies and resources.

J. is a 5-year-old boy born to a 15-year-old mother and 16-year-old father. The paternal grandmother insisted that they have the child. He is an only child and has lived with his parents and his paternal grandmother, who is his guardian and is largely responsible for raising and disciplining him. The family lives in a large urban area. J. frequently visits the Native American reservation where his grandmother was born and lived during her teenage years. J.'s mother is of Hispanic background and was born in the United States. His father is Native American. His father completed high school, is enrolled in college, and works as a computer technician. His mother has completed high school and works as a store clerk. Both parents are frequently away from home. J.'s grandmother has a sixth-grade education and has never worked. She believes that J.'s parents are irresponsible. She was divorced 2 years ago. J. greatly misses his grandfather, with whom he had a special relationship (the grandfather assumed the role of "father") and now never sees. He also has no contact with his maternal grandparents. He feels that his grandfather left because he (J.) was getting into trouble. An uncle, 2 years older than J., also lives in the home. J. and his uncle fight constantly and will not speak to each other for a week or more. English is the main language spoken in the home. However, J. and his grandmother often speak to each other in a Native American dialect that J. speaks more fluently than English. They also frequently practice Native American rituals together.

J. is currently enrolled in a Catholic school and is in kindergarten. His school reports are good and he has become familiar with the alphabet and the sounds of many letters. However, he gets into frequent fights (a concern for the teacher) and has few friends. He also says that he hates school. He tends to be very passive, fears making mistakes, and worries that he will disappoint his parents and grandmother. His parents have high educational goals for their son and hope he will attend college. This goal is not shared by his grandmother, who does not believe in formal education. The grandmother is the one called by school personnel when they need to speak with J.'s guardian. She does not respond and knows little about his progress in school except through his report cards.

Home:

J.	–	Negative relationship with uncle
	+	Relationship with grandmother
Mother	–	Disagrees with her mother about educational goals
Father	+	Relationship with son
Grandmother		Head of household
	–	Disagrees with daughter and son-in-law about educational goals and discipline
	–	Divorced and has no contact with former husband
Uncle	–	Fights with J.

Cultural and religious practices:
- Native American (J., grandmother, father)
- Hispanic (mother)
- English and Native American dialect spoken at home.
- Native American rituals practiced by grandmother and J.
- Grandmother believes that these will deter evil spirits.
- Parents want J. to have discipline of Catholic school.
- Parents attend Catholic church irregularly.
- Grandmother believes that this contradicts their beliefs.
- Grandmother brings J. to visit friends on reservation in summer.

School:
- Attends Catholic school.
- Good grades; has learned how to read simple words.
- Poor peer relationships, with frequent fights.
- Grandmother ignores school contacts; believes outside help is shameful; believes J. gets into trouble to get attention.

Peers:
- No friends in school (fights) or neighborhood.
- Friends on reservation.
- Grandmother is currently his best friend.

Grandfather:
- Has moved away and has lost contact with J.
- J. had a very close relationship with grandfather and greatly misses him.

FIGURE 5.2. Schematic description of a child within his ecosystem.

8. Plan change, including goals and the individuals/agencies responsible for achieving these goals.
9. Detail steps for implementation and evaluation.

Like Hobbs (1978), Cantrell and Cantrell (1985) suggest making a schematic representation of the interacting environmental factors for a particular child that can be used in diagnosis. Through such a diagram, assessors can determine the relative importance of key influences on the child. This *ecological map* (or *eco-map*, for short) should indicate not only key others in a child's life, but also the nature (positive and negative) of the child's interactions with these key individuals, as well as intervention sources and strategies across settings. There are many ways of presenting eco-maps. See Chapter 8 for an alternative approach.

Bailey (1989) also suggests the straightforward procedure of making a diagram of the ongoing situation for a child of concern. For example, if observers are interested in a socially withdrawn child's free-play activity, a diagram can be made of the child's position, objects available, objects played with, other individuals present, and the nature of interactions. These diagrams can help assessors analyze space arrangements in relationship to the child, as well as the nature of the child's play activity.

Thurman and Widerstrom (1990) describe a sequence of steps to help assessors determine the fit between the characteristics of the child and his or her environment. Some of these steps overlap with those of Cantrell and Cantrell, but Thurman and Widerstrom stress different points.

1. Identify the major environmental settings that are important in the child's life.
2. Develop an inventory of critical tasks in those settings with which the child needs to comply to meet success.
3. Assess the child's competence to perform those tasks.
4. Assess motivational variables (i.e., contingency structures) and other factors that affect the child's ability to perform tasks.
5. Assess the child's tolerance of the environment.
6. Determine which of the child's behaviors and/or characteristics are beyond the environment's level of tolerance.
7. Identify objectives for each component of the child–setting interaction that, when accomplished, will lead to increased ecological congruence.
8. Identify strategies for accomplishing objectives.
9. Monitor the effectiveness of interventions.

Important Dimensions of Preschool Environments for Observation

Many elements make up preschool children's learning environments. *Physical and structural dimensions* include the amount of space; classroom design; arrangement of space into activity areas (e.g., areas for housekeeping and sand/water play); noise; physical equipment and materials available (books, pencils, paper, toys); and the placement of equipment and materials in the room. *Interpersonal dimensions* include the ratio of adults to children, and the mix of children with and without disabilities. *Interaction components*, such as engagement and reinforcement, must also be considered. Finally, *instructional characteristics* that influence child behaviors include the nature of transitions; regularity of routines; the nature of language exchanges; emergent literacy activities in reading, writing, and mathematics; teacher and staff training; and many others. Each of these elements contributes to the "quality" of classrooms/settings, which is so important for child development, learning, and behavior.

Physical and Structural Dimensions

Whenever possible, assessors need to visit children's classrooms or daycare centers and focus on physical and structural factors as well as on the children. Heller and Edwards (1993), for example, found that the high noise levels often found in childcare centers affected the listening ability of preschool children and their language learning (e.g., comprehending the speech of others). To combat noise, these researchers suggest that caregivers be aware of their own intonation patterns and (1) present speech within close proximity of a child; (2) encourage the child to look at the speaker to gain visual cues; (3) seat children away from typical noise sources, such as ventilation ducts; and (4) give visual or auditory cues when about to give a message.

Smith and Connolly (1980) noted that the amount of space available affected the amount and kind of physical activity in which preschool children engaged, but not social or aggressive behavior. The amount of play equipment available had several effects: With more equipment, children played in smaller groups; children used popular items extensively and neglected less popular items; with less equipment, there was less sharing, but also less aggressive activity. Other findings from this study are presented below.

Lawry, Danko, and Strain (2000) present useful recommendations to modify a classroom's physical and structural environment to prevent behavior problems, such as running in the classroom and fighting. Examples of environmentally inappropriate and appropriate classroom organizations are presented in Figure 5.3.

Interpersonal, Interactional, and Instructional Dimensions

Considerable attention has been directed in the research literature not only to classroom organization, but to the interpersonal dimensions, interactions among individuals, and instructional characteristics that influence behavior. Research relating to how these characteristics of preschool environments affect child behavior and development has been summarized by Bailey (1989); Dunst, McWilliam, and Holbert (1986); Moore (1987); Paget and Barnett (1990); Smith and Connolly (1980); Weinstein (1979); and Wohlwill and Heft (1997), among others. Zentall (1983) and Harrower and Dunlap (2001) detail some of the effects of these environmental conditions on children with autism and with hyperactivity. A summary of key instructional characteristics in particular is presented in Table 5.1.

Smith and Connolly (1980) reported the results of a 3-year observational study on the effects of the childcare environment on child behavior, which corroborated many of the findings reported in the reviews cited above. This study took place in the industrial city of Sheffield, England, with 24 children from varied home backgrounds between 2 and 4 years of age, in each of two play groups. Children were engaged in free play, choosing their own activities, both with and without staff direction. The major findings of this study, in addition to those noted earlier about space and play equipment, were as follows:

1. *Number of children in the group.* The size of the group affected both the nature of play and the interactions among children. In large groups there was more table play, time when children engaged in no activity, and play among same-sex pairs; in small groups there was more fantasy play and cross-sex friendships.

Classroom A: Environmentally Inappropriate

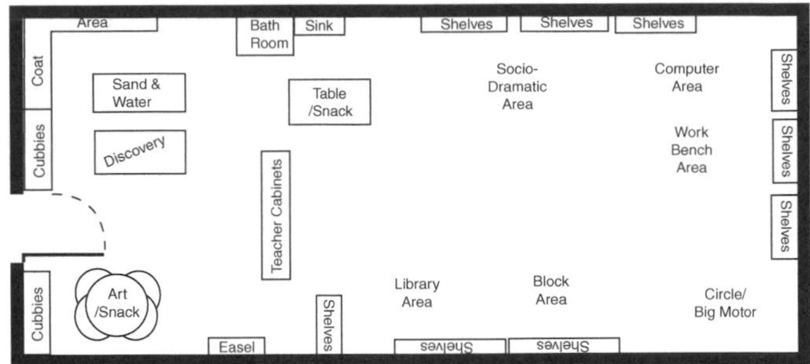

- Art area not near water source
- Toys too close to circle time area
- Quiet centers neighboring noisy areas
- No visual boundaries for play areas
- Unlabeled shelving
- Undefined personal space in circle
- Snack tables far from each other, limiting social interactions
- Space conducive to running
- Cluttered walls

Classroom B: Environmentally Appropriate

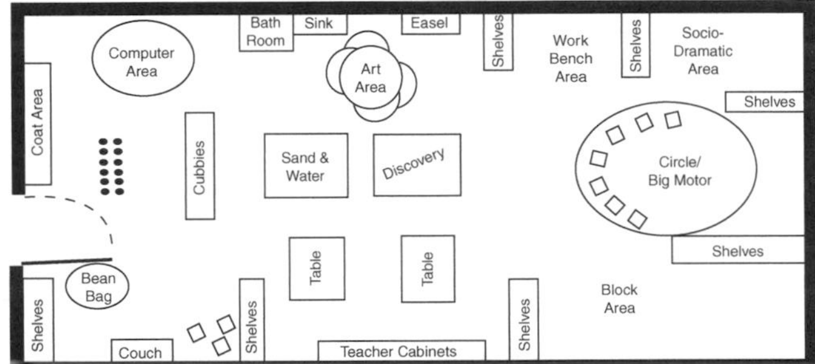

- Visual cues for lining up near door
- Communication pictures pertinent to play area posted for nonverbal children
- Cubbies labeled with photos and names of each child to promote independence
- Shelving labeled to promote independent clean up
- Poster of classroom rules on wall
- Hooks limiting the number of children in each area
- Limited visual stimuli on walls
- Personal visual schedules posted
- Picture of play area at entrance to play area
- Classroom schedule posted
- All shelving/cabinetry low to ground
- (3' high) for staff to see into all areas

FIGURE 5.3. Bird's-eye view of environmentally inappropriate and appropriate classrooms. From Lawry, Danko, and Strain (2000). Copyright 2000 by the Division for Early Childhood. Reprinted by permission.

2. *Structured versus free-play activities.* With structured activities, children spent more time at fewer activities with adults and less time with peers. There were also less physical activity and less fantasy play than in free play. There was increased attention span in activities, and some increase in aggressive interactions with other children.
3. *Variations in staff–child ratio.* High child–staff ratios reduced the amount of contact staff members made with individual children, and more of children's incoming verbal contacts went unanswered. Conversations were shorter and more staff verbalizations were prohibitions.

TABLE 5.1. Instructional Characteristics to Be Considered at the Preschool Level

- High-quality instructional practices are used, including clear directions and support (scaffolding) of behaviors to be learned in relationship to the child's competence.
- Activities heighten interest and encourage children to try new things and interact with others.
- Teachers/caregivers communicate expectations, provide helpful corrective feedback, and reinforce children's attempts.
- Teachers/caregivers model problem-solving behaviors.
- Behavior is managed by using consistent approval and disapproval techniques, and small accomplishments are rewarded.
- Routines are clear and consistent.
- Materials are arranged to encourage independence.
- Outreach and interaction take place between home and school.
- Language is modeled by adults in the preschool setting (e.g., adults use rich language when interacting with children, ask questions, use diverse narrative forms).
- Basic relational concepts needed to follow directions and engage in classroom activities are presented in the context of everyday experiences.
- The classroom environment is least restrictive and fosters the skills needed to mainstream children into regular classrooms (e.g., attention to tasks and appropriate interactions with peers).
- Instruction is focused on emerging literacy and writing (e.g., book reading across genres, cognitively challenging discussions, literacy materials available in free-play areas, rhyming games, discussion opportunities).
- Instruction is focused on numbers and quantitative reasoning (e.g., counting, number identification, simple addition and subtraction, math concepts).

Smith and Connolly (1980) raised a number of important interpersonal and interactional implications, based on the results of their study. For example, social behavior is less frequent in more crowded conditions, and more aggressive behavior may occur. Although the adult–child ratio may be highly regulated in some preschool contexts, such as Head Start and accredited preschool programs, financially strapped state and school districts may have prekindergarten or kindergarten programs that place 25 or more children in a classroom with one teacher and possibly one assistant. The assistant may or may not be well trained. The main benefits of better staff ratios are likely to be in terms of cognitive and linguistic stimulation. Adults can provide a model of appropriate language through their everyday conversations with children, as well as through more directly teaching vocabulary through repeated storybook reading. For example, the FACES study of factors that affected the performance of 3,200 children who entered Head Start in 1997 (U.S. DHHS, 2001) found that children in classrooms with richer teacher–child interactions and more language learning opportunities (as assessed using the Early Childhood Environment Rating Scale [ECERS], discussed below) had higher vocabulary scores, and that children in classrooms with lower child–adult ratios showed greater gains in vocabulary scores over the Head Start year. And children in classrooms rated higher in learning materials spent more time in interactive play. Better staff–child ratios may also encourage children to persist and encourage engagement in desired activities. If improving these ratios is not possible, assessors, teachers, and parents may need to organize volunteer storybook reading and other activities, such as older children or college students coming into the classroom.

As the preceding paragraph suggests, child engagement is also affected by the environment and is an important issue for assessors. According to Bailey (1989), the term *engagement* refers to "the extent to which children are actively and appropriately involved with materials, people, or activities in the environment" (p. 106). Bailey concludes that documenting child engagement is a fundamental measure of environmental effectiveness. McWilliam and Bailey (1995) review research that identifies variables influencing engagement. These include incidental teaching, seamless transition between activities, accessible toys, carefully sequenced activities, adult involvement in play activities of young children, and teaching problem-solving skills (see Hart & Risley, 1975; Karnes, Johnson, & Beauchamp, 1989; Krantz & Risley, 1977; and Montes & Risley, 1975). McWilliam and Bailey (1995) present useful operational definitions for types and levels of engagement and demonstrated a relationship between age groupings on engagement. One scale appropriate for use at the preschool level is the Daily Engagement Rating Scale (McWilliam, Galant, & Dunst, 1984).

Extensive research has been conducted on many other aspects of the environment that influence children's learning and behavior. Several useful instruments are available to assess the global quality of early childhood environments, and these are reviewed in later sections. Other instruments, such as the *Code for Instructional Structure and Student Academic Response* (CISSAR; Stanley & Greenwood, 1981) and the *Abbreviated CISSAR* (Greenwood & Carta, 1987), are complex measures that are used in research investigating the influence of environmental factors on behavior and achievement. Although these two instruments are more appropriate for school-age populations and for judging the effectiveness of interventions (they will not be described in detail here), outcomes of their use can inform intervention.

A number of publications by the NAEYC provide guidelines for developing observational procedures (see NAEYC, 1991, NAEYC/SDE, 2003; Bredekamp, 1991; Bredekamp & Copple, 1997). These guidelines urge that assessment be related to curriculum, cover all developmental domains, support children's learning and development, be used to adjust curriculum and communicate to parents, reflect typical activities, and use an array of tools. The NAEYC and the National Association for Family Day Care (NAFDC) have developed observation rating instruments linked to quality criteria used in the accreditation process (see Harms & Clifford, 1993, for an overview). Bailey (1989) points out that while guidelines such as these were developed with a focus on programs serving normally developing preschool children, they apply to programs serving children with disabilities as well. He also recommends that criteria for evaluating the environments of children with disabilities be specified.

OBSERVATIONAL PROCEDURES USED FOR DEVELOPING INTERVENTIONS

Selected observational instruments that are used in developing interventions for young children's learning environments are presented in this section and in Appendix 5.1. While some instruments are more comprehensive than others, no one instrument covers all of the important features of these environments highlighted in the research—and there are some notable gaps, as the summary and checklist presented at the end of this chapter indicate. Assessors need to be aware of these gaps (e.g., literacy activities that are cognitively challenging) and develop comprehensive procedures to cover all key aspects of environments relevant to the question at hand, as they consider possible instructional and behavioral interventions. Therefore, multiple assessment procedures, including interview formats, checklists, rating scales, and observation schedules, may need to be developed to provide the necessary information about the interaction of environmental characteristics with child behavior. In addition to the physical arrangement of classrooms and the teacher–child ratio, assessors need to request information about (1) activities emphasized, (2) children's typical daily schedule, (3) the circumstances under which children are most successful or encounter problems with daily routines, and (4) the nature of play interactions.

Preschool Assessment of the Classroom Environment (PACE)

The PACE (McWilliam & Dunst, 1985b) is a 70-item rating scale used when teachers request assistance in intervention planning. The main content of the scale covers four broad categories of the classroom environment, each with two to five subcategories, for a total of 14 components. The four broad categories and their components are as follows:

1. *Program Organization*—program management, integration of children with and without disabilities, parent involvement.
2. *Environment Organization*—physical environment, staffing patterns, classroom scheduling, transitions.
3. *Instruction*—child growth and development, curriculum, plans for intervention, method of instruction, behavior management.
4. *Program Outcomes*—program evaluation plan, child engagement.

Each subcategory includes five items that are rated on a 5-point scale; points along the scale are roughly defined as ranging from 1 ("Not at all" or "Never") to 5 ("Always" or "Almost always"). An example in the area of curriculum is "Curriculum meets the individual needs of the children." A final section of the scale includes child engagement (6 items), child behavior (12 items), and caregiver behavior (10 items). The PACE was designed to be used in classrooms or other learning environments with children ages birth–6 years. Administration includes three steps: (1) observing the classroom environment; (2) interviewing all persons responsible for the overall management of the classroom; and (3) reviewing written materials. The observation needs to be carried out over a 2- to 4-hour span, in order to sample the range of activities, events, and routines typical of a particular classroom. Steps for using the PACE for purposes of intervention planning include (1) a self-evaluation of classroom environment completed by the teacher/caregiver requesting technical assistance, using the Needs Evaluation for Educators of Developmentally Delayed Students (McWilliam & Dunst, 1985a), which includes the same 70-item areas as the PACE, but stated in terms of degree of help desired by the teacher or caregiver; (2) completion of the PACE by an independent observer; (3) discussion with the teacher/caregiver, based on the results of 1 and 2; (4) development and implementation of a technical assistance plan; and (5) monitoring of changes in child behavior/functioning that result.

Validity for the PACE was established through a pilot study of 20 preschool programs serving only nondisabled, only disabled, or a mix of children in rural and western North Carolina. In addition to the PACE, information was collected on child behavior characteristics and caregiver styles. A significant correlation resulted between the 14 PACE components, caregiver, and outcome variables, which the authors believe demonstrates that the classroom ecology affects both caregiver and child behavior. Outcomes revealed that the program organization components were most closely related to the measures of child behavior characteristics; environmental organization components to the measures of child engagement; and instructional components to the measures of caregiver interaction styles. Observer agreement was determined in 5 of the 20 settings. Overall median agreement was 82% for PACE, 82% for caregiver styles of interaction, 81% for child engagement, and 84% for child behavior characteristics.

The PACE represents a comprehensive observation process that integrates information from multiple sources and covers important instructional components and interactions of preschool environments for children with and without disabilities. The rating scale is clearly presented, and ratings are based on the impressions of raters after 2–4 hours of observation and an interview. The technical data presented are based on a limited sample and restricted geographic area, however; assessors will need to collect technical data at the local level. PACE was not developed for use with a particular referred child.

Ecobehavioral System for Complex Assessment of the Preschool Environment (ESCAPE)

The ESCAPE (Carta, Greenwood, & Atwater, 1985) was designed to provide detailed information about the classroom program received by a target student, but it may prove to be more useful in developing interventions than in making decisions about individual students, as noted below. ESCAPE is one of three observational systems (CISSAR, MS-CISSAR, and ESCAPE) developed by Greenwood and his associates to evaluate classroom instruction in which ecological factors (use of instructional time and student engagement) have the same priority as student behavior. All three observational systems require observers to follow an individual child for an extended period of time (two hours or more) and use laptop computers to record data (supported by low-priced software). Use of the three systems is seen as feasible in large-scale research projects. ESCAPE consists of 101 codes within 12 subcategories (6 ecological, 3 teacher, and 3 student). The "ecological" subcategories include designated activity, activity structure, task materials, location, grouping, and composition of handicapped and nonhandicapped students. The "teacher" subcategories include teacher definition, teacher focus, and teacher behavior. The "student" subcategories include appropriate target behaviors, inappropriate (competing) behaviors, and talk (verbalizations). ESCAPE involves momentary time sampling of multiple events (three subcategories every 15 seconds; all 12 subcategories every minute). Observation is carried out for approximately 20 minutes at a time, with tape recorder signals every 15 seconds. Extensive training is required; observers are considered proficient with at least 70% agreement. Outcomes involve both molar and molecular descriptions of classrooms and behaviors.

Carta et al. (1985) describe results of a pilot study using the ESCAPE in which three students from each of four classrooms in each of four schools were observed over the course of the entire school day (except bathroom time and nap time). The results indicated that more than 20% of a typical day was spent in transition, followed by play (20%), preacademic activities (10%), and language activities (1%). Play, snack, fine motor, and self-care activities were most closely related to a total engagement score. Student time spent in preacademic activities and level of engagement over the day were correlated with later academic achievement, supporting the validity of the instrument. The lack of time spent in language activities is noteworthy, given the importance of language development to later success in school.

In a more recent study, Le-Ager and Shapiro (1995) used the ESCAPE along with the Assessment Code/Checklist for Evaluating Survival Skills (Atwater, Carta, & Schwartz, 1989)—a time-sampling system of student–teacher interactions during group instruction, independent work, and transition activities—as part of a template-matching strategy to develop an intervention to facilitate the transition between preschool and kindergarten for preschoolers with disabilities. Observations were recorded for two index (target) children who had disabilities (generally speech and language) or were "at risk" from each of three Head Start programs (assigned to intervention, assessment-only, and control groups), and two successful children from each of four regular kindergarten classes likely to receive the Head Start children the following year. The observations allowed the researchers to create ecobehavioral profiles (templates) of the instructional environments for both groups. An intervention program targeting independent seatwork tasks, which did not occur in the preschool environments but occurred daily in kindergarten, was then developed in collaboration with the preschool staff. The independent work tasks involved art and writing materials. Instructions and modeling were done as a large group, with students responsible for completing work independently. Children in the intervention group were observed after the 8-week intervention and again during their kindergarten year. The performance of these children was closer to that of the kindergarten index children than to that of children in the assessment-only group, who were not exposed to independent seatwork activities during their preschool year. Moreover, during their kindergarten year, none of the index children in the intervention group were referred for special education services (while two children from the nonintervention groups were). These findings provide important support for focusing on environmental intervention at the program level and for developing skills and behaviors during the preschool years that lead to success in kindergarten. Bearing in mind that the demands of kindergarten can vary greatly, the assessment team can be instrumental in gathering observations regarding expected behaviors in the district's kindergartens, and in identifying essential behaviors to be incorporated into intervention planning at the preschool level.

Bramlett and Barnett (1993) indicate that while ESCAPE is "one of the best recent examples of an ecobehavioral pre-school code" (p. 51) that can be used to assess early intervention effectiveness, the complexity of the procedure may limit its use for clinical decision making. We agree with this conclusion. A preschool assessor is not likely to participate in the extensive training needed to use this scale appropriately, or to have the time needed to obtain the comprehensive observational sample necessary for data gathering. Furthermore, the scale might not focus on the behaviors of concern for a particular referred preschool child. ESCAPE, however, can be very important for research (such as that cited above) that leads to intervention planning, and preschool assessors should keep track of this information.

OBSERVATIONAL PROCEDURES USED FOR PROGRAM EVALUATION, TRAINING, AND RESEARCH

A number of instruments that focus on characteristics of early childhood environments produce information that can be used for program evaluation, teacher training, and research.

Early Childhood Environment Rating Scale—Revised Edition (ECERS-R)

The ECERS-R (Harms, Clifford, & Cryer, 1998) is a rating scale developed for use in a broad variety of preschool settings (Head Start, religious setting, childcare, preschool, and kindergarten) serving children from 2–6 to 5–11 years of age. The scale represents a major revision of the original ECERS, reflecting current definitions of developmentally appropriate practice to assess the overall quality of these settings. The scale can be used by outside observers for program monitoring, evaluation, improvement, and research, as well as by teachers for self-assessment. This scale consists of 43 items organized into seven areas: (1) Space and Furnishings, (2) Personal Care Routines, (3) Language–

Reasoning, (4) Activities, (5) Interaction, (6) Program Structure, and (7) Parents and Staff. Ratings are made along a 7-point scale, with clear behavioral descriptors for rating points of 1, 3, 5, and 7, specific guidelines for use of midpoint ratings. Ratings are made by observers (often trainers) and need to be based on a minimum of 2 hours of observation and inspection of materials, plus time to interview the teacher about indicators not observed. With each item, space is provided for specific comments. A score sheet that can be copied from the manual is provided to record indicators by item. A sample item is presented in Figure 5.4. The ECERS-R yields a classroom environment profile based on the seven subscale scores, which are plotted on a chart to show areas that are relatively strong or weak. The same profile can be reused at a later point to measure improvements. An updated edition (Harms, Clifford, & Cryer, 2005) provides an expanded score sheet and additional notes for clarification.

A section is included in the manual for training researchers to use the scale in research and program evaluation. The training activities suggested should be useful for training in general. A training package for assessors, which includes a videotape and workbook, is also available. A Spanish edition of the scale is now available as well (Harms, Clifford, & Cryer, 2002). The ECERS-R maintains the same conceptual framework as the original ECERS and takes into account the NAEYC accreditation criteria (NAEYC, 1984) and program quality criteria (Bredekamp & Copple, 1997). It was field-tested in 45 classrooms in 35 centers, after which revisions were made to improve reliability. A second field testing in 21 classrooms across SES groups yielded interobserver reliabilities of 86.1% across indicators. Internal scale consistencies are acceptable and range from .71 (Parents and Staff) to .88 (Activities) for subscales and .92 for the total scale. Observer agreement on the entire scale was .92. The content validity of the original ECERS was supported by conducting an extensive literature review, by having seven nationally recognized experts in early childhood education rate each item in terms of its importance to early childhood programs, and by collecting ratings from two sets of observers (one group of child development professionals, the other of individuals who had no child development background and were trained in the use of the scale). Observations were made along with those of trainers (who had worked with the teachers observed, but received little training in the use of the scale) in 18 classrooms to determine the scale's ability to distinguish between classrooms of varying quality. Rank-order correlations of .74 and .70 were obtained for each group, respectively. These past studies and the long research history of use have attested to the value of the ECERS-R. Good predictive validity was supported by Peisner-Feinberg and Burchinal (1997) and Whitebrook, Howes, and Phillips (1990).

Numerous studies supporting the utility of the original ECERS have been reported (Bailey, Clifford, & Harms, 1982; Bjorkman, Poteat, & Snow, 1986; Cryer, 1999; Harms & Clifford, 1983; McCartney, 1984; McCartney, Scarr, Phillips, Grajek, & Schwartz, 1982; Peisner-Feinberg et al., 1999). The study by McCartney et al. (1982) was based on daycare centers in Bermuda providing services to infants and preschoolers. A total of 156 children were tested in the centers, and their parents were interviewed in their homes. A total quality score, based on the first six dimensions of quality included on the ECERS, was used as an index of center quality. Interrater reliability with the ECERS was .82 (McCartney, 1984). Although many aspects of children's development were found to be moderately to highly related to differences in their daycare environments, language used by daycare providers played a particularly important role. Children at the better-quality centers, particularly those with high levels of caregiver speech, scored higher on measures of language development (McCartney et al., 1982). Only 4 of 43 items on the ECERS focus on language-related materials and interactions.

Inadequate 1	2	Minimal 3	4	Good 5	6	Excellent 7
1.1 Very few books accessible. 1.2 Staff rarely read books to children (Ex. no daily story time, little individual reading to children).		3.1 Some books accessible for children (Ex. during free play children have enough books to avoid conflict). 3.2 At least one staff-initiated receptive language activity time daily (Ex. reading books to children,* storytelling, using flannel board stories).		5.1 A wide selection of books† are accessible for a substantial portion of the day. 5.2 Some additional‡ language materials used daily. 5.3 Books organized in a reading center. 5.4 Books, language materials, and activities are appropriate** for children in group. 5.5 Staff read books to children informally (Ex. during free play, at naptime, as an extension of an activity).		7.1 Books and language materials are rotated to maintain interest. 7.2 Some books relate to current classroom activities or themes (Ex. books borrowed from library on seasonal theme).

LANGUAGE-REASONING

15. Books and pictures

Notes for Clarification

* Reading may be done in small groups or in larger groups depending on the ability of the children to attend to the story.

† A wide selection of books include: variety of topics; fantasy and factual information; stories about people, animals, and science; books that reflect different cultures and abilities.

‡ Examples of additional language materials are posters and pictures, flannel board stories, picture card games, and recorded stories and songs.

** Examples of appropriate materials and activities include simpler books read with younger children; large print materials for child with visual impairment; books in children's primary language(s); rhyming games for older children.

Questions

(7.1) Are there any other books used with the children? How is this handled?

(7.2) How do you choose books?

FIGURE 5.4. Sample item from the Early Childhood Environmental Rating Scale—Revised Edition (ECERS-R). From Harms, Clifford, and Cryer (1998).

A version of the ECERS, which eliminates the "Adult Needs" Scale and modified 11 of 32 items to reflect kindergarten activities, was used in the research of Bryant, Clifford, and Peisner (1991). These researchers collected observational measures of classroom practices, principal questionnaires, and teacher questionnaires for 103 kindergarten classrooms in North Carolina, sampled to be representative of school size and region. Three hours of observation were conducted in each classroom, using the modified ECERS and an observation measure developed for the study, the Checklist of Kindergarten Activities (CKA; Peisner, Bryant, & Clifford, 1988). The CKA assesses areas that are important to kindergarten according to the NAEYC position statement, but that are not included on the ECERS. It consists of two subscales: an Activities subscale, consisting of 32 yes–no items that cover six areas of teaching activities (language, cognitive, socialization, self-esteem, disposition to learn, and physical); and a Materials subscale, consisting of 21 yes–no items about whether specific materials are present. Interrater agreement data, collected by one of the investigators revisiting 11 schools, yielded correlations of .97 for the total score (.89–.95 on subscales) for the modified ECERS and .95 for the CKA (.86 Activities; .96 Materials). Internal consistency (coefficient alpha) on the modified ECERS was .90 for the overall score and ranged from .31 (Personal Care Routines) to .86 (Language–Reasoning) for subscales. Outcomes of the study, which used a criterion score on the ECERS of 5 ("good" on each item) to indicate developmentally appropriate practice, revealed great variability across classes. Only 20% of the classes met this criterion; another 20% scored between 4.5 and 4.9. This type of outcome has been reported across studies using the ECERS and ECERS-R, with fewer than half of the programs achieving a "good" to "excellent" rating (Espinosa, 2002).

Cassidy, Hestenes, Hegde, Hestenes, and Mims (2005) examined the psychometric properties of the ECERS-R with a large sample (1,313 preschool classrooms) in childcare facilities across the state of North Carolina, as part of the licensing process. These programs were striving for higher ratings, and thus the data were reported to probably represent only the higher quality programs in the state. The results indicated that a 16-item version of the ECERS-R can serve as a relatively good proxy for the full scale. These 16 items loaded on two factors (Activities/Materials and Language/Interactions) that accounted for 69% of the variance. The 2 factor-based scales correlated moderately (r = .46) with each other, and .75 and .79, with the full 43-item ECERS-R scale, and strongly (r = .90) when combined with the full ECERS-R scale. Cassidy et al. indicate that the 16-item combination of 2 factors would serve as a better proxy for the full scale than randomly chosen subsets of items suggested by other researchers (Beller, Zellman, & Le, 1996; Perlman, Stahnke, Butz, Stahl, & Wessels, 2004). Since the ECERS-R is increasingly used across states for regulatory purposes, a shortened scale may translate into less observation time. The authors suggest that future research is needed to examine the relationship of this shortened scale with child outcomes.

Palsha and Wesley (1998) describe a model for preparing community-based consultants to work with the staffs of early care and education programs to improve the quality of their early childhood environments. They used the ECERS-R as one of their measures. As a result of the model, all participating staff members improved their ratings, with the most change occurring in the areas with the lowest ratings. These researchers also indicated that there was still room for improvement, and that change is a slow process. They recommended ongoing support over an extended period to ensure further increases in quality.

From our perspective, the ECERS-R is the best measure available of general early childhood learning environments that an assessment team might consider when planning large-scale screening programs. The information yielded might help team members in considering various classroom options for children, particularly those making a transition from Head Start or other early intervention programs. Outcomes might be used as well to work with teachers to modify their practices. Additional attention needs to be given to teachers' key activities related to emergent literacy in reading, writing, and mathematics, as well as to the scope of books and writing materials available. Only 4 of the 43 ECERS-R items are addressed to Language–Reasoning. Programs may be rated as "good" based on the outcomes of this scale, and still lack the literacy activities that are needed for success in kindergarten (Commissioner's Office of Research and Evaluation & Head Start Bureau, 2001b; Espinosa, 2002; McGill-Franzen et al., 2002).

This same criticism is made by Sylva et al. (2006) who have developed a new scale, the *Early Childhood Environment Rating Scale—Extension* (ECERS-E; Sylva, Siraj-Blatchford, & Taggart, 2003) to assess curricular aspects of quality stressed by the English National Early Childhood Curriculum. This supplement to the ECERS-R has 4 subscales consisting of 18 items that include Literacy (e.g., adult reading with child, sounds in words); Mathematics (e.g., counting, shape/space); Science/Environment (e.g., science resources, food preparation); and Diversity (e.g., planning for individual needs, race and gender equality). Sylva et al. (2006) present data on 2,857 children from 141 randomly selected centers from 5 regions of England representing social and ethnic diversity to support predictive validity. Data on children's cognitive and language abilities and social-behavioral development were collected when they were 3–5 years of age. The ECERS-E, in contrast to the ECERS-R, was a significant predictor of children's scores on pre-reading, general mathematical concepts, and nonverbal reasoning. The ECERS-R, in contrast to the ECERS-E, was found to be more related to social-behavioral development than to cognitive development. Sylva et al. (2006) concluded that, depending on the preschool practices emphasized in a particular setting, both scales can be used to assess quality in relation to its effectiveness in enhancing children's development. With the current greater emphasis on developing early literacy competencies in the preschool, a future revision of the ECERS-R could take these concerns into account.

A similar observational instrument focuses on settings for younger children. The *Infant/Toddler Environment Rating Scale—Revised Edition* (ITERS-R; Harms, Cryer, & Clifford, 2002) has been developed to assess daycare settings. This instrument is summarized in Appendix 5.1, as are two other scales by Harms and colleagues: the *Family Day Care Rating Scale* (Harms & Clifford, 1989a) and the *School-Age Care Environment Rating Scale* (Harms, Jacobs, & White, 1996).

Another series of broad-based procedures to judge the quality of preschool programs and their capacity to facilitate learning and development in children has been developed by Abbott-Shim, Sibley, and associates. Each of these profiles follows the same checklist format of statements rated as "observed" or "not observed," based on direct observation, interview (teacher report), and review of written documentation. A code for data source is suggested for each item.

Assessment Profile for Family Day Care/Early Childhood Programs

The *Assessment Profile for Family Day Care* (Abbott-Shim & Sibley, 1987) was developed to serve as part of the accreditation process by the NAFDC. The profile includes 194 yes–no items grouped into seven subscales that examine dimensions of childcare: Indoor Safety, Health, Nutrition, Indoor Play Environment, Outdoor Play Environment, Interacting, and Professional Responsibility. The profile is completed by the service provider, by a parent not using that provider's care, and by a representative of NAFDC. Information on reliability and validity was not reported.

The *Assessment Profile for Early Childhood Programs* (Abbott-Shim, Sibley, & Neel, 1992; Abbott-Shim & Sibley, 1992) is an observation checklist developed for the purpose of program evaluation. The profile consists of 87 yes–no items organized into five scales (Learning Environment, Scheduling, Curriculum, Interacting, and Individualizing) that examine environments and practices to reflect the criteria of recognized accreditation groups. The profile covers multiple aspects of early childhood organization, availability of learning materials, classroom activities, and teacher behaviors. This checklist was designed to be administered three times a year. An explanation is provided to clarify each item, and 6 of the 87 items are directed at children with special needs. Observational judgments are based on three methods of data collection: observation of classrooms, document review, and teacher interview. Content validity was established through review of literature, cross-referenced with NAEYC accreditation criteria, and reviewed by professionals. It was field-tested in 90 childcare centers in Atlanta. Concurrent validity with the ECERS was documented in two extensive studies (Abbott-Shim, 1991; Wilkes, 1989). Subscale correlations were moderate to good, and the total scale correlations were good (.74, Abbott-Shim, 1991; .64, Wilkes, 1989). Split-half reliability (Spearman–Brown) ranged from .81 to .99 and Cronbach's alpha from .87 to .91 across scales, based on data from 174 classrooms.

A time-sampling method is recommended for collecting data across classrooms. This involves four cycles of 15-minute observations in each of three classrooms, for a total of 1 hour of observation per classroom. The authors recommend 10 hours of training, including practice observation, and a criterion of 85% rater agreement. Research studies, involving a large number of sites, are documented in the appendix. Across studies, rater agreement ranged from 89.5% to 97%. Observers do not interpret data; rather, feedback can be requested from Quality Assist, Inc. This feedback includes number and proportion of criteria met, scaled score (based on 75 items), and *SEM*. The scale, however, can be modified to meet program needs, as was done in the Head Start FACES accountability study (Commissioner's Office of Research and Evaluation & Head Start Bureau, 2001b).

Although the Assessment Profile for Early Childhood Programs covers key aspects of classroom arrangements and instructions, many of the instructional behaviors are broad and may be hard to judge (e.g., item 1 under "Curriculum is individualized" is "Teacher led activities focused on specific skills the child is currently mastering and is neither too difficult nor too simple"). Observers may not have enough observational time to complete items thoughtfully. There is also no emphasis on the teacher as a language model. The dependence on Quality Assist, Inc. for overall scoring and interpretation is a further drawback.

Classroom Assessment Scoring System

The CLASS (Pianta et al., 2007) is a multifaceted observational system developed to assess classroom quality in preschool through upper elementary school. (A system for secondary school is in process.) Ten dimensions of classroom quality are observed that result in positive student outcomes based on theory and an extensive review of the research literature. Dimensions focus on interactions among teachers and students and are organized into three broad areas of classroom quality that are common across grades: emotional support, classroom organization, and instructional support.

Emotional support focuses on those factors that foster children's social and emotional functioning in the classroom. These factors include Positive Climate, Negative Climate, Teacher Sensitivity, and Regard for Student Perspectives. Emotional support for students presenting behavioral and emotional problems relates importantly to academic progress (Hamré & Pianta, 2005).

Classroom organization covers the areas of Behavior Management, Productivity (management of time to maximize time spent in learning activities), and Instructional Learning Formats that lead to self-regulated student behavior. For example, positive behavior management leads to greater participation and engagement in learning and greater academic progress.

Instructional support covers the areas of Concept Development, Quality of Feedback, and Language Modeling. An additional area is Literacy Focus at the prekindergarten and kindergarten levels.

Use of CLASS requires the following:

1. Observation that starts at the beginning of the child's school day and continues for about 3 hours. The observer will have discussed with the teacher the day's schedule prior to beginning the observation.
2. Coding then proceeds using 30-minute cycles. During each cycle, users observe a classroom activity for 20 minutes and record their observations for 10 minutes. Four to 8 cycles are then obtained. A score sheet is provided to make notes reflecting the key aspect of each dimension during every cycle. During the 10 minutes of recording, numerical ratings are made for all of the class dimensions. Codes are based on the behavior of all of the adults in the classroom during each cycle. The CLASS has also been validated for coding videotapes of classrooms.
3. Detailed criteria are provided for scoring each dimension at each point using a 7-point range. Clearly it takes extensive training to become familiar with the behaviors included at each point in the dimensions. Master coded tapes are essential.
4. A composite score is obtained by averaging across cycles to arrive at a single score for each dimension. There are composite scores for the 3 domains covered by CLASS.

CLASS requires in-depth training for appropriate use. (Training is offered through the CLASS website: www.classobservation.com.) Training plus regular reliability checks and refresher/drift segments once a year are recommended.

CLASS has been validated in over 2,000 classrooms. The data indicate that (1) across studies there was considerable variability for all dimensions except Negative Climate; (2) the CLASS dimensions are moderately to highly correlated with each other; (3) correlations between preschool studies and a studies of behaviors in third-grade classrooms were moderate to high; and (4) confirmatory factor analysis based on six studies indicated that factor loadings were moderate to high. Scores are reported to be highly stable across time as assessed in preschool and third grade. Criterion validity with the CLASS-Preschool with the ECERS-R Interactions and Provisions scale are good and interrater agreement, based on students coding five 20-minute classroom segments, is high.

CLASS is an example of an excellent research and training system. Findings indicate that the quality of classrooms can change as children progress through the grades, that gains associated with quality prekindergarten teacher instruction are maintained through kindergarten, and that interactions between teachers and children, particularly instructional interactions, are key to positive development. Training materials for teachers, with a web-based support site are available (www.myteachingpartner.net).

Environmental Considerations for Children with Disabilities

Rogers-Warren and Wedel (1979) make empirically based recommendations concerning classroom arrangements for children with disabilities. These researchers are careful to note the minimal research base available regarding the interaction of such children with their environments, and the need for additional empirical research. Adults (teachers, caregivers, aides) are viewed as the most important components of these children's learning environment, because they are largely responsible for determining all other aspects of the environment (selecting and arranging materials, devising schedules, grouping children, and monitoring behavior). Rogers-Warren (1982), in a later article, describes the learning environment as consisting of two interacting components: *physical components* (actual space, arrangement of activity areas, furniture, play and work materials, activities of the program and their sequence, number of staff and students, types of students [disabled and/or nondisabled], groupings of staff and children) and *social components* (behaviors of adults and children). She describes environmental arrangements to support specific behaviors that are typically important aspects of intervention with disabled preschoolers, and she details procedures in eight areas. Important features of these areas that need to be considered during observation and intervention planning are summarized below. These same concerns continue to be important today.

1. *Promoting social interactions*. Simply placing children with and without disabilities in the same classroom is not sufficient for encouraging modeling and direct contact. More direct teacher interventions may be needed, such as pairing disabled and nondisabled children of differing skill levels, using prearranged seating plans, and providing nondisabled children with specific training for imitating and interacting with their disabled peers. The materials available are also important. For example, block play, manipulative floor play, and materials that require two players encourage conversation, joint activity, and social interaction among children.

2. *Facilitating language learning and communication*. Care providers need to use activities that encourage their interaction with children and support generalization of newly learned communication skills. Using materials with a group of children, after using them in a one-on-one situation, is one way to teach generalization. If the goals include building basic communication skills and promoting frequent verbalizations, a highly responsive environment with a greater number of teachers is required. If a goal is to increase peer interaction, it is better to limit the number of teachers.

3. *Arranging instructional settings to promote learning*. Group size is an important consideration. For example, children with mental retardation often learn better in small groups where skills can generalize than in one-to-one training sessions. Children without disabilities also participate less when the group size is too large. In research on seating arrangements (which covered only nondisabled preschoolers), seating children around the teacher, with space between children, increased attention; by contrast, seating children all on a rug decreased attention. Finally, consistent scheduling promotes attention to a task.

4. *Arranging the schedule and classroom to facilitate behavior management*. Problematic behaviors can be prevented by reducing waiting time, providing overlapping activities, and allowing children to move on to the next thing when they are ready. It is important to establish clear boundaries for materials and activities, in order to reduce cross-traffic interaction and let children know where certain activities are accepted. When behavior modification is used, the area the child is taken from must be attractive. Time out is more effective when the area used is consistent.

5. *Building independence and facilitating transitions.* It is important to give children the opportunity to determine their behavior and manage some of their own materials. Teachers need to provide accessibility to things frequently needed (bathrooms, play materials, etc.). Color-coding materials and storage areas will increase independence during cleanup. Allowing a child to keep some materials in a locker or cubby, to help set up for snack time, and to maintain a consistent routine facilitates independent functioning. For highly limited children, teachers can increase interaction with the environment by putting things within reach and so forth. Facilitating transitions can be accomplished by changing the setting slowly to let children acclimate to new activities.

6. *Facilitating appropriate child behavior.* When dividers are necessary, it is important to increase the opportunities for interaction by using low dividers. It is also important to assign teachers to zones rather than to children, so that they spend more time teaching and the children can move to different activities as they are ready. All materials staff members need should be placed near their areas, so that the time away from children is minimal. Finally, it is helpful to post goals, as well as cues, for each child. A pictorial schedule of the day's activities is helpful for all young children. We have found it helpful to use laminated picture clip art for this purpose. Pictures of the day's activities are posted on Velcro vertically from top to bottom. As each activity is completed, the picture is removed so that children know at what point they are on the schedule.

7. *Evaluating environmental arrangements.* A necessary step is to evaluate environmental arrangements in relationship to all children and staff members. Critical child behaviors to review include the use of materials, as well as any inappropriate behaviors. Critical staff behaviors to review include staff presence with the children, engagement with the children, and other nonteaching activities. Data gathering can include time sampling in each activity area; scanning each adult and child in a predetermined order for 3 seconds and recording behavior; and completing a checklist of behaviors, activities, and procedures that are in effect during a specific time. Teachers or staff members should take turns collecting data.

8. *Meeting the special needs of specific children with disabilities.* Rogers-Warren provides a checklist for evaluating the extent to which the setting meets the needs of particular children.

OBSERVATIONAL PROCEDURE THAT FOCUSES ON LEARNING ENVIRONMENTS AND INSTRUCTION FOR A REFERRED STUDENT

Although various observational instruments for problem solving, intervention planning, and program evaluation have been described above, few systematic observational procedures have been developed that focus on learning environments for a referred child. One such procedure is The Functional Assessment of Academic Behavior (FAAB), developed by Ysseldyke and Christenson (2002). This approach builds on The Instructional Environment Scale–II (TIES-II; Ysseldyke & Christenson, 1993–1996).

FAAB is a comprehensive system using multiple methods (observation, interview, and analysis of student work) and information collected from multiple sources (parents, teachers, and students). Although it is not focused on preschool below the kindergarten level, the areas covered by this scale will help observers focus on important components of preschool environments that might be modified. It was developed to provide information for prereferral intervention, instructional consultation, and collaborative intervention planning centered on the referred child's instructional needs, as well as to identify important home supports and ways to involve the students' parents or guardians. Specifically, the scale is intended to be used for these purposes: to (1) describe the learning environments (school and home) of referred children, in order to understand the interaction of these environments with the children's academic and/or behavioral problems; (2) design appropriate instructional interventions for individual children; (3) inform consultation with teachers and parents; (4) identify problems in skill development, student cognition, or mental processing for planning prereferral interventions; and (5) monitor changes in the quality of instruction. It is not necessary to use all parts of the system with all students. Rather, users should choose forms that address the needs of the student about whom they are concerned. There are 5 core forms to be used with the FAAB. They are as follows:

1. The Instructional Environment Checklist (consists of 23 support-for-learning components that are associated with academic success for students).
2. The Instructional Environment Checklist: Annotated Version (delineates the indicators for each of the 23 support-for-learning components).
3. The Instructional Needs Checklist (provides information on the teacher's observation of the student under different instructional conditions).
4. Parental Experience With Their Child's Learning and Schoolwork (provides information about the parents' [caregivers'] perspective on the student's responses to instruction and learning).
5. The Intervention Documentation Record (provides an efficient way for educators to keep track, across school years, of the interventions that have been implemented and their effectiveness).

Six additional forms are provided to assist in data collection. These forms were used in TIES-II, but they may be optional, depending on the needs of the student. They are as follows:

1. The Observation Record (for direct observation in the classroom).
2. The Student Interview Record (a standard set of questions for student interview, which can be supplemented as needed).
3. The Teacher Interview Record.
4. The Parent Interview Record.
5. The Supplemental Teacher Interview Questions (completed by the teacher in order to gather information about instructional conditions that affect student performance).
6. The Supplemental Student Interview Questions (completed by the student in order to gather information about his or her experience with learning. FAAB provides a checklist of alterable variables associated with positive academic performance. These variables fall into 3 distinct categories: (1) Instructional Support for Learning, which occurs in classrooms in school; (2) Home Support for Learning, which occurs in the home or in the community; and (3) Home-School Support for Learning, which represents the degree of continuity across home and school and the quality of the home-school relationship and the support for student learning).

There are a total of 23 support-for-learning components that fall within 3 contexts: (1) 12 classroom components (instructional support for learning); (2) 5 home components (home support for learning); and (3) 6 home-school relationship components (home-school support for learning).

The 12 instructional areas are as follows:

1. Instructional Match (between the student's characteristics and needs and the instruction delivered).
2. Teacher Expectations (and communication of these to the student).
3. Classroom Environment (classroom management, productive use of time, class climate).
4. Instructional Presentation (clarity of directions, nature of presentation of materials, practice, checking for student understanding).
5. Cognitive Emphasis (including teaching and modeling of thinking skills and problem-solving strategies).
6. Motivational Strategies (techniques used by teachers to heighten student interest and effort).
7. Relevant Practice (sufficient time and opportunities for both guided and independent practice).
8. Informed Feedback (specific immediate feedback that models, prompts, and cues).
9. Academic Engaged Time (the extent to which teachers present and monitor instruction and foster student engagement).
10. Adaptive Instruction (instruction that is modified to accommodate the student's needs).
11. Progress Evaluation (frequent, direct measures of the student's progress toward specified objectives, the outcomes of which are communicated to the student and are used to monitor the effectiveness of instruction and adjust teaching).
12. Instructional Planning (including task analysis of curriculum and assessment focused on determining the student's instructional level).

The 5 home-support components are these:

1. Expectations and Attributions (what parents expect from their child's school performance).
2. Discipline Orientation (methods parents use to monitor their child's behavior).
3. Home Affective Environment (emotional tone in the home, particularly between parents and child).
4. Parent Participation (in meaningful activities related to their child's schooling).
5. Structure for Learning (routines, monitoring out-of-school time, availability to provide assistance).

The 6 home-school support components are these:

1. Shared Standards and Expectations (level of expected performance held by parents or caregivers for the student).
2. Consistent Structure (overall routine and monitoring provided by parents or caregivers).
3. Cross-setting Opportunity to Learn (learning options available both at school and out-of-school time).
4. Mutual Support (guidance, communication and interest shown by parents or caregivers).
5. Positive Trusting Relationships (degree to which adult-child relationship is positive).
6. Modeling (parents or caregivers demonstrating desired behaviors and commitment toward learning and working hard).

Through the mutual problem solving achieved through collaborative consultation with school personnel and family members, interventions are developed that consider the roles of parents and teachers as well as the student. Steps of the collaborative intervention planning process are detailed in the manual. Users need to be trained in assessment (including observation, interviewing, and collaborative consultation), as well as to have knowledge about effective instruction and home influences on school performance.

Technical data were presented to support interrater reliability and content validity of the original TIES. Interrater reliability was based on 28 observers watching tapes of two teachers instructing elementary-age students. Reliability coefficients for the 12 TIES components ranged from .83 to .96 and exceeded .90 on all but two components. Thirty-three pairs of observers observing the same student for 1 hour yielded group agreement of 76.2% (Thurlow, Ysseldyke, & Wotruba, 1988). Content validity was supported through a review of the research literature by component area. Supportive references are listed for the correlates of academic achievement, as informed by home and school factors. Concurrent validity ratings in relation to the *Basic Achievement Skills Individual Screener* (Psychological Corporation, 1983) was provided by the TIES components. Ratings for students with mild disabilities, in both general and special educational settings, were also provided.

The "student learning in context" model of assessment detailed by Christenson and Ysseldyke (1989) helps assessors move from a primary focus on identifying student characteristics that affect learning, to viewing learning as a complex set of interactions among student, teacher, instructional, family, and school characteristics. The targets of intervention can then involve all of these factors.

From our perspective, FAAB is one of the few observation systems that integrates both home and school environmental variables into the assessment process for a referred child. It is, however, directed to children in grade 1 and above, although its use is appropriate at the kindergarten level; thus several developmentally appropriate teaching practices for preschool children, as well as typical instructional activities for preschool classes prior to grade 1, are not included. Further drawbacks are the time and training needed to carry out this comprehensive observational system. The observer needs extensive background in observation, interviewing, and consultation skills. Nevertheless, since the theoretical framework and content is informative for preschool assessors, FAAB has been presented in some detail. Multiple useful reproducible forms are presented in Ysseldyke and Christenson (2002).

SUMMARY AND COMMENTS FOR FUTURE PRACTICE

Observing environments is of vital concern for early childhood assessors, who are now mandated by IDEA 2004 to consider situational variables in evaluating young children with suspected disabilities and developing IEPs. Both the school and the family (a subject discussed in Chapter 8) play critical roles in the development and well-being of preschool children. Aspects of educational environments that assessors using observational procedures need to consider have been summarized in this chapter, along with the major measures available. A number of these aspects should be particular concerns for observers, because they are not covered well in existing measures. These include modeling of language; the ability of caregivers to form strong attachments with children; the provision of activities to foster emergent literacy, as well as the teaching of basic relational concepts needed to follow directions and engage in instructional activities; and caregivers' ability to reinforce and promote emotional and social growth, creativity, and independence. As Espinosa (2002) states, current measures of preschool quality do "not adequately capture the enriched language, early literacy, and mathematical and scientific learning that can occur during the preschool years" (p. 4). Attention to these areas has been addressed in England by the work of Sylva et al. (2003). Attention to these neglected issues is needed during observation for a referred child, as well as in-service training activities.

Where appropriate, assessors need to use the outcomes of their observations to help modify the physical arrangements of classroom environments, as well as instructional practices. They should also be used as necessary to provide follow-up guidance that will help teachers and other caregivers improve their overall effectiveness. Since multiple aspects of preschool, childcare, or kindergarten environments influence different aspects of child functioning, no one scale will be able to capture the complexity of these interactions. Rather, the assessment question needs to drive the forms of observational assessment needed. Important considerations to be taken into account when assessors are incorporating environmental observation into the assessment process include the following:

1. The data for most published observational measures of learning environments are based on one observation session (lasting perhaps from 2 to 4 hours). Although this procedure may capture such factors as teacher–child ratio and classroom arrangements, it may or may not capture the typical interaction patterns of teachers or caregivers with particular children. Assessors need to interview the teachers or other caregivers to determine whether the observed interactions were typical. When children are brought to a clinic setting, it may not be feasible to observe them in a preschool setting. However, it is usually possible to interview the teacher or other care providers and use checklists to cover important features of the instructional environment for the referred child.

2. Since most currently available scales (with the exception of FAAB, CLASS, ESCAPE, and CISSAR) provide only broad, general pictures of classroom environments, more in-depth measures need to be developed to understand the interaction between environmental factors and the behavior of an individual child at the preschool level. A series of tasks similar to those included on the FAAB need to be developed at the preschool level. Comparing a child presenting with special needs to a randomly selected comparison child or a larger group of children is particularly useful, since the interaction of environmental variables with child behavior is likely to differ for these children.

3. Some scales, such as the PACE, are part of comprehensive systems. These systems entail observations of both parents and teachers, interviews, and the use of structured observational procedures and work samples. This comprehensive approach will provide the most detailed understanding of environmental effects on children. Assessors, however, need to consider whether the outcomes yield enough payoff to justify the time needed for training, carrying out the procedure, and analyzing results. They also need to consider whether these systems provide the most useful data for their particular assessment purposes.

In summary, excellent environmental rating scales are available for purposes of teacher training and global program evaluation. However, although observing environments for a referred child is stressed in the literature as essential, it is often not carried out for a number of reasons. First, this is a time-consuming activity for time-pressed assessors; second, realistic instruments have not been developed for use at the preschool level. However, observation of the environment is a critical link between child assessment and intervention. Changes may be needed in the organization of the setting and/or in the nature of teacher–child or parent–child interactions to facilitate positive behavior and learning for the child.

The following is a checklist of observational activities to help assessors account for environmental factors that might influence the behavior of a referred preschool or kindergarten child. These are reasonable for assessors assigned to a preschool setting or to the primary grades. Assessors at a clinic need, if possible, to observe in both the home and school (as is done with preschool children assessed at the clinic at Teachers College, Columbia University). If not, telephone interviews with teachers and the use of rating scales and checklists need to be part of standard practice.

1. Observe the situations likely to encourage or hinder desired child behaviors, and consider the following:
   - In what ways do the physical arrangements of the environment facilitate or interfere with children's behaviors? Draw a diagram of the room arrangements, and write specific descriptions of the context.
   - What activities and materials are most likely to elicit desired child behavior across developmental areas of concern, such as language or social interaction? This information can be obtained through an interview or on a questionnaire.
2. Observe the effect of instructional activities, teacher behaviors, and intervention strategies on desired child behaviors, in the context of typical children in the group. Review the curricular materials and approaches used. In particular, look at activities that focus on language and literacy, child engagement, interactive play, and other activities important for a child to be successful in kindergarten.
3. Interview the teacher or other caregiver to check out your observations and to elicit their observations.
4. Prepare an eco-map for the individual child of concern, highlighting interactions with key individuals and the positive and negative impact (valence) of these interactions within and across key settings.
5. When possible, collect repeated observations on the outcomes of modification of the physical environment, instructional activities, or behavioral intervention, in order to build a database on intervention effectiveness with children from diverse cultures and those presenting special needs. Consider the interactions between the learning environment characteristics listed in Table 5.2 and the following child behaviors or characteristics:
   - Engagement/time spent with materials.
   - Attention to teacher/caregiver directions.
   - Ability to hear what teachers/caregivers are saying.
   - Access to materials (especially for children with disabling conditions).
   - Access to teachers/caregivers.
   - Interaction with adults present.
   - Interactions with peers.
   - Independence.
   - Creative play.
   - Use of language to meet needs.
   - Tolerance/ability to comply.
   - Unacceptable behaviors.

TABLE 5.2. Summary of Important Dimensions of Learning Environments

Structural and physical dimensions

- Amount of physical space available; density; center size
- Classroom design, including the layout of physical space and organization of space into well-defined activity areas/zones so as to encourage attention and discourage behavior problems
- Range of equipment and materials to encourage exploration and problem solving by children from diverse backgrounds and with disabilities
- Background conditions, such as noise, lighting, and color
- Availability/placement of materials (especially for children with special needs)

Interpersonal dimensions

- Staff–child ratio
- Group size
- Mix of children with and without special needs
- Opportunities for children to interact with adults and with peers
- Outreach to home, and parent involvement[a]

Interaction dimensions

- Frequency and quality (valence) of interactions with adults
- Frequency and quality (valence) of interactions with peers
- Management of problem behaviors
- Techniques used to encourage motivation and engagement
- Feedback interactions and reinforcement of desired behaviors
- Adult–child conversations rich in language

Instructional dimensions

- Types of teaching methods used
- Activities across all development areas
- Activities that encourage appreciation of diversity
- Appropriate activities for children with disabilities
- Instructional features that encourage engagement, development of language, emergent literacy, social interaction, independence, and problem solving
- Adult scaffolding as needed; appropriate pacing
- Consistent schedule
- Activities that are child-focused (not merely drill and practice)
- Observation and intervention procedures/activities as ongoing processes
- A training component for staff that provides opportunity for feedback on performance
- Teacher directions are simple (consisting of no more than two behaviors to be followed and one qualifying adjective)

[a] Parent involvement should include the following: consultation and involvement in decisions and interventions; carrying out activities at home; reinforcing desired behaviors; talking/interacting with children; and modeling literacy and problem-solving behaviors. High expectations by parents for their child's success in school are also important.

APPENDIX 5.1. Review of Measures

Measure	**Assessment Profile for Early Childhood Programs. Abbott-Shim, Sibley, and Neel (1992), Abbott-Shim and Sibley (1992).**
Purpose	Evaluating programs and developing recommendations for improving quality.
Areas	Five subscales: Learning Environment; Scheduling; Curriculum; Interacting; and Individualizing.
Format	87-item checklist in yes–no format. Observational judgments are based on three methods of data collection: observation of classrooms, document review, and teacher interview.
Scores	Proportion of criteria met; scale scores.
Age group	Infancy through school age.
Time	One hour of direct observation per classroom, plus review of documents and teacher interview.
Users	Trained observers.
Norms	Not available.
Reliability	Split-half, .87–.91; interrater, .89–.97.
Validity	Content, established; concurrent, established.
Comments	Feedback can be requested from Quality Assist, Inc.; this includes number and proportion of criteria met, scaled score, and *SEM*. Although this measure covers key aspects of classroom arrangements and instruction, many of the instructional behaviors are broad and difficult to judge. Observers may not have enough observational time to complete items. There is no emphasis on the teacher as a language model. The dependence on Quality Assist for overall scoring and interpretation is a major drawback.
References consulted	RTI International (n.d.). See book's References list.

Measure	**Assessment Profile for Family Day Care. Abbott-Shim and Sibley (1987).**
Purpose	Serving as part of the accreditation process of the National Association for Family Day Care (NAFDC).
Areas	Seven subscales that examine dimensions of childcare: Indoor Safety; Health; Nutrition; Indoor Play Environment; Outdoor Play Environment; Interacting; and Professional Responsibility.
Format	194-item checklist in yes–no format.
Scores	Not detailed.
Age group	6, 15, 24, and 36 months.
Time	Not available.
Users	The profile is completed by the service provider, by a parent not using that provider's care, and by a representative of NAFDC.
Norms	Not available.
Reliability	Information not available.
Validity	Information not available.
Comments	Feedback can be requested from Quality Assist, Inc.
References consulted	RTI International (n.d.). See book's References List.

Measure	**Classroom Assessment Scoring System (CLASS): Preschool (Pre-K Version). Pianta, La Paro, and Hamré (2007).**
Purpose	Assessing classroom quality for purposes of research, program evaluation, and professional development.
Areas	Ten dimensions of classroom quality are observed that are organized into three broad areas of classroom quality: Emotional Support (Positive Climate, Negative Climate, Teacher Sensitivity, and Regard for Student Perspectives), Classroom Organization (Behavior Management, Productivity, and Instructional Learning Formats), and Instructional Support (Concept Development, Quality of Feedback, and Language Modeling). Literacy Focus is an additional dimension included under Instructional Support at the prekindergarten and kindergarten levels. The degree of Student Engagement is also rated.
Format	Each dimension consists of 4–7 items that are rated on a 7-point scale, ranging from uncharacteristic to highly characteristic. Clear behavioral descriptions are provided for points along the scale.
Scores	Scores for the three domains and for Student Engagement.
Age group	Prekindergarten and kindergarten. (Materials are available for other grade levels.)
Time	3 hours.
Users	Educational professionals trained in use of the scales.
Norms	Not reported.
Reliability	Interrater agreement, based on students coding five 20-minute classroom segments was .87. Agreement in ratings (within 1 point) was from 78.8 to 96.9 across dimensions.
Validity	Content, construct, and predictive, supported through research findings. Criterion validity with the CLASS-Preschool with the ECERS-R Interactions scale ranged from .45–.63 and with Provisions scale from .33–.36.
Comments	CLASS is an excellent research and training system to rate the quality of teacher–student interactions. Outcomes can be used for research and teacher training. Excellent training materials are available as well as web-based support.

Measure	**Early Childhood Environment Rating Scale—Revised Edition (ECERS-R). Harms, Clifford, and Cryer (1998).**
Purpose	Assessing the overall quality of a broad variety of preschool settings (Head Start, church, day care, preschool, and kindergarten).
Areas	Seven subscales: Space and Furnishings; Personal Care Routines; Language–Reasoning; Activities; Interaction; Program Structure; and Parents and Staff.
Format	43-item, 7-point rating scale, with clear behavioral descriptors for rating points of 1, 3, 5, and 7.
Scores	Seven subscale scores; global scores based on the average of all items.
Age group	2–6 to 5–11 years.
Time	Minimum of 2 hours of observation and inspection, plus time to interview teacher.
Users	Outside observers or program staff.
Norms	Criterion-referenced (no normative data available).
Reliability	Internal consistency, .92; interrater, .92.

Validity	Content (for original ECERS): Supported by rank-order correlations of .74 and .70 for each of two groups. See text for details.
Comments	A section is included in the manual for training researchers to use the scale in research and program evaluation. A training package that includes a videotape and workbook is also available. The ECERS-R is an excellent measure of general childhood learning environments, which the assessment team might consider when planning large-scale screening programs. The information yielded might help in considering classroom options for children. Outcomes might be useful in modifying teaching practices. An expanded response form (Harms, Clifford, & Cryer, 2005) is available.
References consulted	Paget and Schwarting (2001); Sakai, Whitebrook, Wishard, and Howes (2003). See book's References list.

Measure	**Family Day Care Rating Scale. Harms and Clifford (1989a).**
Purpose	Assessing the quality of care in home-based settings.
Areas	Subscales include: Space and Furnishing (for care and learning); Basic Care; Language and Reasoning; Learning Activities; Social Development; Adult Needs.
Format	40 items across the subscales, plus a supplementary section consisting of 8 items; 1–7 rating scale.
Scores	Total score per subscales and an average score (total subscale score divided by number of items scored).
Age group	Preschool.
Time	2 hours.
Users	Multifunctional: Caregivers for self-assessment; agencies for monitoring; researchers.
Norms	Field-tested at 150 Los Angeles family daycare locations.
Reliability	Internal consistency, .70–.93; interrater (19 family daycare homes in North Carolina), .84; interrater (a second study in Michigan), .83.
Validity	Content: Based on ECERS, supported by a correlation of .80 with home visitor ratings.
Comments	The scale was developed to be consistent with the Child Development Associate and the NAFDC credentials.
References consulted	Harms and Clifford (1989b); Iverson (1992). See book's References list.

Measure	**Functional Assessment of Academic Behavior (FAAB). Ysseldyke and Christenson (2002).**
Purpose	Assessing how instruction will be planned, managed, delivered, and evaluated using multiple methods (observation, interview, and analysis of student work) and multiple sources (parents, teachers, and students). Useful for prereferral intervention, instructional consultation, and collaborative intervention planning around the instructional needs of a referred child.
Areas	All areas of academic learning. Content, in part, based on The Instructional Environment Scale–II (TIES-II) (1993–1996).

Format	Consists of five core forms: The Instructional Environment Checklist, The Instructional Environment Checklist: Annotated Version, The Instructional Needs Checklist, Parental Experience with Their Child's Learning and Schoolwork, and The Intervention Documentation Record. Six additional forms are provided to assist in data collection, including the Observation Record, Student Interview Record, Teacher Interview Record, Parent Interview Record, Supplemental Teacher Interview Questions, and Supplemental Student Interview Questions. Forms are selected to address the assessment question.
Scores	Not reported.
Age group	Grades K–12.
Time	Not applicable; evaluation based on a multistep process.
Users	Educational professionals trained in observation and interviewing.
Norms	Not available.
Reliability	Interrater reliability for the original TIES ranged from .83 to .96 and exceeded .90 on all but two components.
Validity	Content supported through research findings.
Comments	FAAB is a unique observation system that integrates environmental information from both the teacher and family into the assessment process for a referred child. Multiple reducible forms are provided. This system is directed largely at children in grade 1 and above, although it may be used at the kindergarten level. Thus, a number of developmentally appropriate teaching practices for preschool children are not included. In order to carry out this comprehensive observational system, background in observation, interviewing, and consultation is important.
References consulted	Boehm review.

Measure	**Preschool Assessment of the Classroom Environment (PACE). McWilliam and Dunst (1985b).**
Purpose	Using multiple sources to plan interventions for children with and without disabilities.
Areas	Program Organization; Environment Organization; Instruction; Program Outcomes.
Format	70-item, 5-point rating scale based on observation of classroom environment, interview of all persons responsible for classroom management, and review of written materials.
Scores	Summary ratings.
Age group	0–6 years.
Time	2- to 4-hour span for observation.
Users	Trained observers.
Norms	Not available.
Reliability	Based on a pilot study of 20 preschool programs serving both disabled and nondisabled children in North Carolina, overall median agreement was 82% for PACE, 82% for caregiver styles of interaction, 81% for child engagement, and 84% for child behavior characteristics.

Validity	A significant correlation resulted between the PACE components, caregiver variables, and outcome variables. Outcomes revealed that the program organization components were most closely related to measures of child behavior characteristics; environmental organization components to measures of child engagement; and instructional components to measures of caregiver styles.
Comments	PACE is a comprehensive observation process integrating information from multiple sources and covering important instructional components and interactions of preschool environments for disabled and nondisabled children. The technical data presented are based on a limited sample and restricted geographic area; assessors will need to collect technical data at a local level. When PACE is used for purposes of intervention planning, these steps should be followed: (1) self-evaluation of classroom environment completed by teacher/caregiver, using Needs Evaluation for Educators of Developmentally Delayed Students (same items as PACE, stated in terms of help desired by teacher); (2) completion of PACE by an independent observer; (3) discussion with teacher/caregiver, based on results of 1 and 2; (4) development and implementation of technical assistance plan; and (5) monitoring of changes in child's behavior based on changes in caregiver interactions.
References consulted	Boehm review.

Measure	**School-Age Care Environment Rating Scale. Harms, Jacobs, and White (1996).**
Purpose	Assessing center-based and nonparental care programs for school-age children.
Areas	Six subscales: Space and Furnishings; Health and Safety; Activities; Interactions; Program Structure; Staff Development.
Format	49 items; 7-point rating scale from "inadequate" to "excellent."
Scores	Total score and average score.
Age group	5-0 to 12-0 years.
Time	2 hours.
Users	After-school agencies.
Norms	Criterion-referenced; normative data not available.
Reliability	Internal consistency, .95; interrater, .83.
Validity	Content, good; Construct, good.
Comments	The manual is clear, with helpful step-by-step instructions on what to do when not sure about scoring. There is also a useful section in the manual on steps for training observers. Scoring criteria are clear and easy to understand, with space provided to record specific observations. The manual emphasizes using the scale to improve programs rather than simply to judge them.
References consulted	Harms, Jacobs, and White (2000); Kieth and Michaels (2001). See book's References list.

Chapter 6

Screening Practices and Procedures

A FOCUS ON DEVELOPMENTAL SCREENING

The term *screening* is used in a number of ways by early childhood specialists. These can range from using a brief measure to identify children potentially at risk for later school difficulty and in need of in-depth evaluation, to using a comprehensive measure to plan learning experiences based on children's strengths, strategies, and areas needing development. Screening with preschool children serves at least four assessment purposes:

1. *Developmental screening*—a continuum of preliminary activities used to identify children in need of more in-depth evaluation, and to plan initial learning experiences and forms of early intervention.
2. *Readiness screening*—procedures used to determine a child's preparedness to engage in the curricular activities of kindergarten or first grade.
3. *Instructional screening*—procedures used to guide instructional planning (including a general overall picture of a child's strengths and areas needing development), as well as to obtain information relative to specific teaching goals (often at a beginning point of instruction, following an instructional unit, and continuing throughout instruction).
4. *Selective screening*—an initial step for selection/entrance into special programs or acceptance into private schools.

These screening purposes result in different, often overlapping outcomes and lead to confusion in reviewing the related literature and in applying the term. None of the forms of screening, however, should be confused with diagnosis. *Diagnosis* (frequently referred to as *comprehensive evaluation*) involves procedures used to (1) determine whether a problem exists and, if so, its nature; (2) understand the causes of problems, along with child strengths and strategies; (3) understand environmental constraints and facilitators; (4)

specify specific strategies for intervention; and (5) help parents and teachers set appropriate expectations for rate of learning.

This chapter consists of two major sections. The first section focuses on developmental screening and general screening issues; the second section details steps for developing and carrying out a screening program. The next chapter covers screening for early academic preparedness (commonly referred to as *readiness*) and instructional screening. Many of the issues and procedures discussed in these two chapters are appropriate for screening for entrance into special programs or private schools, although this topic is not addressed specifically in this book.

DEVELOPMENTAL SCREENING

Purposes and Scope of Developmental Screening

At the preschool level, perhaps the most prevalent type of screening cited in the literature is developmental screening, the goal of which is to early identification of children who have problems or who are likely to be most vulnerable to learning or behavioral difficulties during their primary school years. Developmental screening involves comparing a child's skill acquisition across developmental domains with normal developmental patterns, in order to determine whether the child is functioning within normal limits for his or her age. As noted earlier, developmental screening is an initial step of an assessment process that identifies children in need of prereferral intervention and ongoing observation or in-depth evaluation, and that may eventually lead to referral for special educational services. Developmental screening, however, does not tell us the kind of problem a child has or the kind of program he or she needs.

As Meisels and Provance (1989, p. 31) point out, "Tests do not have magical properties. They are only as good as the people using them," and no single test result can be effective in early identification. Therefore, it is necessary to look not only at the qualities of tests that have been developed for the purposes of developmental screening, but also at how they are supplemented by other approaches within the context of local screening policies and intervention options.

Broad-scale developmental screening was called for by the original IDEA (Public Law 101-476) and continues to be mandated by IDEA 2004. Each state must provide a free and appropriate public education (FAPE) to all children ages 3–21 with disabilities residing in the state. As part of this, each state must ensure that all children with disabilities are identified and provided with an opportunity for a FAPE, including children who attend private schools, are homeless, or are wards of the state. States typically meet their obligation by early outreach to identify severely disabled children in the first years of life, and then seek to identify milder or later-onset disabilities by screening all children before or at the beginning of kindergarten (and at any point by parental request). The definition of what constitutes "developmental delay" is determined by each state (which in turn may delegate this responsibility to local school districts), and delay is measured by appropriate diagnostic instruments and procedures in one or more of the following areas:

1. Physical development (including tests of vision and hearing), motor development, and health.
2. Cognitive development (including verbal and nonverbal measures of concept development, reasoning, memory, general information, and problem solving).

3. Communication (including receptive and expressive language development and speech and articulation, such as reproducing sounds and words; repeating words, phrases, and sentences; and intelligibility of speech).
4. Social and emotional development (social competence, internalizing or externalizing problems).
5. Adaptive development and self-help skills.

Presently, however, many developmental screening procedures focus on the cognitive, physical, motor, and language behaviors of young children. Lacking in many procedures is attention to potential behavioral, attention, and socioemotional difficulties. To begin to address these behavioral and socioemotional areas, some screening devices (e.g., the Early Screening Inventory—Revised [ESI-R; Meisels, Marsden, Wiske, & Henderson, 1997) are accompanied by parent questionnaires or include brief observation checklists. Other tests have been developed that may be used with developmental screening tests that cover social and emotional development (such as the Ages and Stages Questionnaires: Social–Emotional). School districts also must make sure that children are screened in a fair and unbiased manner; every effort must be made to screen children in their native language and mode of communication. Materials and procedures used to assess children with limited English proficiency (LEP) need to be used in a manner to ensure that they measure the extent to which a child has a disability, not the degree of the child's LEP. Here lies a major problem: Few measures are available in languages other than English, and in some cases Spanish.

Since the goal of developmental screening is to identify children who will profit from early intervention in order to prevent later learning or behavioral difficulties, it is important that preschool screening procedures not only survey those factors that relate to later difficulties, but also provide information of immediate relevance to preliminary intervention planning, focus on strengths as well as areas needing development, and consider environmental factors that impede or foster development. Considering both environmental and family risk and protective factors is essential to the multifactor ecocultural model of assessment advanced in this text (see Chapter 2). Up to the present time, however, most developmental screening programs have focused largely on the child, instead of on the complex interplay of multiple risk factors and buffers across the environments the child experiences, when planning the next steps in the assessment–intervention process.

From our perspective, developmental screening needs to cover the following factors:

Factors	Information sources
Family	
• Risk factors	• Interview
• Protective factors	• History (questionnaire)
• Perceived strengths and needs	• Questionnaires, rating scales
• Interactive styles with the child	
• Cultural background expectations	
Child	
• Strengths	• History (questionnaire)
• Areas needing development	• Observation of classroom environment when possible
• Strategies/styles	• Interview
• Test outcomes	

Interaction patterns • Parent–child • Child–child • Child–screener • Child's response to adults' supports/ scaffolding, reinforcement	 • Brief game or task with parent • Observation of child interacting with other children • Observation in natural settings • Observation checklist
School practices • Program features • Instructional practices • Teacher beliefs (e.g., "Older girls do better") • Supports/scaffolding • Sensitivity to diversity • Organization of classroom	 • Records • Teacher questionnaire/checklist • Observation • Interview
Prior interventions • Nature of intervention • Transition activities • Parent involvement in prior programs	 • Records • Parent interview • Interview/questionnaire with key others

Strategies for assessing family strengths and needs are covered in Chapter 8. Although collecting these data at the time of developmental screening is more costly than may be allowed by current practices, it is critical both in assessing possible risk and in planning intervention. The evidence to date clearly suggests that assessors need to focus on multiple risk and protective factors, not only on child factors, in making long-term predictions of risk status. The long-term outlook for a child who is at risk and lives in poverty, whose mother has a substance addiction and less than a 12th-grade education, and whose teacher has rigid beliefs about child development is grim. A more positive long-term outlook is possible for a child who is at risk and lives in poverty, but whose mother cares warmly for him or her, provides consistent routines, and has completed high school, and whose teacher seeks to match instruction to child needs.

Developmental Screening Measures

Obviously, no one brief, easily administered, easily interpreted instrument or battery can tap the complex interaction of factors that contribute to a child's possible risk for later problems in school performance. Yet a great deal is expected from the brief sample of child behavior gathered during developmental screening. The outcomes of this sample generally lead to the following decisions: "Refer for in-depth evaluation," "Rescreen," or "No problem." The need for in-depth evaluation to identify children who might need special education services is costly for school districts and involves a great deal of concern on the part of parents. Therefore, considerable attention has been addressed to the technical qualities of screening tests. The goal is to use measures that have high degrees of predictive accuracy, including few *false positives* (children referred who do not demonstrate problems later) and few *false negatives* (children missed who demonstrate learning or behavioral difficulties later). The focus on the technical qualities of measures, however, often fails to take into account the scope and effectiveness of home and school intervention, the quality of instruction, teacher attitudes, subsequent learning demands, other risk factors, and the quality/inclusiveness of the criterion measures selected. In addition to questions about technical qualities, these questions need to be raised when a measure is being selected:

1. What areas are covered by the screening measure used? How extensive a behavior sample is obtained in each area (such as the number and scope of the items included)?
2. In what ways is the screening measure supplemented by observation or other procedures, such as parent questionnaires and interview?
3. Will those individuals responsible for the screening program engage in systematic evaluation of their screening model? Is the information used in a prediction matrix? What is the point of prediction (end of kindergarten, first grade, second grade, later)? What associated information is collected?
4. How are environmental/instructional constraints and facilitators measured and accounted for in prediction?
5. What are teachers' prevailing beliefs about children who encounter difficulty?
6. How lenient/stringent are the cutoff criteria?

Guidelines for Selecting Screening Procedures

A large number of screening measures have appeared in recent years and are used across states; however, the quality of these is variable and in some instances poor. Some lack normative data, validity or reliability information that substantiate their accuracy over a brief period of time. Essential characteristics of good screening instruments (both developmental and readiness) have been described by numerous experts in the field (Bagnato, 1984; Bracken, 1987; Emmons & Alfonso, 2005; Flanagan & Alfonso, 1995; Glascoe, 1991; Gredler, 1992; McCauley & Swisher, 1984; Meisels & Atkins-Burnett, 2005; Salvia & Ysseldyke, 2004; Zeitlin, 1976) and are detailed in the AERA et al. (1999) *Standards for Educational and Psychological Testing*. These characteristics are presented in Table 6.1.

Furthermore, since many test authors state multiple objectives, instruments need to be evaluated in relationship to each of these objectives. Many instruments available for developmental screening provide insufficient technical documentation and limited normative or field data particularly if they are locally developed (see Chapter 3). Even instruments with adequate psychometric properties may not lead to appropriate educational programming. Several widely used screening instruments that cover multiple developmental domains are summarized in Appendix 6.1, including the following:

- American Guidance Service (AGS) Early Screening Profiles (ESP; Harrison et al., 1990)
- Battelle Developmental Inventory, Second Edition (BDI-2) and its Screening Test (Newborg, 2004)
- Denver Developmental Screening Test II (Denver II; Frankenburg et al., 1990)
- Developmental Indicators for the Assessment of Learning—Third Edition (DIAL-3; Mardell-Czudnowski & Goldenberg, 1998)
- Early Screening Inventory—Revised (ESI-R; Meisels et al., 1997)
- FirstSTEp: Screening Test for Evaluating Preschoolers (FirstSTEp; Miller, 1993)

These instruments are representative of the major published instruments that are currently available. From our perspective, the ESI-R, DIAL-3, AGS ESP, and FirstSTEp are

TABLE 6.1. Characteristics of a Good Screening Instrument

1. The primary/auxiliary purpose(s) of the instrument is (are) stated explicitly: developmental screening, readiness screening, and/or enhancing instructional decisions. Consider the specific areas that are included.
2. Empirical documentation of reliability is presented. Depending on the purpose of the measure, test–retest reliabilities need to be at least .80 for referral for comprehensive assessment, .90 or greater for high-stakes decisions such as placement in a special class, and .50–.60 for research purposes; agreement among assessors should be .80 or greater.
3. Empirical documentation of validity is presented, with a correlation of .60 with other diagnostic measures for predictive validity and .70–.80, depending on the purpose of the measure (i.e., developmental screening or instructional screening), for concurrent validity.
4. The instrument has a sensitivity of .80, based on studies documenting the percentage of children who are referred as a result of screening test outcomes and are found to have actual problems when given diagnostic tests or later in their schooling.
5. The instrument has a specificity of .90, based on studies of children who are correctly identified without delays on the screening measures and who continue not to have delays later on.
6. There is a clear description of the groups included in the standardization population, suggesting a good match with the local population (if not, local norms may need to be collected).
7. An adequate sample size is reported in the manual (100 subjects per age group are considered a minimum for developmental screening tests).
8. Measures of central tendency and variability are reported for norm-referenced tests.
9. Children with disabling conditions are included in the standardization sample, or special studies are reported in the manual.
10. The instrument has an adequate floor (sufficient range of easy items with which children can meet success in subtests) to differentiate children 3 years of age and above who have developmental difficulties from those who do not.
11. Items are culturally appropriate; translations with normative data are available.
12. Items appeal to young children (not necessarily to the assessor).
13. Recommendations for assessors' qualifications, type of training, and supervision are given; training materials are available or training activities are suggested.
14. Test administration, scoring, and interpretation are relatively easy.
15. Information/recommendations for intervention planning are provided for parents, teachers, or other specialists.
16. Information relevant to monitoring progress or the effectiveness of intervention is provided.

the most useful for developmental screening of children ages 3–5. It is important for assessors to note in their review of these tests that tasks covering the same area (e.g., stringing beads) may be presented at very different levels of difficulty (large beads vs. small beads). Screening instruments focused on the particular developmental area of language are covered in Chapter 10.

Assessors need to be mindful as well of the caution that even instruments with adequate psychometric properties may not lead to appropriate programming. Therefore, the focus of developmental screening should not be primarily on the test instrument, but on multiple determinants and a multistep process. Developmental screening needs to be considered as a repeated feedback loop (Boehm & Sandberg, 1982) that is carried out over time.

Challenges to Developmental Screening

Early childhood professionals have been struggling for a long time with the challenges inherent in developmental screening. Some of the classic work was done in the 1980s. The challenges remain largely the same today. Lichtenstein and Ireton (1984) indicate that the model of early identification and intervention is predicated on three assumptions: that (1) early intervention produces a significant positive effect; (2) children with developmental problems can be accurately identified early in the course of their problems; and (3) early identification/intervention can be implemented without prohibitive costs. These authors also address the limitations of these assumptions, including scanty evidence regarding the long-term effects of intervention; the tenuous nature of predictions as to whether children ages 3–5 will experience problems in school; and cost issues that vary with national priorities (and, we might add, state and local priorities). If early programs are effective in resolving or lessening early learning and behavior problems, even if they do not prevent them, these programs must be considered as successful from both a personal and an economic perspective.

Despite the research to support the utility of early identification of children at risk for difficulties (Harrison, 1992; Schonkoff & Meisels, 2000), there is conflicting evidence regarding the predictive utility of early developmental screening—not only due to the variability in the procedures used, but for the following reasons:

1. There is tremendous variability across school districts in referral rates of children as having possible problems. In a statewide study conducted by Thurlow et al. (1986), referral rates ranged from 0% to 86% of children screened.
2. There is great variability in the information collected at the time of screening and teacher ratings at the end of kindergarten. For example, Gallerani et al. (1982) studied the relationship of information gathered at the time of screening of children entering kindergarten with the end-of-year ratings of kindergarten teachers of readiness for first grade. The screening procedures resulted in 75.9%, 73.9%, and 47.8% correct identifications for those classified as "not ready for any reason," "not ready for academic reasons," and "not ready for emotional/social reasons," respectively; thus they still left considerable room for error.
3. Approaches to prediction at the preschool level of later school achievement differ greatly. Tramontana, Hooper, and Selzer (1988), for example, reviewed 74 longitudinal studies (1973–1986) on preschool prediction of later academic achievement. Of those studies reviewed, the approach to prediction varied: 20% of studies focused on one area of functioning, 33% used a single test measure, and 40% used test batteries or a combination of measures. Criterion measures were generally found to be narrowly based, with reading the first and math the second most emphasized area of achievement. Little attention was given to multimethod assessment, to differentiating global abilities into component skills, to behavioral or emotional functioning, or to predicting achievement past the first grade. Across the studies reviewed, significant predictive relationships of measures administered in kindergarten with early elementary school achievement were found for preacademic skills such as letter naming, IQ, language abilities, visual–motor skills, finger localization, and behavioral measures of attention, with measures of general ability accounting for the bulk of the prediction results. Predictive outcomes varied according to the academic criterion assessed, grade level when evaluated, age of child when initially tested, and other demographic variables. In an earlier review of 15 studies (Mercer et al.,

1979a), the accuracy of prediction (hit rates) was 75% for single test measures, 79% for test batteries, and 80% for teacher ratings.

4. The predictive usefulness of many traditional tasks included on screening measures is low. Simner (1983) reviewed more than 20 studies that employed 23 behavior inventories or screening tests plus teacher/examiner ratings as they related to school achievement in grades 1 through 3. Overall, Simner found low predictive utility for many of the traditional warning signs included on these measures, and concluded that individual signs such as hopping or skipping are ineffective for identifying children in kindergarten who later encounter academic difficulty. Gross and fine motor coordination; peer acceptance and cooperation with adults; basic language skills (e.g., the ability to define words or name colors, parts of the body, or common objects); and auditory discrimination of similarities showed only a marginal relationship with subsequent school performance. In contrast, warning signs obtained from the same studies that correctly identified 70%–80% of those children who later encountered difficulty included attention span/distractibility; memory span for remembering and following directions; memory for details and general content; verbal fluency/spontaneous use of precise words (the capacity to convey abstractions); interest and eagerness to participate; letter and number identification skills; and printing of individual numbers and letters. While Simner focused on the predictive utility of the signs individually, he did not focus on the predictive utility of clusters of signs, of total batteries, or on the usefulness of these signs for program planning and intervention. Rather, he suggested that brief surveys should focus on those signs with stronger predictive value.

Additional issues that should lead to caution in the use of screening outcomes have been identified (i.e., Adelman, 1982; Emmons & Alfonso, 2005; Gredler, 1992; Keogh & Becker, 1973; Lichtenstein & Ireton, 1984; Lidz, 2003; Meisels, 1987, 1999; Meisels & Atkins-Burnett, 2005). These include limitations in the accuracy of screening procedures that relate to problems with the measures used; variability of child behavior across developmental areas; the small sample of child behavior generally collected; appropriateness of materials across cultures; assessors' limited training or experience with young children; the nature of the screening situation; and the availability of adequate follow-up services and appropriate intervention options. In particular, a child's first formal educational assessment experience is likely to occur under less than ideal conditions. For example, children brought to a new environment may find the situation frightening, confusing, or highly stimulating. In addition, these children may be accompanied by parents who are concerned about outcomes. The particular tasks used or format of presentation may be unfamiliar, and young children are generally assessed by one (or more) adults with whom they are unfamiliar. Nevertheless, major decisions are based on this screening.

Moreover, the specific screening procedures used are dictated by economic resources, and often also by the availability of appropriate personnel—an issue detailed later in this chapter. Screening is costly for tax-driven school districts, which often need to settle for less than ideal procedures. Clearly, more comprehensive observation-based screening procedures would allow for a broader sample of all children's functioning, would provide information about the key environmental contexts of home and school, and would yield more helpful information to both teachers and parents for intervention planning.

Increasing attention is also being addressed to the prediction accuracy of screening measures in general (Algozzine, Schmid, & Mercer, 1981; Emmons & Alfonso, 2005; Gredler, 1992; Harrison, 1992; Lichtenstein & Ireton, 1984; Meisels, 1999; Nagle, 2000). The typical risk prediction matrix used is illustrated in Figure 6.1, Part A. Issues

Part A: The typical risk prediction matrix

Screening test outcomes	Functioning at the end of K, grade 1, or grade 2	
	Encountering learning/behavioral problems	Progressing normally
At risk	Children with problems correctly identified (true positive)	Children identified as at risk who do not have problems (false positive = overreferral)
Not at risk	Children with problems missed (false negative = underreferral)	Children not identified as at risk who are progressing normally (true positive)

Part B: Influencing factors

- Specific cutoff criterion used
- Scope of screening procedures
- Range of child functioning covered
- Normal variability in children's performance from day to day
- Environmental influences of home and school (i.e., multiple risk and protective factors)
- Cultural differences in child development practices
- Language differences
- Intervention effectiveness
- New learning demands that change with time
- Teacher beliefs and expectations

FIGURE 6.1. The typical risk prediction matrix and influencing factors that need to be taken into account. (See also Chapter 3.)

influencing outcomes that are not accounted for through this approach, such as environmental influences and intervening intervention activities, are summarized in part B of the figure (see also Chapter 3). Procedures to address these issues include (1) use of a "rescreen" category, (2) home and/or school prereferral interventions, (3) ongoing observation as children participate in kindergarten activities in consultation with parents and teachers, (4) frequent rescreening with subsequent adjustment of activities to meet child needs, and (5) consideration of home and school stressors and buffers.

Teacher ratings are often cited as an important component of the screening process, but they do not necessarily resolve issues regarding prediction of risk. Coleman and Dover (1993) have considered risk status based on teacher ratings and caution that classification matrices need to be analyzed carefully. Total accuracy rates may be misleading, in that many children who encounter difficulty may still be missed. These researchers present the results of a 6-year study in which four cohorts of children (n = 1,306) from a major metropolitan area in Tennessee were rated by teachers on the Risk Screening Test (Coleman & Dover, 1989) during the spring of the kindergarten year, and were tracked in grades 3–6 as to whether or not they received special education services in addition to speech therapy. Data were collected from school records, including Stanford Achievement Test scores and Otis–Lennon IQ scores (administered in grade 2). The Risk Screening Test consists of a 34-item, 6-point rating scale covering five factors: School Competence, Task Orientation, Social, Behavior, and Motor. Although overall accuracy was high (96.76% nonrisk, 78.72% risk), false negatives were 21.28%. Teacher ratings using the Risk Screening Test missed one in five children later placed in resource classrooms. More than 50% of these false negatives were girls who were socially competent in kindergarten. In contrast, a large proportion of the false positives were boys. The false positives tended to be children with lower achievement in the regular classroom, who, according to these researchers, might have benefited from prereferral intervention.

Critical Issues When Screening Is Conducted

Whatever the specific purposes of screening are, assessors need to be mindful of several critical issues that can influence outcomes. These issues are summarized in the sections that follow.

The Timing and Follow-up of Screening

Insufficient attention is often directed to the immediate follow-up to screening. Frequent points for screening include the spring prior to kindergarten entrance or entrance into first grade; late summer prior to entrance into prekindergarten; the early months of the school year; or the end of prekindergarten or kindergarten. If screening occurs during the spring semester prior to kindergarten entrance, such as in April or May, a number of problems often arise. For example, what developmental progress does a child age 4–10 years in May make over the course of the summer (by September, he or she is 5-3 years old)? Does this child present the same "at-risk" or "borderline" picture? Has significant progress occurred in a particular area? Has the family received a report filled with terminology that parents or other caregivers do not understand? Has the family been provided with ideas for enriching a child's experience, along with suggested areas for ongoing observation? If screening occurs just prior to school entrance during late summer or during the first few weeks of school, the lag of the summer period is avoided. However, some schools feel that they have inadequate time to hire teachers or plan programs for children.

From our perspective, the most desirable time for developmental screening is during the course of the kindergarten year *if necessary resources have been dedicated to prereferral programming and intervention*. Vision, hearing, and health screening should occur at the beginning of the year, and screening should be available at parents' request, consistent with the mandates of IDEA 2004. At this point the child has been observed over time by the teacher (working, as needed, with consultants in the classroom context). Prereferral intervention strategies have been tried, including curriculum modifications, additional teacher supports or assistance, and parent education. Children still encountering difficulty are referred for in-depth evaluation in the areas identified. A process of ongoing assessment has been initiated with immediate relevance to instruction. Curriculum-relevant tests can provide teachers and specialists with information relevant to beginning points for instruction or intervention, which can be confirmed or rejected through ongoing observation. *The need for large-scale developmental screening as it is currently practiced would be eliminated*. Parent input can be gained through interview or parent report measures such as the Ages and Stages Questionnaires. Throughout the kindergarten year, children encountering difficulty can be identified and referred. Figure 6.2 summarizes the typical and proposed outcomes of developmental screening. Meisels and Atkins-Burnett (2005) present an excellent figure that summarizes the screening process.

Definition of "At Risk" or "Developmental Delay"

The definition of what constitutes being "at risk" or having "developmental delay" is left up to states and districts by IDEA 2004. States are not required to classify children ages 3–9 into disability categories to receive services, although some states require the use of

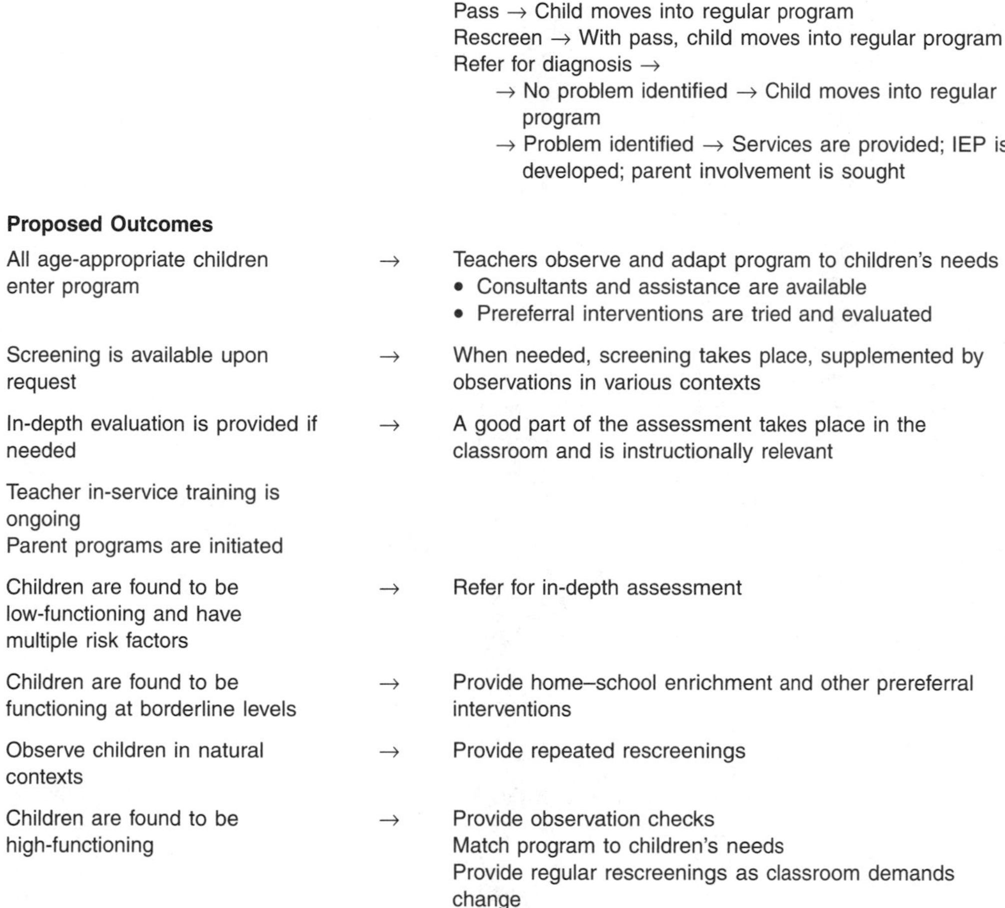

Typical Outcomes		
Screening takes place	→	One of the following outcomes: Pass → Child moves into regular program Rescreen → With pass, child moves into regular program Refer for diagnosis → → No problem identified → Child moves into regular program → Problem identified → Services are provided; IEP is developed; parent involvement is sought
Proposed Outcomes		
All age-appropriate children enter program	→	Teachers observe and adapt program to children's needs • Consultants and assistance are available • Prereferral interventions are tried and evaluated
Screening is available upon request	→	When needed, screening takes place, supplemented by observations in various contexts
In-depth evaluation is provided if needed	→	A good part of the assessment takes place in the classroom and is instructionally relevant
Teacher in-service training is ongoing Parent programs are initiated		
Children are found to be low-functioning and have multiple risk factors	→	Refer for in-depth assessment
Children are found to be functioning at borderline levels	→	Provide home–school enrichment and other prereferral interventions
Observe children in natural contexts	→	Provide repeated rescreenings
Children are found to be high-functioning	→	Provide observation checks Match program to children's needs Provide regular rescreenings as classroom demands change

FIGURE 6.2. Typical and proposed outcomes of large-scale developmental screening.

disability designations for children to receive special education services. Therefore, political and economic forces along with geographic location are likely to interact with the definition of possible delay and the provision of services. As detailed in Chapter 3, commonly used standards include the following:

- Falling 2 *SD* below the mean in one developmental area (the bottom 2.3% of children).
- Falling 1.5 *SD* below the mean (the bottom 6.7% of children) in two or more developmental areas.
- Falling into the lowest quartile in a developmental area, or below 75% of one's age group.

Thus the cutoff established will determine who receives further assessment. If a stringent referral rule is established (–2 *SD*), the probability is increased that children will be missed—particularly those with mild to moderate problems, who may later encounter more serious problems. In contrast, a more liberal referral rule (–1 *SD*) will result in an increase in overidentification of children as at risk and in need of in-depth evaluation. For financially strapped districts, the cutoff decision presents a problem. For example, those children falling between 1.0 and 1.5 *SD* below the mean, who may profit the most from intervention and who can benefit from additional support, attention, and parent involvement, may be missed. It may be this group of children who are most affected at the grades where new curricular demands are made, such as decoding at grade 1, the introduction of multiplication and division during grade 3, changing teachers by subject matter area that often occurs at grade 4, or the cognitive demands of arithmetic word problems encountered at grades 3 and 4. The "misses," who are identified later, may have missed a crucial year or more of early intervention. Furthermore, as Harrison (1992) points out, agencies use different criteria in arriving at decisions as to who will be referred, including falling below the cutoff on global measures, in one particular area of development, or in two or more areas of development. Meisels (1991) addresses two other concerns: (1) difficulty in interpreting the meaning of *SD* units if a district uses more than one test, since the use of different standardization groups may result in defining different children as eligible; and (2) the fact that delays defined in terms of percentages, such as being in the lowest 25% of one's age group, differ in meaning as a child increases in age and their knowledge repetoire is greater. Some early childhood specialists (Shonkoff & Meisels, 1991) consider the use of psychometric criteria to determine eligibility a questionable practice altogether. They also point out that tests *sample different behaviors in the same domain*, differ in the variability of the standardization sample, and often are not sufficiently precise to make fine distinctions regarding delay.

Developmental Screening: Summary

Developmental screening involves using brief, easily administered measures to assess a child's status across all major developmental areas. Outcomes indicating that a child might be "at risk" for later learning or behavioral difficulties lead to an important safety net of in-depth evaluation. Developmental screening, however, needs to be considered as a process that involves ongoing observation and is confronted by a number of challenges. Particular points of concern include the following:

1. Overinterpretation of the outcomes must be avoided. Since screening generally involves very brief measures, the information obtained can be viewed only as preliminary and should *not* be misused for purposes of diagnosis and labeling. It does not identify the kind of problem a child has or the type of program a child needs.

2. Screening procedures in general are child-focused and do not cover environmental factors. Applying a multifactor ecocultural model to screening will substantially affect outcomes: It not only will improve the identification of children in need of services, but also will broaden the scope of possible interventions to include families and schools.

3. The technical quality of many screening instruments is poor, including low reliability levels, insufficient validity documentation, and limited normative data. Some of these concerns have been addressed in the revisions of widely used instruments. The predictive utility of the tests used needs to be a major consideration. Across studies, criterion measures in general involve measures of achievement and not behavior or the child's emotional state. Except at the extremes, prediction is only as good as the intervention. However, most predictive studies do not detail the nature and extent of the intervening instruction or other intervention variables. Indeed, if early intervention is successful,

one would hope for poor long-term prediction. The goal would be to "shoot down" the prediction. Furthermore, the cognitive demands of learning tasks change as children progress through school, necessitating repeated, ongoing screening. It may not be possible to predict at age 4 or 5 those problem-solving skills required to be a successful learner at age 8, or the challenges children will encounter as the demands of the curriculum change.

4. Many individuals involved in screening have not had experience with young children or families from diverse backgrounds. A 3- or 4-hour training session is not sufficient to develop such fundamental knowledge. Training needs to be carefully planned and carried out over time, so that assessors have acquired criterion-level skills.

5. Definitions of what constitutes risk differ across school districts and states or provinces. The same problem may or may not be viewed as a problem across settings (Adelman, 1982).

ESTABLISHING AND CARRYING OUT A SCREENING PROGRAM

Many of the issues that need to be accounted for in developmental screening apply as well to readiness screening, covered in the next chapter. The issues that are most troublesome, some of which can be addressed by using the procedures described in this section, include the following:

1. General acknowledgment in the field of the need for engaging in ecologically sound procedures and practices. Due to time and budgetary constraints, most screening programs focus largely on child factors, particularly deficits.
2. An overemphasis in the field on the statistical qualities of single measures or batteries, instead of looking at a predictive decision matrix based on multiple measures that encompass both child and environmental factors.
3. The fact that accurate long-term prediction of child learning outcomes from single tests or batteries is problematic for children who do not fall at the extremes of the distribution.
4. A limited, although emerging, research base to provide guidance on developmental patterns among culturally diverse groups.
5. Lack of screening measures in languages other than English, and increasingly in Spanish.

Implementing an Early Childhood Assessment Policy

Each school system needs to adopt an early childhood assessment policy that takes into account federal, state, and local requirements to find children with disabilities; sources of funding; past services; community characteristics; and available resources. In order for any screening program to be successful, the school system needs to be supportive of a flexible early childhood curriculum that incorporates all child development areas, as well as parent support services at all levels of the educational process. Time also needs to be spent on reviewing local teachers' beliefs, biases, expectations, curricular practices, and perceptions, especially in regard to diversity, delays, and disability. As an outcome, this review might lead to ongoing staff development activities. The overall policy adoption process should result in a written account of the district's early childhood assessment philosophy, objectives, and procedures.

The Planning Phase

Large-scale developmental or kindergarten developmental screening needs to be planned systematically. A planning committee headed by a designated coordinator needs to be established to develop and monitor the purposes, objectives, delivery plan, and outcomes of the screening program. The planning committee generally consists of an administrator, an early childhood specialist/teacher, a language/speech specialist, a social worker, a nurse or physician, at least one parent, and a psychologist. It is desirable to have a parent (or parents representing the major cultural constituents of the district) as a member of the planning team to reflect parents' concerns, to make sure that a comprehensive description of each child is gained, to understand the concerns of the different cultural groups served, and to foster the collaborative activities of the program. Developing a plan to carry out screening involves multiple steps, which will be detailed next.

Step 1: Considering Population and District Characteristics

In developing a screening program, policy concerns, demographic variables, intervention options, and funding sources all need to be considered. Specifically, the following factors need to be taken into account:

1. Characteristics of the population to be served, such as educational levels, SES, cultural diversity, and size and diversity of language communities. If there are large numbers of children from culturally diverse groups, it is important to consider the child development and child-rearing practices of these groups (see Chapter 9).
2. In the case of kindergarten screening, the number of elementary schools, total kindergarten-age population, average class size, and staffing patterns. School systems also need to deal with the logistics of outreach.
3. Types of preschool programs available, their location, and the number of children involved. In addition, the planning team should consider the programs that have served the population ages 0–3, to determine the children's present status and continued need for special services.
4. Support staff available to assist in assessment, availability of trained bilingual professionals, and the scope and need for training of others to participate in the screening process.
5. Local policy reflecting the degree of commitment to early intervention and maximizing its effectiveness. Some districts are highly committed; other may either have few resources or are not focusing on this age group.
6. Projected number of children to be identified as determined by cutoff criteria, along with the range of intervention programs/services available within the school and through local and regional agencies.
7. Transportation needs.
8. Financial resources from the state, district, and other sources.
9. Colleges, universities, and agencies that might provide personnel as advisors or participants in the screening process, as well as providers of intervention options.
10. Space requirements and screening locations, including, if possible, those in which families and children from particular cultural/language groups might feel more at ease (e.g., shopping centers, religious settings, work spaces, community centers).

Step 2: Arriving at a Local Definition of "At Risk" or "Delay" and Steps for Arriving at Screening Decisions

As noted earlier, the percentage of children identified as being "at risk" differs across states and districts. Local districts therefore need to determine the number of children they can serve in relation to state and local financial means, the availability of different forms of intervention, and their willingness to engage in prevention programs. However, since the largest groups of "at-risk" children are likely to be those who are environmentally at risk because of socioeconomic or second-language influences (Harrison, 1992), many districts will be working with children who are culturally and/or linguistically different from current mainstream groups or who come from impoverished backgrounds. If this is likely, a district may seek to engage in systematic prereferral enrichment for children and education programs for parents prior to referral for in-depth assessment, except for children who encounter severe problems. Such an approach is consistent with the two-stage screening approach detailed by Lichtenstein and Ireton (1984).

Step 3: Laying Out the Screening Budget

The screening budget needs to take into account the projected number of children for whom intervention is possible, intervention options, and parent education programs, as well as the cost of the assessment process. Financial supports available through federal, state, and local resources need to be determined, along with possible supports from local colleges, universities, and social service organizations. In relation to the screening process itself, the following need to be considered:

- Cost of test materials, bearing in mind that they should be up to date, attractive to children, culturally fair, and cover most developmental areas.
- Observation approaches, including those of naturally occurring behavior.
- Usefulness of assessment outcomes for intervention planning, whether or not a child is referred for further assessment.
- Extent and type of training required to administer, score, and interpret the procedures selected.
- Payment to screeners (if not part of full-time staff).
- Administrative support for scheduling appointments, letter writing, telephone calls, typing reports, follow-up, and so forth.
- Costs for advertising, preparing video examples of the screening process, preparing other outreach activities (visuals, fliers, etc.), and preparing of activities booklets for parents.
- Need for translations or bilingual assessors and other helpers sensitive to cultural diversity.
- Creation of local norms where needed. Good tests should not be eliminated simply because the reported norms do not match local population characteristics.

Step 4: Considering Points of Parent Involvement

Parent involvement is critical throughout all phases of the assessment process, from planning to intervention. In addition to their input and concerns about their children, parents can serve as a members of the planning and/or screening team, as evaluators of the screening process, and as facilitators of intervention. The assessment team needs to be aware of parents' potential questions about screening and things parents need to know about the screening process, such as services available, necessary steps to obtain services, and personnel to contact both before and after screening. These questions and concerns, along with types of parent input, are listed in Figure 6.3.

The long-term goal needs to be to establish a collaborative relationship between parents and school, in which lines of communication are open and participation is encouraged. Although parents want to do the right thing for their children, many do not know how to go about doing it and may be unfamiliar with what is expected by schools. Research (Goldenberg & Gallimore, 1991; Reynolds et al., 2004; Snow et al., 1991) indicates, however, that various forms of parent involvement (e.g., attending school meetings, PTA meetings, and open-school nights, and otherwise making contact with teachers) relate both to child achievement in school and to teacher expectations. Teachers, for example, often hold higher expectations for children whose parents are involved. Schools clearly have to reach out to parents by providing parent education programs and by encouraging parent volunteers and observation in classrooms (a practice encouraged in many Head Start programs, but often avoided by kindergarten teachers who are concerned about being observed).

Parent input
- Granting permission for screening/assessment
- Providing developmental information:
  - Developmental milestones
  - Health history
  - Results of previous evaluations
  - History of any special services received
  - Current description of the child
  - Current concerns
- Providing information about family structure and perceived needs and resources
- Participating in screening and/or feedback
- Confirming accuracy of findings or providing contrasting observations
- Providing ongoing observations
- Participating in prereferral activities

Typical parent questions
- "What is normal for a child of this age?"
- "Is my child having trouble?"
- "Why? What is the cause? What did I do wrong?"
- "Who can provide support or more information?"
- "What must I do next? What remedies are possible?"
- "What activities can I be carrying out at home?"

Things parents need to know about screening
- What screening consists of
- What the process consists of, including where and when it will take place and when they will receive the results
- How confidentiality will be respected
- How results will be communicated
- What they need to do to help their child, and how to go about doing this
- Specific names/recommendations, if referrals are made to other agencies or if the child is referred for in-depth evaluation

FIGURE 6.3. Parent input during and after screening, typical parent questions, and things parents need to know about screening.

Step 5: Developing the Screening Team

Although state and district regulations vary as to who is included on screening teams, all states require a multidisciplinary approach for identifying children to be served under IDEA 2004. Thus most districts include members of children's IEP teams, as well as other relevant professionals. Typical members of the core screening team are usually, though not always, the same as the members of the planning team; they usually include at least one parent, a school psychologist, a social worker, a teacher or early childhood specialist, a healthcare professional, other specialists (e.g., a speech clinician, audiologist, occupational therapist, and/or physical therapist), and (where needed), a bilingual professional or trained paraprofessional. One member of the core team is designated as the coordinator. A support team will carry out many aspects of the actual screening and may include teachers, administrators, parents, and other volunteers. In all cases, the composition of the team needs to address the diversity and needs of the community served. Whatever the exact composition of the team, it is important for all team members to recognize the important contribution of different disciplines. Screening efforts can be carried out in various ways: Each team member can work independently (a multidisciplinary approach); members can work independently, but can share outcomes and develop recommendations together (an interdisciplinary approach); or members can work collectively, with active consultation and knowledge about each other's fields (a transdisciplinary approach). Through a transdisciplinary approach, each member of the team has a specific role, but all members of the team (not just a specific professional), seek to observe behaviors that represent the major developmental domains. In the screening procedures that we detail in step 6, we recommend establishing four to five observation points throughout the activities where each team member can record observations (i.e., children's use of language, attention, physical abilities, and interaction with others) across developmental areas.

Step 6. Establishing Screening Procedures and Selecting Measures

As we have emphasized throughout this chapter, screening is a comprehensive *process* that involves looking at multiple risk and protective factors for children, families, and learning environments. The planning team selects screening instruments and procedures accordingly, using guidelines for evaluating tests such as those detailed in Chapter 3. Team members must do the following:

1. Review instruments to determine whether there is a match between the stated objectives of the test being considered for use and the objectives of the local assessment team.
2. Review information regarding the scope and technical qualities of assessment materials.
3. Consider, in relationship to local population characteristics, whether modifications or translations need to be made and whether local norms need to be collected (bearing in mind the caution by Meisels and Atkins-Burnett [2005] caution that it is better to collect more data on reasonably good existing measures than to create a local instrument).

Although a single screening measure may require 15–30 minutes to administer, the full screening process—including vision and hearing screening, parent input and initial feedback, and observing the child engaged in natural activities (play, warm-up)—is going to require between 60 and 75 minutes. Fortunately, developmental screening also has the safety network of in-depth evaluation when a "refer" decision is reached. This safety network, however, does not extend to those children who are missed and might benefit from intervention. Frequent points of observation and rescreening are necessary to identify these children.

INFORMATION OBTAINED FROM PARENTS OR GUARDIANS

Information regarding children's development, health, current functioning, and home history is generally obtained by questionnaire or interview with family members. The questionnaire is often sent to families prior to the screening day, in order for parents to have time to reflect as they complete the questionnaire. However, filling out forms may be an unfamiliar activity for many families, such as those from other cultures (especially new immigrants). Families with low-level reading skills may find this an impossible task. Thus, for many families, it is preferable to fill out the questionnaire in the context of the interview. Each interview needs to be conducted by an individual skilled in interviewing and sensitive to cultural diversity and background, such as a social worker or a school psychologist. Where possible, the interview should be conducted in a parent's home language (again, if possible, with an interviewer from the same culture), in order to get the best possible sample of information and to help put the parent at ease. In districts where families speak many languages and dialects, interpreters may be needed to obtain family information. Interpreters need to be appropriately trained (see Chapter 9).

Parents, guardians, or other primary caregivers are experts about their children. In addition to providing information about children's overall development and medical history, preschool and childcare experiences, and prior interventions, parents can (1) provide detailed information about children's cognitive, language, motor, social, and emotional development; (2) describe the children's present level of functioning, attention span, behavior, interests, and strengths; (3) provide observations of typical behavior at home; and (4) raise their own concerns. It is also important to obtain information about the individuals a child comes into contact with daily in the home (and a schedule of a typical day during the week and weekend). Furthermore, the presence or absence of key protective factors that operate across socioeconomic backgrounds should be ascertained. These factors include (1) a regular, caring relationship with a particular individual (e.g., a grandparent or other caring adult); (2) regular daily routines; (3) monitored TV watching; (4) family storybook reading; and (5) hopes/positive expectations for the child (e.g., that the child will complete high school). It is also useful to learn whether a parent has been involved in a parent program or has volunteered in a preschool program. A sample interview/questionnaire format incorporating these factors is presented in Appendix 6.2.

Finally, it is important to obtain information regarding how the family perceives its strengths and needs. A number of forms have been developed for this purpose; these are summarized in Chapter 8.

INFORMATION GAINED THROUGH CHILD MEASURES

1. *Vision and hearing.* When developmental screening takes place upon request, a child may be referred to the family physician or a clinic for screening of health, vision, and hearing. During large-scale developmental screening, it is a widespread practice to have a nurse or audiologist be a member of the screening team and assess vision/hearing at the time of screening. This assessment should occur early during the overall screening process, since vision and hearing problems will affect all other forms of functioning.

2. *Testing procedures.* Instrument selection will have occurred during the planning phase. Since no one instrument will accomplish all screening purposes, measures including tests, checklists, rating scales, and other forms of observation need to cover multiple domains and observation opportunities. Observational information and informal measures need to be coupled with standardized measures (Glascoe, 1991).

With children from LEP or bilingual backgrounds, screeners will also need to determine what language each child speaks and how proficient each child is in English (see Chapter 9). Therefore, a longer screening time might be needed than is generally allocated to assess such a child in both the primary home language and English, to pick up what the child has learned in preschool settings. Alternate screening procedures may need to be used, such as using structured observation while the child is at play. The norms of standardized testing may not apply.

OBSERVATION POINTS DURING THE SCREENING PROCESS

There are many observational opportunities during the screening process, and the data obtained at these points can be incorporated into the screening outcomes. One possible approach is to collect specific observations at each phase of the screening process and from each member of the screening team. These observations can then be combined and used, along with other information, to arrive at a screening decision. The types of observational information that can be collected are presented below in the context of the screening day for a child. Children and parents arrive in groups of three or four, and each parent and child are greeted.

1. Children receive name tags and go to play area	5–10 minutes (serves as warm-up)	Observation point 1 • Motor behavior • Spontaneous language forms/content • Separation from parent • Emotional tenor • Activity level • Interaction with other children • Materials used
2. Vision/hearing screening	10 minutes	Observation point 2 • As above
3. Parent interview + 4. Child screening	20–30 minutes each (these take place concurrently)	Observation point 3 • As in point 1, except now the focus is on the adult–child interaction • Attention • Compliance • Need for adult assistance/praise
5. Brief parent–child task (snack)	10 minutes	Observation point 4 • As above (optional, but desirable)
6. Exit contact		Check out parent concerns; indicate date when next contact will be made

The order of activities 2–5 can be varied to maintain the flow of children and parents through the process. A trained aide can make sure that children are in the right places at the right times, collect and collate observation sheets, and give them to the assessor or exit interviewer.

Step 7: Working Out Details (Physical Arrangements, Schedules, Childcare, and Transportation Plans)

The location for screening should be as culturally friendly and child-friendly as possible, with good lighting and ventilation; child-sized furniture should be available. Possible distractions should be minimized (e.g., noise, distracting objects, mirrors, etc.). Testing materials should be out of sight except for the tasks at hand.

In many locations, arrangements will need to be made to bring parents and children to the screening site. Since screening may entail a hardship for many families (lost work time, distance), as many components of the process as possible (ideally, all) should be carried out at this location, including vision and hearing screening. On-site childcare arrangements will be necessary for many families.

Step 8: Training the Screeners

High-quality training of all individuals involved in screening is critical. This is particularly true when paraprofessionals, volunteers, and teachers who have worked mainly with older children are involved. Areas that need to be considered in training screeners are summarized below.

1. *Background characteristics of the population to be screened.* If culturally diverse groups are to be served, it is important for assessors to be aware of the cultural expectations for children in these groups, the kinds of behaviors that might be displayed by children and their parents during screening, and the types of concerns parents might raise during interviews. For example, children from economically disadvantaged or immigrant families may not have been socialized into sitting still, playing with blocks, cutting with scissors, and so forth. These issues are detailed in Chapter 9. If large numbers of children from a particular cultural group are to be screened, training should also include culturally relevant expectations of appropriate behavior on the part of the assessors. For example, screeners may need to consider alternative ways of posing questions. In addition, all members of the screening team need to spend time exploring their own attitudes, beliefs, and biases with regard to diversity. Whenever possible, members of the major cultural groups served should be involved both with training and in the screening itself.

Screeners also need to explore their conceptions of bilingualism. They need to realize, for example, that second-language learning develops in a similar pattern to first-language learning in English, and that proficiency in English takes considerable time—18–36 months with preschoolers (Duncan, 1989). Characteristics typical of children learning a second language, which do not necessarily occur when a child speaks their own language, include frequent requests for repetitions, pauses before speaking, articulation difficulties, word-finding problems, and code switching or mixing. Other issues related to bilingualism are detailed in Chapter 9, along with a checklist for making the screening environment culturally friendly.

2. *Overview of the screening procedures to be used.* This overview needs to describe screening as a process, to summarize the specific procedures selected, and to give the rea-

sons for their selection. Assessors should check that all major areas of a multifactor ecocultural approach are covered (child factors, family and learning environment factors, and the child's interactions with others, such as adults and peers). The organization of the screening day needs to be described in detail, including timing, number of children to be covered, responsibilities of team members, and so forth.

3. *Overview of the variability of child functioning across developmental areas.* This overview should cover the typical range of functioning to be expected across all areas of development, the fact that development is uneven, and the possibility that some children who do not face difficulty at the time of screening may encounter difficulties later. Furthermore, children may spontaneously exhibit a behavior that is not later elicited through direct questioning. This information needs to be noted on the protocol and taken into consideration when a decision whether or not to refer is being made. Therefore, screening outcomes need to be used in conjunction with observations from observers throughout screening and from parents, and to be followed by ongoing observation in the classroom. Examples that illustrate preschool children's normal short attention span, are helpful. For instance, it is quite typical for these children to move around, touch objects, and do what they want. Thus screeners need to be comfortable with young children's behavior, and to learn useful techniques to refocus their attention.

4. *Establishing rapport.* Procedures for establishing rapport need to be detailed, in order to put children and their caregivers at ease in an unfamiliar setting. These activities are extremely important with young children, some of whom are unfamiliar with the kinds of questions/materials used and are not willing to be compliant with the assessor. Furthermore, little children swiggle and do not have long attention spans, as noted above; allowing some warm-up time and breaking up tasks into small chunks will help address these problems. The screeners need to get used to children moving around and accommodate children's different response styles. Here are some procedures that can foster rapport with children and families:

- Begin with straightforward, easy items.
- Smile and be friendly with the child, use the child's name, make a positive comment about something (e.g., a shirt or barrette), and appreciate his or her attempts. Do not focus on inappropriate behaviors. With caregivers, be friendly, but act as a professional they can respect.
- With a very young child, begin the screening day with a brief period of play involving a familiar object or activity. With an older preschooler, solving a simple puzzle or drawing can be used as a brief warm-up activity. Cognitive behaviors, motor functioning, and other child responses can be observed during the warm-up period.
- As noted above, be responsive to the child's physical needs and attention span—take a brief break, move back to easier items, praise a child's efforts, engage the child in everyday conversation—but also keep the flow going.
- Reassure the child (and caregiver) that the experience will be enjoyable. In this context, possible opening remarks might be practiced during training.

5. *Training in observation.* Screening procedures include astute observation, not only the administration of a test. (Specific suggestions regarding observation of the child are given in Chapter 4.) Training needs to focus on the range of observations that can be made during screening and on ways of recording these observations systematically. Training videotapes are very useful. Observations by all members of the team need to be

collected and compared, as noted earlier. Important aspects of observation that need to be covered in training include making objective observations; separating observations from inferences; and supporting observations with brief, specific accounts of behavior. These key aspects need to be practiced, using typical local examples.

6. *Engaging in professionally appropriate behavior.* Because confidentiality is of utmost importance, talking about children or referring to families by name outside the screening situation needs to be avoided. This may present a challenge for volunteers who interact daily with the families involved. A second issue is the importance of adhering to procedures specified in test manuals. The rationale behind standardized testing and objective scoring needs to be discussed.

7. *Handling special problems.* The team needs to learn how to handle emergencies and special problems, such as a sick child or an abusive parent. Local safety procedures and regulations need to be covered. Here the screeners also need to be sensitive to their own reactions to the situation. If a screener feels that a child is too ill or that there is too much going on to get a good sample of behavior, another screening session may need to be scheduled.

8. *Practice in the administration of tests/procedures.* Individuals who will administer the screening tests/procedures need ample time for practice. During practice sessions, screeners should do the following:

- Go over the administrative procedures and layout of materials, and then read through the written materials and review test items. This can occur prior to a practice session.
- Practice administration of the test and procedures with each other. Ample time should be allowed for questions and answers as screeners learn to use the materials.
- Either receive feedback on the practice administration from a trained person, or engage in a supervised discussion of the results following the administration.
- Practice scoring against a videotape, if screeners will be doing the scoring.
- Cover techniques for improving reliability, particularly when behavior checklists and rating scales are used.
- Practice techniques for providing feedback to parents and for responding to their concerns.

Some screening tests, such as the ESI-R (Meisels et al., 1997), detail procedures for training in the manual or are accompanied by videotaped illustrations of test administration. In many cases, however, districts will need to create their own training videos.

The areas that need to be covered in screening, and the specific procedures to be used, require at least 1½ days and preferably 2 days of training. The half-day training session often allocated for this purpose is insufficient. The goal is for screeners to be totally familiar with the procedures used, so that they can present materials with a natural flow, pay total attention to each child, enhance rapport, and also act as observers. A sample schedule for training screeners is presented in Figure 6.4.

Step 9. Observing Classroom Environments and Instructional Procedures, and Exploring Intervention Possibilities

As detailed in Chapter 5, the settings in which children may be placed need to be observed, in order to determine the fit for individual children. It is also important to consider the strengths and the drawbacks of available intervention possibilities. For example,

Prior to day 1, send participants preliminary materials (and, where appropriate, screening materials that can be read beforehand).

Day 1

Session 1

Whole group

- Define what screening can and cannot accomplish, and the assessment process used in the system.
- Discuss the diverse cultural and language populations to be served, and how their cultural styles and child-rearing practices might affect screening.
- Discuss the typical range of child behaviors across developmental areas, using videos if available.
- Discuss the kinds of behaviors young children are likely to display during screening, and techniques to refocus attention.

Small groups

- Conduct an exercise to explore attitudes and beliefs about diversity; brainstorm ideas for making screening culturally friendly.
- Discuss procedures to be used with non-English-speaking or bilingual children and families.

Session 2

Whole group

- Focus on specific instruments and procedures used, and explain why they were selected.
- Show a training video.
- Discuss material layout, administrative, and scoring procedures.

Small groups

- Have screeners practice giving the tests/measures to each other, using the procedures detailed.
- Give screeners sample protocols to score, if they will be doing the scoring.
- Answer questions.
- Request screeners to administer procedures to a child (one not to be screened) for practice, with the opportunity for discussion on day 2. All screeners need to study the materials at home and be prepared to ask questions.

Session 3

Whole group

- Overview essential features of observation.
- Detail procedures for conducting and recording objective observations, and for completing rating scales if they are used.

Small groups

- Have screeners practice observational techniques, using the procedures selected by the district. Show a video or demonstrate typical examples. Discuss agreements and disagreements.
- Assign an observation exercise to be carried out at home.

Day 2

Session 4

Whole group

- Discuss ways of establishing rapport with children, using actual examples.
- Discuss how to handle special problems.

Small groups

- Discuss practice test administration and observation exercise carried out at home.
- Engage in activities for establishing and maintaining rapport. Use typical examples.

Session 5

Whole group

- Discuss ways to establish rapport with parents in general, and in relation to particular cultural groups represented locally. Use video examples if possible, or demonstrate typical scenarios.
- Discuss conducting information-gathering and feedback interviews.

Small groups

- Role-play establishing rapport with different kinds of parents (reticent, highly anxious, etc.).
- Have screeners practice techniques for gathering information, responding to parent concerns, and providing feedback.

Session 6

Whole group

- Overview the whole process to be used, who exactly is responsible for what, organization of materials, and other logistical details.
- Emphasize the need for engaging in professionally appropriate behavior.
- Evaluate the training days.
- Provide suggestions for further reading and practice.

FIGURE 6.4. Sample schedule for training screeners.

what classroom arrangements are possible? What resources (e.g., consultants or a support team) are available to teachers for engaging in prereferral intervention? Are regular in-service training sessions scheduled, in which consultants and teachers can present their ideas or can discuss problematic behaviors?

The Outreach Phase

Outreach procedures are essential to identify preschool children with disabilities or those who are at risk of developing later learning or behavior problems. These procedures have several potential targets and purposes. First, the general public needs to be alerted that early intervention can better prepare children for school learning, and in so doing can help to resolve problems and maximize each child's potential. Second, outreach needs to help parents understand the normal milestones across developmental areas, the normal variability in behavior on the part of young children, and possible signals for seeking help. Third, outreach needs to focus on locating and informing particular families with young children who might benefit from a district's programs. These purposes can be accomplished as follows:

1. *Informing the public about the importance of early intervention and the availability of services.* General publicity can present the screening program as fun, nonthreatening, and an experience with positive benefits. This presentation can be accomplished through notices, brochures, newspaper articles, TV and radio public service announcements, and posters and fliers placed in locations parents are likely to frequent.
2. *Educating parents about normal child development and signals for seeking help.* Presentations and workshops can be developed that describe normal development across key areas, including the kinds of unevenness to expect and the kinds of problems that may indicate a need for help. The desirability of early intervention and how it relates to children's later school experiences can be presented, along with description of what screening is all about, its purpose, and how it is conducted. Some families need more outreach than others. A videotape of a typical screening using local procedures may help alleviate fears. It is important to detail how results are to be used, as well as to emphasize that they are confidential and that decisions will involve parent input. Timelines, transportation concerns, and contact procedures can be addressed.
3. *Informing families with young children about the availability of screening.* Specific contacts by phone or letter (in the parents' home languages; see below) need to be made with parents of young children identified through hospital records, information from pediatricians, and social service agencies. Despite public announcements, such parents may still be unaware of services—particularly if they are new to the community, if they do not speak English, if they have low-level reading skills, or if they are homeless. To reach these parents, a team can be sent into the community and work through community social service, health, and religious groups.

In developing outreach activities, the languages and backgrounds of families to be served need to be considered. Notices and letters may need to be translated into several languages. Since the language of testing itself is often complex and frightening to parents, the wording of letters and forms needs to be simple and inviting. The book *Developmental Screening in Early Childhood: A Guide* (Meisels with Atkins-Burnett, 1994) presents a number of sample forms to be used for the purpose of outreach.

Conducting the Actual Screening and Integrating the Results

Screening is conducted, using the procedures developed during the planning phase. Next, the screening team needs to put all the information together in arriving at screening decisions and next steps. In addition, the team needs to determine the environmental factors that impede or facilitate development in both the school and/or childcare setting and the home. If multiple risk factors are present, efforts need to be directed not only at the child, but also at modifying these environmental factors through parent and/or teacher education. If children come from culturally and linguistically different backgrounds and lack the experiential base to succeed in school, effort may need to be directed toward providing the experiential base, not toward labeling the children. A caring teacher may be the path to helping children gain desired skills and behaviors.

The multiple observations collected during different points of the screening process need to be summarized and integrated. These can be used either to confirm the screening test results or to counterbalance these results. For example, if a child uses good expressive language during the warm-up activity and with the parent, but "clams up" with the screener, the observations should probably outweigh the brief sample obtained on the screening measures. If the parent presents contradictory observations, these differences need to be explored during follow-up.

Communicating Results to Parents

Most parents will have questions when they leave the screening session and want to know how their children performed. Although some screening programs are set up to provide feedback regarding results that day, members of most screening teams need to consult with each other first, with the result that outcomes are not immediately available. Nevertheless, some feedback at the time of screening is necessary, so that parents do not leave with great anxiety about the next steps of the process. During this initial feedback, parents can be provided with a general impression of the day, but should be told that the team needs to meet and review all of the information collected. However, parents need to leave knowing when they will be contacted and reassured if there is great concern. Leaving with some simple activities they might carry out at home may help reassure some parents.

The full results are generally communicated by letter, phone call, or personal contact at a later date, as soon as possible after screening. Ideally, a follow-up interview is set up—particularly if rescreening is suggested, if prereferral activities are recommended, or if further assessment is the next step. Particular attention needs to be given to parents' worries when the recommendation is in-depth evaluation. They may be concerned about what they did wrong and will want to know what they can do. The month or more that can elapse until the in-depth assessment is scheduled is likely to be a time of great anxiety. Some parents will want recommendations for outside referral services. In some cultures it is important that not only the parent(s) be present, but also other individuals influential in decision making about education and receipt of special services, such as a grandparent. Team members should also consider possible cultural differences in views about child development and disabling conditions.

Whatever the circumstances, the team needs to communicate screening outcomes with care to parents. Meisels with Atkins-Burnett (1994) and the Ohio Department of Education (1989) provide sample letter formats. These letters usually thank parent(s) for participating and report whether the child is progressing normally, whether rescreening is suggested (if the child was ill the day of screening, encountered special problems, or performed at a borderline level), or whether the child demonstrated difficulty during screening and needs to have an in-depth evaluation. Such letters need to be written without jargon and in simple language, especially when it is likely that parents have low-level reading skills; when parents do not read English or have LEP, letters should be written in the parents' home language. The use of understandable language is particularly important when a child needs to be rescreened or has encountered difficulty. If rescreening or referral for in-depth assessment is recommended, a time frame needs to be suggested, along with suggestions for activities that can be carried out at home. For children needing further attention, the next steps need to be spelled out in detail, including places, times, phone numbers, and contact persons.

Many districts follow letters with a telephone call (if parents have no telephone, other arrangements are made); this provides parents with an opportunity to ask questions and help plan next steps. It also helps to personalize the process, and allows parents to voice whether or not they agree with the outcomes and provide additional observations.

Other procedures include a general follow-up session available to all parents, where the meaning of results is discussed and activities are suggested. From our perspective, some information needs to be provided to all parents beyond "pass," "rescreen," or "need for further assessment." It is useful as well to include a checklist in the written summary explaining which skills a child has, are emerging, or need to be developed. Some districts have developed booklets of activities across developmental levels that all parents receive and that are personalized for each child. Individual districts could create such a booklet reflecting the diverse cultures represented and local interests.

Follow-Up and Prereferral Intervention Phase

For children who demonstrate extreme difficulty, referral for in-depth assessment is generally the next step. An alternative practice allowed by some states is for children to be placed in diagnostic classrooms prior to referral. This practice allows for observation over time by teachers, specialists, and parents. Prereferral interventions need to be directed not only at children, but also at parents and teachers (e.g., removing environmental barriers, changing beliefs and expectations, modifying instructional practices, and improving home–school communication).

The follow-up to screening can be approached in a number of ways for children falling at borderline levels or performing somewhat below developmental expectations. One approach is for these children to be placed in enrichment classes where activities are geared to their needs. Since parent education is an appropriate activity/intervention for many of these children, parents can be given the opportunity to join existing programs. Or a local facilitator can develop workshops that engage parents in developmental and early literacy activities with children or assist them in handling behavioral problems. Under these circumstances, a working relationship is developed with the parents. Additional information can be gained through parent and teacher consultation. Regular and ongoing observation reports may be set up in conjunction with the preschool or kindergarten program. Rescreening can take place after a defined period of time, and observations collected in natural settings can be used to guide intervention and/or further assessment.

The Evaluation Phase

Evaluation of the screening program needs to (1) account for the screening process as a whole, (2) review specific screening procedures, and (3) examine screening's effectiveness in relationship to individual children and families. In order to address these issues, the following evaluation steps might be considered:

1. Determine the effectiveness of procedures for finding children and preparing parents for the screening day. This can be done through parent interviews or a simple questionnaire covering how parents found out about the program, whether procedures were clear, whether their questions were answered, and how they would improve outreach.
2. Relate the outcomes of the parent interview/questionnaire to findings obtained through screening measures and observation points, along with the percentages of children moving on to diagnosis, to prereferral interventions, and to particular developmental problems.
3. Keep track of parents who are involved in parent programs and activities, and the progress made by their children.
4. Keep track of children referred for services in grades K–2, and relate these findings back to screening outcomes and prereferral interventions. Differentiate the types of special services used (class tutoring, resource room, speech therapy, etc.).
5. Compare the number of referrals to those in previous years when the program did not exist or when a different program was in place.
6. Relate screening to achievement and/or child behavior at the end of kindergarten, grade 1, and grade 2 as determined by achievement measures and teacher reports gained through ratings. Take into account instructional practices, teacher expectations, and the quality of the teacher–student relationship.
7. Hold a debriefing session with the screening team, if possible. If this is not possible, distribute a questionnaire to obtain team members' feedback and recommendations for improving the process.
8. In relationship to the measures and procedures used, plan for reliability checks with regard to administration and scoring of instruments and observer agreement. If the number of children is small, consider readministration of selected measures after a brief interval.
9. To the degree possible, engage in program evaluation to identify instructional and home environmental factors that contribute to child functioning and how these factors relate to success in the local school's program. This can be accomplished through periodic team discussion of child progress and maintaining a database as children progress through the early grades.
10. Account for intervening teacher factors and changes in instructional environments when addressing the longer-term accuracy of screening outcomes.

Refer to Lichtenstein and Ireton (1984) for detailed information regarding evaluation of a screening program.

SUMMARY

Large-scale developmental screening is a process that consists of multiple steps and measures to encompass both child and environmental factors. Demographic and sociocultural risk and protective factors that affect the child at home, as well as the quality of the child's past and near-future instructional environments, need to be accounted for systematically in deciding which children should be referred for in-depth evaluation and which children and/or families would profit from prereferral interventions and/or enriched learning opportunities.

Establishing and carrying out a developmental or readiness screening program entails multiple activities that have been detailed in the second portion of this chapter. These include the following:

- Establishing an early childhood assessment policy.
- Designating a coordinator and planning the screening process (especially training of the screening team).
- Engaging in outreach to parents and the community.
- Conducting the actual screening, including multiple steps and observation points.
- Integrating information and providing feedback to parents.
- Conducting follow-up and initiating of prereferral parent and child interventions.
- Evaluating the effectiveness of the screening process.

In addition, a systematic process of ongoing observation, frequent rescreening, enriched learning opportunities, and teacher education are necessary parts of the process. The interaction of these multiple factors in the long-term well-being of children needs to be documented through ongoing research. Such research, despite limited budgets, is also a school district's responsibility as it implements national and state mandates and serves families and children.

APPENDIX 6.1. Review of Measures

Measure	(AGS) Early Screening Profiles (ESP). Harrison et al. (1990).
Purpose	Identifying children with possible disabilities and other developmental problems. It also identifies gifted children and those who are in need of a comprehensive diagnostic assessment; screens children in transition from one program to another; provides a brief evaluation of program effectiveness; and has research applications. Specific sections can be used for particular screening needs.
Areas	Three profiles: Cognitive/Language (four subtests: Verbal Concepts, Visual Discrimination, Logical Relations, and Basic School Skills); Motor (Gross and Fine); and Self-Help/Social (Communication, Daily Living Skills, Socialization, and Motor Skills). Four surveys (Articulation, Home, Health History, and Behavior Survey) can also be administered. The 7 components can be used independently or in any combination.
Format	Test tasks, rating scales and parent/teacher questionnaire.
Scores	Standard scores, percentile ranks, NECs, stanines, and age equivalents.
Age group	2-0 to 6-11 years.
Time	Testing, 15–40 minutes; parent/teacher questionnaire, 10–15 minutes.
Users	Teachers or specialists; training materials include blackline masters in the manual and a videotape.
Norms	Data collected on 1,149 children. Grouped into four geographic regions, racial/ethnic groups (white, black, Hispanic, and other), gender, and SES groups (measured by parent educational attainment).
Reliability	Interrater, .80–.99 (for the Motor profile); test–retest, .84 (for total screening and parent questionnaire composite; .56–.82 for the domain screening indices).
Validity	Concurrent validity, .76 (average correlation with comparable areas in Vineland Adaptive Behavior Scale); .66 (correlation with motor profile with Bruininks–Oseretsky Battery); .68–.84 (correlation with cognitive and language domains of the Kaufman Assessment Battery for Children). Predictive validity, .56 (Stanford Achievement Test after 1 year); .56 (grades in reading); .37 (grades in math); .58 (Otis–Lennon IQ). Sensitivity, .53–67; specificity, .86–.88.
Comments	The manual provides all testing materials, explicit instructions for administration, and scoring sheets that are clear and easy to follow. The Verbal Concepts subtest includes colorful and engaging pictures for young children. The Visual Discrimination and Logical Relations subtests, on the other hand, have small, black-and-white pictures that are crowded onto one page. Many items are similar to those included on intelligence tests. Some items involve many concepts and involve a heavy memory load. The Basic School Skills subtest jumps rapidly in difficulty level. The test is available only in English. The authors indicate that if a child does not speak English, the Cognitive/Language subtests may be administered in the child's native language. Profiles consist of activities that include interaction with and manipulation of materials that a child is likely to find fun and inviting. Although the test is relatively easy to administer, deriving index scores is very complex. Excellent training materials are provided, including an instructional video. Reviewers have found that the AGS ESP features many high technical qualities, resulting in a reliable and comprehensive addition to early childhood identification and service delivery. However, technical adequacy is lacking for the Motor profile and Behavior Survey. Finally, the fact that test–retest scores range from .56 to .82 produces significant variability in decisions.

References consulted	Barnett and Telzrow (1995); Emmons and Alfonso (2005); Meisels and Atkins-Burnett (2005). See book's References list.

Measure	**Battelle Developmental Inventory, Second Edition (BDI-2) and its Screening Test. Newborg (2004).**
Purpose	Identifying the developmental strengths and opportunities for learning of typically developing children and those with disabilities in preschool, kindergarten, and primary education programs; assessing of children "at risk" in any developmental area; general screening; team assessment and development of IFSPs or IEPs; and progress monitoring.
Areas	Five areas are included that can be used individually or in combination: Personal–Social (data gained primarily through caregiver interview and observation) describes the child's awareness of and interactions with others; Adaptive (data gained through caregiver interview and observation) describes child's self-care behaviors; Motor (gained through observation of child's gross- and fine-motor activities such as sitting, walking, running, stacking and tossing objects, writing and drawing); Communication (assesses receptive and expressive language abilities by having child respond to interrogatives, follow verbal commands, match words to definitions, and engage in sustained conversation with the examiner); Cognitive (notes child's ability to attend to events and objects, locate hidden items in a picture, note differences in given stimuli, categorize, and repeat sequences). Items administered depending on child's age level.
Format	The BDI-2 offers two types of assessment, the full assessment and the screening test. Structured administration, interview, and observation. Available in Spanish and English. Basal and ceiling rules.
Scores	Domain, subdomain, developmental quotients, scaled scores, percentiles, confidence intervals.
Age group	Birth to 8-0 years.
Time	For full BDI-2, 1 hour (Ages under 2 or over 5) and 1½ hours (ages between 2 and 5). For Screening Test, 20–30 minutes).
Users	Professionals.
Norms	Data gathered from over 2,500 children between birth and 7-11 years of age. The normative sample closely matches the 2000 U.S. census (education level based on 2001 data; norm intervals of 3 months, ages 24 months and older.)
Reliability	Reliabilities for the BDI-2 meet or exceed traditional standards for excellence at the subdomain, domain, and full test composite levels.
Validity	Concurrent and criterion data obtained using the original BDI, the Bayley Scales of Infant Development—Second Edition, the Woodcock–Johnson III, the Denver II, the PLS-4, the Vineland SEEC, and the WPPSI-III.
Comments	The BDI-2 provides updated test items from the original BDI, with increased awareness of multicultural diversity and ethnic differences among children. It also has updated artwork with colorful, child-friendly materials; easier administration and scoring with starting points for each age range; more useful normative information for practitioners to make accurate decisions regarding a child's developmental level; and the addition of computer scoring. The test covers a broad age range, allowing repeated use to document progress. The BDI-2 Screening Test consists of 100 items from the BDI-2; two items in each domain at ten age levels. Instead of norming the Screening Test, the authors used the norms and reliability and validity data derived from the BDI-2 so that it is not possible to know whether the Screening Test yields reliable data.

	Glascoe and Byrne (1993) found the BDIST to have good sensitivity, but overreferred children. These data are not yet available for the revision. There are many concerns for use of the Screening Test out of context of follow-up by the appropriate section of the BDI-2. These include lack of test–retest reliability, validity data, inadequate ceiling and floor for the domain scores, and inadequate item gradients.
References consulted	Berls and McEwen (1999); Boehm review; Glascoe et al. (1992). See book's References list.

Measure	**Child Development Inventory (CDI). Ireton (1992).**
Purpose	Identifying children with developmental problems by obtaining information from parents.
Areas	Social, Self-Help, Gross Motor, Fine Motor, Expressive Language, Language Comprehension, Letters, Numbers, and General Development.
Format	300-item checklist with yes–no format.
Scores	The score for each of the eight scales is the number of yes responses; the General Development score is derived by adding the yes responses to select items from each of the scales; each scale's score is then plotted on the profile sheet; mental age and chronological age are used to determine strengths and weaknesses.
Age group	1-3 months to 6-3 years.
Time	30–50 minutes.
Users	Professionals.
Norms	Data collected on 568 primarily white children from Minneapolis–Saint Paul.
Reliability	Internal consistency, .33–.96.
Validity	73% of children enrolled in an early intervention program had CDI profiles that were delayed in one or more areas. The CDI scores (Letters, Numbers, and General Development) of beginning kindergarten students had correlations ranging from .56 to .69 with their reading scores in first grade.
Comments	The manual provides detailed descriptions of the items in each scale and the scoring procedures. Parents must possess at least grade 7–8 reading level in order to complete the CDI. The compositionally narrow and small norm group is perhaps the biggest weakness for this instrument; examiners working with their children who differ substantially from the normative group are encouraged to develop local norms. Further validity evidence is needed to support that the test measures what it claims to measure. Evidence from the reliability studies and from the norm sample indicates that the instrument is more appropriate for identifying developmental problems in children below the age of 5-5.
References consulted	Kirnan, Crespo, and Stein (1998). See book's References list.

Measure	**Denver Developmental Screening Test II (Denver II). Frankenburg et al. (1990).**
Purpose	Identifying developmental problems in children.
Areas	Five areas included in scoring. Starting points correspond to the age sector indicated on the response form for each of 4 areas: Personal–Social (getting along with people, and caring for personal needs); Fine-motor–Adaptive (eye–hand coordination including (starting at age 3): stacking blocks; thumb

	wiggling; drawing a person; copying a circle, cross, and square; manipulating small objects; problem solving); Language: hearing, understanding and using language including (starting at age 3): naming colors; counting; opposites (analogies); and defining words; and Gross Motor: sitting, walking, jumping, and (at age 4 and above), hopping balancing, and heel-to-toe walking.
Format	125-item rating scale with "pass," "fail," "no opportunity," and "refusal" responses; Criteria are given for determining whether a child's development is "normal," "questionable," or "abnormal." Assessed through observation, direct interaction with child, and parent report. The number of items administered depends on the child's age and ability.
Scores	Percentile ranks.
Age group	2 weeks to 6 years.
Time	20–25 minutes; 10–15 minutes for abbreviated test.
Users	Users should be properly trained and pass the proficiency test before using the Denver II for clinical purposes. A 2-day training workshop is suggested as outlined in the technical manual.
Norms	Data collected on 2,096 children representative of the population of Colorado.
Reliability	Interrater, 99.7%; test–retest (7–10 days), .89.
Validity	Concurrent not addressed by the authors, because they feel that there are no tests in some of the areas assessed by the Denver II. Other types not provided. As reported by Glascoe et al. (1992), sensitivity was .50 or .83 and specificity was .43 or .80, depending on the scoring method. Only items in the language domain were helpful in discriminating children with difficulties. Another study (Greer et al., 1989), which pooled results from five studies, found good specificity of .94 but poor sensitivity of .20.
Comments	This test is easily to administer and user-friendly. The authors provide a number of guidelines for the identification of children who need further diagnostic assessment and intervention. The new Language items and Personal–Social items for children between the ages of 4-5 and 6 strengthen the test. The standardization sample has an overrepresentation of Hispanic infants and an underrepresentation of black infants. This measure has a number of psychometric weaknesses. Specifically, the test has low sensitivity and it does not identify many children with developmental problems. Nevertheless, it has a certain appeal to health providers because of its pragmatic and easy-to-use features. The authors strongly encourage training and periodic training evaluation of those who use the measure. A Spanish version is available. The authors caution that the Denver II provides a brief overview of functioning and should not be used to predict later learning or emotional problems.
References consulted	Glascoe and Byrne (1993); Greer, Bauchner, and Zuckerman (1989); Meisels and Atkins-Burnett (2005); U.S. DHHS (n.d.). See book's References list.

Measure	**Developmental Indicators for the Assessment of Learning—Third Edition (DIAL-3). Mardell-Czudnowski and Goldenberg (1998).**
Purpose	Identifying young children with developmental delays and those who are in deed of a further diagnostic evaluation.
Areas	Three developmental areas directly assessed: Motor (catching bean bag; jump, hop, and skip; constructing models with blocks; thumbs and fingers to touch thumb in sequence; cutting lines and shapes; copying shapes; writing name); Conceptual (body parts; color names; rapid color naming; counting; understanding positional and descriptive concepts; sorting and identifying

	shapes); and Language (providing name; age, birthday, and gender; naming objects on Dial; telling what common objects do; reciting alphabet, naming letters, identifying sounds of letters; saying rhyming words; responding to comprehension questions). A rating scale and parent questionnaire for the Self-help and Social Development domains are available but are not included in scoring.
Format	Tasks individually administered to child generally at separate stations for the Language Development, Conceptual, and Motor areas; rating scale and parent questionnaire for the self-help and social development areas. An abridged (10-item) version (Speed DIAL) also available. Both forms available in English and Spanish.
Scores	Raw scores, scaled scores, percentile ranks. Parent questionnaires scored separately.
Age group	3-0 to 6-11 years.
Time	Full DIAL-3, 30 minutes; Speed DIAL, 15 minutes.
Users	Professionals with formal education in child development and standardized tests and trained screeners.
Norms	Data collected on 1,560 children grouped into four geographic regions and four ethnic groups (white, Hispanic, black, and other).
Reliability	Internal consistency, .87 (Full DIAL-3); .80 (Speed DIAL); test–retest, .88 (full DIAL-3), .84 (Speed DIAL).
Validity	Correlation between full DIAL-3 and Speed DIAL was .94. Correlations between the Social Development and Self-Help areas ranged from .23 to .31. The full DIAL-3 and the AGS ESP had correlations ranging from .38 to .63. Correlations of the Speed DIAL and the AGS ESP ranged from .42 to .64. The full DIAL-3 and the Battelle Developmental Inventory Screening Test had correlations ranging from .25 to .55. Correlations between the Speed DIAL and the Battelle Developmental Inventory Screening Test ranged from .35 to .63. For total sensitivity of .83 and specificity of .86 compared to performance on the Differential Ability Scales.
Comments	Materials are colorful and attractive to children. Tasks are presented on clocklike dials with one item exposed at a time. Very clear directions for administration and scoring. Training materials are included in the testing kit. The measure was normed on a separate sample of 605 Spanish-speaking children. The English and Spanish versions have the same dials and manipulatives except for the Articulation dials. The floor may not be low enough to discriminate between younger children with poorly developed skills. Interpretations limited to "potential delay" or "OK." Lack of evidence supporting the five cutoff points indicated. Evidence of predictive validity is missing. The DIAL-3 appears to be a stronger and better instrument than earlier editions. The authors have addressed concerns and incorporated changes suggested by earlier reviewers.
References consulted	Cizek (2001); Emmons and Alfonso (2005); Fairbank (2001a); Meisels, with Atkins-Burnett (2005). See book's References list.

Measure	**Early Screening Inventory—Revised (ESI-R). Meisels, Marsden, Wiske, and Henderson (1997).**
Purpose	A developmental screening instrument for children ages 3–6 years. It identifies young children at possible risk for school failure.
Areas	Two forms: ESI-P for children ages 3 years to 4-6 years and ESI-K for ages 4-6 to 6 years; both forms consist of 25 items that assess 3 main areas: Visual

	Motor/Adaptive, Language and Cognition, and Gross Motor. Tasks for both levels in the Visual Motor/Adaptive area include Block building, Copy forms, Draw a person, and Visual-Sequential Memory. Tasks in the Language and Cognition area include Ability to Reason and Count, Verbal Expression of Object Qualities, Verbal Reasoning (analogy questions), and Auditory Sequential Memory (digit span). Tasks in the Gross Motor area for the ESI-P include Jump, Walk on a line, Balance, and Hop, and for the ESI-K include Balance, Hop, and Skip. A parent form that consists of four sections (information on the child, the child's family, the child's school history, and overall development can be used but it is not included in the scoring.)
Format	Individually administered; can be used in a variety of settings.
Scores	Total score. Cutoff scores provided by 6-month intervals; a rescreen category is included.
Age group	3-0 to 4-6 years (P); 4-6 to 6-0 years (K).
Time	15–20 minutes
Users	Teachers, specialists, or trained paraprofessionals or volunteers. Examiner should have knowledge of child development. Training tapes and a training manual are available
Norms	Norms for the ESI-P and ESI-K were established separately. The ESI-P standardized norms were developed with a sample of 977 children drawn from 16 preschools or childcare programs from five states; approximately half of the sample was male and white. The ESI-K data are based on 5,034 children enrolled in 60 classrooms in 10 states with approximately equal numbers of males and females; 70% were white.
Reliability	For the ESI-P, interrater reliability was .99 based on 35 tester pairs; test–retest was .98 for two different examiners, collected 7–10 days apart. The ESI-K demonstrated an interrater reliability of .97 based on 586 tester pairs; test–retest coefficient was .87 for two different examiners, collected 7–10 days apart.
Validity	There are no available data for concurrent validity for either the ESI-P or the ESI-K. The ESI-P predictive validity, .73 (4–6 months later with McCarthy Scales of Children's Abilities); ESI-P sensitivity, .92; specificity, .80. The ESI-K predictive validity, .73 (7–9 months later with McCarthy Scales of Children's Abilities); ESI-K sensitivity, .93; specificity, .80.
Comments	The ESI-R is easy to administer, and training materials are readily available. The manual is comprehensive and online scoring is available. An excellent tool for developmental screening. Has been described as "the gold standard" (Paget, 2001, p. 452). Available, but not normed, in Spanish.
References consulted	Emmons and Alfonso (2005); Meisels, with Atkins-Burnett (2005); Paget (2001). See book's References list.

Measure	**FirstSTEp: First Screening Test for Evaluating Preschoolers. Miller (1993).**
Purpose	Identifying young children who may have developmental delays or school-related problems, and who are in need of a comprehensive assessment. It is also a short companion to the MAP (see below).
Areas	Three profiles: Cognition, Communication and Motor (12 subtests). Optional Social Emotional Scale, Adaptive Behavior Checklist, and Parent/Teacher Scale outcomes are part of the composite score. Subtests presented as games include: Cognitive Domain: Money Game (quantitative reasoning), What's Missing? (picture completion), Which Way? (visual positioning in space), and a Put

	Together Game (problem solving); Language Domain: Listen Game (auditory discrimination), How Many Can You Say? Game (word retrieval), Finish Up Game (word association), and Copy Me Game (sentence and digit repetition); and Motor Domain: Drawing Game (visual–motor integration), Things With Strings Game (fine-motor planning), Statue Game (balance), and Jumping Game (gross-motor planning). Areas included on the optional four-point rating scale for the Social–Emotional Domain include Task Confidence, Cooperative Mood, Temperament and Emotionality, Uncooperative/Antisocial Behavior, and Attention/Communication Difficulties. In the Adaptive Functioning Domain areas assessed include Daily Living, Self-management and Social Interaction, and Functioning Within the Community. A third optional scale, the Parent–Teacher Scale, was developed to obtain information relating to the child's performance outside of the testing session. Available only in English.
Format	Test tasks, rating scales, and parent/teacher questionnaire.
Scores	Composite, domain; standard scores, percentile ranks.
Age group	2-9 to 6-2 years. Separate forms are available for ages 2–9 to 3 years, 3–9 to 4–8 years, and 4–9 to 6–2 years.
Time	15–20 minutes.
Users	Professionals familiar with child development; trained volunteers.
Norms	Data collected on 1,433 children in seven groups, stratified by geographic region, community size, race/ethnicity, parent education level, age, and gender.
Reliability	Test–retest, .93; split-half, .89; interrater, .91.
Validity	Composite score correlates with the MAP total score at .71. There is a correlation of .82 between the composite score and the WPPSI-R Full Scale IQ; .61–.76 (language domain) with the Test of Early Language Development, 2nd ed.; .29–.56 with the Vineland Scales of Adaptive Behavior. Sensitivity, .72 (language domain) to .85 (cognitive domain). Specificity, .76 to .83 (Language domain).
Comments	Most materials are included in the test kit except 15 pennies, a nickel, a quarter, a ruler, a roll of masking tape, and a stopwatch. Administration is quick and relatively easy; the majority of the items are interesting to children at this age and are presented as "games." Five of these games, however, are timed, requiring considerable practice on the part of the examiner and possibly putting some children at a disadvantage. Some directions (e.g., "jumping") contain multiple concepts and behavior steps that may be difficult to follow. Requires scoring as one goes through the test, but the scoring is at the end of each subtest, requiring either much flipping back and forth or extreme familiarity with the test. Detailed instructions are provided in the manual. Many of the items were derived from the MAP. There is a section in the manual that discusses the theoretical and empirical development of the MAP. Overall, this measure meets technical standards expected for a screening measure. It will identify those students possibly at risk in need of further testing, plus some false positives. However, timing factors and the basic concept load in test directions are important considerations.
References consulted	Emmons and Alfonso (2005); Meisels and Atkins-Burnett (2005). See book's References list.

APPENDIX 6.2. Parent Interview/Questionnaire

Child's name:

Address:

Phone:

Date of birth:

Interviewer:

Date:

Parent address and phone (if different from child's):

Place(s) of work:

Names of other children in family	Ages

What languages do you speak at home?

Who are the people who live in your household? What languages do they speak?

Does your child have close relationship with someone at home or in the family or community? Describe briefly.

Who takes care of your child during the week? Weekends?

During your child's early years, did any of the following apply?

- Was your child born prematurely? If so, how much? Were there any problems?
- Has your child had ear infections (seldom/often)?
- Does your child have any other health problems?
- Was your child in other programs, such as nursery school, Head Start, religious programs? If so, how long?
- Names of programs and schools:

How does your child get along with adults?

Does your child play with other children? Get along with them?

Has your child received any special services up to this point? If so, describe briefly.

Does your family work with other agencies? Which ones?

Are there any medical circumstances in the family that might affect your child?

Are there other family circumstances that might affect your child?

Have you participated in any parent workshops or programs?

Describe a typical weekday for your child, beginning when the child gets up:

How would you describe your child's development overall, compared to the development of other children the same age you know?

How does your child behave when angry or when things do not go his or her way?

How do you respond to your child when he or she misbehaves?

Does your child have special qualities/talents? Please describe.

Do you have particular concerns or questions?

Chapter 7

Assessment of Early Academic Learning

Attention to preschool children's preparedness for school was underscored by the first of six national educational goals formulated by former President Clinton and the nation's governors in 1991 to improve educational opportunity and achievement by the year 2000 (National Educational Goals Panel, 1991). This goal—"By the year 2000, all children in America will start school ready to learn"—has focused attention on the importance of providing all children with the necessary physical, language, cognitive, social, and other learning experiences to prepare them to cope effectively with the demands of their early years of formal schooling. The lack of financial resources has made the objectives attached to goal 1, such as "All disadvantaged and disabled children will have access to high-quality and developmentally appropriate preschool programs to help them prepare for school," difficult to achieve. For example, the quality of many programs continues to be rated as only "fair" or "poor" (Hirsh-Pasek et al., 2005).

A major change in current educational practice is the pressure for accountability (Meisels, Steele, & Quinn-Leering, 1993). This pressure is currently reflected in the standardized testing mandated in Head Start and by the NCLB Act of 2001. According to the NCLB legislation, children need to have learned how to read by the end of grade 3, as measured by standardized achievement tests. The NCLB mandate has led to a "trickle-down" of academic expectations to kindergarten and an escalation of curricular demands. What formerly was expected of first-grade students is now often expected of kindergarten students, with a focus on literacy and mathematics proficiency. The NCLB Act provides funding, under Reading First grants, to states and districts for comprehensive professional development and ongoing assessment of students' progress in grades K–3 toward mastery of the scientifically based essential components of reading. There are also Early Reading First grants to provide high-quality early education to preschool children at risk for reading problems, especially low-income children. Many schools thus engage in readiness screening in order to determine the extent to which children have mastered the underlying skills deemed to be prerequisites for school learning. The outcomes can be used for multiple purposes—to group children for purposes of instruction, to plan instruction, or to exclude children from kindergarten or first grade. These issues, along with issues related to instructional screening, are addressed in this chapter.

The first major section of the chapter focuses on readiness screening. The issues covered in this section include difficulties with various definitions of readiness; the content of typical screening measures versus developmental screening tests; the widespread practice of readiness screening; problems pertaining to transitional programs and retention; reviews of two widely used screening instruments; the importance of teacher/parent attitudes, curriculum-relevant assessment, and sensitivity to cultural context; tasks tapping various aspects of emergent literacy; and group-administered tasks of academic preparedness. The second major section focuses on instructional screening: three forms of performance-based assessment (criterion-referenced, curriculum-based, and work sampling); strategy assessment; and the role of the assessor in modifying tasks. Thus we cover the spectrum of early childhood academic assessment, from traditional test-based assessment procedures to currently advocated alternative approaches to assessing learning and behavior.

SCREENING FOR READINESS OR PREPAREDNESS

The Concept of Readiness: Definitions and Difficulties

As suggested above, many issues related to readiness for entrance into kindergarten or first grade are areas of controversy. These include (1) decisions to exclude some children from kindergarten; (2) decisions to retain some children in kindergarten or place them in transition classrooms; (3) the trend toward pushing academic activities typical of first grade down to younger and younger children; and (4) the near-exclusive focus on child functioning, rather than taking into account home and school environmental factors in planning instruction. Indeed, the term *readiness* itself is an elusive construct (Meisels, 1999; Shepard & Graue, 1993). What exactly marks the state of a child's being ready for kindergarten or first grade? According to Nurss (1987), the term *readiness* needs to be used to describe preparation for what comes next and involves both the child and the instructional situation. Scott-Little, Kagan, and Frelow (2006) indicate that the concept of *readiness* has taken on increased significance as policymakers have recognized the importance of specifying the knowledge and skills children need to learn or develop during the preschool years. Through their content analysis of 46 early learning standards documents developed by state-level organizations published since 1999 and available for review in January 2005, these researchers detail how states have defined school readiness. Results of their review indicate that not all key areas of development are emphasized and that states vary widely in the standards they emphasize. The language and cognitive domains are emphasized across states, although some of the areas within these domains identified as important by the research literature (such as vocabulary development) are less emphasized, or omitted. These researchers also identified several important areas of children's development that have limited emphasis or have been omitted from some of the early learning standards such as (1) physical well-being and motor development, (2) social and emotional development, and (3) approaches to learning, such as curiosity and persistence. The extent to which a child is "ready" or prepared for the work of kindergarten and first grade thus depends not only on the child and the child's prior experiences, but on how states define readiness and on the *nature of the kindergarten or first-grade program*. That is, the program needs to be ready to accommodate the needs of the child. According to the National Center for Education Statistics (1994, p. 7), "When viewed in the context of developmental principles, readiness can be conceptualized most meaningfully as the convergence of schools that are prepared to accommodate children who are similar in age but are at different stages of development." This position recognizes that readiness is multifaceted and reflects the latest position statement of NAEYC (2003).

Since the readiness construct is often used to make critical decisions about entering kindergarten or first grade, there is considerable debate about the appropriateness of the construct altogether. Despite the caution of Nurss (1987), the common use of the term *readiness* is misleading, in that it focuses largely on the child and presumes that each child must reach a defined point (often developmentally inappropriate) for schooling or for instruction. Children's preschool experiences, however, are likely to differ based on their culture, SES, health, and geographic location. From our perspective and that of other early childhood specialists, assessment needs to tap the scope of children's early academic learning and behavioral preparedness for schooling, rather than their "readiness," in order to guide educational planning and early intervention. Meisels (1999) delineates competing definitions of readiness that affect assessment practices: (1) those based on the child's level of maturation; (2) those based on the child's past experiences ("what the child can do and how the child behaves"—p. 47); (3) those based on the skills and abilities the school and community expects, which vary greatly; and (4) those that recognize a reciprocal relationship between the child and the school. We endorse this last definition.

Gredler (1987, 1992, 2000) points out that two differing theoretical positions have dominated approaches to early childhood education since the 1960s and have had an important influence on readiness screening as it is currently practiced. The first position, influenced by the work of Arnold Gesell and his collaborators at the Yale Child Study Center in 1928, views development as controlled primarily by a child's biological maturation, with environmental factors having little effect. The practice related to this maturationist position that continues to be used to determine whether it is appropriate for a child to be enrolled in kindergarten or first grade is to assess whether the child has reached the *developmental age* needed to perform the tasks typical of kindergarten or first grade. If the child is viewed as not having reached this benchmark, the recommendation often made to parents is to delay school entrance until the child has gained the necessary skills; such a delay is sometimes referred to as "the gift of time" (Gesell Institute of Human Development, 1982). This practice is based on the belief that entering school "developmentally too young" is the cause of later problems. Some parents choose to delay school entrance so that their child will be better prepared for the demands of schooling or will be a "leader"—a practice sometimes referred to (in an athletic metaphor) as "redshirting."

Delaying school entrance, however, has not proven in general to be successful and may even lead to behavioral problems during adolescence (Byrd, Weitzman, & Avinger, 1997). They tend to fair less well on behavior problems, self-concept, peer acceptance, and teacher ratings (Graue & DiPerna, 2000), may develop poor attitudes to school, and are less likely to be well liked by peers (Marshall, 2003). Critics of this position (Graue & DiPerna, 2000; Gredler, 1980, 2000; Kagan, 1990; Marshall, 2003; Meisels, 1999; Rafoth, Dawson, & Carey, 1988; Shepard & Graue, 1993; Shepard & Smith, 1986, 1989) point out that another year prior to kindergarten or prior to entrance into first grade is not sufficient to resolve differences in performance. Furthermore, as May et al. (1994) observe, delayed school entrance and extra-year programs miss children in need of early intervention and "serve to obstruct the inclusion of students into schools with their non-disabled peers" (p. 297) and may deprive children of those social interactions that promote learning (Graue & DiPerna, 2000). Rather, a flexible, enriched instructional program is needed to meet these children's needs. The skill levels assessed by readiness tests may not reflect how much a child can benefit from kindergarten; in fact, those children with lower initial skill levels may profit more than those with higher levels (Shepard & Graue, 1993). Delay of schooling may thus increase the discrepancy between these two groups' early academic performance. Children who demonstrate special needs, or who come from low-income or other backgrounds that provide limited experiential opportunities, may be at a particular disadvantage if schooling is delayed. An extensive study of Head Start programs that serve children from low-income backgrounds documents considerable gains in preparedness for schooling on the part of these children (Commissioner's Office of Research and Evaluation & Head Start Bureau, 2001b).

The second theoretical position is based on children's *chronological age*; it is simply the belief that older children will do better. This belief is commonly held by many teachers and parents, particularly with respect to boys and for children whose birth dates are near the cutoff date for entrance into kindergarten. This belief, however, again places the focus on children: Children are expected to meet the school's expectations. Using chronological age as the gauge for school entrance introduces other issues as well. First, research does not support chronological age alone as a predictor of success or failure (Carlton & Winsler, 1999; Gredler, 1978, 1992; Meisels, 1987, 1999; Shepard & Smith, 1989; Shepard & Graue, 1993; Stipek, 2002). Gredler (1992), in a review of the literature regarding common school practices, indicates that raising the entrance age *does not decrease* the percentage of failures later on; younger children perform as well as older children. Second, the chronological age at which children begin kindergarten varies by state and community. The majority of states and communities set a child's reaching the age of 5-0 years by September 1 as the cutoff date for kindergarten entry, but this can range to December 1 of an academic year. Third, Gredler (1980, 1992) and Shepard and Smith (1985, 1986, 1987) note that no matter what age is set as the cutoff for kindergarten entrance, there will always be a group of children who are the *youngest*. The youngest children in a group are usually less successful at first than the oldest. However, while statistically significant, the achievement differences between these two groups are not very large (7–9 percentile points). Furthermore, there are few or no differences in achievement between the oldest and youngest children who perform above the 75th percentile. Rather, the differences result from children who are below the 25th percentile of their respective age groups (Shepard & Smith, 1985); that is, a combination of youngness and low ability is at work here. The small disadvantage of youngness also disappears by about third grade. Finally, within any age group there is considerable variability.

In sum, the combination of redshirting, national standards, and high-stakes testing has led to a curriculum "push down," in which the first-grade curriculum is now becoming the kindergarten curriculum. Although some children are able to meet these standards, many others experience failure at an early age. Kindergarten students are frequently expected to be well on their way to reading, if not actually reading, by the end of the kindergarten year. This has led some families to seek tutoring and extra services for their children. In some kindergartens, children are being drilled and taught, often in developmentally inappropriate ways. In some schools art, music, gym, and even recess are being put on the back burner so that more time can be devoted to academic work (Tyre, 2006).

The practice of redshirting also creates an older group of students in kindergarten, sometimes a spread from 5-0 years to 6-11 years or more, if children have been retained. Parents may be fearful that their children will fail, and as a result, hold them back (Graue

& DiPerna, 2000). Meisels (1992) proposed that we are witnessing the emergence of a four-tiered kindergarten in which the first tier is composed of regular age-appropriate children, the second tier is composed of students retained in kindergarten, the third tier is composed of students who are extra-year students in transitional programs, and the fourth tier is composed of those who have been redshirted. In this situation sound pedagogical principles cannot be followed.

There is also concern that the gap between class and race will be widened through the practice of redshirting. Families with financial means will be able to provide higher-quality resources to their children while they remain out of kindergarten (Stipek, 2002); many families do not have such resources.

Typical Readiness Measures versus Developmental Screening

Typical readiness measures focus in large on physical/motor, language, prereading, and socioemotional skill acquisition. Skills generally covered on readiness tasks have been detailed by many researchers (Abbott & Crane, 1977; Anastasi, 1988) and are summarized in Table 7.1. Of note is the often significant overlap in the content of instruments used for purposes of developmental screening, instructional screening, the assessment of readiness, and in-depth assessment. The differences among these types of instruments lie in the theoretical orientations and purposes of users—determining preparedness for school, identifying developmental problems that require special intervention, or planning instruction. Despite the broad overlap in content, Meisels (1987) believes that developmental screening instruments and readiness tests are not interchangeable, since poor performance on a readiness test may largely reflect limited prior experience rather than an impairment that affects the child's *ability to acquire knowledge* (which developmental screening tests are designed to tap). Furthermore, when developmental screening reveals a possible problem, there is the important safety net of in-depth evaluation. When a child does not pass a kindergarten readiness test or is deemed "not ready" to cope with the demands of first grade, *there often is no safety net*. In addition, many parents have not

TABLE 7.1. Skills Areas Included on Readiness Tests

Visual discrimination	Recognition of similarities and differences in letters, numbers, and forms; letter identification
Auditory discrimination	Identification of target sounds of letters, blends, and words; recognition of similarities and differences in sounds and words presented by the assessor
Verbal comprehension	Understanding words and sentences presented aurally; ability to follow directions
Vocabulary	Recognition of word units and comprehension of words
Recognition of symbols	Naming letters, numerals, and geometric forms
Reproduction of symbols	Copying letters, numerals, and geometric forms
Quantitative concepts	Adding simple quantities presented in pictorial or symbolic form; telling when a group of objects has *more* or *less*
General information	Knowledge of personal information (name, address, age, birthday, etc.), body parts, and so forth

Note. These are skills generally acquired during prekindergarten and kindergarten.

been prepared to be advocates for their children and may accept a school's recommendation without question (they may not be fluent in English, may not be familiar with American schools, and/or may not be aware that they have a voice in the decision). Thus readiness screening often results in what Shepard and Smith (1986) refer to as "high-stakes" decisions. These researchers emphasize, "The more crucial the decision for an individual child, the greater are the demands for test validity evidence and due process" (p. 83), and point out that readiness tests are not sufficiently accurate to remove children from their normal peer group. In addition, the content covered by readiness tests does not include many areas that are essential for success in kindergarten, such as the ability to work independently, pay attention, follow directions, communicate one's needs, and get along with others. The distinction between these two types of tests' purposes, however, is often difficult to ascertain or is ignored (Shepard & Graue, 1993), or efforts to call attention to the distinction may be futile (Lichtenstein & Ireton, 1984).

The Widespread Practice of Readiness Screening

Despite the problems with readiness testing prior to kindergarten and first grade that have been noted above, it continues to be a widespread practice. Citing the survey of early childhood specialists and testing specialists conducted by Gnezda and Bolig (1988), Shepard and Graue (1993) indicated that such testing occurred in all but three states, with tests such as the Brigance Diagnostic Inventory of Early Development—Revised (Brigance, 1991), the original Battelle Developmental Inventory (Newborg, Stock, Wnek, Guidubaldi, & Svinicki, 1984), the Denver Developmental Screening Test II (Frankenburg et al., 1990), the Developmental Indicators for the Assessment of Learning—Revised (DIAL-R; Mardell-Czudnowski & Goldenberg, 1998), and the Gesell School Readiness Test (GSRT; Ilg & Ames, 1972) as the instruments most frequently used. A survey in New York State by May and Kundert (1992) found that 33% of the districts surveyed used locally developed measures, 30% used developmental screening measures, 28% used skill-oriented measures, and 20% used informal observation (some districts used more than one approach).

A more recent survey (Costenbader, Rohrer, & Difonzo, 2000) of 385 public and private school districts in New York State responding to a questionnaire (out of 775) revealed the following: 30% used locally developed instruments (including parts of other measures), Human Figure Drawings, the Peabody Picture Vocabulary Test—Third Edition (Dunn & Dunn, 1997), and the Developmental Test of Visual–Motor Integration (Beery, 1997). The most widely used standardized instruments were the DIAL-R (Mardell-Czudnowski & Goldenberg, 1998) in 26% of districts, the Brigance K and 1 Screen for Kindergarten and First Grade—Revised (Brigance, 1997) in 16%, and the GSRT (Ilg et al., 1978) in 13%. (It should be noted that the DIAL-3 is a developmental screening test used to help identify children at possible risk for later learning problems and does not cover instructional areas related to the content of early childhood classrooms. See Chapter 6 for a review.) As an outcome, about 50% of districts referred children identified as "unready" through screening for further evaluation. Children were listed for further monitoring in kindergarten in 24% of districts. Another 19% advised parents to delay school entry for an additional year (Costenbader et al., 2000). The number advised to delay schooling was considerably lower than the 45% so advised in the study reported by May and Kundert (1992).

Screening is also initiated at different times in different districts, often beginning as early as the April prior to the start of kindergarten (Morado, 1987); during this 3- to 5-month gap, significant growth may occur, or stimulating at-home activities could have been suggested. Moreover, districts report the use of different types of staff members to carry out screening (Costenbader et al., 2000; Morado, 1987).

Transitional Programs and Retention: Practices and Problems

In the study reported by Morado (1987), teachers rated 27 selected learning activities in terms of their importance for children who attended regular kindergarten and developmental (extra-year) kindergarten, as well as the extent to which eight social behaviors were typical. Findings indicated that the range of learning activities differed in these two types of kindergartens. For developmental kindergartens, 18 activities were rated as important, versus 24 for regular kindergarten classrooms in which more academically oriented activities were included. In addition, children in regular classrooms were judged as socially mature, whereas those in developmental classrooms were judged as socially immature. Morado concluded that inappropriate practices were used in some school districts to delay entrance into first grade by 1 year, and that there was an overreliance on testing for placement. This conclusion is still valid today.

Controversy regarding readiness for beginning the reading instruction typical of first grade follows a similar pattern. Mason and Sinha (1993) argue that the acquisition of reading ability has been misunderstood, and that this misunderstanding leads to such erroneous practices such as delaying instruction in reading concepts until children reach a predefined maturation level and possess a prescribed set of prerequisite skills. Repeating kindergarten, participating in a year-long pre-first-grade experience, or repeating first grade is often recommended as the course of action for those children who lag behind. Despite the warnings of Nurss (1987) cited earlier, the practice of both kindergarten and first-grade retention is widespread, with as many as 40–60% of children retained in some districts (Gredler, 2000; Shepard & Smith, 1989). In Collier County, Florida, for example, of the 2,227 students retained in 2004 in grades K–10 (5% of the total school population at these grade levels), 207 were retained in kindergarten and 304 in grade 1—almost 20% of the retainees (Parker, 2005). Another district in Florida (Miami–Dade County) was reported to retain 37% of children.

Clearly, many school districts still believe that with another year of development or placement in a transition classroom, children will have developed the necessary skills to be successful in first grade and beyond. Research, however, does not support this practice. Based on their review of 16 controlled research studies conducted between 1984 and 1988 on the effects of extra-year programs prior to first grade, Shepard and Smith (1989) concluded that (1) kindergarten retention *does not boost* the subsequent academic achievement of children who spend the extra year in kindergarten, versus those equally at risk who go on to first grade; (2) a social stigma is often attached to retention for children; and (3) kindergarten retention fosters inappropriate demands in first grade, such as being able to decode successfully at the beginning of first grade. These researchers urge, rather, that teachers need to adapt their curricula and instructional practices. Professional groups such as the NAEYC (Bredekamp, 1987), the National Association of State Boards of Education (1988), the National Association of Early Childhood Specialists in State Departments of Education (1987), and the NASP (Shakel, 1987) have all endorsed the view and urge that retention at the kindergarten level is *not* a viable option for most young children. As Rafoth et al. (1988) point out, retention is a costly and largely ineffective way to deal with academic failure. Assessors need to identify alternative solutions and begin this process early during the kindergarten year.

Long ago, DeHirsch, Jansky, and Lanford (1966) urged that educators should not wait passively for maturation to occur, but that instruction should match the needs of the child. Instructional practices thus need to be questioned. For example, do they result in locking children into a full extra year of schooling through placement in transition classrooms so that they are a year behind their peers, or are there provisions so that children can rejoin their peer group following the year of placement in a transition class? (Such provisions are very unusual and generally involve enriched, personalized learning experiences—e.g., a program tied to the specific needs of children, tutoring, or a summer program.) If they do not rejoin peers, they are spending the equivalent of 2 years in kindergarten—1 year of which may represent a watered-down curriculum or a focus on isolated skill-and-drill practice, rather than on the kinds of extended experience with stories or with the sounds of language that they may need most. In addition, 3 years instead of 2, are needed to move through kindergarten and first grade.

Increasingly, research supports the outcome that children who stay in the regular kindergarten classroom despite a recommendation for retention or placement in a transition classroom make progress by the end of second grade. Furthermore, retention is often based on a teacher's decision, without extensive review (Gredler, 1992; Mason & Sinha, 1993). This practice often entails retaining a disproportionate number of males, particularly African American males (Shepard & Smith, 1989; Gredler, 1992). A more proactive process would be for schools to review their teaching practices and place children in smaller classes that provide adaptive learning experiences, allocate funds for classroom aides, provide for small-group tutoring that might take place within the context of the classroom, and actively seek to involve parents.

Mantzicopoulos (2003) documented that after children made the transition from Head Start to kindergarten, flexible programming tied to individual needs contributed to successful completion of kindergarten, as well as multiple contextual factors. These factors included the extent to which schools (1) were structured to promote continuity of the educational experiences when Head Start children moved into kindergarten, and encouraged parent involvement in school activities. In a sample of 261 Head Start children, Mantzicopoulos found that promoted children had higher achievement scores and were rated by their teachers as better behaved and more socially competent. Furthermore, children in kindergarten classrooms that stressed the links among school, families, and community were more likely to be promoted. Parent-reported involvement in school activities and satisfaction with the school program were also positively related to promotion. In contrast, lower parent estimates of children's adjustment to school were related to nonpromotion. Mantzicopoulos (2003) concluded that a child-focused skill deficit paradigm provides an insufficient view of nonpromotion. The family–school connection and parents' support for children's school-related efforts are essential factors for success in kindergarten. These findings underscore the need for intervention efforts that emphasize continuity in programming from preschool to kindergarten, work with teachers to use developmentally appropriate instructional practices, and develop supportive links with families.

Factors to Examine before Retention Is Considered

If retention is a possibility, it is essential to find out the following:

- What skills (expected early reading, writing, and counting skills) and behaviors has the school set as benchmarks? Are they reasonable?
- Why is the child having difficulty in achieving these skills?
- What behaviors are of concern to the teacher (not paying attention, inability to sit and listen, moving around a lot, difficulty following directions, interacting inappropriately with other children, etc.)?

- Is there a mismatch between the child's learning style and the teacher's degree of flexibility and warmth?
- If the child has been placed in a crowded classroom with little personal attention given to individualized instruction, how does the child respond? If poorly, to what extent might this poor response be due to lack of environmental support?
- What is the extent of outreach to encourage parent involvement throughout the year?
- How involved and satisfied are the parents with their child's schooling?
- Are problems with hearing, vision, or health present? If so, have these problems been addressed?
- Are the language differences typical of children learning English as a second language (ESL) perceived as deficits?

It is also important to find out what interventions have been tried—including alternative instructional strategies such as cooperative learning, individualized instruction, peer tutoring, and curriculum-based assessment approaches that have shown positive results for low-achieving children (Rafoth et al., 1988), as well as supplemental programs such as adult tutoring, summer enrichment activities, and intergenerational literacy programs. Depending on the answers to all these questions, and if ongoing consultation with early childhood specialists and early intervention activities have not been successful in producing change, the next step should be referral for comprehensive evaluation and individualized program planning.

State and local policies and mandates will, by necessity, influence what procedures early childhood assessors use. If the local system's belief is that holding a child out of school for an extra year or placing a child in a transition classroom will have positive benefits, an assessor may be required to follow those mandates. Assessors such as special educators, school psychologists, and speech–language specialists, however, need to advocate for children identified as "unready" (May et al., 1994; Rafoth et al., 1988), work to change local policies, and work with teachers to provide enriched early experiences and explore alternatives to retention. If the first year in kindergarten was not successful, for most children another year will not pay off in long-term benefits if other intervention activities have not taken place. It can be expected that just as there is wide variability in the rates at which children develop across developmental domains, there will be wide variation in how they develop their school-related skills. And if successful teaching strategies are not identified, the children will not learn.

Current Readiness Screening Tests and Practices: Further Comments

In summary, not only do currently used readiness screening tests themselves have many limitations, but these tests are too often overinterpreted and misused. The technical adequacy and purpose of some tests may be adequate to help guide instruction, but not adequate to serve as the basis for a placement decision that removes a child from the normal peer group. School district personnel also often miss the point well articulated by Nurss (1992, p. 275): "It is not the intention of informal teacher observation or formal tests of any type to be the sole criterion for grading the child, for making decisions about retention or promotion, or for evaluating the teacher or the school. Any such use of these data is inappropriate and can have disastrous results for children." The NCLB Act of 2001 stresses that assessment should be based on current empirical knowledge, with particular attention to the processes of learning. Assessment needs to be an ongoing and dynamic process that focuses on the essential components of reading (such as phonemic awareness, print awareness, letter knowledge, and vocabulary development), writing, and mathematics. This mandate is particularly relevant to the area of readiness testing and the content of the assessment measures used. It is also essential to monitor the effectiveness of the approaches used. Few schools, however, monitor early readiness screening practices, and most do not collect longitudinal data when children have been placed in transitional classrooms or retained (Gredler, 1992; Rafoth et al., 1988; Shepard & Smith, 1989). Results of the few controlled studies to date are inconclusive, and most do not follow children as they move through second and third grades. They do not detail the nature of instruction or intervention. This situation is changing with NCLB mandates.

Since the GSRT continues to be used and incorporated by some districts into early identification programs, as noted above, it is described in some detail in the section that follows. The Brigance K and 1 Screen—II, also widely used, is then described. Several other widely used tests used to contribute to readiness decisions are summarized in Appendix 7.1.

The Gesell School Readiness Test: An Example of Inappropriate Readiness Screening

The GSRT (Ilg & Ames, 1972; Ilg et al., 1978) is based on the assumption that a child's developmental age, as opposed to chronological age or environmental experience, is directly related to his or her ability to master school tasks. It is further assumed that children who lack maturity to comply with the tasks presented will not succeed in school, and that children need to have a maturation age of 7 to be successful in grade 1 (Gesell Institute of Human Development, 1982). The GSRT is derived from the Gesell Preschool Test and spans ages 2½–6. It consists of 52 tasks organized into eight subtests, which represent two developmental domains, adaptive and language. These subtests are Cubes, Copy Forms, Incomplete Man, Writing Names, Writing Numbers, Animals (naming as many as possible in 1 minute), Interview (personal information), and Interests. The GSRT takes 20–30 minutes to administer. Subtest developmental ages are determined using norms, which in turn are used to generate a Developmental Profile. Overall developmental age is estimated subjectively by the examiner, using the Developmental Profile. No specific cutoff scores are provided (Bradley, 1992). Extensive training is required to administer the GSRT.

Normative data for the GSRT were collected in the 1940s on a small (n = 80), largely white, above-average-SES population; the norms are out of date and not representative of the population today. Reviewers (e.g., Bradley, 1985, 1992; Costenbader et al., 2002; Gredler, 1992; Lichtenstein, 1990; Meisels, 1987) have consistently cautioned that the GSRT *does not meet technical standards for reliability, validity, or normative information.* Few studies have reported reliability information. In one study by Lichtenstein (1990), test–retest reliability was .73, and interrater reliability among trained examiners was .71. Thus there is considerable room for examiner error if results are used to exclude or retain children. A number of more recent studies have detailed negative outcomes. For example, May and Welch (1986) studied all students (n = 152) in a suburban district in grades 3–6 still enrolled in the district who had the Gesell Preschool Test administered prior to kindergarten, the GSRT administered at the end of the kindergarten year, and the GSRT administered again at the end of the first-grade year. The test results were examined in relationship to month of birth and gender. The criterion measure was the Stanford Achievement Test (SAT) administered in the spring of grades 2, 4, and 6. Although all three administrations of the Gesell tests were sensitive in predicting differences among children from different birth date groups, these differences diminished as children aged, with younger children appearing to catch up. Furthermore, the results did not support the recommendation of delayed school entrance for young boys.

Banerji (1992a) investigated the factor structure of the GSRT and pointed out that it possesses the properties of a developmental screening test rather than a readiness test, the purpose of which is to identify curriculum-related strengths and weaknesses. In another study, Banerji (1992b) reported the questionable usefulness of the GSRT in making placement decisions. Correlations of developmental age scores with first-grade achievement as measured by the SAT were reported as modest (.29–.39), but not sufficient to enable classification of "mature" and "immature" students. Banerji also addressed the efficacy of two-year placements for those students identified as "immature" or "delayed" in this study, and found that extra-year placements did not improve the relative rank order of low-performing students on first-grade SAT achievement. That is, it did not allow them to "catch up" with their peers even when they were a year older.

Finally, Shepard and Smith (1989) and Shepard and Graue (1993) have described the large overlap in the content of the GSRT with IQ tests and indicated that the resulting decisions are problematic. First, the GSRT does not measure curriculum-related content. Second, IQ tests are administered by highly trained individuals and must be used in the context of other assessment information. These researchers indicate that the GSRT is often administered by minimally trained individuals who can readily misinterpret outcomes. Furthermore, the test is often not used in the context of other assessment information, and this may be particularly problematic for children who have had limited learning opportunities. In summary, the GSRT lacks up-to-date norms, has insufficient technical data, and should not be used to make placement decisions. Yet this test continues to be widely used, as indicated in the study reported by Costenbader et al. (2000) cited earlier.

The Brigance K and 1 Screen—II

Another widely used screening measure is the Brigance K and 1 Screen—II. This is a criterion-referenced, curriculum-referenced, and norm-referenced instrument that includes a basic skills test, supplementary assessments (used to assess more capable students), a screening observation form, a teacher rating form, and a parent rating form. Items were derived from the Brigance Diagnostic Inventory of Early Development—Revised (Brigance, 1991) and the Brigance Comprehensive Inventory of Basic Skills—Revised (1999), which are more comprehensive tests. Two age levels are covered: 5-0 to 5-11 years for the K Screen, and 6-0 to 6-11 years and up for the 1 Screen. The K Screen has 12 subtests: Personal Data Response, Identifies Body Parts, Gross-Motor Skills, Color Recognition, Visual–Motor Skills, Draws a Person, Prints Personal Data, Rote Counting, Numeral Comprehension, Number Readiness, Reads Uppercase Letters (alternative-Reads Lowercase Letters), and Synatx and Fluency. The 1 Screen also has 12 subtests: Personal Data Response, Recites Alphabet, Visual Discrimination, Reads Lowercase Letters, Auditory Discrimination, Phonemic Awareness and Decoding, Listening Vocabulary Comprehension, Word Recognition, Draws a Person, Prints Personal Data, Computation, and Numeral in Sequence. The number of items on these subtests contribute differentially to the total score of 100. At the first-grade level, for example, two items in Computation contribute 10% of the score and Reading Lowercase Letters contributes 13% of the score. How these score assignments is determined is not detailed. In addition, as noted above, parent and teacher rating forms (for grades K–2) are available.

The stated purpose is to obtain a broad sampling of a student's skills and behaviors for one or more of the following reasons: identifying students to be referred for more comprehensive evaluation to determining the existence of a disability or the need for special education; determine most appropriate initial placement or grouping of students; assisting the teacher in program planning; and complying with mandated screening requirements. This is an easy and quick screen to use, which contributes to its appeal. However, it *must* be used with other measures; its use alone could lead to high-stakes decisions (e.g., whether a child should start school) based on a very small amount of data. (Of course, no single measure should be used as the *sole* basis for such a decision, as noted earlier.) For example, naming 10 colors contributes 10% to the child's score on the K Screen. If these colors are introduced at home or preschool, the child might be familiar with their names. If the child has not been introduced to them, he or she might learn them readily once they are introduced. The *Technical Report for the Brigance Screens* details a process for collecting data from the screen and associated rating forms and school records for review and decision making, such as placement in programs for the gifted or Title I Reading. The outcomes of the K Screen, therefore, thus, can lead to instructional planning or more comprehensive evaluation, but should not be used to recommend delayed school entrance.

Although the procedures for using the screens available for different age levels are well presented, technical data are minimal. To find such data, the *Technical Report for the Brigance Screens* (Glascoe, 2005) needs to be purchased separately. Both the 2005 and 2001 data presented in the *Technical Report* for restandardization of the Brigance Screens were collected at four geographic locations with small subsamples (95, 86, 180, and 411 children age 3, age 4, in kindergarten, and in first grade, respectively). The overall sample was largely white. Data regarding predictive validity, interrater reliability, and test–retest reliability are lacking in the test manual. In the *Technical Report for the Brigance Screens* (covering the screens at all age levels), Glascoe (2005) indicates that the screens have good concurrent and discriminant validity. Reliability data are minimal and are, in large part, based on the Brigance Diagnostic Inventory of Early Development—Revised. This is a major gap in data, considering that this screening test is widely used in decisions about whether or not a child is ready to start school. A study by Mantzicopoulos and Maller (2002) with Head Start children found no evidence to support the use of the Brigance scores as described in the *Technical Report* for identifying "at-risk" children. Spanish-language directions are provided as are considerations for children who are not fluent in English or who have developmental problems.

The Role of Teacher and Parent Attitudes, Beliefs, and Expectations

Teacher attitudes, beliefs, and expectations, along with the delivery of instruction, are all likely to influence children's performance. Therefore, teacher and classroom variables are as important as child variables in evaluating a child's preparedness for kindergarten or first grade. In a study by Fedoruk and Norman (1991), 21 first-grade teachers randomly selected from six elementary schools in a large Canadian city were presented with 86 descriptor cards describing characteristics associated with first-grade students' success and failure, generated from the research literature. Teachers were asked to rank the cards on a 9-point continuum, according to how strongly they felt these characteristics contributed to a student's academic success or failure. The wide range in ranking these descriptors vividly illustrated how differently teachers reacted to certain student characteristics: Some of the same characteristics that were irrelevant or mildly important to some teachers were moderately or very important to others. Such differences were seen as contributing to problems of over- or underidentification of potential learning problems in first grade. The authors concluded that first grade is not a standard experience for all young children, and that vastly different prerequisite competencies may be expected or required in different classrooms.

Another issue relates to teacher attitudes and expectations regarding poor and minority students, who are disproportionately targeted for retention or enrolled in special education (see "Sensitivity to Cultural Context," below). If these children have not been enrolled in Head Start programs, they may come to school without many of the experiences that kindergarten and first-grade teachers expect. Not only teachers' attitudes, beliefs, and expectations, but those of parents, play a role in children's preparedness for school. For example, Burchinal et al. (2002) found that African American children from more authoritative families had enhanced reading skills. In addition, as Meisels (1999) details (citing the work of Graue, 1992), parents' beliefs and expectations will affect school practices, and the skills required will vary from one school to another. In some schools, it is expected that children will learn how to read and write by the end of kindergarten, and some parents place great pressure on schools to fulfill these expectations. This is happening in more and more schools, in part because of the NCLB Legislation.

Curriculum-Relevant Assessment

Assessment that is congruent with the curriculum and informs instructional planning is of particular concern to kindergarten and first-grade teachers. Many procedures that were widely used in the past to screen for kindergarten entrance or for beginning reading instruction have been challenged for focusing on isolated skills in a decontextualized format that does not represent book and print awareness as emphasized by emergent literacy programs (Stallman & Pearson, 1990). Many of the measures included on Stallman and Pearson's list, however, have been updated and provide curriculum-relevant information in an organized way. Many curricular materials and reading programs currently combine an emergent literacy perspective with some emphasis on explicit instruction (see, e.g., Carnine, Silbert, & Kame'enui, 1997). Early childhood researchers (e.g., Genishi, 1992; Meisels, 1999; Salinger, 2001; Stallman & Pearson, 1990; Teale, 1990) recommend that informal observational assessment within natural contexts should replace group standardized measures as the first step in assessment. They believe that standardized tests yield little information that helps guide teachers regarding particular child needs and teaching strategies. Others recommend "a flexible approach to assessment," along with a "dramatically improved teacher knowledge base" (Garcia & Pearson, 1991, p. 254). Such a knowledge base needs to include knowledge of the cognitive processes that underlie early reading and mathematics, as well as the use of methods documented by the research literature as effective when presenting instruction (such as scaffolding, adequate practice across contexts, feedback, and reinforcement) (Hirsh-Pasek et al., 2005; Peverly & Kitzen, 1998; Scarborough, 2001).

From our perspective, a balanced approach may best serve children across settings. The results of tests of academic preparedness administered early during the school year can help provide an initial overview or survey of child functioning across multiple learning areas. The overview can be refined through ongoing teacher observation (including systematic recording of children's behavior, checklists of skills attained, and work samples), consultation with specialists, prompting responses using scaffolding techniques, and ongoing adjustment of instructional experiences. Under these circumstances, comparing a child's functioning with that of the standardization group can help a teacher understand those broad areas where the child might need assistance and begin to explore the reasons why the child lags behind peers. These screening results, however, should not be used to limit instruction to isolated skills; this is the crux of the issue. Results need to be used to help teachers evaluate the extent to which students have mastered instructional goals, identify areas of needed instruction, and reconsider the effectiveness of their own instructional activities—not to narrow their curriculum to those areas covered by the test. Many other behaviors are needed (e.g., attention, curiosity, and ability to get along with others) for children to be successful learners. These behaviors can all be observed and fostered in early childhood settings.

Based on the information presented thus far in this chapter, assessors need to avoid (1) basing so-called "readiness" decisions on a single instrument; (2) excluding children from regular kindergarten or first grade on the basis of readiness tests; and (3) using measures with inadequate technical support. Assessors should insist on (1) using outcomes of readiness tests (which we prefer to call *preparedness*) that assess children's knowledge of areas related to the curriculum as a "first pass" for planning instruction; (2) using multidimensional approaches, including criterion-referenced tests and work products; (3) conducting observations over time for children when there is some concern; and (4) working closely with teachers to address their concerns, modifying the presentation of instruction as needed, and charting progress. Furthermore, assessors need to become familiar with the curricula used at the early childhood level, with classroom arrangements and teacher interaction styles, and with the range of possible enrichment activities that might inform intervention.

Sensitivity to Cultural Context

Of particular concern in the assessment of early skills is the need to be sensitive to cultural context. As Heath (1983) has so poignantly demonstrated, schools too often look only for the experiences of middle-class children, and leap to conclusions that children from other sociocultural backgrounds lack essential skills. Heath (1983, 1986), for example, detailed the different language and social interaction characteristics of adult–child talk in three communities in the Piedmont region of North and South Carolina: one middle-class, one white working-class, and one black working-class. She found that there were large differences in the frequency of adult–child conversations in these three communities, as well as in the kinds of conversational forms the adults used. Thus children came to school with very different types and degrees of oral language practice. Some had more practice than others in less formal language, and some had greater practice in those language forms used in school. Such differences are likely to be misinterpreted, with the outcome that children who have less practice in school-related language forms may be viewed as lacking so-called "readiness" when indeed they may be quite ready to learn.

Pellegrini (1991) would concur with Heath; he is critical of the "at-risk" concept as it relates to early literacy and believes that it should be eliminated. He goes on to argue that the reasons for "at-riskness" of many non-mainstream-culture children versus those from the mainstream culture are "the contextual similarities of literacy events in home and school" (p. 282) for mainstream-culture children and the lack of such similarities for non-mainstream-culture children. If the contexts are familiar, children may be able to infer or generalize the rules of the game. Thus, as Garcia and Pearson (1991) caution, "Because of differences in language and/or literacy experiences, children from diverse backgrounds frequently are placed in transitional kindergarten or first-grade programs where they are exposed to the same type of activities that are measured on readiness tests in an attempt to get them 'ready' to read" (p. 257). As a consequence, these children may not be exposed to activities thought to promote emergent literacy.

Since emergent literacy is so central to children's preparedness for instruction in kindergarten and first grade, we focus attention on this issue in the next section to help assessors determine the scope of their procedures. Many of the procedures recommended may be described as *curriculum-based*—a topic to be discussed in detail later in this chapter.

Tasks Tapping Forms of Emergent Literacy

Numerous researchers have described how significant aspects of literacy develop during the preschool years, as children become aware that written language makes sense. The works of Adams (1990), Bradley and Bryant (1985), Clay (1966, 1972, 1979, 2002), Goodman (1986), Goodman and Altwerger (1981), Goswami (2001), Mason (1992), Neuman and Dickinson (2001), NICHD Early Child Care Research Network (2005), Rathvon (2004), Scarborough (2001), Schatschneider, Fletcher, Francis, Carlson, and Foorman (2004), Teale and Sulzby (1986), Torgesen (2002), Wagner and Torgesen (1987), and Whitehurst and Lonigan (1998, 2001), among others, serve as a basis for our views on the assessment of emergent literacy skills. We review this research very briefly as the context for considering key behaviors of children who are in the process of becoming literate.

Clay (1972) urged that terms such as *reading readiness* and *prereading* be avoided, and focused on the importance of the early childhood period for the *emergent literacy* of reading and writing. Clay (1966) used the term *emergent literacy* to refer to those reading behaviors used by a child prior to independent reading, and those scribbles and invented writing activities used prior to conventional writing. Scarborough (2001) details the multifaceted nature of reading acquisition, in which readers need to coordinate many component skills. Scarborough refers to these as "strands" that are woven together during the course of becoming a skilled reader, and stresses that these strands develop in an interactive manner. These interactive components include those involved in language comprehension and word recognition, and are illustrated in Figure 7.1. In an extensive review of the research literature regarding prediction of reading achievement from measures administered during kindergarten, Scarborough (1998, 2001), identified those involved in processing print and in gaining oral language proficiency as most predictive. Preschool children's language abilities are a particular area of concern (NICHD Early Child Care Research Network, 2005; see Chapter 10).

The presence of many emergent literacy skills is *inferred from observed* child behaviors—for example, when a child asks what a sign "says" or scribbles a menu during play. According to Mason (1992), entering kindergarten children's understanding of language—including the abilities to define and classify words, and to use and remember book language—predicts decoding in kindergarten and comprehension at the end of grade 1. An enormous literature now exists regarding these factors (see, e.g., Neuman & Dickinson, 2001; Rathvon, 2004).

Aspects of emergent literacy identified by researchers are presented by Clay (2002) and are embedded in tests such as the Concepts about Print Test (Clay, 2002), the Dynamic Indicators of Basic Early Literacy Skills (DIBELS; Good & Kaminski, 2002), and the Test of Early Reading Ability—Third Edition (TERA-3; Reid, Hresko, & Hammill, 2001) (see Appendix 7.1 for a summary of selected measures). Rathvon (2004),

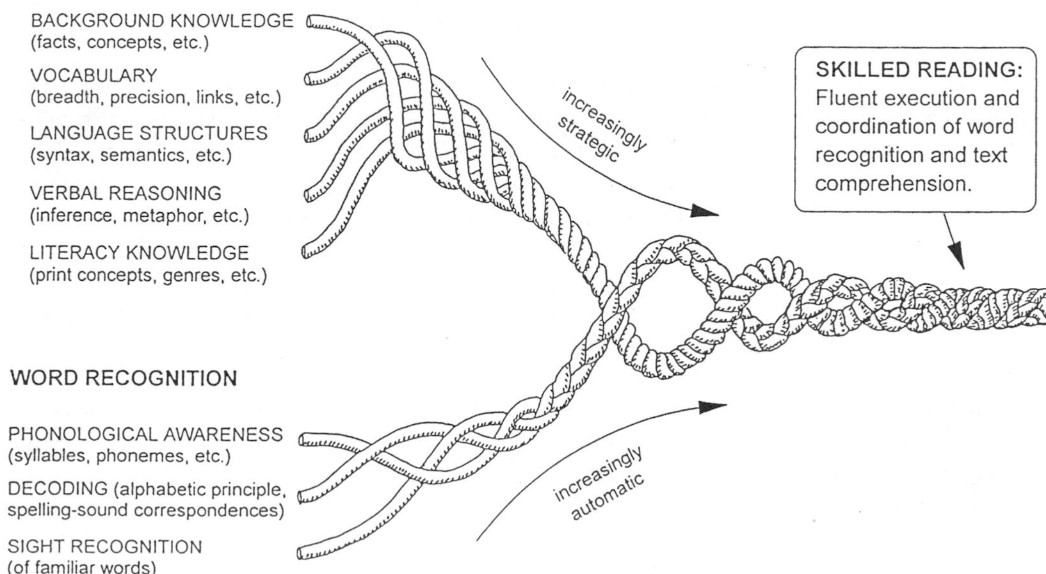

FIGURE 7.1. Illustration of the many strands that are woven together in skilled reading. From Scarborough (2001). Copyright 2001 by The Guilford Press. Reprinted by permission.

in her comprehensive text *Early Reading Assessment*, presents detailed reviews of 42 recent tests with psychometric soundness and usability that measure aspects of early reading acquisition in children in grades K–2. Many of these measures also cover younger age levels as well. The research base for the areas assessed is presented by Rathvon, along with critical issues in early reading assessment.

The sections that follow briefly highlight essential skills that develop prior to formal instruction in first grade.

Phonological Processing and Word Identification Skills

Current studies reflect a growing consensus that problems with fluent word identification and phonological processing (including problems with phonemic awareness, verbal short-term memory, and rapid automatized naming) are associated with reading difficulty (Casey & Howe, 2002; Felton & Pepper, 1995; Goswami, 2001; Holland, McIntosh, & Huffman, 2004; Scarborough, 1998, 2001; Snow, Burns, & Griffin, 1998; Torgesen, 2002; Wasik, Bond, & Hindman, 2006). Assessment of these skills at the preschool level is informative for purposes of both early identification and early intervention. Such identification and intervention are especially important, because it has been well documented that reading problems occurring by the end of first grade tend to persist, despite remediation (Johnston & Allington, 1991; Juel & Leavell, 1988; Kaminski & Good, 1996; Torgesen & Burgess, 1998). Therefore, assessing early literacy skills before children begin to learn how to read in a formal sense is an important preventive measure (Kaminski & Good, 1996). According to Kaminski and Good, such assessment needs to include both the identification of children who are not making progress in the acquisition of early literacy skills, and ongoing evaluation of the effectiveness of intervention. Torgesen (2002) indicates that intervention for children who have difficulty with regular classroom instruction needs to be more intensive, explicit and supportive than that usually provided by a classroom teacher.

Aspects of such explicit instruction are detailed by Baker, Kameenui, Simmons, and Stahl (1994). Since phonological processing skills are so important for success with reading, assessors involved in screening children in kindergarten and first grade need to screen for possible difficulty with these skills (Casey & Howe, 2002; Berninger, Thalberg, DeBruyn, & Smith, 1987; Holland, McIntosh, & Huffman, 2004). According to Whitehurst and Lonigan (2001), "Poor phonological processing skills are the hallmark of poor readers" (p. 16). In kindergarten, such assessment needs to cover phonemic awareness, letter–sound knowledge, and vocabulary (Torgesen, 2002). Commonly used developmental screening measures may miss children who may later show difficulties in learning to read (Scarborough, 1998). Phonemic awareness involves the awareness of the sound structure of words; it (1) helps students understand how the alphabet represents language, and (2) enables students to compare the order and identity of sounds in spoken words with the sequence of letters (spellings) in written words. These skills are closely related to the child's growing vocabulary and create "an implicit need for making comparisons between similar sounding words" (Goswami, 2001, p. 111). This leads to what Goswami refers to as "restructuring" or fine-tuning the phonological characteristics of words. Restructuring is likely to occur with words that children have encountered many times and with words with similar-sounding "neighbors."

In addition to observation during routine activities and maintaining portfolios of children's work (see below), two assessment approaches are suggested in the research literature: "dynamic" test–teach–test activities, and the use of standardized tests. Good and Kaminski (2002) and Kaminski and Good (1996), in presenting their series of measures known as the DIBELS, indicate that the rationale and procedures of these indicators parallel those of curriculum-based measurement as described by Deno (1989). These researchers identified three areas of early basic skills at the kindergarten level vital to acquisition of reading skill in the early grades that need to be considered during assessment. These include (1) phonemic awareness (the ability to manipulate the phonological components of words, including segmenting a word into its component phonemes [c/a/t]) and pronouncing words after the initial phoneme is removed ([c/at]); (2) letter naming in combination with phonological awareness and letter–sound awareness; and (3) language development, including receptive and expressive vocabulary and rapid naming retrieval ability. (See Good & Kaminski, 2002, 2003; and Kaminski & Good, 1996, for evidence supporting the psychometric characteristics of this approach.)

Between kindergarten and first grade, children make rapid gains in phonological processing, particularly phonemic awareness (Chafouleas, Lewandowski, Smith, & Blachman, 1997). Chafouleas and Martens (2002) found that segmentation tasks were the most sensitive phonemic awareness tasks at kindergarten for measuring growth in phonological awareness, followed by rhyming and sound providing if the segmentation task is too difficult. In grade 1, segmentation tasks again are most sensitive to growth, followed by blending and deletion tasks.

Kaminiski and Good (1996) investigated the reliability, validity, and sensitivity of three measures that can be used repeatedly to serve as dynamic indicators of the early literacy skills of kindergarten and first-grade children, based on the local curriculum: (1) Phonemic Segmentation Fluency in two- and three-phoneme words from the local curriculum (18 forms of 10 randomly selected words); (2) Letter-Naming Fluency in 1 minute

(18 forms of randomly ordered uppercase and lowercase letters); and (3) Picture-Naming Fluency in 1 minute (18 forms of 48 common nouns). Subjects included cohorts of kindergarten and first-grade children. Children in the experimental group were administered the DIBELS measures two times a week for 9 weeks, while those in the control group were administered these measures at the beginning and end of the 9 weeks. Each of the DIBELS measures used in kindergarten was related to success in learning to read. There were significant differences between kindergarten and first-grade children, with first-grade children scoring better on all three measures. For kindergarten children, measures were moderately to highly reliable and were significantly correlated with the criterion measures. At the kindergarten level, the outcomes suggested that phonemic segmentation measures reflected change over time. Changes were not reflected in either letter-naming or picture-naming fluency over the 9-week period. The authors suggested two hypotheses: that the measures were not sensitive to skill changes over time, or that the measures were sensitive but the students did not change much in 9 weeks. Finally, these researchers recommended that the DIBELS measures be used in conjunction with other assessment procedures, to determine intervention effectiveness such as observation of children's prereading skills during routine classroom activities. Kindergarten and first-grade benchmarks for using DIBELS measures are detailed by the authors.

The latest version of the DIBELS (Good & Kaminski, 2003; see also their website, http://dibels.uoregon.edu, for the latest updates) includes the following tasks at the kindergarten level:

1. Initial Sound Fluency (children's ability to identify and produce initial sounds in orally presented words—"what sound does (picture name) have?" The benchmark is 20–25 initial sounds correct by mid-kindergarten.
2. Phonemic Segmentation Fluency (children's ability to produce individual sounds within three and four phoneme words). The benchmark is 35–45 correct by spring of kindergarten or fall of first grade.
3. Nonsense Word Fluency (measures letter–sound correspondence and the ability to blend letters together to form unfamiliar "nonsense" words; measured at mid-kindergarten and again at first-grade level). The benchmark is 50 correct per minute mid-first grade.
4. Oral Reading Fluency (reading connected text in grade level material for 1 minute; an established reader at first grade can read 40+ words per minute using a standardized set of passages calibrated for each grade level. The test is used mid-first grade through third grade. Letter Naming Fluency (the rapid naming of upper- and lowercase letters) is also measured at the kindergarten level with children scoring in the lowest 20% considered at risk. Note that the child is asked to "tell me the names of as many letters as you can," not "as fast as you can," although the child sees the examiner using a stopwatch. Alternative form reliability data are available, as well as concurrent validity in relations to the Woodcock Johnson Readiness Cluster score [data retrieved from http://dibels.uoregon.edu?dibels_what.php]).

Casey and Howe (2002) present useful information that school psychologists can use to help kindergarten teachers carry out these procedures and they provide specific intervention activities as well.

The DIBELS is widely used as an assessment tool that has proven useful to assess and monitor students' development of early literacy skills (Coyne & Harn, 2006). Strong evidence regarding the validity and reliability is documented by Coyne and Harn (2006), Good and Kaminski (2003), and Kaminski and Good (1996). DIBELS has appeal and is widely used for a number of reasons detailed by Pearson (2006): (1) its simplicity and ease of use for monitoring student progress; (2) it provides accountability data in relation to the curriculum championed by the National Reading Panel (2000), which is aligned with NCLB legislation; and (3) pressure on the part of federal or state reviewers to use this approach to monitor progress in the Reading First program. In the Reading First program, the DIBELS is administered three times a year, either by the teacher or another individual, often unfamiliar to the child. DIBELS, however, only measures a limited portion of reading—phonemic awareness, phonics, and fluency. It does not measure receptive vocabulary development and whether the reader comprehends. Unfortunately, this narrow focus has become a blueprint for instruction in many states and communities, shaping curriculum in counterproductive ways as teachers are required to build instruction around scores and are evaluated based on the scores pupils receive (Goodman, 2006). This translates into extensive time spent in kindergarten on drill and practice using speeded tests to meet the benchmarks set by states that are linked to performance on the DIBELS. The many critics of this approach (Goodman, 2006; Manning, Kamii, & Kato, 2006; Paris, 2005; Pearson, 2006; Seay, 2006) argue that curricular activities focused on narrow skills such as these do not promote children's progress as readers and take time away from many other skills that need to be fostered in kindergarten. It also places great pressure on kindergarten children to respond quickly and does not take into account the syntax and complexity of text, where children need to slow down and think.

Research supports a number of other approaches. In a longitudinal study conducted by Felton (1992), the best combination of predictive measures collected in kindergarten (via standardized tests) for reading achievement in third grade included tasks tapping general ability, rapid naming of letters, and phonemic awareness (deletion of initial consonants). This combination accounted for 41% of the variance in reading outcomes. With IQ removed, rapid naming of letters, a deletion task, and a phonological task (measuring auditory discrimination, working memory, and segmenting and sequencing sounds within words) resulted in an overall hit rate of 80%; only 3% of students identified as not at risk in kindergarten were missed. Felton and Pepper (1995) also indicate that prediction of children at risk for milder reading problems is difficult, and that preschool children with speech or language problems plus phonological processing difficulties are particularly at risk for reading problems. These researchers describe a number of tools useful for early identification of difficulty in phonological processing, word identification and attack, and rapid naming. Tasks of phonological processing appropriate for children in kindergarten or younger identified include subtests from such tests as the Kaufman Survey of Early Academic and Language Skills (K-SEALS; Kaufman & Kaufman, 1993), the Lindamood Auditory Conceptualization Test—Revised (LAC-R; Lindamood & Lindamood, 1991), the Test of Auditory Analysis Skills (TAAS; Rosner, 1975, 1979), and the Test of Phonological Awareness (TOPA; Torgesen & Bryant, 1994). More recent measures include the Comprehensive Test of Phonological Processing (CTOPP; Wagner, Torgesen, & Rashotte, 1999) and the Pre-Reading Inventory of Phonological Awareness (PIPA; Dodd, Crosbie, McIntosh, Teitzel, & Ozanne, 2003). (See Appendix 7.1 for details.) Some of these measures, however, are not designed for repeated measurement (Chafouleas & Martens, 2002), since only one form is available. Preschool assessors can thus either use available standardized measures or develop their own measures, using procedures such as the one developed by Kaminski and Good (1996). Goswami (2001) cautions, however, that a child's performance will vary depending on the cognitive demands made by different tasks. Knowledge of the letters of the alphabet is essential and is the best indicator of reading achievement (Adams, 1990). Children who know letters will have greater success in learning the sounds those letters represent (Mason, 1980).

Important related instructional activities at the preschool level include informal tasks where children's attention is directed to the sounds of spoken language and to auditory discrimination through exploration and discovery, not through drill alone (Felton & Pepper, 1995), although Goswami (2001) cites evidence that direct instruction in alphabetic orthography contributes to achievement in reading and spelling. Kindergarten and first-grade intervention activities that have been successful in improving children's later reading are described by Mason and Sinha (1993), and instructional activities for teaching phonological awareness are presented by Baker, Kameenui, Simmons, and Stahl (1994), Casey and Howe (2002), and Mason and Pepper (1995). Torgesen (2002) recommends explicit and comprehensive teaching of component skills for children at possible risk or displaying weakness, including a greater number of teaching–learning opportunities per day, more repetition in order to solidly establish critical skills, and careful sequencing and practice so that skills build gradually. Torgesen is also careful to point out that additional resources are needed for teachers to have time available for more preventive instruction—a crucial point for financially stressed districts.

Emergent Literacy in Writing and Mathematics

The assessment of children's use of language in written form is often not included in the screening conducted at the Kindergarten level. However, written language is an important aspect of literacy (Holland, McIntosh, & Huffman, 2004; Richgels, 2002; Snow et al., 1991; Sulzby, 1985, 1986; Whitehurst & Lonigan, 2001). Sulzby (1985), in her study of kindergarten children's writing, found six categories that covered children's productions: drawing, scribbling, letter-like forms, well-learned units, invented spelling, and English orthography. Sulzby (1986) cautions, however, that these categories should not be treated as a developmental ordering, since different tasks presented to children result in different kinds of representations. While Sulzby's longitudinal research with 5- and 6-year-olds was not intended to develop a formal assessment technique, several of its findings have important implications for observational screening: (1) Emergent writing skills develop before formal instruction; (2) these writing skills are task-dependent; and (3) children will use lower-level skills to serve higher-level skills. Thus assessors might find it useful to ask children to produce "writing" during preschool screening, such as their own names. "Journal writing" often begins in kindergarten, if not earlier.

Ginsburg (1997b) would urge as well that we consider a child's emergent mathematical understanding—an area often neglected in the literature on emergent literacy. However, children's concepts of number and time (e.g., *more*, *less*, *before*, *after*; number order; one-to-one correspondence) begin to unfold during their preschool years as well. Instruction in these concepts is often part of the kindergarten program, and the concepts are also likely to be covered in early school achievement measures. Many of the same concerns that apply to the assessment of reading and writing in kindergarten apply to mathematics as well, such as "speeding up" the curriculum by introducing in kindergarten cognitive or learning skills formerly introduced in grade 1 or above. Rather, the teacher needs to play a critical role in designing, conducting, interpreting, and integrating their observations of children using mathematic concepts while teaching children, and using flexible instructional approaches. The Test of Early Mathematics Ability—Third Edition (TEMA-3; Ginsburg & Baroody, 2003) assesses many of these concepts (see Appendix 7.1).

Group-Administered Tests of Academic Preparedness

A number of group-administered achievement test series have forms appropriate for use with preschool populations. These include the Gates–MacGinitie Reading Tests, the Iowa Tests of Basic Skills (ITBS), the Metropolitan Readiness Tests—Sixth Edition (MRT-6), the California Achievement Test, and the Stanford Early School Achievement Test—Fourth Edition (SESAT). (See Appendix 7.1 for details about the ITBS, MRT-6, and SESAT.) These tests all contain similar tasks (such as word analysis, vocabulary, language comprehension, sound recognition, listening, etc.); are in general technically sound (Gredler, 1992; Meisels, 1999); have been standardized on large, representative groups of children; and can provide instructionally relevant information in addition to norm-based information. However, tests such as these have been criticized for focusing largely on isolated subskills; they do not provide opportunities for children to integrate skills, and do not tap "real" instances of performance that can be gained through observing children engaged in classroom tasks. Appropriately used, however, these tests can survey groups of children across many areas and provide insight into areas where instruction is needed. This is particularly important when teachers are responsible for large numbers of children. Tests such as these are also important for purposes of accountability as mandated by the NCLB legislation. It must be noted, however, that these tests require multiple sessions to administer and generally are not scored by teachers. (Teachers may not have the ability to review outcomes in detail.)

Readiness or Preparedness Screening: Summary

If screening of children's academic preparedness for kindergarten or first grade is to be worthwhile, assessors need to engage in a process in which (1) children's skills are surveyed early in the school year, along with the strategies (e.g., attention, memory) they use to solve problems; (2) progress is monitored after instruction; (3) attention is paid to understanding the classroom environment and instructional practices; (4) assessment is conducted at the end of the school year or unit of instruction, to monitor progress and provide direction regarding summer intervention activities; and (5) families are involved so that they support early school learning. Tests must be used as part of an *ongoing* process in which observation is key to monitoring children's progress in order to plan instructional experiences, not to sort children in or out of kindergarten or first grade or limit the scope of instruction. A second outcome is to support teachers as they assume greater roles in carrying out ongoing screening in the contexts of their classrooms. Assessors may need to press for additional administrative support for such activities as workshops for teachers and parents, specialists' spending time in classrooms, and greater involvement of *well-trained* classroom help.

The process of becoming a competent reader is multidimensional and begins during the child's preschool years with parents and caregivers reading aloud to children, asking questions about stories, and having children talk about and retell stories. Such activities help children understand story organization and enhance their understanding about the concepts of print. Playing rhyming word games, along with alphabet books, can help children during the early years understand the relationship between letters and sounds (the alphabetic principal) (NAEYC/IRA, 1998). Snow, Burns, and Griffen (1998) detail the developmental accomplishments of literacy acquisition (pp. 60–62) from birth to grade 3. This detailed listing is an excellent source for the assessor's observations. Literacy development (and assessment) needs to focus on other areas of the curriculum as well, including mathematics, writing, and social–emotional and physical development. States have standards and guidelines regarding expected outcomes in these areas by grade level that can be accessed through the Internet. Scott-Little, Kagan, and Frelow (2006) provide a comprehensive overview of these standards. A useful resource for teachers and assessors is *Making Early Learning Standards Come Alive* (Gronlund, 2006). This book details activities that can be used to foster the learning standards indicated across different states.

Children need to have the fundamentals for successful reading by the end of first grade. If not, they will fall increasingly behind in all curricular areas. Many will also develop problems with behavior, motivation, and self-concept. The assessment process therefore needs to begin in prekindergarten and kindergarten. As Hirsh-Pasek et al. (2005) emphasize, assessment needs to be empirically based and focus not only on what children have learned, but also on how children learn and the strategies they use to solve problems. This information in turn can better inform instructional practices and intervention activities.

To conclude this section and illustrate many of the points made, an example of a model kindergarten screening program used by the Hawthorne School (Hawthorne, New York) is presented in Figure 7.2.

FORMS OF INSTRUCTIONAL SCREENING

Instructional screening that directly observes the performance of children engaged in everyday tasks is critical for the purpose of informing curriculum development, including detailing the materials, activities, and strategies that need to be considered in teaching. The ideal outcome is to adapt teaching expectations and goals to child needs. Instructional screening informed by current research is an ongoing process that helps to (1) identify what a child already knows; (2) identify areas of knowledge a child needs to acquire, and establish learning objectives; (3) identify the strategies a child uses to solve problems; (4) identify whether an instructional activity is appropriate for a child; and (5) match instruction to a child's individual needs by monitoring the development of desired skills or behaviors. Thus instructional screening can help determine the beginning points of teaching (and prevent unnecessary repetition), build upon areas of strength, and identify areas needing development. Those children encountering great learning difficulties over time can be referred for comprehensive assessment, with attention directed as well to the levels of adult support or help needed to foster development.

It is important at this point to distinguish between brief screening measures (which often are highly problematic) and detailed curriculum-referenced measures or developmental scales (which have often been developed by the same authors). In general, these detailed measures are excellent references for teachers and early interventionists. The Gesell Developmental Schedules (Ames, Gillespie, Haines, & Ilg, 1979) as contrasted with the GSRT; the Battelle Developmental Inventory, Second Edition (BDI-2; Newborg, 2004), from which the BDI-2 Screening Test was derived; and the Brigance Inventory of Early Development—II (Brigance, 2004) as contrasted with the Brigance K and 1 Screen for Kindergarten and First Grade (Brigance, 1997) are a few examples.

Depending on the assessment question, curriculum-referenced information (instructional screening) is often more meaningful and directly relevant to intervention than the global information yielded from many norm-referenced tests (NRTs), and it is increasingly the form of assessment used at the preschool level. Such instructional screening

Time	Parent outreach	Assessment activities
March prior to kindergarten	Registration for kindergarten.	Parents are given a preschool questionnaire to be filled out by the preschool teacher (if the child attends preschool). This covers socioemotional/preacademic development. (To be returned to school principal.)
April	Parent orientation day.	A Kindergarten Profile Form (translated as needed) is distributed to be completed by parents. This covers general information about the child and family. (To be returned to principal.)
May	Child–parent orientation day. Parents are provided with information about program, busing, and time frame for September.	Children are assigned in groups of 10 to spend time (45 minutes) in a classroom with teacher-directed activities (manipulatives at table, circle time, draw-a-person, shared book reading). An aide/specialist observes/completes a checklist for each child. Later in the day, teachers meet with support staffers and school psychologist to debrief and record information on a placement card for each child.
June–July		Principal meets with teachers, school psychologist, reading specialists, and English-language-learning teacher to integrate all information collected and assign children to teachers.
August	Placement letters are sent to parents (teacher assigned). School day, bus transportation procedures, early start day are reviewed.	
September of kindergarten	Letters welcoming children and parents to early start day are sent.	Early start day (7:30). Teacher meets with individual students and parents for individual assessment, using the Hawthorne Kindergarten Inventory.
Mid-September	*Back to School Parent Handbook* and teacher handouts are distributed (translated as needed).	
October–November	Parent conferences; Parents as Partners Workshops (hands-on activities; demonstrations of reading, language, and mathematics strategies used by teachers; suggestions for at-home reading and language activities; meetings with parents/caretakers at home; suggestions for character education activities); Parent Resource Center.	Boehm Test of Basic Concepts–3 (Boehm-3) administered by teachers; Developmental Reading Assessment (DRA; Beaver, 1997); Hawthorne Kindergarten Inventory; Gates–MacGinitie Reading Tests for children at possible risk; ongoing observation by teachers; ongoing staff conferences throughout the academic year; provision of early intervention activities as needed.
December–January–February	Parents as Partners Workshops.	Ongoing assessment; Hawthorne Kindergarten Inventory; DRA.
March–April–May	Parents as Partners Workshops.	Ongoing assessment; Hawthorne Kindergarten Inventory; Boehm-3; DRA.
May		Kindergarten and first-grade teachers review overall achievement for each child (in language, math, writing, DRA reading level, language concepts); support services a child receives; health concerns; need for counseling; whether or not to keep certain children apart or together the next year; teacher comments/concerns; any parent concerns or requests.

FIGURE 7.2. The Hawthorne School parent outreach and early assessment program. Based on Amoruso et al. (2004) and the materials distributed.

needs to be considered both at a particular screening point and as an ongoing process that builds on teacher observation and on informal as well as formal tasks. Thus curriculum-related screening must focus on both the learner and on the presentation and content of instruction. Specific outcomes of instructional screening at different points in the school year follow. The Boehm Test of Basic Concepts—Third Edition (Boehm-3; Boehm, 2000a) and its preschool version (Boehm, 2001) are presented as examples.

1. Early in the year, instructional screening can be used to identify what a child already knows or needs to learn when beginning a particular learning sequence. An analysis of the child's errors as detailed on the response form allows assessors to generate hypotheses and develop learning objectives. Thus it helps establish a baseline from which to plan and monitor the effectiveness of instruction and the child's learning. The Boehm-3: Preschool (3–5 years, individually administered) or Boehm-3 (grades K–2, group-administered) can be used early in the school year to survey a large number of basic relational concepts that have been documented to be important to following teacher directions or the content of instruction (e.g., for emergent literacy in reading, *top–bottom*, *beginning–end*, *right–left*, *first–last*, *before–after*); to mathematics (more–less, equal, before–after); to following directions used in tests or other assessment activities (e.g., *same–different*, *over–under*); and to thinking. The spatial, quantitative, dimensional, and temporal concepts included are also necessary components of higher-level cognitive tasks, such as ordering, making comparisons, and classifying (Boehm, 2000b). A brief group-administered measure such as the Boehm-3 is an efficient means of identifying initial instructional objectives for individual children or the class as a whole. A section of the response form for parents details their child's performance on all concepts and presents activities that can be carried out at home. Instructional activities are indicated in *The Boehm Resource Guide for Basic Concept Teaching* (Boehm, 1976) and in the test manual.

2. As an ongoing process, instructional screening enables teachers to track progress in relation to the curriculum and to determine the effectiveness of teaching activities and interventions, as well as the amount and type of adult support needed to achieve desired outcomes. An observational guide has been built into the Boehm-3 test materials to assist teachers in observing basic concept use across learning contexts. For example, children may know the temporal use of *before* and *after*, but not the spatial or quantitative uses. Thus basic concept learning is more than vocabulary learning. The use of basic concepts across contexts, and their use for following directions of increasing complexity, need to be goals of instruction (Zhou & Boehm, 2004).

3. As in other areas of learning, it is also important to consider the cognitive processes required for complying with instructions that include basic concepts. In order to follow the instruction "Put all the red blocks that are little in a pile," the child needs to pay attention to the spoken direction, remember all components of the instruction, scan the objects presented, focus on critical elements, recall from memory the key components, and act on this information. Teachers or assessors can use a strategy interview with children who encounter difficulty to understand where the difficulty occurs (see "Strategy Assessment" later in this chapter). A large research literature documents the development of individual basic concepts.

4. Toward the end of the year, instructional screening (e.g., readministration of the Boehm-3, using the alternate form) can be used to evaluate the effectiveness of the instructional program, the concepts children have learned, and their ability to generalize these concepts across contexts, as well as those that need additional practice.

Instructional screening takes many forms that focus on the child's performance; collectively, these are referred to as *performance-based assessment*. As defined by Airasian (1991), performance-based assessment involves "assessments in which the teacher observes and makes a judgment about a pupil's skill in carrying out an activity or producing a product" (p. 252). In what follows, we present three different forms of performance-based assessment: criterion-referenced tests (CRTs), curriculum-based assessment (CBA), and portfolio assessment.

Types and Characteristics of Performance-Based Assessment

One of the characteristics of both CRTs and CBA is task analysis. The work of Gagné is fundamental to these approaches (Gagné, 1965, 1978, 1987).

Criterion-Referenced Tests

CRTs are instructional screening instruments that, as their name indicates, are used to compare the child's skill mastery to an established criterion rather than to the performance of other children. Skill areas (e.g., writing one's name or engaging in one-to-one correspondence) are broken down into task-analyzed subskills that are ordered by difficulty, with criteria specified for successful performance. This task breakdown allows the teacher and other interventionists to ascertain the level of a child's mastery and instructional needs before proceeding to the next skill or behavior, to set learning objectives, and often to establish an IEP if the child has a documented disability. Many procedures used, however, cover mainly the performance aspects of task analysis, without specifying the learning processes required or the environmental supports needed (Howell, 1986). Gagné (1978) has indicated that instruction needs to be planned to support the processes of learning, and to take account of both the *internal* conditions of the learner (e.g., information-processing skills and long-term memory) and *external* conditions (relevant environmental stimulation and feedback). To achieve this end requires a learning analysis, which involves (1) identifying the learning outcomes desired for a specific task the learner needs to acquire; (2) analyzing tasks to reveal the component steps that lead to the desired learning outcome and their sequence, taking into account both internal and external conditions; (3) further analyzing each component step when needed, based on prior learning, to reveal the essential prerequisite subskills that need to be incorporated into the new learning performance; and (4) as needed by the learner, further breakdown of the prerequisite skills.

A learning analysis also involves identifying which external conditions critical for effective learning need to be incorporated into instruction. These may include (1) stimulating recall to activate retrieval of previously learned information that can be incorporated into new learning; (2) providing guidance to support the encoding process (including ways of presenting the material, eliciting responses, and providing reinforcement); and (3) providing the necessary contextual cues and practice opportunities over time to enhance retention and transfer. The assessor needs to evaluate criterion-referenced materials to determine the extent to which problem-solving strategies are embedded or need to be added.

Many types of CRTs are used by schools at the early childhood level. CRTs, however, do not necessarily differentiate children who have completely mastered a skill or desired behavior from those who have achieved only partial mastery (Sattler, 1988). Fundamental issues include who sets the goals and establishes the criterion level, and the extent to which the criterion level is meaningful and related to the instruction received. The criterion levels used to indicate mastery are generally determined locally and may not always reflect useful criteria. For example, "Mastery of one-to-one correspondence 80% of the time" may meet the criterion level established, but it still indicates that the objective is not fully met. In addition, CRTs often do not tap into the strategies and processes a child uses to arrive at responses or the kind of adult assistance that is needed for the child to be successful.

Although the purpose and use of many CRTs may be different from those of NRTs, there are often few differences in their format and content (Calfee & Hiebert, 1991; Garcia & Pearson, 1991; Stallman & Pearson, 1990). In both types of tests, the child's performance is still compared with a preestablished standard or specified objective. Thus users need to consider whether the test content sufficiently matches the curriculum to be useful for success in teaching and can be translated into instructional objectives (Shinn, Rosenfield, & Knutson, 1989).

Curriculum-Based Assessment

A particular form of CRT is CBA, which directly links assessment of specific curriculum activities with intervention (Bagnato, Neisworth, & Munson, 1989, 1997; Hintze, Christ, & Methe, 2006; Neisworth & Bagnato, 1988; Shapiro, 1987, 1990, 2004; Shinn, 1989b; Shinn et al., 1989). CBA is intended to be of assistance to teachers and children during classroom instruction. CBA provides continuous assessment of instruction based on the local curriculum. A frequently cited definition of CBA is that provided by Deno (1987): "Any . . . measurement procedures that use direct observation and recording of the student's performance in the local curriculum as a basis for gathering information to make instructional decisions" (p. 41). This definition is the basic premise from which a variety of CBA models have been derived. Although these models share the same basic definition, their purpose and outcomes vary in accordance with the design of the model. Shinn et al. (1989) present the theoretical and practical similarities and differences of four commonly used CBA models. They note four common principles of CBA (citing Frisby, 1987): "a) student assessment in classroom instructional materials, b) short-duration testing, c) frequent and repeated measurement, and d) graphed data to allow for monitoring of student progress" (p. 301). These authors indicate that not all models meet all four of these principles, and that they differ in their focus on the level and/or content of instruction. Models also differ in their assumptions and address different aspects of educational decision making (including instructional planning, evaluation of student progress, and eligibility decisions), each of which requires different supportive documentation. Shinn et al. (1989) indicate that all models point to the need for skill on the part of assessors in devising tasks and in translating objectives into useful test items. Hintze, Christ, and Methe (2006) have explored these issues further with an example applied in the area of early reading.

CBA is intended to be used repeatedly over time to track small changes in a child's performance, and thus to provide teachers or other interventionists with ongoing feedback about the effectiveness of their instruction or interventions. No single model of CBA is comprehensive enough to answer all the critical questions related to issue of evaluation, remediation, and level of instructional placement. The assessor needs to be clear about his or her assessment purpose, and to differentiate the strengths and weaknesses of various forms of CBA. Learner processes and strategies are not directly addressed in any of the models, although they are essential to understanding the sources of error and developing appropriate intervention. Shinn et al. (1989) indicate that while all models have utility for curriculum planning and monitoring progress, only standardized curriculum-based measurement (CBM) can be used for making eligibility decisions. They also stress that high-quality educational assessment needs to be tied to effective educational interventions. And effective interventions involve other factors in addition to CBA, including student learning abilities, motivation, the nature of the curriculum, and the quality of instruction. Hosp and Fuchs (2005) present an excellent example of CBM in reading across the early grades.

However, as Shapiro (1996, p. 62) points out, most CBA models other than the one developed by Shapiro and Lentz (1986) "do *not* incorporate significant efforts at evaluating the academic environment along with the child's skills" (emphasis in original). Shapiro (1987, 1990, 1996, 2004a) presents an integrated model (behavioral assessment of academic skills), which ties together the various models of CBA and which addresses the instructional environment along with instructional content. Shapiro (1996, 2004a) indicates that behavioral assessment is directly compatible with CBA and leads directly to developing interventions. Students are directly tested on materials they are expected to learn, with errors seen as reflecting real deficits in performance (Shapiro, 1996). Performance is directly linked with curriculum, so that teachers can focus on skills that have not been mastered. Students can be retested frequently without practice effects.

Shapiro (1996) also indicates that the link between assessment and remediation in academic subjects is not straightforward; he states, "The critical issue in selecting the appropriate behaviors for assessment is the functional relationship between the assessed behavior and remediation strategies designed to improve the skill" (p. 47). In other words, the focus should be on skills that are sensitive to remediation. Reproducible forms, charts, and case examples are presented in Shapiro (2004a, 2004b).

Shapiro's work is largely directed to students in the elementary grades, but the principles he sets forth are applicable at the preschool level as well. At the preschool level, it is important to ascertain (through teacher interview and classroom observation) information such as that presented in Table 7.2. A recent, well-researched approach, the *Classroom Assessment Scoring System* (Pianta, La Paro, & Hamré, 2006) begins at the preschool level. This system reviews essential interactions between teachers and students (Emotional Support, Classroom Organization, and Instructional Support) that can be modified through preservice training or other intervention activities. (See Chapter 5 for details.)

PRESCHOOL APPLICATIONS OF CBA

A number of researchers have focused specifically on the application of CBA at the preschool level. In their useful book *Linking Developmental Assessment and Early Intervention: An Authentic Curriculum-Based Approach*, Bagnato et al. (1997) distinguish between two forms of CBA used at early childhood levels: (1) scales containing items taken directly from a particular curriculum, which are referred to as *curriculum-embedded*; and (2) scales containing items that cover tasks that are common to many developmental curricula, which are referred to as *curriculum-referenced*. According to these authors, characteristics of CBA at the preschool level include (1) objectives that are developmentally task-analyzed and sequenced to reflect increasingly sophisticated competencies; and (2) a test–teach–test format to monitor progress. Mastery criteria must be clearly stated, must make sense in reference to the child's needs, and must be verifiable across observers. These last points are particularly relevant at the preschool level, where

TABLE 7.2. Relevant Information at the Preschool Level for Performance-Based Assessment

Instructional goals and activities

- What are the teacher's instructional goals across learning areas?
- How does the teacher believe instruction should be presented?
- What is the typical daily schedule? What activities are included?
- What kinds of emergent literacy activities are fostered (e.g., activities that focus on phonological awareness, print awareness, comprehension of story events, emergent writing, mathematical concepts)?
- How is mastery assessed and recorded?

Transition

- How does the target child respond during transitions from one activity to another?
- What does the teacher do to facilitate transitions?

Teacher directions

- How well does the child comprehend and follow teacher directions?
- How complex are teacher directions (i.e., how many steps and qualifiers are involved)?
- What is the pacing of instructions? Are directions repeated with key points emphasized to focus attention?

Interactive behavior

- To what extent does the child participate in classroom activities?
- How does the child interact with peers?
- How does the teacher facilitate social interactions?
- How are behavior problems typically handled?
- What is the child's attention span like?
- What does the teacher do to foster attention and interest in classroom activities?

Language behavior

- What is the child's use of language like?
- Is the child able to express thoughts and needs?
- To what extent does the teacher model a rich vocabulary and diverse language forms?
- How does the teacher modify instructions to address the needs of children experiencing difficulty?

Creativity and problem solving

- To what extent does the child display interest in new tasks and use creative strategies to solve problems?
- How does the teacher model the use of creative strategies in problem solving?

developmental progressions may be broadly defined (e.g., 3-month, 6-month, or 1-year intervals), and thus are too broad to provide feedback on children's learning progress.

It requires great thought and care to conduct and interpret CBA in a systematic and well-organized manner. Bagnato et al. (1989, 1997) present a systematic process for linking preschool assessment with curriculum and for integrating assessment information in order to inform intervention strategies across developmental domains. The linkage process described also allows for the use of NRTs for prescribing developmental objectives when NRTs assess the same skills as those covered in the curriculum. Bagnato et al. (1989) detail seven criteria for selecting developmental scales to be included in a prescriptive assessment battery: (1) a developmental base, (2) a multidomain profile, (3) a multisource sample, (4) curricular links, (5) adaptive options, (6) ecological emphasis, and (7) technical support. Using an Evaluation Rating Form based on these criteria, these authors present detailed overviews of developmentally based infant and preschool instruments that are compatible with developmental curricula. Bagnato et al. also present descriptions of multiple-task-analyzed developmental curricula to which assessment can be linked. Many of these curricula have updated forms. Assessors, however, need to be mindful of Fewell's (1984) caution that many popular developmental and behavioral checklists vary widely in quality, content, length, administrative requirements, purpose, reliability, and validity. Fewell points to some of the problems, including inappropriately ordered skill sequences, gaps in skill sequences, and bulkiness for practical use (to which we might add sequences that are not sufficiently fine-tuned or appropriately ordered to address the diverse needs of children with cognitive, language, sensory, or motor disabilities).

TECHNICAL CONSIDERATIONS REGARDING CBA

Many forms of CBA are appropriate for all children, as well as those presenting special needs. Important questions that need to be raised when one is considering their use include "Is the measure appropriate to the child's developmental level?" and "To what extent are the tasks that a measure taps developed within the curriculum within a similar developmental age range?" When appropriately used, CBA can help teachers and assessors gain perspective on how children learn, enhance children's motivation, accommodate a wide range of competence, and enhance communication with families (Meisels, Dorfman, & Steele, 1995; Bagnato & Neisworth, 1991). However, technical data for CBA approaches are often not reported. In particular, data on reliability and validity, other than content validity, are usually not provided (Shinn, 1989b). As stated by Messick (1995), the principles of validity apply to all forms of assessment, including performance-based assessment. Messick (1995) states the issue clearly: " . . . validity, reliability, and fairness are not just measurement principles; they are *social values* that have meaning and force whenever judgments and decisions are made" (p. 5; emphasis in original). (See also Chapter 3.)

SUMMARY: THE ADVANTAGES AND DISADVANTAGES OF CBA

In summary, the primary purpose of CBA is to collect data that can be used to modify instruction or behavioral intervention. Advantages of CBA cited in the literature include the following:

1. CBA brings assessment and programming together, and yields information about what a child can and cannot do within a specific learning domain.
2. Since CBA uses curriculum objectives as assessment items, content validity is assured.
3. CBA facilitates monitoring of student progress and provides a basis for program accountability, since changes resulting from instructional intervention can be documented.

4. CBA can help identify the educational problems of students with disabilities, as well as of those progressing according to age expectations.
5. CBA is useful to the extent that *the curriculum and teaching represent high-quality instruction* (Peverly & Kitzen, 1998). For example, Peverly and Kitzen point out that the research literature in the area of reading calls for high-quality instruction to include both meaning-based and code-based instruction. Young children need both to develop knowledge about language and to have sound–symbol skills available that will later help them to decode words quickly. Both of these sets of skills are necessary for listening and reading comprehension. At the preschool level, these are developed through activities, teacher questions, and interactions that get children to think about story events, predict outcomes, summarize, make inferences, interpret the information presented in pictures, learn rhymes, learn letters and their sounds, and so forth. The Analytic Framework for Coding Teacher Talk during Storybook Reading (McGill-Franzen et al., 2002) is an excellent example of teacher–child exchanges during storybook reading that are more or less cognitively challenging. The question for the assessor is the extent to which preschool curricula include these activities.

Limitations of CBA cited in the literature include the following:

1. CBA alone is not sufficient to serve the many diverse purposes of assessment. As a tool for making instructional decisions, CBA has proven to be valid, but most forms of CBA are not suitable for making eligibility decisions.
2. Not only are the methods that teachers use to design CBA unclear (Fuchs & Fuchs, 1986); there is no uniform approach with consistent, identifiable sets of procedures (Shinn, 1989b), although this situation is changing (Coyne & Harn, 2006; Hintze, Christ, & Methe, 2006).
3. CBA often fails to detail the kinds of adult supports a child needs and does not provide an indication of a child's work style or strategies.
4. Users of CBA, with the exception of those who follow Shapiro's model, often fail to account for how the interplay of environmental factors affects performance.
5. Data supporting the technical adequacy of CBA approaches are often not reported, with the exception of content validity, a situation that is now changing, with researchers presenting data regarding reliability and concurrent and predictive data.
6. CBA is no better than the curriculum on which it is based. The curriculum or teaching practices used may be the cause of some children's difficulties, not just the children's performance.
7. Users of CBA often fail to consider the cognitive processes needed to solve instructional tasks.

Portfolio Assessment

Portfolio assessment, a third form of performance-based assessment, involves observing children's behaviors and work samples in order to evaluate their progress. Portfolio assessment takes place through the ongoing activities of classrooms. Traditional grading and assessment practices are often replaced with documentation of student performance through anecdotal records, checklists, samples of students' work, and other documents that a teacher or student think are important to get a clear picture of a child's progress (Genishi, 1992). Portfolio assessment has as its overarching goals to determine the extent to which classroom activities facilitate learning objectives for individual children, to evaluate teaching effectiveness, and to modify objectives and teaching strategies as needed. Portfolio assessment involves the following key aspects:

1. *Monitoring children's mastery of specified curricular goals as an ongoing process by keeping daily records of observed behaviors and by collecting children's work products.* For young children, portfolios might include photographs and audio or video recordings of the children's art, block constructions, language, and motor behaviors, along with actual "writing" samples or art products. Observations can be contributed by parents as well as by teachers. Children can also actively participate in identifying items to be placed in portfolios, and can comment on observations and entries. Teachers use the information yielded to evaluate the effectiveness of their activities and to modify their plans and objectives, as noted above.
2. *Evaluating children's work samples in relationship to specific goals.* Mastery of goals is often recorded on skill checklists. The extent to which these checklists break down tasks into their component parts and detail the criteria for attaining a specified standard of performance is variable. Skills may be very broadly described (e.g., "Uses scissors with control" or "Follows two-step directions") and may not be sufficiently detailed to detect the progress made to the overall goal for children presenting special needs. Checklists therefore need to be reviewed with regard to the needs of the children served.
3. *Using portfolios as a means to foster ongoing communication with parents.* Parents can be requested to offer information about behaviors often seen at home to be included in the child's portfolio. Project Synergy (Wright & Borland, 1993), for example, uses "Let-Me-Tell-You-about-My-Child Cards" (sent in the appropriate home language) to encourage parents to contribute their perceptions and experiences to their child's portfolio. Teachers use pocket-sized "Notable Moment Cards" to record behaviors reflective of the child's development. The use of portfolios allows parents and teachers to reflect on what and how the child is learning without using jargon, and to consider useful instructional activities to foster the next steps of learning.

Various issues affect what materials are included in portfolios and how effectively portfolios are used:

1. Are teachers prepared to maintain and store large amounts of children's work?
2. Which individuals at school contribute to portfolios (classroom teachers, ESL teachers, speech–language specialists, school psychologists, special educators, others)?
3. What training is provided regarding how to create and use a portfolio? Are specific procedures and aids detailed? Are there examples of typical portfolios, so that teachers may see examples of work illustrating tasks in each developmental area? Guidelines for judging merit should be included, as well as for assessing children's self-selected choices. How are teachers' observational skills refined?
4. What support is provided by the school for ongoing training and for regular weekly meetings of the portfolio team?
5. What in-class supports (e.g., adolescent mentors) are available for children who evidence difficulty or who demonstrate particular strengths?

A number of projects and procedures at the early childhood level involve the use of portfolios. Although space does not permit us to describe all these in detail here, the Work Sampling System, Fourth Edition (Meisels, Jablon, Dichtelmiller, Dorfman, & Marsden, 1998) is presented as a model.

THE WORK SAMPLING SYSTEM

The Work Sampling System documents and assesses children's skills, as well as their behavior, knowledge, and accomplishments across a wide variety of domains throughout the school year. It systematizes teacher observation by guiding these observations with specific criteria and well-defined procedures. The Work Sampling System consists of three complementary elements:

1. *Developmental Guidelines and Checklists*. Eight checklists cover seven domains (Personal and Social Development, Language and Literacy, Mathematical Thinking, Scientific Thinking, Social Studies, The Arts, and Physical Development and Health). These checklists provide teachers with a set of observational criteria as a basis for their judgments, and are organized by age level. Teachers' observations are recorded three times a year to help document each child's growth and progress. Explicit rationale and examples are given in the guidelines for each performance indicator.
2. *Portfolios*. Portfolios contain a purposeful collection of children's work that illustrates their efforts, progress, and achievements throughout the year. A structured approach is used to collect samples for the portfolio, with at least five items collected on three occasions over the year representative of five of the core domains (Language and Literacy, Mathematical Thinking, Scientific Thinking, Social Studies, and The Arts; Social Development and Physical Development are not included), plus individual items of interest. Individual items reflecting the special characteristics and talents of the child are also included. Portfolios help document qualitative differences among children's work accomplishments on multiple occasions across a wide variety of classroom activities. By participating in the collection of material to be placed in portfolios, children play an active role in their own learning and in evaluating the quality of their own work.
3. *Summary Reports*. Completed three times a year by a teacher, these reports are brief summaries of each child's classroom performance, summarized from the portfolio, checklists, and observations. The checklists and the accompanying guidelines provide the teacher with a framework for structured observations. In addition to serving as a forum to communicate information to parents, the Summary Reports provide information about each child's progress that can be used by administrators and others concerned with documenting children's educational accomplishments.

The teacher, the child, the child's parents, and the school administration are all participants in the process. The Work Sampling System can be used with children as young as 3 through grade 5. Evidence of the reliability and criterion validity of the system is provided. The checklists and Summary Reports are reported to have high internal reliability, to have moderately high interrater reliability, and to predict performance on individually administered NRTs accurately (Meisels, Liaw, Dorfman, & Nelson, 1996).

ISSUES AND QUESTIONS IN PORTFOLIO ASSESSMENT

Issues related to portfolio assessment include the burden on teachers for maintaining up-to-date records for all children across developmental areas, the frequent subjective appraisal of the quality of children's work, and the question of who sets the standards for evaluating the quality of the work. Hiebert, Hutchinson, and Raines (1992) point out that little attention has been directed to collecting information about teachers' abilities to integrate alternate assessments into an already full agenda. Examining data collected from two teachers in a suburban school district that had eliminated all standardized testing until the end of grade 3, these researchers found that the results for the two teachers differed. One teacher was directed in her use of alternative assessment procedures, while the other made no connections between instructional activities and assessment. Clearly, alternative assessment procedures require special dedication and competence on the part of teachers. Some will use the method well; others will not. The authors concluded that for portfolio assessment to become an enduring part of school practices, its use must go beyond the classroom, be part of the school's policy, and be clearly articulated to parents. Assessment data need to be seen by parents and teachers as specific, useful, and understandable. A school also needs to be dedicated to providing supports to teachers, including in-service training, consultant time, and time to maintain up-to-date portfolios for all children.

The use of alternative assessment procedures such as portfolio assessment requires many talents on the part of a teacher, including good organization, observation skills, discipline in regular note taking for individual children, and skills for integrating information from multiple sources. These talents may be hard to exercise when a teacher is working with large numbers of children (especially children who come from diverse cultural/language backgrounds), when time is limited, and/or when behavior management is a major issue. Furthermore, all of the burden cannot fall on the shoulders of the teacher. It is essential that educational consultants, specialists, and school psychologists serve as resources to the teacher, assist in the observation process, and be available when a particular child's progress is of concern. Finally, one thing that is often missing from portfolio assessment is documentation of what the teacher does to elicit responding (such as modeling, enlarging on, and reinforcing responses), to enhance retention of information, and to encourage transfer.

Although the scores generated by NRTs and CRTs, along with the information yielded from CBA and portfolios, help in generating general diagnostic hypotheses or in adjusting instructional content, they do not necessarily provide insight into the specific reasons for a child's learning problems. The strategies that children use to solve problems, and the kinds of adult supports they need to be successful, are often neglected areas in assessing preschool children. In the two sections that follow, we consider strategy assessment and the role of the assessor in modifying tasks—approaches that can be used across all areas of functioning with preschool children.

Strategy Assessment

Strategy assessment focuses on how children think, how they approach tasks, how the strategies they use fit along the continuum of development suggested by the research literature, and what their errors mean. According to Siegler (1988, 1996, 1998), assessing thinking and reasoning can help us understand the processes that underlie children's performance and may be useful for developing interventions. Siegler points to an important phenomenon: "that even young children often use diverse strategies to solve a given class of problems, and that these diverse strategies contribute positively to their ability to adapt to changing task and situational demands" (1998, p. 15) A programmatic line of research by Siegler shows that children use multiple strategies on a wide variety of educational tasks over a short period of time. The interviewer needs to be guided by an understanding of the complexity of individual tasks based on a review of developmental research.

Ginsburg (1986) refers to the process we describe here as *cognitive analysis*, which he defines as the discovery and measurement of specific cognitive activities used by the child in academic performance. Insights about these activities are gained through an interview, which in this text we refer to as the *strategy interview*. The strategy interview is based on the clinical interviewing methods set forth more than 70 years ago by Piaget (1929), the work of Vygotsky (1978), and the work of Ginsburg (1986, 1997a). The assessor's aim in this interview to use open-ended questions to explore children's understanding, and then to get children to explain what they are doing and thus provide insight into what they are trying to do. We have discovered that with appropriate probes, children as young as 3 can tell us a lot about what they are doing (Boehm, 1990). Assessors can learn more about this technique by reading the multiple examples in Ginsburg's (1997a) book *Entering the Child's Mind*, by practicing the technique, and by reviewing audiotapes or videotapes of such exchanges. This method has a number of essential components (Ginsburg, 1986, 1997a):

1. Tailoring an engaging task to the child's needs and being interested in how the child solves problems. The assessor needs to be sensitive to the child's affect, and to change the task as necessary (either to simplify it for the child or to allow the child to reveal his or her thought processes).
2. Using open-ended questions to explore the child's thinking processes and strategies, and considering hypotheses about what the child is doing (and thus what the meaning of errors and correct responses may be).
3. Determining what methods of solution were used. The child is requested to give reasons for his or her answers, whether right or wrong; the assessor focuses on how the child arrived at these solutions and what he or she means by the explanations. At the same time, it is important to praise the child's attempts, even if they are unsuccessful (e.g., "Give it a try" or "You really worked hard on that one").
4. Testing hypotheses with such questions as "How did you know?", or giving the wrong answer and letting the child tell the assessor what was done wrong—in other words, making the child the expert.

As this list suggests, the interview begins with open-ended questions and gradually moves to more specific, focused questions. It then moves to testing hypotheses by coming up with alternative ideas about what is happening. Thus the assessor is able to determine the child's levels of competence as well as problems (e.g., with counting, one-to-one correspondence, or understanding the concepts *before* and *after*). The assessor uses language suitable for the child's level of understanding and modifies wording until the child understands what the task involves. These guidelines are particularly important for the preschool assessors, who may not give children enough time to respond or may not reword questions enough times to get at understanding. Little children often pause a lot or say they don't know, when in fact they have specific ideas about the problems presented. Strategy probes can help identify children's approaches to problems, their reasoning, their areas of competence, and the meaning of many of their errors. Very frequently, these errors are similar across children as they acquire knowledge in a particular learning area. The sensitivity of the individual assessor and the ability to probe children's responses without revealing errors are central to the success of this approach.

The Role of the Assessor in Modifying Tasks

The focus on strategies children use and on the adult's role in the assessment process is not new. The pioneering work of Elsa Haeussermann is particularly useful in understanding the role of the assessor in modifying tasks to understand the capabilities of children with severe disabilities, such as cerebral palsy. In her classic book *Developmental Potential of Preschool Children*, which remains an excellent resource, Haeussermann (1958) details a structured interview along with multiple areas of observation. Various possible modifications are described for children whose performance falls outside the range of the test items, or whose physical conditions make items inaccessible to direct contact. These modifications are particularly useful for assessors and include the following:

- Reducing choices and restoring choices.
- Using pantomime and gesture in the presentation of questions.
- Using materials that involve sound, such as blocks that make sounds.
- Assisting the child manually.
- Motivating the child (e.g., the child can eat a cookie if he or she can find it; the child can play with the surprise hidden in a box).
- Modeling the behavior for the child.
- Providing larger objects.
- Asking the child to follow commands, using objects.
- Engaging in game-like tasks, such as hide and find.

Methods for cross-checking modifications are also suggested.

Jedrysek, Klapper, Pope, and Wortis (1972) adapted Haeussermann's materials and methods for children 3–6 years of age without physical disabilities. Their adaptation involves using a series of graded probes to explore how a child arrives at a solution. Learning skills are covered in five areas of functioning: (1) physical functioning and sensory status, (2) perceptual functioning, (3) competence in learning for short-term retention, (4) language competence, and (5) cognitive functioning. Within each area, items are arranged in order of increasing difficulty, culminating in a level of mastery for each functional area viewed as appropriate for entrance into grade 1. Jedrysek et al.'s items are coreferenced to Haeussermann's items. Their predetermined series of probes includes the following:

- Breaking the task apart and demonstrating it.
- Making the task more concrete by naming it.
- Demonstrating the task nonverbally, using objects familiar to the child.
- Providing additional tactile and kinesthetic stimuli (e.g., letting the child feel objects).
- Using three-dimensional forms.
- Training with the task further broken down.

- Observing unguided play with related materials.
- Focusing the child's attention and giving the child additional chances.

Successive items can be used after a period of training, allowing the assessor to explore the effects of training on the skills investigated. The assessor's dual activities of probing and teaching are also integral to dynamic assessment, which is reviewed in Chapter 11.

Instructional Screening: Summary

The various forms of performance-based assessment, including portfolio assessment, have common goals (Chittenden, 1991). These include focusing on the work of the student in relation to the curriculum, enhancing teacher and student involvement in evaluation, and satisfying the demands for accountability prompted by school reform. Portfolios and other performance-based methods also make teachers accountable for their teaching methods and utilize the teachers' unique position in watching the developmental progress of their children (Genishi, 1992).

Instructional screening can play an important role in helping teachers individualize their teaching activities—but it must not be used to track children into programs that delay their movement from prekindergarten to kindergarten, or to first grade. Clearly, it needs to be an ongoing process in the context of other activities that motivate children to explore their environments and express their ideas. The many assessment forms that can be used to achieve this end—including NRTs and CRTs, ongoing observation and CBA activities, and collecting portfolios of children's work in a systematic manner—should not be pitted against each other. Rather, these multiple forms of assessment need to be used to understand children's preparedness for the learning tasks to come and to provide instruction or intervention matched to their strengths and needs. The strategy interview and task modification can be built into this process.

A number of key questions relate to the effective use of instructional screening, some of which may be useful in developing interventions:

1. How comprehensive and flexible is the teacher's curriculum? For example, to what extent is it linked to one philosophy or one curricular approach (such as phonics or whole language), and to what extent does the teacher adapt instruction to each child's needs?
2. How good is the teacher at observing and recording the day-to-day behaviors of the many children in his or her class, and maintaining up-to-date records or portfolios with information integrated from multiple sources? The assessor may be able to help the teacher develop a workable record-keeping system, or to conduct workshops that cover this issue. Adequate help is needed in the classroom for adequate record keeping to be a realistic outcome.
3. To what extent does the teacher model desired behaviors related to student learning, use strategies that break down tasks, and provide needed supports to assist children to focus attention and acquiring learning goals? Again, a teacher workshop can be developed to provide multiple examples, and/or consultants can be made available in the classroom.
4. How much support does the school provide in terms of classroom help, outreach to parents, and ongoing training for parents and teachers? Assessors need to be involved with training programs, know the curriculum, keep up-to-date with related empirical evidence, spend time in classrooms, and gain the confidence of teachers.

SUMMARY

This chapter presents a review of approaches to assessing the preparedness of children as they enter kindergarten and first grade. Because of the dramatic increase in high-quality research on early development, early childhood specialists have a much better understanding of the skills and behaviors children need to be successful in school and how to assess them. We believe most children should enter kindergarten at an age-appropriate level and urge that resources be made to help those children who have not been in preschool to gain the experiences needed to be successful in kindergarten and first grade. These activities need to take place in the context of the regular classroom, through summer programs, and through parent involvement. This places a tremendous burden on teachers who need to have the support of their local administration and the availability of consultants as they adapt their curriculum to meet child needs. Except for some short-term gains, the practice of "redshirting" has proved to be in large part unsuccessful. There are possible long-term negative effects, and it is an area of inequity for many minority students who do not have access to quality preschool programs.

The assessment–teach–assessment (or instructional screening) approach we recommend, when appropriately used, can help teachers adjust their curriculum to meet student needs through a broad variety of activities that break down tasks, understand how children arrive at their responses and that mistakes make sense, model desired behaviors, and provide students with the supports and reinforcement they need in order to be successful. These activities need to be engaging and build on the strategies children use to solve problems.

This chapter has reviewed many approaches assessors can use to achieve this end, including the appropriate use of those that are norm based and curriculum based. The area of academic preparedness is critical to parents and to teachers and administrators who need to be responsive to the demands of NCLB. Quick, speeded testing is not the answer, although it is very appealing. Assessment approaches need to be more responsive to the needs of the child and lead to developing intervention approaches that build on the rich literature on learning, not only as it relates to reading, but also to writing, mathematics, and the child's socioemotional development. Thus, the assessment of early academic learning is a dynamic, ongoing process that informs parents and teachers about what to do next and provides administrators with a broad spectrum of data to document progress.

APPENDIX 7.1. Review of Measures

Measure	**Battelle Developmental Inventory, Second Edition (BDI-2). Newborg (2004). See Chapter 6, Appendix 6.1.**

Measure	**Boehm Test of Basic Concepts—Third Edition (Boehm-3). Boehm (2000a).**
Purpose	Assessing "students' understanding of 50 important concepts they need to know to be successful in school" (p. 1), and helping to identify children at potential risk for learning difficulty.
Areas	Basic relational concepts relevant to school learning, including size, position, quantity, classification, direction, time, and general (other).
Format	Group-administered; 50 items on each of two forms (Forms E and F). Students mark correct answers in picture booklet in response to verbal instructions.
Scores	Percentage correct, performance range, percentiles. No percentiles available when test is used out of age range.
Age group	Grades K–2. May be used to test students out of range as well.
Time	Up to 45 minutes; may be administered in two sessions.
Users	Teachers and other assessors.
Norms	Fall and spring norms available for grades K–2. Sample was representative of 1998 U.S. census data in terms of race/ethnicity and geographic region. Gender was distributed evenly. Fall norms based on sample of >11,000 children (*n* = 6,055 English-speaking); Spring norms based on sample of >7,000 children (*n* = 4,544 English-speaking). Special education students who were mainstreamed in regular classes were included. Schools were selected to be representative in terms of district size, SES, urban–rural location, and geographic region. An extensive bias review was conducted, which utilized an expert review panel and statistical analysis.
Reliability	Internal consistency, .80–.91; *SEM*, 1.14–2.43; test–retest (2–14 days), .80–.84 (Form E) with an overall reliability of .80, and .70–.88 (Form F) with an overall reliability of .89; alternate-form (*n* = 216 second graders, 2–14 days, counterbalanced design), .83.
Validity	Content validity indicated by method of item selection; items were chosen through a review of children's printed materials, reading and math curricula, and concepts frequently used in teachers' directions. Evidence of validity based on a comparison of the Boehm-3 with other variables is available for the Boehm-R, the Metropolitan Achievement Tests—Eighth Edition, the Metropolitan Readiness Tests—Sixth Edition, the Otis–Lennon School Ability Test—Seventh Edition, and a longitudinal study of the Boehm-3 (from fall to spring).
Comments	This measure is easy to administer and score. The examiner's manual is easy to follow and provides all directions in both English and Spanish for both forms of the test. Pictures are all in full color and include children of several races/ethnicities and children with disabilities. Improvements upon previous edition include color illustrations, a fourth choice to reduce guessing, and updated norms. A Spanish edition was standardized with the English edition. A teacher report and observation form and a parent report form are included. Test results are useful to document progress as a result of teaching or intervention. The concepts included are often those used in the directions of other preschool tests.
References consulted	Bain (2005); Hawkins (2005); Keller (2005). See book's References list.

Measure	**Boehm Test of Basic Concepts—Third Edition: Preschool Version (Boehm-3: Preschool). Boehm (2001).**
Purpose	Assessing young children's understanding of basic relational concepts relevant to early childhood learning.
Areas	Basic relational concepts of size, direction, position, time, quantity, classification, and general (other, such as same–different).
Format	Individually administered. Child responds to verbal instructions by pointing to a picture (one of four options) on an easel. Each concept is presented twice to determine the child's understanding across contexts.
Scores	Percentage correct, performance range, percentiles. No percentiles available when test used out of age range.
Age group	3-0 to 5-11 years.
Time	15–20 minutes; may be administered in two sessions.
Users	Teachers and other assessors.
Norms	Data collected on 660 children (equal numbers of girls and boys). Representative of 1998 U.S. Census data in terms of race/ethnicity, geographic region, and parental educational level. Extensive bias review was conducted, which included review by an expert panel and statistical analysis.
Reliability	Internal consistency, .85–.92; *SEM*, 2.08–2.88; test–retest (2–21 days), .90–.94.
Validity	Content validity suggested by method of item selection, which included a review of children' s printed materials, math and reading curricula, and concepts frequently used by teachers when giving instructions. Evidence also provided by correlations with the Boehm-3 and the Bracken Basic Concept Scale—Revised. A clinical study was conducted with two age groups (3-0 to 3-11 years and 4-0 to 5-11 years). Children were matched by age, gender, race/ethnicity, and parent educational level. Mean scores differed for children with and without receptive language disorders. (The author cautions against use of this information alone as evidence to support the measure's diagnostic utility.)
Comments	This measure is easy to administer and score. The examiner's manual is easy to follow and provides all directions in both English and Spanish for both forms of the test. Pictures are all in full color and include children of several races/ethnicities and children with disabilities. A teacher summary and observation form and parent report form are included. The examiner's manual includes a useful chapter on planning interventions. The concepts assessed include those important to early childhood learning and are often included in the directions to other preschool measures. Improvements in new edition include updated norms; extension of age range to 5-11; overlapping items with Boehm-3; a fourth response option to reduce guessing; and updated illustrations.
References consulted	Graham (2005); Malcolm (2005). See book's References list.

Measure	**Bracken Basic Concept Scale—Revised (BBCS-R). Bracken (1998).**
Purpose	Measuring receptive language, vocabulary, and basic concepts in children to identify delays or disorders; school readiness screening; and clinical and educational research.
Areas	Diagnostic Scale covers educational concepts in 11 subtests or concept categories: Colors, Sizes, Texture/Material, Direction/Position, Letters, Comparisons, Quantity, Self-/Social Awareness, Numbers/Counting, Shapes, and Time/Sequences. The first six subtests constitute the School Readiness

	Composite Score, which is used to assess children's knowledge of those "readiness" concepts traditionally taught in preparation for formal education.
Format	Individually administered. Children are shown pictures and required to identify which of four pictures represent a concept. Ceiling and basal rules apply.
Scores	Scaled scores, standard scores, percentile ranks, concept age equivalents, and normative conceptual classifications. Subtest scores, total test scores, and School Readiness Composite Score are available.
Age group	Diagnostic Scale, 2-6 to 7-11 years; Screening Test, 5-0 to 7-0 years.
Time	30 minutes plus for full measure; 10–15 minutes for School Readiness Composite.
Users	Professionals trained in administration and interpretation of educational instruments. Can be administered by paraprofessionals under appropriate supervision.
Norms	Data collected on 1,109 children stratified on the basis of age, gender, ethnicity, geographic region, SES, and community size. A Spanish version is available, with separate norms based on 109 Hispanic children proficient in English.
Reliability	Split-half for subtests, .78–.98; split-half for total test, .96–.99; internal consistency, .76–.80; test–retest for subtests, .78–.88 (with the exception of Sizes at .67), and a median of .81 and .94 for the total test.
Validity	Items are used very often in preschool and on primary tests given to young children. Thus the author claims the BBCS-R has good content validity. This measure correlates significantly with the Boehm-R, the Token Test, the Kaufman Assessment Battery for Children Achievement Scale, and the Peabody Picture Vocabulary Test—Revised.
Comments	The test is easy to administer and score. The test correctly identified the presence or absence of developmental delay 74%–76% of the time, with 4%–13% incorrectly identified. The manual provides a thorough discussion of administration and scoring, interpretation, uses in remediation, development and standardization and technical characteristics. The BBCS-R is useful in assessing basic concept knowledge at the preschool, kindergarten, and first-grade levels. A Spanish edition is available with field data based on a small sample. Useful as a criterion-referenced measure.
References consulted	Nellis (2001); Solomon (2001). See book's References list.

Measure	**Bracken School Readiness Assessment (BSRA). Bracken (2002).**
Purpose	Assessing academic readiness by evaluating a child's understanding of 88 important foundational concepts in several categories.
Areas	Colors, Letters, Numbers/counting, Sizes, Comparisons, and Shapes.
Format	Individually administered measure with six subtests making up a school readiness composite. Concepts are presented orally in complete sentences and visually in a multiple-choice format. Pointing and short verbal responses are acceptable ways of answering.
Scores	Percent mastery scores, standard scores, percentile ranks, and interpretative labels (very delayed to very advanced).
Age group	2-6 to 7-11 years.
Time	10–15 minutes.
Users	Teachers, trained professionals.

Norms	This instrument is composed of the first six of the 11 subtests of the revised Bracken Basic Concept Scale. Data for the English standardization sample included 1,100 children (2-6 to 8-0 years of age), stratified by age, gender, ethnicity, region, and parent education, with 50 children at 3-month age intervals from 2-11 to 6-0 years. Data collected for the Spanish version used 193 children, with ages ranging in number from 16 children at 2-0 years to 40 children at 7-0 years.
Reliability	Split-half reliability (Spearman-Brown), .78–.97 with an average of .91; test–retest (based on 114 children retested after 7–14 days), .88; internal consistency for the Spanish version, .72–.95.
Validity	Concurrent validity with the revised BBCS-R is high (.81 corrected for restriction of range); WPPSI-R (.85, .76, and .88 for Verbal IQ, Performance IQ, and Full Scale IQ, respectively); and the Differential Ability Scales (/69, .72, and .79 for the Verbal Ability, Nonverbal Ability, and General Conceptual Ability scores, respectively.) Correlations with the PPVT-III, Boehm-R, and PLS-3 are presented. Specificity was between 82–90% for 71 children when identifying students nominated for retention. No validity studies using Spanish children were reported in the manual.
Comments	The BSRA is composed of the first six subtests of the BBCS-R. Test materials include a stimulus book, which includes colorful drawings that seem appealing to children, and an administration manual. The test includes English and Spanish versions. Directions provided for the BSRA are clear and easy to follow. Psychometric information for the test is adequate for the English version but limited for the Spanish version. Overall, the BSRA is valuable in assessing the needs of preschool children and making decisions about early school entrance and retention.
References consulted	McKnight (2005). See book's References list.

Measure	**Brigance Inventory of Early Development—II. Brigance (2004).**
Purpose	Determining the developmental or performance level of the infant or child, and identifying his or her strengths and weaknesses through the use of skill assessment and a comprehensive record-keeping system. It can also be used to identify instructional objectives and obtain data that can be used as part of an assessment to support a diagnosis or referral.
Areas	Perambulatory Motor Skills, Gross Motor Skills, Fine Motor Skills, Self-Help Skills, Speech and Language Skills, General Knowledge and Comprehension, Social and Emotional Development, Readiness, Basic Reading Skills, Manuscript Writing, and Basic Math. Each broad skills area is further divided into a number of subskills.
Format	A criterion-referenced (and norm-referenced) measure based on parent interview, observing the child, asking the child to perform tasks, engaging the child in conversation, and teacher interviews. Items are not normed; rather, skills were assigned developmental ages by referencing several texts in which age norms for the skills are published. Methods used to assess skills include interview, observation, and asking the child to perform tasks and to engage in conversation.
Scores	Quotients, percentiles, age equivalents, instructional ranges, adaptive behavior score.
Age group	Birth to 7 years.
Time	15–20 minutes.

Users	Examiners who have knowledge of child development and are familiar with the procedures in the manual; requires little specialized training.
Norms	Criterion-referenced instrument and standardized in five skill areas: Expressive Language, Academic/Cognitive; Daily Living/Self-Help; and Social–Emotional.
Reliability	Internal consistency, .99; test–retest (*n* not defined) ranged from .28 (Picture Vocabulary) to .84 (Number Comprehension); interrater reliability ranged from .40 to 1.00. Not presented in the test manual.
Validity	Not presented in the test manual; content based on a review of curriculum practices, current pupil texts, and popular developmental scales.
Comments	Easy to use and score. Covers a broad range of behaviors and skills associated with early childhood development. The developmental age scores are not intended to be used rigidly, but to serve as guidelines. Follow-up assessments can be conducted to assess whether instructional objectives have been met. Lacks information regarding reliability and validity. Analyzes a child's performance across 98 skill sequences within 11 domains; many of the skill sequences lack the necessary detail to provide assessments that are precise enough to identify preschool children with severe difficulties. Most effective when used with children with mild to moderate difficulties. Computer-based programs are available. Materials needed can be purchased as a kit or gathered locally.
References consulted	Glascoe (2002); Penfield (1995). See book's References list.

Measure	**Brigance K and I Screen—II. Brigance (2005).**
Purpose	Screening instrument used to obtain a broad sampling of child's skills and behaviors to identify children with a disability or who may need special placement; identifying most appropriate initial placement; assisting teacher in planning a more appropriate program for a child; and complying with mandated screening requirements.
Areas	Assesses Fine-Motor Skills (i.e., drawing symbols and writing name), Gross-Motor Skills, Body Awareness (i.e., naming body parts), General Knowledge (i.e., names of colors), and Language Development (i.e., word recognition). Skills are divided into two age groups, kindergarten and grade 1; there are also parent and teacher report forms: the social–emotional scales (ages 2-0–5-11 years) and the reading readiness scale.
Format	Individually administered; however, there are a list of alternative administration procedures. It is recommended that the examiners set up stations (a table and two chairs) for large groups of children. It is also recommended that children be tested twice a year—once in the fall then again in the spring.
Scores	Total score out of 100, standard scores, age equivalent, and percentiles.
Age group	Kindergarten (5-0 to 5-11 years), and First grade (6-0 years+).
Time	15–20 minutes.
Users	Teachers, paraprofessionals, or other professionals, such as physical therapist, nurse, or physician.
Norms	Norms were derived from 1,366 children (ages birth to 6-0+ years) in 27 states (95, 86, 180, and 411, ages 3-0 to 6-0+, respectively).
Reliability	Information on test–retest, internal consistency, and interrater reliability are contained in the *Technical Report for the Brigance Screens—II* (Glascoe, 2005).

Validity	Support for content validity presented in original screens, by extensive use in the field, and age-related trends in scores. Other validity data can be found in the *Technical Report for the Brigance Screens—II*. Identifies 81% (range = 70–91% across all ages) of children with disabilities, 84% (range + 81–100% across all ages) of children with advanced development, and 84% (range + 72–94% across all ages) of children with typical developments.
Comments	Manual is clear and comprehensive. There are explanations and examples of the criteria for the items. Although the manual is concise and user-friendly, minimal data are reported regarding the technical characteristics of the test. Users need to purchase the *Technical Report* that covers all of the screens and is often difficult to understand. A strength of the assessment is that it obtains information from parents, teachers, and other relevant professionals. A major difficulty with this test is that each stimulus page contains numerous stimulus items. For example, the Visual Discrimination skill test for first graders contains 10 rectangular boxes of four words or letters per box. It would have been preferable to have fewer stimulus items per page. The data sheets, or record forms, are in triplicate and seem too small for the amount of information contained on them. There is not enough room for the examiner to quickly record responses and note behavioral observations within a skill area during testing. The measure is available, but not normed, in Spanish. A training video is available as well as informational presentations at publisher's website.
References consulted	Brigance Screens web page; Emmons and Alfonso (2005); Watson (1995). See book's References list.

Measure	**Comprehensive Test of Phonological Processing (CTOPP). Wagner, Torgesen, and Rashotte. (1999).**
Purpose	Assessing phonological awareness, phonological memory, and rapid naming in order to identify individuals performing below their peers in phonological processing ability.
Areas	Three composites include Phonological Awareness, Phonological Memory, and Rapid Naming. The preschool version of the CTOPP includes seven core subtests and one supplementary subtest. The core subtests are elision, blending words, sound matching, memory for digits, nonword repetition, rapid color naming, and rapid object naming. The supplementary subtest is blending nonwords.
Format	Individually administered; 60 items across three subtests make up the phonological awareness composite; 39 items across two subtests make up the phonological memory composite; 144 items across two subtests make up the rapid naming composite; 18-item supplementary subtest is also included.
Scores	Standard scores, composite scores, percentiles, age equivalents, grade equivalents.
Age group	5-0 to 6-11 years for the first version. A second version is available for ages 7-0 to 24-11 years.
Time	30 minutes.
Users	Must have training in assessment, test statistics, and phonological ability testing.
Norms	1,656 individuals in 30 states during 1997–1998. Sample sizes for 14 age groups ranged from 76 to 155 (13 samples represented each age, 5-0–17-0 years, separately; ages 18-0–24-0 years comprised a single sample of 112 respondents). It appears that respondents were not randomly selected, but a

	comparison to U.S. school population estimates for the targeted year revealed close matches for the resulting percentages of CTOPP examinees across the four regions, gender and age, ethnicity, and other SES indicators.
Reliability	Internal-consistency reliability (Cronbach alphas) estimates were reported for all nonspeeded subtest scores and alternate-form reliability estimates were reported for speeded subtest scores. Across age groups, these ranged from .77 to .95; test–retest reliability (2-week interval) for 32 individuals aged 5-0–7-0 years, .68 to .97; interrater reliability for 30 completed CTOPP batteries for ages 5-0–6-11 years, .95 to .99.
Validity	Validity was assessed with content validity (including item rationale, item response theory, and differential item functioning analysis), criterion-related validity, and construct validity. Content validity tests indicated that the subtests are a good measure of phonological processing. Construct validity was supported using confirmatory factor analyses. A three-factor solution for the normative sample of children ages 5-0–6-0 years yielded the composite/subtest make-up of the CTOPP for the younger version. Criterion-related validity examined the correlations between the CTOPP and the WRMT-R with 216 kindergartners yielded coefficients for the composite scores of .71, .42, and .66 one year after the CTOPP was given in kindergarten. When later assessed in first grade with the CTOPP and then compared to their WRMT-R composites a year later in second grade, coefficients values were .80, .52, and .70. Concurrent validity ranged from .00 to .75 with the Lindamood Auditory Conceptualization Tests, the WRMT-R, the GORT-3, and the WRAT-3 across age levels. Predictive validity ranged from .21 to .72 with the Lindamood Auditory Conceptualization Tests, the WRMT-R, the GORT-3, and the WRAT-3 across age levels.
Comments	The test materials include a stimulus book, technical manual, and audiocassette for presenting sounds in various subtests. Test administration instructions are well written, with detailed examples. The examiner needs to be comfortable in scoring verbal responses. A sample answer audiocassette would be a useful addition to the revision of the test. Overall, CTOPP subtest scores appear to provide reliable and valid indicators of phonological awareness, phonological memory, and rapid naming for individuals of ages 5-0 through 24-11 years. Additional studies are needed to replicate the observations reported for individuals with learning and speech-language disabilities.
References consulted	Wright (2001). See book's References list.

Measure	**Concepts About Print Test. Clay (2002).**
Purpose	Providing knowledge about children's awareness of print and its uses. One of six tasks included on the Observation Survey of Early Literacy Achievement—Second Edition (Clay, 2002); developed to inform instruction and monitor progress.
Areas	Print conventions, book orientation, vocabulary, upper and lowercase letters, and punctuation marks.
Format	24 items individually administered; the examiner reads one of four small picture books aloud. Verbatium directions provided for each item. Two of the books are available in Spanish.
Scores	Stanines, mean, standard deviations.
Age group	5-0 to 7-0 years.

Time	10–15 minutes.
Users	Teachers, trained professionals.
Norms	Data collected on 796 New Zealand children (2002) and 109 American children (1990–1991).
Reliability	Test–retest reliability, .73–.89; Split-half reliability, .84–.88. Reliability data collected on a study of 106 Ohio urban children.
Validity	Correlations with other measures range from .64 to .79 in studies carried out in New Zealand more than 20 years ago.
Comments	Developed by the founder of the Reading Recovery Program. The assessment can be customized to the individual, but it is time-consuming to administer. Updated local norms on American children need to be developed. Moderate to strong predictor of reading achievement in the early grades. Limited reliability and validity evidence. A training tape is available.
References consulted	Clay (2002); Rathvon (2004). See book's References list.

Measure	**Developmental Profile—Second Edition (DP-II). Alpern, Boll, and Shearer (1986).**
Purpose	Assessing a child's strengths and weaknesses and measuring a child's progress in order to develop an individualized education plan or determine eligibility for receiving special education services.
Areas	Physical, Self-Help, Social, Academic, and Communication.
Format	186-item inventory across five areas of functioning which can be administered either individually or in a group format. Can be administered as a direct test or by interviewing parents, teachers, or others who are well acquainted with the child. (Norms were gathered through parent interviews only.)
Scores	Age scores, ratio IQ equivalency score for Academic scale only.
Age group	Birth to 9-5 years (0 through 7-0 years for normally developing children).
Time	20–40 minutes.
Users	Trained professionals.
Norms	Data derived from the original standardization study and do not reflect the items in the current revision. The original sample consisted of 3,008 children from 0 to 12-6 years from Indiana (91%) and Washington (9%) assessed during the early 1970s. Only normally developing children were included in the standardized sample. The standardization group is biased in that the sample is disproportionately urban, middle-class, and Midwestern; although blacks are adequately represented, other minority groups (e.g., Asians and Hispanics) are not; sample sizes for children ages 1-7 to 2-0 and 2-1 to 2-6 are smaller (n = 91 and 95, respectively) than other age levels.
Reliability	Test–retest reliability (2–3 day intervals with 11 mothers) was assessed with the original version of the scale. The small sample size limits generalization of the results. Internal consistency reliability coefficients, .78–.87 for each of the five subtests (with a sample of 1,050 children ages 3–5 years); interscorer reliability data were adequate.
Validity	Concurrent validity measured with correlations between criterion measures (e.g., Binet, Slosson Intelligence Test, Learning Accomplishment Profile) was satisfactory. Predictive validity was not measured. Factor-analytic studies investigating the structure of the DP-II have not been conducted.

Comments	The DP-II represents a revision of items based upon feedback from users rather than a restandardization. These revisions include deleted items above the age of 9-6 years, clarification of some directions, and removing sexist items and language. The psychometric properties of the DP-II are lacking in reliability and validity studies. The identification of children needing special education services (i.e., the primary objective of the DP-II) requires a technically sound norm-referenced instrument. Unfortunately, the DP-II is simply technically inadequate for the task. May be administered and scored by hand or using computer program.
References consulted	Huebner (1989). See book's References list.

Measure	**Dynamic Indicators of Basic Early Literacy Education—Sixth Edition (DIBELS). Good et al. (2002–2003).**
Purpose	Benchmarking or monitoring the development of prereading and early reading skills.
Areas	Initial sound fluency (ISF), letter naming fluency (LNF), phoneme segmentation fluency (PSF), nonsense word fluency (NWF), oral reading fluency (ORF), oral retelling fluency, word use fluency.
Format	Individually administered battery of early literacy tests that measure phonemic awareness (K–1), letter knowledge (K–1), decoding skills (K–2), oral reading fluency (1–.3), and vocabulary knowledge and expressive language (1–3); 20 alternate forms are available; benchmark versions are to be given three times per year to all primary grade students, and the progress-monitoring forms are to be used more frequently with children who are at risk of failure.
Scores	Raw scores, developmental benchmarks.
Age group	Grades K–3.
Time	1–3 minutes for each individual subtest.
Users	Properly trained teachers or professionals. Website includes video clips of each subtest being administered appropriately.
Norms	A representative standardization sample is not available for the DIBELS. An online system allows comparison with 300 school districts, 600 schools, and 32,000 children.
Reliability	There is no technical manual for this test. Reliability data are extensively detailed on the DIBELS website. Test–retest reliability ranged from .92 to .97.
Validity	Strong predictive and concurrent validity evidence when compared to the Woodcock-Johnson Reading Mastery Test and other measures with reported coefficients of .80 for ORF, .58 for NWF, .44 for PSF, and .55 for ISF. The predictive validity coefficients were .47 for PSF, .53 for ISF, .66 for ORF, and .68 for NWF (see also website).
Comments	The DIBELS tests have made individual assessment practical for classroom purposes since the tests take very little administration time, are inexpensive to purchase (forms also can be downloaded from the Internet), the alternate forms allow for frequent monitoring of progress, and the results are designed to help teachers shape instruction for individual children. In addition, the DIBELS helps fulfill requirements mandated by the federal Reading First Program. As a screening tool, the DIBELS does a fine job of evaluating letter name knowledge, phonemic awareness, and oral reading fluency; however, it does not adequately measure reading comprehension and vocabulary knowledge. The psychometric evidence suggests higher reliabilities and concurrent and predictive validities

	than is typical of screeners. However, the online database (used as a comparison sample) is part of an ongoing process where schools enter their own data into the database, leaving plenty of room for error. At the kindergarten level there is an overemphasis on speed.
References consulted	Goodman (2006); Rathvon (2004); Shanahan (2005). See book's References list.

Measure	**Gesell School Readiness Test (GSRT). Ilg and Ames (1972).**
Purpose	Evaluating maturational factors affecting a child's learning, and determining appropriate grade placement.
Areas	Two developmental domains: adaptive and language.
Format	Nine subtests: Interview, Paper and Pencil Test, Cube Tests, Copy Forms, Incomplete Man, Right and Left, Monroe Visual Tests, Naming Animals, Home and School Preferences.
Scores	Cutoff points.
Age group	2-6 to 6-11 years.
Time	20–30 minutes.
Users	Extensive training is required to administer the GSRT.
Norms	Data collected in the 1940s in North Haven, Connecticut, on a small (n = 80), largely white, above-average-SES population. Norms are out of date and nonrepresentative of the population today.
Reliability	Reviewers have consistently cautioned that the GSRT does not meet technical standards for reliability, validity, or normative information. Lichtenstein (1990) found that test–retest reliability was .73 and that interrater reliability among trained examiners was .71.
Validity	Reviewers have consistently cautioned that the GSRT does not meet technical standards for reliability, validity, or normative information (see above).
Comments	The GSRT lacks up-to-date norms, has insufficient technical data, and should not be used to make placement decisions.
References consulted	Bradley (1985); Gredler (1992); Lichtenstein (1990); Meisels (1987). See book's References list.

Measure	**Iowa Tests of Basic Skills (ITBS). Hoover, Hieronymous, Frisbie, and Dunbar (1996).**
Purpose	Assessing the basic skills needed by a student to progress satisfactorily through school, so that instruction can be improved.
Areas	Core Battery (Listening, Word Analysis, Vocabulary, Reading Comprehension, Language, Mathematics); Complete Battery (Core Battery + Social Studies, Science, and Sources of Information); Survey Battery (Reading, Language, and Mathematics).
Format	Multiple-choice; available in levels 5–14 (roughly corresponding to age); Forms K (Braille or large-print edition), L, M.
Scores	Percentiles, grade equivalents.
Age group	Grades K–8.
Time	130–310 minutes for Complete Battery, 100 minutes for Survey Battery.

Users	School personnel.
Norms	Separate norms for high- and low-SES areas, Catholic private schools, large cities, and international students; local norms can also be computed. Norms based on 136,934 students in Catholic and non-Catholic schools. The number of schools participating was not indicated.
Reliability	Internal consistency, .85–.92.
Validity	Criterion, .75; concurrent, mid-.80s. No information on validity on listening tests, language tests, and writing assessments.
Comments	The test claims to be culturally fair. Reliability for writing section is modest. The newly developed Reading, Language, and Mathematics sections have no information regarding interpretation or technical information. Reliability is questionable. There is a penalty for guessing, so it should be stated in the examinees' directions that only educated guesses should be made.
References consulted	Brookhart (1998); Cross (1998). See book's References list.

Measure	**Kaufman Survey of Early Academic and Language Skills (K-SEALS). Kaufman and Kaufman (1993).**
Purpose	Measuring children's language skills, preacademic skills, and articulation.
Areas	Vocabulary; Numbers, Letters, and Words; and Articulation. The Vocabulary subtest is composed of 20 receptive and 20 expressive items. Numbers, Letters, and Words consists of 20 items that assess number skills and 20 items that assess prereading and reading skills. This subtest assesses long-term memory, number facility, visual perception of objects and symbols, and early language development.
Format	Individually administered. All ages begin with same item on the subtests, and discontinue after five consecutive item scores of 0.
Scores	Standard scores, confidence intervals, composite scores.
Age group	3-0 to 6-11 years.
Time	15–25 minutes.
Users	Professionals with experience working with young children.
Norms	Data collected on 1,000 children across geographic areas in the United States representative of a wide range of ethnicity and SES. Children with disabilities were not systematically represented.
Reliability	Test–retest, .87–.94 (twice within a month); split-half, .94.
Validity	Concurrent, correlated substantially with standard scores on individually administered tests (average correlation in the low .80s). Predictive, against teacher ratings (average falls around .60).
Comments	Administration and scoring are clear and straightforward. Detailed information is provided regarding interpretation of results. Unclear in manual whether this is intended to be a screening measure or a diagnostic measure. Caution is appropriate when interpreting outcomes because of limited item coverage in all areas. Appropriate only for children whose primary language is English.
References consulted	Ackerman (1995); Ford (1995); and Turk (1995). See book's References list.

Measure	**Learning Accomplishment Profile—Diagnostic Edition (LAP-D). Nehring et al. (1992).**
Purpose	Assisting in the formulation of developmentally appropriate instructional objectives and strategies for young children by identifying a child's mastery level across three domains of functioning.
Areas	Three developmental domains: Cognitive, Language, and Motor domains, which are divided into subscales: Cognitive (counting, matching); Language (comprehension, naming); Fine Motor (writing, manipulation) and Gross Motor (body movement, object movement).
Format	LAP-D is one of four tests available. The others in the series include the LAP-D Screen, the LAP-R, and the ELAP; may be administered in station or individual format; each item is marked with a plus (+) if the child exhibits the criterion-referenced behavior, or a minus (–) if the skill is not demonstrated by the child.
Scores	Percentile ranks, normal curve equivalents, age equivalents, *T*-scores, *z*-scores.
Age group	2-6 to 6-0 years.
Time	45–90 minutes.
Users	Teachers, trained professionals.
Norms	Data collected on 792 children with seven 6-month age groupings, 2-5–6-0 years of age, across 10 locations throughout the United States. The sample was based on the 1990 U.S. census and stratified by sex and race.
Reliability	Internal consistency, measured by split-half, .80.
Validity	Construct validity coefficients, .10 to .56; concurrent validity coefficients, .49 to .87 with the BDI and the DIAL-R.
Comments	The LAP-D includes a test kit with materials for each individual subscale. The materials are colorful and packaged in individually labeled bags by subscale making it easy to prep for administration. Overall, the LAP-D can be used as part of a multidisciplinary assessment to determine eligibility or in planning and monitoring a child's progress. However, its limitations should be noted. While the LAP-D includes a variety of test items in three developmental domains, it fails to address the areas of adaptive behavior and social–emotional functioning. Furthermore, because many of the objectives are based on specific test items, they are narrow in focus and do not address more functional skills. Finally, the psychometric data for the LAP-D needs updating. The norms are over 10 years old and the norming sample is relatively small. Additional information for reliability and validity need to be included as part of a restandardization of the instrument.
References consulted	Spenciner (2005). See book's References list.

Measure	**Lindamood Auditory Conceptualization Test—Revised. Lindamood and Lindamood (1991).**
Purpose	Measuring speech sound discrimination and perception of number, order, and sameness or difference of speech sounds in sequences.
Areas	Isolated Phoneme Patterns, Sounds with a Syllable Pattern, Total.
Format	20 phoneme sequences and responses, and 12 orally presented syllable patterns.
Scores	Total.
Age group	Preschool children and over.
Time	10–35 minutes.

Users	Not specified; a training tape accompanies the test.
Norms	Data collected on 660 students in K–12 of the Monterey, California Public schools, who represented a wide range of ethnicity and SES.
Reliability	Test–retest, .96.
Validity	Predictive, .66–.81 (when scores were compared to the Wide Range Achievement Test.
Comments	No data are provided regarding the performances of ethnic minorities and low-SES students. Examiner variability may affect the obtained results, says one reviewer. Data presented in the manual are based on theory, not on controlled research.
References consulted	Bountress (1985); Cox (1985). See book's References list.

Measure	**Metropolitan Readiness Tests—Sixth Edition (MRT-6). Nurss and McGaurvan (1995).**
Purpose	Assessing basic and advanced skills important in beginning reading and mathematics, in order to assist with curricular planning.
Areas	Beginning Reading Skill Area (Visual Discrimination, Beginning Consonants, Sound–Letter Correspondence, Aural Cloze with Letter); Story Comprehension; Quantitative Concepts and Reasoning; Prereading Composite.
Format	Two levels; individual administration for level 1, and group administration for level 2.
Scores	Performance ratings, stanines, NCEs (mean and *SD* not reported), scaled scores, standard scores (level 1 only).
Age group	Pre-K through grade 1.
Time	85 minutes per level.
Users	Classroom teachers and administrators.
Norms	Normative sample reported to be representative of 1990 U.S. census; however, no breakdown by grade.
Reliability	Internal consistency, .90.
Validity	Limited evidence of validity.
Comments	The MRT-5 was said to have numerous deficiencies, including outdated material, technical inadequacies, possible confusion for target audiences, possible detrimental use for children in schools, and lack of validity evidence for some of the major issues of the scale. No evidence that test content is relevant for any group. Lack of information regarding content selection or appropriateness for children from diverse backgrounds. Review cited below notes: "Unusable unless locally validated." These same issues apply to the MRT-6.
References consulted	Kamphaus (2001); Novak (2001). See book's References list.

Measure	**Pre-Reading Inventory of Phonological Awareness (PIPA). Dodd, Crosbie, McIntosh, Teitzel, and Ozanne (2003).**
Purpose	Assessing phonological awareness in young students.
Areas	Rhyme Awareness, Syllable Segmentation, Alliteration Awareness, Sound Isolation, Sound Segmentation, and Letter–Sound Knowledge.

Format	Individually administered. There are six subtests; each item within a subtest has three possible score values: 1 for each correct response, 0 for an incorrect response, and NR for no response.
Scores	Percentile ranges.
Age group	4-0 to 6-11 years.
Time	25 minutes.
Users	Speech–language pathologists, teachers, and paraprofessionals.
Norms	Norms are based on data that reflect the 2000 U.S. census. Subtest percentile ranges for 6-month intervals (six age groups) are provided.
Reliability	Moderate to high levels of test–retest, internal consistency, and interscorer reliability were found.
Validity	Evidence of validity based on test content, internal structure, and relationships to other variables.
Comments	The clarity of the materials is commendable. The record forms are extremely user-friendly, and the stimulus book is colorful and engaging. Unfortunately, the information regarding standardization procedure is sparse, and the rationale behind test seems to lack support from other studies. The 2003 revision includes U.S. normative data.
References consulted	Inchaurralde (2005); Schwarting (2005). See book's References list.

Measure	**Stanford Early School Achievement Test—Fourth Edition (SESAT). Harcourt Brace Educational Measurement (1996).**
Purpose	Measuring a child's cognitive abilities from time of entering kindergarten to middle of first grade. A downward extension of the Stanford Achievement Test Series.
Areas	Level 1: Sounds and Letters; Word Reading; Total Reading; Mathematics; Listening to Words and Stories; Total for Basic Battery; Environment; Total for Complete Battery. Level 2: Same as Level 1, plus Sentence Reading.
Format	Group administration.
Scores	Percentile ranks, stanines.
Age group	Grades K–1.5.
Time	Level 1, 2 hours, 15 minutes; level 2, 2 hours, 50 minutes over multiple sessions.
Users	School personnel.
Norms	Norms collected on a sample representative of the 1992–1993 census.
Reliability	Internal consistency, .78–.98; Test–retest, not reported.
Validity	Content validity supported. As with previous editions of the SESAT, the only validity coefficients reported are those with the Stanford Achievement Test subtests and the Otis-Lennon School Ability Test—Seventh Edition (OLSAT-7) with which it is conormed.
Comments	Some conflicting information given in the manuals in the interpretation section; Lack of sufficient reliability and validity information; Difficult for children with physical disabilities that affect their writing capabilities. Adequate for screening purposes.
References consulted	Salvia and Ysseldyke (2004). See book's References list.

Measure	Test of Early Reading Ability—Deaf or Hard of Hearing (TERA-D/HH). Reid, Hresko, Hammill, and Wiltshire (1991).
Purpose	Measuring children's ability to "attribute meaning to printed symbols, their knowledge of the alphabet and its functions, and their knowledge of the conventions of print."
Areas	Total Early Reading.
Format	44 items, scored correct or incorrect; can be adapted using American Sign Language.
Scores	Percentiles, *T*-scores, NCEs, standard scores, stanines.
Age group	3-0 to 13-11 years.
Time	20–30 minutes.
Users	Professionals with knowledge of assessment, interpretation, and communication methods employed by students.
Norms	Data collected on 1,146 children with hearing impairments across 29 states and Washington, DC. Sampling seemed adequate.
Reliability	Internal consistency, .87–.97; test–retest (2 weeks), .83.
Validity	Criterion, supported; Construct, supported.
Comments	Test manual states, "To ensure optimal performance, any item can be repeated or reworded if the concept being tested appears unclear"; this calls the standardization of the test into question. Limited set of items appropriate for children under 6 years of age. "Floor" was not easily established. Although many children with hearing impairments have multiple disabilities, there was no information regarding other handicapping conditions in the normative sample. Adaptation of TERA-2. Manual gives means but not *SD* of standardization sample.
References consulted	Rothlinsberg (1995); Stavrou (1995). See book's References list.

Measure	Test of Early Reading Ability—Third Edition (TERA-3). Reid, Hresko, and Hammill (2001).
Purpose	Measuring children's ability to attribute meaning to printed symbols, their knowledge of the alphabet and its function, and their understanding of the conventions of print.
Areas	Three subtests: Alphabet, Conventions, and Meaning.
Format	80 items on each of two forms (Forms A and B).
Scores	Age and grade equivalents, percentile scores, standard scores for each subtest, and an overall Reading Quotient.
Age group	3-6 through 8-6 years.
Time	15–30 minutes.
Users	Professionals with formal training in assessment, basic statistics, administration, and interpretation.
Norms	875 school-age children from 22 states, representative of the 1999 U.S. census (matched with regard to race, gender, ethnicity, SES, urban–rural location, education level of parents, disability status, and geographic region). Participants took both forms of the test.

Reliability	Internal consistency, .83–.95; test–retest using alternate-form procedures (reported on a small group of 30 children ages 4-0–6-0 years), .94–.98; interrater reliability, .99; alternative-form reliability, .82–.92 across the six age groups.
Validity	Content focuses only on print-related skills and does not include phonemic awareness skills. Criterion-related validity was high in relation to the TERA-2 (.85–.98), and moderate in relation to other measures. Discriminant validity are not presented below second grade.
Comments	Some items are strangely classified (e.g., pointing to a number is an Alphabet item, and matching an uppercase letter with its lowercase representation is a Convention item). MMY "extreme professional caution in interpreting [the instructional target zone on the protocol] is urged." Ceiling rules, but some tests do not seem to increase in order of difficulty. Test user must create six stimulus items, such as pasting a coupon to a card; although suggestions are made, this calls the standardization of this test into question. There are also questions as to how to score some test items; the manual gives no help. Test does not provide specific information that would place child in an early reading curriculum. Diagnostic validity is limited by inadequate floors. Criterion-related validity data are lacking for children in preschool, kindergarten, and first grade.
References consulted	deFur (2001); Smith (2001); Rathvon (2004). See book's References list.

Measure	**Test of Early Mathematics Ability—Third Edition (TEMA-3). Ginsburg and Baroody (2003).**
Purpose	Measuring progress, evaluating programs, screening for readiness, discovering the bases for poor school performance in mathematics, identifying gifted students, and guiding instruction and remediation.
Areas	Numbering Skills, Number-Comparison Facility, Numeral Literacy, Mastery of Number Facts, Calculation Skills, and Understanding of Concepts.
Format	72 items on each of two parallel forms. Basal and ceiling rules apply.
Scores	Standard scores, percentile ranks, and age and grade equivalents.
Age group	3-0 through 8-11 years and older children who have learning problems in mathematics.
Time	45 minutes.
Users	Professionals with formal training in assessment, basic statistics, administration, and interpretation.
Norms	The standardization sample is composed of 1,228 children (637 took Form A; 591 took Form B). The characteristics of the sample generally approximate those in the 2001 U.S. census, with the South and females overrepresented and the West underrepresented.
Reliability	Internal consistency, all above .92; immediate and delayed alternate-form, in the .80s and .90s. Test–retest reliability with an interval of 2 weeks, .82 for Form A and .93 for Form B.
Validity	Many validity studies are described with moderate to strong relationships between the TEMA-3 and other measures.
Comments	The TEMA-3 is easy to administer and score. However, only a comprehensive score is provided. Subscores would be useful to determine areas of relative

	strength and weakness. Assessors need to review individual responses—a time-consuming task—in order to obtain this information. A book of remedial techniques (assessment probes and instructional activities) for improving skills in the areas assessed by the test, as well as numerous teaching tasks for skills covered by each TEMA-3 item, are included. Bias studies are now included that show the absence of bias based on gender and ethnicity.
References consulted	Bliss (2006); Crehan (2005). See book's References list.

Measure	**Test of Phonological Awareness—Second Edition: PLUS (TOPA-2+). Torgesen and Bryant (2004).**
Purpose	Measures young children's awareness of individual sounds in words.
Areas	Phonological awareness of individual phonemes in spoken words and understanding of the relationship between letters and phonemes in English.
Format	Two 10-item subtests. A Kindergarten version and an Early Elementary version each contain two subtests.
Scores	Standard scores and percentiles.
Age group	Kindergarten, 5–6 years; Early Elementary, 6–8 years.
Time	30–45 minutes (Kindergarten version); 15–30 minutes (Early Elementary version).
Users	Examiners with clear speech and dialect similar to that of students being examined.
Norms	Data collected on 1,035 students (Kindergarten version) and 1,050 students (Early Elementary version). The demographic characteristics matched the school-age population in relation to the 2001 census. Detail is not provided regarding students with limited English proficiency, or diverse home linguistic experience.
Reliability	Internal consistency ranged from .80 to .90; test–retest and interscorer reliability is reported as .80 or greater across all ages.
Validity	Content validity is well supported. Concurrent reported to be moderate. Additional research in the area of predictive validity is needed.
Comments	Assessors must possess speech that is sufficiently clear. Otherwise, the test is easy to administer and score with useful information provided for interpretation of outcomes. The test is useful as a measure of phonological awareness and letter-sound knowledge with students who are standard speakers of English. The test needs to be used with other evidence prior to recommending intervention. Additional validity studies are needed with nonstandard English speakers.
References consulted	Fenton (2005). See book's References list.

Measure	**Woodcock–Johnson III (WJ III-ACH) Tests of Achievement, Preschool Cluster. Woodcock, McGrew, and Mather (2001a).**
Purpose	Providing age-based or grade-based norm-referenced individual achievement scores, which can be used to identify academic strengths and weaknesses, for educational programming, and to monitor progress.
Areas	Twelve of the 22 WJ III-ACH tests are recommended for use with preschool children and can be used with children as young as 2 years of age. Test 1,

	Letter-Word Identification; Test 3, Story Recall; Test 4, Understanding Directions; Test 7, Spelling; Test 9, Passage Comprehension; Test 10, Applied Problems; Test 12, Story Recall-Delayed, Test 13, Word Attack; Test 14, Picture Vocabulary; Test 15, Oral Comprehension; Test 19, Academic Knowledge; and Test 21, Sound Awareness.
Format	Individually administered. Standard and Extended Batteries. Audiotapes are used for standardized presentation of oral material. Alternate forms are available. Accommodations can be made for testing young children, English language learners, and individuals with various difficulties and impairments (including reading, attention, hearing, visual, and physical impairments).
Scores	Raw scores are entered into a computer-scoring program that generates the following norm-referenced scores: grade equivalents, age equivalents, relative proficiency indexes, percentile ranks, discrepancy scores, standard scores.
Age group	For the 12 subtests in the preschool cluster: 2-0 years to adult or 2-0–5-0 years for preschool aged children.
Time	5–10 minutes per test; 60–120 minutes for batteries.
Users	May be administered by those with specific training in administration and scoring, but should only be interpreted by professionals with graduate-level training in relevant areas. Training videos and workbooks are available from the publisher.
Norms	Data collected on 8,818 people in over 100 U.S. communities for the entire WJ-III sample. The preschool sample, children age 2 to 5, but not enrolled in kindergarten, included 1,143 children (259 children age 2, 310 children age 3, and children age 4), all representative of the U.S. population.
Reliability	Internal consistency reliability: Split-half reliabilities were calculated for all but the timed tests and tests with multiple-point scoring systems. Reliabilities for children age 2 and 3, .56 to .98, with almost all of the correlations at the .80-level or above; Test–retest reliability: Studies of test–retest reliabilities for children age 2 and 3 for the timed tests were not described in the technical manual. Nontimed test reliabilities ranged from .57 to .96 for a 1-year interval.
Validity	Achievement clusters yielded correlations in the .70 range.
Comments	The WJ III-ACH Preschool Cluster has sound psychometric properties and recent norms. Examiners can select specific subtests or administer all 12 subtests for preschool children. Administration and scoring is fairly straightforward with the help of stimulus flipbooks containing all instructions and a computer-scoring program. Limitations are the lack of manipulatives and interactions, which may make the test less engaging for preschool children and the inability to substitute a comparable subtest if one is inappropriately administered or spoiled.
References consulted	Cizek (2003); Sandoval (2003). See book's References list.

Measure	**Work Sampling System, Fourth Edition. Meisels, Jablon, Dichtelmiller, Dorfman, and Marsden (1998).**
Purpose	Enhancing instruction and improving learning.
Areas	Checklist domains: Personal and Social Development, Language and Literacy, Mathematical Thinking, Scientific Thinking, Social Studies, The Arts, and Physical Development and Health. Five specific areas of development are assessed: art and fine motor, movement and gross motor, concept and number, language and literacy, and personal and social development.

Format	Three elements: Developmental Guidelines and Checklists, portfolios, and Summary Reports.
Scores	The checklists contain 69 items scored as 1 ("not yet"), 2 ("sometimes"), or 3 ("often"). Subscores for the portfolio are based on children's performance in the five areas of development; each area is scored as (1) "not yet accomplished," (2) "accomplished," or (3) "highly accomplished." Total scores for the Summary Report are based on the results of the checklists, portfolio, and observations.
Age group	Preschool (age 3)–grade 5.
Time	The checklists and Summary Reports are completed three times a year (fall, winter, and spring). Portfolios are considered a continuous measure of performance.
Users	Trained teachers, professionals, or paraprofessionals.
Norms	Criterion-referenced instrument.
Reliability	Internal reliability for the checklists .87–.94; interrater reliability for the Summary Reports .68–.88.
Validity	Concurrent validity was demonstrated when the fall and spring checklists were compared to the Woodcock–Johnson–Revised (WJ-R) (.75 for fall and .66 for spring) and when the spring checklist was compared to the spring Child Behavior Rating Scale (CBRS) (.80). High correlations with the WJ-R and the CBRS were obtained for predictive validity. The concurrent validity of the Summary Reports ranged from .61 to .80.
Comments	Spanish version available. Special considerations for children with disabilities.
References consulted	Meisels, Liaw, Dorfman, and Nelson (1995). See book's References list.

Chapter 8

Family Assessment

Young children are dependent on their families for food, clothing, protection, shelter, comfort, and instruction in cultural etiquette (Whiting & Edwards, 1988). Families teach young children how to communicate (Hart & Risley, 1995, 1999); to understand, express, and regulate emotions (Gottman, Katz, & Hooven, 1997; Sroufe, 1996); and to engage in culturally valued behaviors for their age and gender, in part through assignment of children to various settings (Whiting & Edwards, 1988). The many pressing demands on families and their limited energy means that each family has different priorities, depending on its circumstances, and that some functions may not be met. Table 8.1 outlines the tasks of parents of preschoolers in mainstream North American culture, as well as the resources and stressors that facilitate and inhibit their performance.

Families are embedded within cultures, and cultures and families influence each other reciprocally over time (Rogoff, 2003). This awareness of families' powerful role in shaping early child development, and of the corresponding importance of cultures and cultural institutions in providing essential support for families, has resulted in active efforts over the past decades by researchers, educators, clinicians, and governments to join with families as partners in addressing the educational, psychological, and physical needs of young children (Bronfenbrenner, 1979; Dunst, Trivette, & Deal, 1988; Seligman & Darling, 1997). Representative of these efforts in the United States are the Head Start program, with its long-standing outreach to parents for children from economically poorer families (Zigler & Muenchow, 1992); and IDEA 2004, which expressly involves families as partners with professionals in the development of individualized family service plans (IFSPs) for children with disabilities ages 0–3, and individualized education plans (IEPs) for children ages 3–5. Although assessment of family context is not required by IDEA 2004 for preschool children referred for suspected disabilities, there are compelling reasons for conducting such an assessment, which will be highlighted in this chapter.

TABLE 8.1. Tasks of Parents of Preschool Children, and Factors That Facilitate or Impede Task Completion

Tasks of parents

- Meeting basic survival needs (food, shelter, clothing, temperature, transportation, health care).
- Keeping child safe from psychological and physical harm (close monitoring, use of car seats, elimination of hazards in the home, protection from family violence).
- Giving child sense of acceptance, belonging, and identity (displaying interest in child; comforting child when distressed; making room in home and in parents' minds for child; involving child in community and cultural activities).
- Providing a structured environment to promote physical self-regulation and learning (parental leadership, eating/sleeping routines, contingent enforcement of rules).
- Teaching culturally valued behavior and mores. In North America, this teaching includes the following:
  - Promoting cognitive, academic, and language development (talking with child; reading to/with child; teaching vocabulary and concepts important in schooling; providing toys).
  - Promoting emotional self-regulation and social competence (teaching compliance to adult commands; teaching emotion words; discussing feelings, how to express them, and how to solve problems; supporting sibling and peer relationships and finding peer groups that will promote competent development).
  - Promoting moral development (modeling and discussing empathetic, ethical treatment of others; punishment of inappropriate behavior).

Contextual factors that enable parents to function competently

- Parental emotional and cognitive resources (IQ, education, emotional adjustment).
- Financial stability (steady, secure employment; rewarding work; benefits).
- Social support (spouse/partner, other relatives, friends; community groups; professionals, disability services, and education).

Factors that make it harder for families to perform their tasks

- Workload to care for the child.
- Behavior problems of the child.
- Shame, lack of acceptance of child and/or family when child has a disability.
- Level of coordination involved in getting service needs met.
- Lack of appropriate or high-quality services.
- Closely spaced children (less than 2 years apart).
- More than one child with a disabling condition.

Note. Data from Dunst, Trivette, and Deal (1988); Nihira, Weisner, and Bernheimer (1994); Patterson, Reid, and Dishion (1992); Werner and Smith (1992); and Whiting and Edwards (1988).

PURPOSES OF FAMILY ASSESSMENT

Families of preschoolers may be assessed for a variety of purposes. The approach to assessment and its comprehensiveness depend on the characteristics of a particular family, the skills and training of an assessor, and the setting in which the assessment is conducted. A family assessment can range from a brief screening to assess family resources, stress, and need for information and referrals for a child with mild developmental delays in a family that appears to be coping well, to an extensive evaluation as prologue to intervention in a family coping with a child with multiple disabilities, parental mental illness, poverty, and problems with the law. Despite this wide variability, most assessments that involve families with young children have certain common purposes, and these organize the activities of the assessor.

The first purpose of family assessment is to *build a partnership for promoting the development and education of a child.* Parent–professional relationships can last for years when young children with disabilities are involved. The first encounter is likely to establish the tenor of such a relationship. The quality of the initial parent–professional relationship influences the ability of all parties to work together for the child's benefit, the family's receptivity to intervention, the professional's to input and feedback from the family, and the quality of the later relationship. Some professional practices that promote this partnership include creating a welcoming environment; respecting cultural diversity; showing positive and nonjudgmental interest in the whole family; maintaining confidentiality and keeping agreements; sharing information and resources; and focusing on parents' hopes, concerns, and needs (see Esler et al., 2002, and Fish, 2002, for detailed discussions).

Over the last decade, professionals working with families on behalf of children with disabilities have moved toward a collaborative model of parent involvement. The objectives of this model, as specified by Fine and Nissenbaum (2000), are including parents in decision making, educating parents in decision making, assisting parents as needed therapeutically, and empowering parents to work actively on behalf of their child. The model also promotes a respectful view of family members as knowing what is best for their child and the family as a whole; a constructive team approach to problem solving, with an emphasis on family members' priorities for the child, based on their knowledge of the environment in which the child must function; and an acknowledgment that parents can teach professionals as well as learn from them. (See Doll & Bolger, 2000, and Hanson & Lynch, 2004, for excellent illustrations of this model as applied to families with young children with disabilities.)

A second goal of family assessment is *to gather information essential for case conceptualization and clarification of a diagnosis, if appropriate.* Parents are typically the single best source of information about a child, because they have been with the child since birth (or soon thereafter in the case of adoption), spend the most time with the child, and care the most about the child's well-being. They can provide firsthand information on a child's developmental competence; typical approach to new problems and situations; and typical behavior with adults, with peers, and in the home. A small number of parents are not accurate reporters of their child's functioning, however, and a family assessment can assist assessors in interpreting information from these parents (Kamphaus & Frick, 2002).

A detailed family educational and psychiatric history can clarify a diagnosis, given the heritability of many children's learning and behavioral problems. Family interpersonal and economic factors also play a causal role in the development of some psychopathology and personality problems in children (see Erickson, 1998, for a review). Parent–child problems are the second most common psychiatric diagnosis in the preschool years (Campbell, 2002), and many of the most potent risk factors for poor adult adaptation are family-related factors in early childhood that are susceptible to intervention, such as mother–infant interaction, the spacing of children, health status in early childhood, and reading and academic competence in the early grades (Werner & Smith, 2001).

A third purpose of family assessment is to *gather information essential for intervention with the child* in the school or clinic setting, as well as the home. Family members can tell professionals about their priorities and their needs, and can then work with professionals to create an intervention program that will be effective for them and for their child. Preschool children are highly dependent on their families, and interventions that focus on the family or have a family component at this age are the most effective (Reid, 1993).

Fourth, parenting is stressful; parenting a child with a disability is quite stressful, even for the best functioning families (Seligman & Darling, 1997). An assessment of a child that includes the family can *serve a preventive function by screening* for financial needs, parent–child problems, lack of social support, parent and/or sibling mental health problems, marital/couple difficulties, and common challenges faced by families with a child with a disability. Appropriate services or referrals can then be provided when problems are identified.

Fifth, most families need *information on the diagnosis, formal support services, treatment options, federal special education law, and the regulations of their state* if their child is identified as having a disability. Assessors can inform parents about these issues at the end of the assessment process, and, when necessary, can help them navigate the bureaucracy involved.

Sixth, assessors need *information on family members' interest in and ability to participate in home-based interventions*, if appropriate. Parent training and home-based programs are expensive to offer if families do not benefit, and some families may find the additional stress of an intervention more than they can bear, causing a deterioration in functioning (see Chapter 13 for a discussion of this issue).

In general, family assessments can be divided into three broad categories: (1) assessments where the probable source of the presenting problem lies within the family (e.g., anxiety and acting out in a child exposed to domestic violence); (2) assessments where the family members may need support for a problem that is not directly within their control or responsibility (e.g., the birth of a child with mental retardation) (Brassard, 1986); and (3) assessments where family members have a combination of problems (e.g., a child who is deaf in a physically neglectful family). The assessment model presented in this chapter can be used flexibly with all three types of families. Children from all types of families are eligible to receive early intervention services when they display disabilities or delays in development. Some states also allow children to receive services when they live in environments that place them at risk for delays or for less optimal development. Under the IDEA (2004), parents have the right to refuse to have their child evaluated for a suspected disability.

The purposes of this chapter are to (1) present theoretical models of family assessment and intervention appropriate for assessors working with preschool children referred for suspected learning, behavioral, or emotional disabilities; (2) present a flexible school/clinic-based family assessment and consultation model that draws on aspects of these theoretical models; (3) in the process of presenting this model, review some of the more useful procedures and instruments available; and (4) illustrate how to pull together the assessment data obtained into effective intervention approaches and strategies through a detailed case study. Approaches to families with particular circumstances or suspected disorders are covered in Chapters 9, 12, 13, and 14.

THEORETICAL MODELS OF FAMILY ASSESSMENT AND INTERVENTION

Researchers from four theoretical traditions have developed models of family assessment relevant to assessors of preschool children and their families. The models differ in their understanding of how and why problems develop, and thus in the behaviors that are assessed and targeted for change if a problem is identified. Despite initial differences in theoretical constructs, the models have influenced one another over time and have all been influenced by social science and biosocial research on families and child development, resulting in many shared concepts. The models are presented here to illustrate how theories and the characteristics of families being seen drive models of assessment and intervention, and to enhance assessors' understanding of family functioning. Assessors may find that a particular model is a better fit than others with their setting or with particular clients.

Models Based on Family Systems Theory

Family systems theory evolved out of general systems theory (Bateson, 1979; Bateson, Jackson, Haley, & Weakland, 1956). The family system is viewed as a consistent and complex whole made up of semi-independent parts (individual family members) and evolving together through time. Family therapy focuses on changing the dysfunctional aspects of a family system that are identified when a family experiences stress as the result of an individual member's or members' having or causing difficulties (Minuchin, 1974). The source of stress may be internal (e.g., developmental transition, disabling condition in a family member) or external (e.g., school problems of a child, unemployment of a parent). The therapist enters the family to support or change it in a growth-enhancing way. There are many models of family therapy (see Walsh, 2003, for descriptions) but all have a strong systemic, developmental, and multicultural perspective, making them highly relevant to work with young children and their families. In our opinion, the *family life cycle* paradigm is particularly helpful for early childhood assessors and interventionists.

A number of authors have been credited with the conceptual framework now known as the family life cycle (Duvall, 1977; Haley, 1973; Hill, 1970). This paradigm is based on the notion that the family proceeds through time as a developmental unit, rather than as a collection of individuals with independent developmental progressions. For example, each family member and generation has its own tasks to accomplish and master, but, the stage of each family member affects the successful achievement of different tasks by other family members or other generations (Carter & McGoldrick, 1989). For instance, when a 5-year-old child with moderate mental retardation exhibits delay in mastering basic self-help skills, such as dressing and toileting, this prevents his or her parents from reorganizing as a family with a school-age and increasingly independent child. In such a family, the child's slow rate of development maintains a family organization that is typical of families with toddlers.

Carter and McGoldrick (1989) have defined the *family* as the entire emotional system of at least three, and now frequently four, generations. The nuclear family is one of many subsystems in a larger network that is, according to their model, "reacting to past, present, and anticipated future relationships within the larger three-generational family system" (p. 6). According to Carter and McGoldrick, family stress or anxiety evolves from two sources. The *vertical* sources of anxiety are generationally transmitted patterns of relating and functioning that are usually passed on through intergenerational coalitions, including, "all the family attitudes, taboos, expectations, labels, and loaded issues with which we grow up" (p. 6). The *horizontal* sources are "the stresses that the family encounters as it moves through developmental and historical time" (p. 6). Included here are both normative events (e.g., birth of first child) and non-normative events (e.g., death of a mother with a young child). Carter and McGoldrick contend that all families will become dysfunctional if enough external and developmental stressors are placed on the horizontal axis. Under these conditions, even a small amount of vertical stress will result in disruption beyond that already caused by the pressures along the horizontal axis. A professional using this model assesses general life stress, normative developmental stress, and the extent to which these stressors connect with inherited themes and labels. Figure 8.1 presents Carter and McGoldrick's (1989) horizontal and vertical stressor model.

The family life cycle paradigm outlines the specific emotional processes and second-order changes that a family needs to undergo to move from one stage to the next (see Table 8.2). This outline, however, is based on a late-20th-century, middle-class, European American milieu, and so its elements may differ for individuals of other cultures and SES levels. In addition, families may of course be affected by a child's disability, parental divorce, parental remarriage, immigration, or other fairly common life cycle derailments. (See Carter & McGoldrick, 1989, for descriptions of the life cycle challenges experienced by families who divorce, remarry, or must contend with other tasks by virtue of immigration, poverty, illness, or substance abuse.)

For parents of young children, the chief task is to "move up a generation and become caretakers to the younger generation. Typical problems that occur when parents cannot make this shift are struggles with each other over taking responsibility, or refusal or inability to behave as parents to their children" (Carter & McGoldrick, 1989, pp. 16–17). Carter and McGoldrick highlight two common complaints from families with young children presenting for therapy: Either (1) parents are not accepting the responsibility of behaving as the parents, and thus their children are out of control; or (2) parents are expecting children to behave as adults and are not allowing them to be children with a need for guidance and patience. Treatment focuses on helping parents accept their responsibilities for their stage in the family life cycle and perform the necessary tasks.

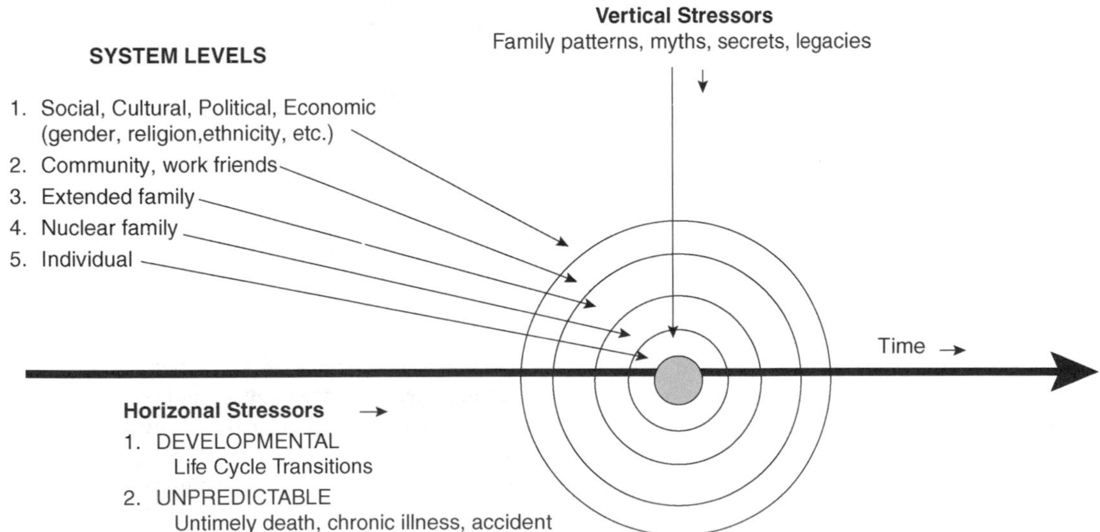

FIGURE 8.1. Model of horizontal and vertical stressors on families. From Carter and McGoldrick (1989). Published by Allyn & Bacon, Boston, MA. Copyright 1989 by Pearson Education. Reprinted by permission of the publisher.

TABLE 8.2. Stages of the Family Life Cycle

Family life cycle stage	Emotional process of transition: Key principles	Second-order changes in family status required to proceed developmentally
1. Leaving home: Single young adults	Accepting emotional and financial responsibility for self	a. Differentiation of self in relation to family of origin b. Development of intimate peer relationships c. Establishment of self to work and financial independence
2. The joining of families through marriage: The new couple	Commitment to new system	a. Formation of marital system b. Realignment of relationships with extended families and friends to include spouse
3. Families with young children	Accepting new members into the system	a. Adjusting marital system to make space for children b. Joining in childrearing, financial, and household tasks c. Realignment of relationships with extended family to include parenting and grandparenting roles
4. Families with adolescents	Increasing flexibility of family boundaries to include children's independence and grandparents' liabilities	a. Shifting of parent–child relationships to permit adolescent to move in and out of system b. Refocus on midlife marital and career issues c. Beginning shift toward joint caring for older generation
5. Launching children and moving on	Accepting a multitude of exits from and entries into the family system	a. Renegotiations of mental system as a dyad b. Development of adult-to-adult relationships between grown children and their parents c. Realignment of relationships to include in-laws and grandchildren d. Dealing with disabilities and death of parents (grandparents)
6. Families in later life	Accepting the shifting of generational roles	a. Maintaining own and/or couple functioning and interests in face of physiological decline; exploration of new familial and social role options b. Support for a more central role of middle generation c. Making room in the system for the wisdom and experience of the elderly, supporting the older generation without overfunctioning for them d. Dealing with loss of spouse, siblings, and other peers and preparation for own death. Life review and integration

Note. From Carter and McGoldrick (1989). Published by Allyn & Bacon, Boston, MA.

Carter and McGoldrick (1989) also note that mothers of young children often pay a heavy price for the fact that North American culture has no societal provision for adequate childcare. If women work, they are often faced with two full-time jobs while their husbands have one. If they stay at home, they may be giving up a career and/or the social contact with peers that work provides; this may make them vulnerable to isolation and depression, especially when caring for multiple young children (Hertzig & Farber, 2003; Lyons-Ruth, Wolfe, Lyubchik, & Steingard, 2003). Maternal depression and couple conflict or divorce are both relatively common at this phase of the life cycle and are often linked (Cummings, Keller, & Davies, 2005). Depression is common in fathers of young children as well (Ramchandani, Stein, Evans, O'Conner, & ALSPAC Study Team, 2005). The relationship between depression and the quality of parenting young children is complex, influenced by comorbid factors and stressors in the family. However, maternal depression has been linked with poorer-quality caretaking (e.g., less cuddling, reading, playing) and lower maternal tolerance for children's behavior. In children, maternal depression has been tied to lower self-esteem, self-efficacy, and emotional regulation (Campbell, 2002), as well as poorer peer relationships, more school problems, and greater risk of later psychopathology (Lieberman, 2004) . Paternal depression in a child's early life is related to the subsequent development of emotional and behavioral problems in early childhood, even after maternal postnatal depression and later paternal depression are controlled for; it has persistent negative effects on children's development (Ramchandani et al., 2005). In terms of divorce, "almost half of all couples with children who divorce will have done so before their first child enters kindergarten" (Cowan & Cowan, 2003, p. 437). Divorce is very distressing to young children and is related to short-term disruptions in functioning and long-term adjustment difficulties (Hetherington & Kelly, 2002; Wallerstein & Lewis, 2004). Thus parental stress and depression and marital/couple dysfunction are important areas to attend to at this stage of the family life cycle.

Special Education/Early Intervention Models

Parent Empowerment Model

Over the last two decades, special education models for early intervention with families of young children with disabilities have been developed largely through the efforts of two research teams. The first team, led by Carl Dunst and Angela Trivette (Dunst et al., 1988), developed a model out of their early intervention efforts with such families in western North Carolina. This model emphasizes creating a sense of empowerment in families through promoting the acquisition of self-sustaining and adaptive behavior that allows families to cope effectively with their children and with their environment. The role of professionals in this model is to shape, encourage, and facilitate whatever development is necessary to allow families to meet their own needs through exploitation of their informal social network in particular, and formal networks to a lesser extent. Dunst and Trivette help families identify and prioritize their needs, and then they assist them in locating the informal and formal resources necessary to satisfy these needs. They have collected research evidence that supports the effectiveness of their model over early intervention approaches directed specifically at reducing deficits and increasing functioning in children. Their studies have been a powerful influence on the development of IFSPs for children ages 0–3 with disabilities.

Family assessment in this model thus involves the use of (1) family needs surveys to be filled out by both parents; and (2) social support surveys that ask both parents which individuals and groups in their informal and formal social networks they perceive as able to provide useful resources currently and in the future, to help them meet and address some of the needs that they have identified and prioritized. A professional then uses this material to establish and prioritize goals and to work with the family members to identify ways in which they personally, and through the trading of services, might meet these needs. The expert provides just enough support to the family members to promote their development as problem solvers, and also provides them with information about the disabilities or about local services that the family members may not have access to themselves. Dunst et al. (1988) have demonstrated that early intervention programs are most useful when they empower parents to meet their own needs and solve their own problems.

Family-Focused Intervention Model

Bailey and Simeonsson (1988), also working in North Carolina, have developed a family assessment model as well. In their family-focused intervention model, the characteristics of effective family assessment are based on the "goodness-of-fit" concept developed by Thomas and Chess (1977) in their longitudinal research. That is, services must be individualized so that they fit each family and are tailored to the particular goals or services that the family members perceive themselves to need. Successful family intervention is the degree to which intervention provides families with what they need to function effectively as developmental environments for their children (e.g., adequate health care, knowledge of child development and how to enhance it).

The characteristics of effective family intervention that Bailey and Simeonsson (1988) have identified include (1) assessing important family domains (child needs and characteristics likely to affect a family's functioning; parent–child interaction and whole-family needs; critical events and their sources); (2) learning about a family's culture and traditions; (3) determining family priorities; (4) tailoring program type to the family; and (5) incorporating routine evaluation of family outcomes.

Both the parent empowerment model and the family-focused intervention model view families of children with disabilities as healthy families coping with unusual stress. Their emphasis on addressing what families need and want, and on allowing families to set their own priorities, is a major advantage. Both programs have developed measures that focus on the needs and demands of families and young children with learning and behavioral problems. Most of their measures are easy to administer and score and are written at a fairly low reading level. They are reviewed later in the chapter.

Psychoanalytically Influenced or Relationship-Oriented Early Intervention Models

Several psychoanalytically influenced researchers have developed assessment and treatment approaches that have been applied to high-risk or maltreating families. Models arising from this theoretical framework assume that a particularly critical caregiver function is to provide the context for a child to develop a model of interpersonal relationships and to learn what to expect of the other and of the self in the relationship. The research generated by this model has tied patterns of caregiving (hostile, rejecting, psychologically unavailable) to impaired child competence at successive ages and to the development of psychopathology. It has also demonstrated a relationship between a mother's emotional and environmental resources and her competence in parenting (Egeland & Farber, 1984), between couple violence and each parent's physical and emotional availability to a child and his or her parenting effectiveness (Erel & Burman, 1995), and between a mother's childhood history of adequate or abusive care (as assessed retrospectively) and the quality and pattern of care she gives her children (Egeland, Jacobvitz, & Papatola, 1987; Main & Goldwyn, 1984; Sroufe, Jacobvitz, Mangelsdorf, DeAngelo, & Ward, 1985).

Assessment focuses on adult models of self and other, specifically models of attachment; child attachment to the primary caregiver; parenting, life, and marital/couple stress; social support; and the adaptive behavior of parents. Parenting competence is evaluated through the use of videotaped parent–child interactions. Sensitivity to the child's cues, developmentally appropriate and sensitive stimulation and instruction, and the presence of hostility are some of the interaction patterns of interest to assessors and interveners using this model.

The treatment approach stresses the importance of developing a long-term therapeutic relationship with the high-risk or maltreating parent(s), if possible. This relationship provides parents with the opportunity to learn new ways of relating to another individual, work through some of the psychological trauma from their own childhoods that may serve as a barrier to a nurturing relationship with the child, and develop the types of behavioral competence that are important to successful functioning as adults and parents in our society.

Fraiberg's (1983) Clinical Infant Mental Health Program, developed in Michigan and replicated in San Francisco with immigrant families (Lieberman, Weston, & Pawl, 1991) and in Rochester, New York, with depressed mothers and their infants (Cicchetti, Toth, & Rogosch, 1999); the University of Minnesota's STEEP Project (Egeland & Erickson, 1990); and the Clinical Infant Development Program (Wieder, Poisson, Lourie, & Greenspan, 1988) are examples of intervention programs that appear to be successful in using this approach to treat high-risk families. Landy and Menna (2006) provide an excellent comprehensive review of such programs (and programs using other models) as well as their own integrated model for providing early intervention with multirisk families. Funding for these programs comes from a combination of federal research and demonstration grants, state and county monies, private foundations, and independent donations.

These models differ significantly from the special education/early intervention models, in that the researchers and clinicians who have worked in these programs begin with the assumption that a family has developed pathological patterns. However, it is assumed that such patterns have been developed because they are adaptive for the environment that individual members of the family and the family as a whole have been living in. The models were also developed as attempts to engage families who are not seeking help, but who have children at serious risk, in a therapeutic process that will ideally allow the families to stay together and to foster the development of these at-risk children. Exquisite sensitivity to a family's feelings and concerns must be carefully balanced with social coercive power to intervene if necessary. As with the special education/early intervention models, most of these models have been developed as the result of federal- and state-funded research projects. The well-trained and highly motivated staffs received ongoing supervision, and they had the opportunity for extensive problem solving and innovative planning in terms of how best to work effectively with these families. (See Sameroff, McDonough, & Rosenblum, 2004, for a recent presentation of this approach.)

Not all psychoanalytic models are focused on families with suspected pathology. Reid (1999) has developed an assessment and treatment model for families of young children with autism. She makes the assumption that having a child with autism in the family is frequently a traumatic experience. She uses her observation of a family in the waiting room and her office, her own countertransference reactions (her analysis of how the child and family make her feel), and interviews across a number of sessions to understand what life is like in this family. She then engages the family as a whole as part of a collaborative treatment team to improve life for the family and for individual members, including the child with autism.

Sameroff (2004) has developed an intervention model involving what he calls the "three R's of intervention": *Remediate* when a child with known organic impairment is unable to elicit a normal caregiving response from the parent (e.g., structural repair of a biological condition); *redefine* when parents' beliefs and expectations do not fit the child (e.g., failure to adapt to disabling condition in the child, or seeing a child as abnormal when he or she is not); and *reeducate* when parents need to be taught how to parent their child (e.g., providing care for a very-low-birth-weight baby, intervening in a multi-problem family). Each of these interventions could be applicable to families varying greatly in their level of adaptive functioning.

Behavioral Family Intervention Models

Behavioral family intervention models are based on social learning theory and applied behavior analysis, but are also influenced by family systems theory. They are appropriate when a child's behaviors need to be increased (e.g., compliance to parent commands) and/or decreased (e.g., dysregulated behavior). Use of these models with families requires training in the relevant theories and techniques. Child clinical psychologists are most likely to be trained in this approach. Many special education and school psychology programs offer training in this area for use with children and in schools, but infrequently with families. The positive behavior supports (PBS) movement (see below) is an effort to draw all of these disciplines into a multicomponent, flexible model of interventions for families of children with severe disabilities. Within these models, assessment focuses on a detailed description of the behavior in context, sometimes using a formal functional analysis of behavior. It tries to identify the reinforcement contingencies for language development and creative play as well as compliance to parental commands, and for noncompliant, antisocial behavior such as hitting and tantrums (Mash & Terdal, 1997). Parental problems that may interfere with competent parenting and intervention effectiveness, such as marital/couple conflict, parental depression, or antisocial behavior, are also assessed to ascertain the need for adjunctive treatments (Fleischman, Horne, & Arthur, 1983; Webster-Stratton & Herbert, 1994).

Three commercially available parenting programs based on this theoretical model have demonstrated effectiveness in treating young children with oppositional defiant disorder (ODD): (1) Helping the Noncompliant Child (Forehand & McMahon, 1981; McMahon & Forehand, 2003); (2) Parent–Child Interaction Therapy (Eyberg & Boggs, 1998; Hembree-Kigin & McNeil, 1995); and (3) The Incredible Years (Webster-Stratton, 1999, 2000). They all include modeling of parenting skills, parent role play, didactic instruction, discussion, and homework assignments to teach parents how to attend to child behavior, reward, ignore, give clear instructions, and administer time out (McMahon & Forehand, 2003). They differ in several respects: whether they are group- or individually administered, whether children participate in the sessions, whether behavioral criteria have to be met, and how many/what types of topics are covered. The Incredible Years has a validated teacher training component and a child component that have been shown to improve the behavior of children with ODD, conduct disorder (CD), or attention-deficit/

hyperactivity disorder (ADHD), as well as nonreferred children in Head Start. It is thus ideal for preventive efforts following screening and prior to referral, or as an adjunct to a parent program for treating ODD (Webster-Stratton et al., 2004).

The family-centered PBS movement, mentioned above, is a systems-oriented behavioral approach to helping "parents and other family members achieve meaningful and durable improvements in the child's behavior and lifestyle and in the quality of family life as a whole" (Lucyshyn, Horner, Dunlap, Albin, & Ben, 2002, p. 8). The model was developed in the early 1990s in an effort to move away from aversive responses to severe behavior problems in children with severe disabilities. It is derived from four theoretical/philosophical foundations: applied behavior analysis, behavioral family therapy, family systems theory, and the community living and family support advocacy movement. The PBS approach focuses on behavior change that results in desired outcomes defined by individuals in the environments in which children function (home, school, community). It involves analyzing a child's problem behavior to identify the function of the behavior for the child, and then testing alternative strategies to meet the child's needs in a way that supports positive behavior. Empirically validated procedures are implemented in the setting in which the problematic behavior occurs, and refinements are made until positive behavior is achieved. There is a major emphasis on teaching parents the skills so that they can eventually design and implement PBS themselves (see Lucyshyn, Dunlap, & Albin, 2002, for a detailed presentation of research support and clinical practice). This is a broad yet flexible model, and it is a promising development in family interventions.

CLINIC/SCHOOL-BASED FAMILY ASSESSMENT AND CONSULTATION

Over the last two decades, family systems theory has had an influence on school psychological practice (Brassard, 1986; Esler et al., 2002; Fine & Carlson, 1992). In this section, we present an adaptation of Brassard's (1986) school-based family assessment and intervention model, tailored to an early childhood setting and practice (see Table 8.3). This adaptation incorporates aspects of the special education/early intervention models, the psychoanalytically influenced models, and the behavioral family intervention models as well. It is important to emphasize that the approach described here is appropriately used as just one component of a comprehensive assessment in a psychoeducational setting.

We view family assessment as a potentially therapeutic intervention that assists families in making decisions and identifying resources and options. We recommend a cautious approach to developing hypotheses regarding families, and suggest that professionals subject their professional observations and interpretations to critical examination. We have found it clinically useful to share an initial draft of our evaluations, including those of the family, with parents or other primary caregivers; we make it clear that the report is based on our tentative analysis, and we ask them for their feedback and commentary. Not only has this saved us from some major misinterpretations, but when our judgments have been accurate, it has resulted in intense and clinically useful discussions among family members (see Brassard, 1986). Parents then choose what information about the family to include in an abbreviated report for schools or other service providers. Although family assessments have not been evaluated for their effectiveness in alleviating distress, research by Finn and Tonsager (1992) suggests that individual psychological assessment of adults can be an effective intervention in and of itself, if care is taken to write reports

TABLE 8.3. Steps in the Family Assessment of a Preschool Child Referred for an Evaluation

Step 1: Building a family–professional relationship.

Step 2: Obtaining a detailed description of the problematic behavior, its context, and its impact on the family.

Step 3: Taking a developmental, health, and educational history of the child.

Step 4: Assessing family history, current functioning, and social support.

Step 5: Screening family for parenting stress, marital/couple problems, family violence, and mental health problems.

Step 6: Reviewing symptoms and severity for diagnoses being considered.

Step 7: Assessing adaptive behavior across developmental domains.

Step 8: Observing parent–child interaction in the clinic and/or the home.

Step 9: Assessing the child's perception of the family.

Step 10: Developing a case formulation from a family perspective.

Step 11: Making a therapeutic presentation of the findings.

Step 12: Co-constructing recommendations/interventions.

in an empathetic fashion and to address clients' concerns at a depth of interpretation that they can understand and accept.

Family measures are not well developed for clinical use. There are now several good paper-and-pencil research measures, completed most often by individual parents (and sometimes by adolescents), that tap family members' perceptions of various aspects of family functioning (e.g., the Family Environment Scale—Third Edition [FES-3]; Moos & Moos, 1994). With several exceptions, however (e.g., the Parenting Stress Index—Third Edition [PSI-3]; Abidin, 1995), those that exist have limited norms and evidence for reliability and validity (Grotevant & Carlson, 1989; Kamphaus & Frick, 2002; Yingling, 2004), and most were developed in the 1980s. In addition, we have not found most of these measures useful for the assessment of families with young children. In part, this is because many family measures reveal individual members' perceptions of static concepts such as communication, which do not capture the culture and full complexity of a family (Deacon & Piercy, 2001); in part, it is because they are designed as a prelude for family therapy, which is not the purpose of assessing families as part of a comprehensive psychoeducational assessment. Thus this chapter focuses on a core of qualitative techniques, observational techniques, some self-report measures, and an observation/interview measure that can be used with any family of a preschool child presenting with learning or behavioral problems. References are given for more specialized family assessments.

We now describe steps and measures in the family assessment of a preschool child referred for a comprehensive psychoeducational evaluation for a suspected or diagnosed disability.

Step 1: Building a Family–Professional Partnership

Initial Contact

In order to set up the initial meeting, we recommend telephoning the family first and getting a brief sense of the referral question from their perspective before agreeing on a time for the initial session and deciding who will participate. We try to gather as much information as possible prior to the initial session with the family, so that we have a preliminary case formulation when we start the assessment of the family and of the child. Professionals differ in how much they want to know about a child prior to the initial interview with the family. Reid (1999) argues that the family members should be allowed to tell their story to the assessor, without the potential bias introduced by the assessor's having first reviewed other evaluations and intervention records. Although we find her approach to assessment maximally sensitive to the family's perspective and supportive of a strong therapeutic alliance, we find it impractical in the assessment-focused preschool and clinic settings in which we work. Because of the time pressures, we often ask parents who speak English to fax or mail back consent for a center/school visit, interview with teachers/caregivers, and review of records; we also send a behavior rating scale for each parent or adult caring for the child (with stamped return envelopes), and we request copies of all prior evaluations if not in school or center files.

If a family is resistant or ambivalent about meeting or participating in an evaluation; perhaps because of a past disappointment with a school/agency or other issues, the resistance or ambivalence will need to be addressed during the telephone interview or first session by listening empathetically to their story, and, if possible, explaining how you would handle the situation if the parents were willing to take a chance on working with you. With reluctant parents, Landy, Menna, and Clipsham (2006) recommend being clear and direct about how the family was referred, who you are, who you work for, what your role would be if they agreed to an evaluation, and what the evaluation might lead to in terms of services if the child qualifies for them. It helps to make clear to the family that a first contact doesn't require a commitment and that they are in control of the process and have the choice to not participate.

Who Should Be Seen

For the initial interview, we prefer to see everyone in the family, if possible. At the very least, we find it essential to interview both parents (if both are involved in the child's life), preferably at the same time. To get both parents to attend, we volunteer to schedule meetings before or after work, or to have a speakerphone in the interview room and call the absent parent at work during the meeting so that he or she can participate. Each parent often has a different perspective, and children tend to interact differently with fathers than they do with mothers. Similarly, we have found that older siblings have useful information to share. Nannies, grandmothers, and other adults living in the home frequently have unique perspectives and important information to offer as well. If it is not convenient for these individuals to attend the initial session, we ask for permission to conduct an interview by telephone or in person at another time. In short, we prefer to interview as many of the important people in a child's life as is possible. Sometimes parents prefer to be interviewed separately because of divorce or separation. Culturally diverse families require a special sensitivity as to who should be seen; see Chapter 9 for a discussion.

Creating a Welcoming Environment or Visiting the Home

This first meeting generally takes place at a school, clinic, or center. It is desirable to arrange the environment to be as welcoming as possible. Parents who did not do well in school themselves, or parents who come from a different cultural or linguistic background, may feel particularly ill at ease in a professional setting. Any efforts that can be made to provide a welcoming environment (e.g., the provision of culturally appropriate beverages and snacks; a friendly, sensitive receptionist; furniture that is inviting; posters that emphasize the value of individuals from many cultures; and signs that are in more than one language) may go a long way to putting parents at ease and making them feel as if they too have a right to participate in the mission or operation or activities of the school, clinic, or center (see the screening environment checklist in Chapter 9, Figure 9.4).

A home visit is another option for the initial session. It is more comfortable for some families to be seen at home, and it allows for an observation of family members in their natural environment. In conducting home visits, we follow the model of social workers—who attempt to dress in as comfortable a manner as possible while still appearing appropriate, and to downplay any class distinctions. Accepting any food or beverages that are offered indicates an acceptance of the family's hospitality.

Conveying Purpose, Defining Role, and Setting Boundaries

The purpose for the interview and the amount of time available for it should be clearly conveyed to the family in the initial telephone call and at the beginning of the interview. In general, interviews with family members are designed to find out what concerns they may have regarding their child; any problems the child may have, and what they have attempted to do about them in the past; information on the child's developmental history, as well as his or her medical, educational, and social background; the family's background; and any expectations for treatment that the family members may have (Sattler, 1988).

The family also needs information on the assessor's role and how long it is going to last. This is particularly true if the professional is going to be involved in a very restricted way with the family. This allows family members to make their own decisions about how much information they wish to share and the amount of emotional energy they may wish to invest in developing a relationship. Similarly, the professional should have a clear idea as well of what's going to be involved and should not encourage family members to share more information (particularly of a sensitive nature) than is in their best interest to share, given limitations on their involvement with a particular professional or institution (Kagan & Schlosberg, 1989).

The limits of confidentiality need to be discussed at the beginning of the initial session, so that family members know what the assessor will share in oral and written form with others and can make informed decisions about what to share with the assessor. Child maltreatment, harm to self, and harm to others are the standard legal imperatives to breach confidentiality in all situations, and these should be reviewed at the start of any professional relationship. However, the confidentiality of other material varies by setting, and the ground rules for sharing information need to be established. In private or community mental health agencies, evaluations and family sessions are typically protected communications between the professional and family; only with the express written permission of the parents will a report, file notes, or assessor impressions be shared with others. In our university clinic, we prepare a report for each family that includes a full family history and case conceptualization. We consult with the family about what should be included in a report to a school or other treating agency. Although we do not change diagnoses or information essential for treatment in the school/center/agency receiving the report, we do remove family information that is not essential if the family asks us to do so. In a school-based evaluation, the assessor has discretion in what to report about the family. However, some developmental information about the child, and all test scores and observations of the child and of parent–child interactions, are reported; whatever is in the report also becomes part of the child's permanent record. In an assessment for child protective services, juvenile justice, or a custody evaluation, no information is confidential in the sense that all relevant information becomes part of the record for purposes of case determination.

Joining with the Family

In the initial interview, the focus should be on the parents' (and other family members') concerns and needs regarding the referred child. Nonjudgmental listening; eliciting and responding to parental concerns and needs; and soliciting parental ideas about the child in a manner conveying that the parents are the expert on their child—all these send a clear message of concern and respect to the parents, and go a long way toward developing a working relationship between the professional and the family. The use of simple English, or the provision of a professional who speaks the family's native language (or, in cases where that is not possible, the provision of a well-trained interpreter), will increase the chances that the parents and the professional will clearly understand one another and communicate effectively.

All of the theoretical models presented earlier advocate as the first step seeking to join with the family members by allowing them to share their concerns and by trying to enter their world. Given the need to tailor assessments and interventions to referral questions, it's appropriate to focus the opening stages of the family interview on clarifying the concerns that have led to a referral. The session can begin with a broad question such as "Why are you here?" when the referral comes from the parents or when the parents have been referred by one agency or another. When the family has been invited in by a referral source, such as the school or clinic, a description of the perceived problem by the referral source is helpful in focusing the group on the initial agenda for the meeting. Here, addressing the question "How do you see the problem?" to first one parent and then the other is a good beginning. This question elicits the family's perspective on the problem, and the questioning is done in a hierarchical order (parents before siblings), which reinforces the leadership of the parents (Karpel & Strauss, 1983, p. 118). Asking the father first, if he is present, often elicits his participation in a way that may not be possible after the mother (often the person most involved with the child) has presented her view.

Step 2: Obtaining a Detailed Description of the Problematic Behavior, Its Context, and Its Impact on the Family

There are a number of ways to gather information about the referral problem, depending on the practitioner's theoretical perspective. From a family systems perspective, many practitioners focus on the onset, severity, and previous family responses to the problem. For instance, Karpel and Strauss (1983) suggest asking for a history of when the problem started, what other things were going on at the time, and what the family considers to be the problem's source or to have precipitated its onset. Severity questions include asking what impact the problem has had on the family and how the problem has developed and changed since its onset. Questions related to family coping address what the family members have done (have they actively confronted the problem or avoided it?); the answers may reflect the family's decision-making ability, motivation for intervention, crisis intervention skills, and so forth, all of which are important observations that will help the practitioner to develop appropriate interventions with the family.

Karpel and Strauss (1983) recommend spending only about the first 15 minutes of the initial interview on the presenting problem, to leave sufficient time for a more global family assessment. They focus the family interview on a family's level of adaptation. They ask not only how the family members have attempted to handle the particular referred problem, but how they have handled past family crises. All past problems (e.g., the birth of a child with a disability, immigration, psychiatric hospitalization) are clinically important, in that they reveal a great deal about individual family members, family themes, and coping strategies at specific stages in the family's development (Carter & McGoldrick, 1989; Karpel & Strauss, 1983).

Once uncovered, past problems can be compared and contrasted to current problems (e.g., if this is the family's second child with a disability, how have the family members dealt with the first?), to explore whether the current crisis could be "acute exacerbation of a chronic family difficulty" (Karpel & Strauss, 1983, p. 147). These comparisons may reveal long-standing family organization, decision-making, and judgment processes.

When family members have received treatment before or survived a significant crisis, it is often useful to ask them what they have learned from the experience. Well-considered, effective responses to crises indicate a favorable prognosis, the presence of resources to resolve problems and issues, and high motivation for treatment or assistance. An inability to answer may indicate an impaired ability to experience or to respond to treatment (for whatever reasons).

In families of children with disabilities, high levels of stress are common. Often it is helpful if the practitioner comments on that and pulls for information about day-to-day pressures that such a family has learned to adapt to and may have minimized. As a way of eliciting information about methods of adaptation, Karpel and Strauss (1983) suggest beginning the assessment in this area by asking for the following information:

> It will help us in dealing with the present problem to learn something about any previous problem the family has experienced or that any members of the family have gone through themselves. Any past situation that has been especially upsetting to the family or puts stress on it would be of interest to us, as would any previous problems that would require professional help. (p. 146)

They end the first session by asking, "Let me ask all of you again, in recent months, have there been any other changes for people in the family as a whole or any other problem areas besides the situations you've mentioned so far?" (p. 131). This question successfully elicits information that family members either have avoided or may have not found or thought relevant.

From a social learning/behavioral perspective, Mash and Terdal (1988) approach the referral problem in a manner that is similar to the family systems approach presented above, but is more specifically targeted toward clarifying the patterns of social rewards and punishments that are maintaining the objectionable behavior. They suggest directing the interview toward answering the following questions: (1) Is there a problem (i.e., is the child's behavior non-normative, and if so, to what extent)? (2) What is the child doing or not doing that's bringing him or her in conflict with the environment or causing problems within the family? (3) What variables potentially control these behaviors?

From a similar theoretical perspective, Webster-Stratton and Herbert (1994) take a less structured approach at first, as their assessments lead directly to longer-term treatment. In their initial assessment, they take great pains to develop a collaborative process with parents—one that fully engages them, so that they won't drop out of treatment when things get difficult. They do this in part by allowing parents to structure their presentation of their concerns, to address the issues that are on their minds, to tell their story, and to make it clear why they have come for help, with minimal interruption and structuring by the assessor/therapist.

Reid (1999) takes a psychoanalytic perspective, but also employs an assessment-to-treatment model (in her case, with families of children with autism). She stresses the importance of using the initial family interview to perceive the family through the family's eyes rather than those of other professionals. To facilitate this, she advocates (as noted earlier) not reading reports from other professionals "to prevent generalized judgments and pressure for certainty" (p. 70), and she uses her observations of the family in the waiting room and in her office to take in the unique characteristics of the child and the impact of the child on the family. She solicits a spontaneous account of the child's developmental history, with the focus on the child's uniqueness and stage of normal development without trying to cloud the picture with a diagnostic label. Only after this has been accomplished does she seek permission to read reports and communicate with other professionals working with the child. In the next stages of assessment, she tries to contain the traumatic impact of autism on the mental health of other family members by having each one describe the effect of the discovery or diagnosis on them. Through observations of the child and her own attempts to interact differently with the child, as well as parental diaries, she searches for new strategies that might improve the quality of family life (e.g., during mealtimes or sleeping). Only after trust has been established does she then look at the family's history independent of the child with autism—using separate sessions for parents and for siblings, appraising both healthy development and distress, and trying to discern what support and interventions might be most appropriate.

In the special education/early intervention models, the focus of the assessment is on getting a general picture of the family by having the parents fill out family needs measures, clarify their needs more precisely through interview, and then prioritize which needs to address first. Once the most pressing need is identified, the assessor explores with the family what must be accomplished to address this need and what all of the underlying concerns related to it might be. Resources needed to address the need are then identified, in part by mapping the family's social network through the use of social support measures (reviewed below). The family members are then helped to generate their own solutions toward meeting their needs through the assistance of their social network, with problem-solving support from the assessor/therapist (Dunst et al., 1988).

A comparison of the four types of models indicates that the family systems practitioner and the psychoanalytically oriented assessor spend relatively little time on the presenting problem, focusing most of the session on assessing the family as a whole. For the social learning/behavior therapist, on the other hand, the presenting problem *is* the focus of the interview. The special education/early interventionist attempts to get a general picture of the family, but then quickly focuses on addressing the family's most pressing concern. Our own belief is that an assessor working with families of at-risk or disabled young children must consider both of these two foci. The presenting problem is the primary focus of the interview; however, the functioning of the family as a whole is essential to understanding the child and making successful efforts to address the problem and engage in interventions. The assessment model presented in this chapter therefore attempts to meld these two approaches: The assessor spends time on each focus, with the proportion of time spent determined by the case conceptualization. If the problematic child behavior is embedded in family dynamics, then understanding the family requires more time than if the family is stressed but coping as well as can be expected with the child's disability.

In observing family dynamics, we attend closely to two aspects of family interaction that we think reflect the overall state of family functioning. The first is the degree to which the family *promotes the development* of individual members and particularly the target child. This can be assessed by asking each parent to describe the child and assessing the degree to which the portrait presented resembles a clearly differentiated awareness of the child as an individual, separate and distinct from the parents' own identities. Parental sensitivity to the child's cues and needs, and awareness of the child's emotional life, can be detected through observing parent–child interactions and through carefully listening to the parents' depiction of the child. Insensitivity to the child's uniqueness, distorted perceptions of the child's functioning, and hostility toward the child are indications of family and parent–child problems.

The *emotional content* of the familial interactional process is important to assess as well. Clear expressions of warmth, caring, interest, and responsiveness to the child's overtures are signs of emotional support and warmth. These should be carefully distinguished from presentations of pseudowarmth (see Crittenden, 1989), in which the parent says warm and caring things with a constricted and false tonal quality. Studies have shown that children as young as 1 year of age detect both positive and negative messages in interactions, and, when there is a discrepancy interpret the interaction on the basis of the negative message (Bugental, Mantyla, & Lewis, 1989; Volkmar & Siegel, 1979).

Table 8.4 describes interview process checkpoints.

TABLE 8.4. Interview Process Checkpoints

Setting up and conducting the initial interview/contact	First session	Succeeding sessions

• Clearly convey purpose.
• Arrange welcoming environment.
• Dress appropriately.
• Be aware of possible issues related to trust, past disappointments.
• Obtain related information:
  • Concerns about child.
  • Problems child might have.
  • Past efforts on part of parents.
  • Child's medical, educational, social history.
  • Expectations for treatment or intervention.
  • Have parents complete a developmental history prior to interview, if possible.
	• If in home, accept family's hospitality.
	• Clearly define your role, explain confidentiality.
	• Know as much as possible about child prior to visit.
	• Focus on the parent(s).
	• Be nonjudgmental.
	• Use simple English or child's home language.
	• Conclude the visit by leaving the family with something useful.
	• Provide a brief summary of what was discussed, next steps, timeline.
	• See the entire family, if possible.
		• Administer and discuss results of family measures.
		• Agree on definition of problem.
		• Set goals and prioritize them.
		• Problem-solve how to achieve goals.
		• Address psychological barriers that prevent empathy with other family members, or solutions.
		• Promote family competence and control.
		• Provide help with problems the family identifies.
		• Use the professional–family relationship to build trust and identify problematic relationship issues.

Step 3: Taking a Developmental, Health, and Educational History of the Child

We use Barkley's (1997a) Clinical Interview—Parent Report Form to organize this section of the interview. It asks for detailed information about parental concerns that have led to a referral; reviews criteria for childhood disorders that may be alternative diagnoses or comorbid diagnoses; gathers information on the parents' child management strategies; and assesses the child's past evaluation and treatment history, educational history, and strengths, as well as the family psychiatric history.

Step 4: Assessing of Family History, Current Functioning, and Social Support

The family's development over time; its cultural, religious, and immigration patterns; its developmental stage at the time of the referral; and the context in which the family and the problem are embedded relate directly to problem analysis and treatment planning. The techniques and measures described in this section fall into three general groups. The first group has to do with the family's history, patterns, and developmental stage; it includes the genogram and family life cycle, and, if the history is a complicated one, a timeline of important family events. The second general group of techniques and measures involves assessment of the current environment (social and physical). This group includes the eco-map, which portrays the family embedded in its context at one point in time; descriptions of the home environment and the neighborhood, which may include actual observations of these; and descriptions of the daily routine of family members. It also includes an assessment of both social support and social stressors, as well as the degree to which the family interacts with the community (and the quality of these interactions). The third group focuses on assessing the family's perceptions of its needs and resources.

As a context for understanding the techniques described in the following section, see the detailed case study beginning on page 266.

Family History, Patterns, and Developmental Stage

The *genogram* is based on the concept of a genealogical family tree or family pedigree. As such, it is a visual description of the family over at least three generations (see Figure 8.2 for a guide to the symbols used in constructing and interpreting genograms, and Figure 8.3 for a case example). The genogram provides considerable information quickly by naming all family members, their biological and emotional relationships to one another, and their psychological and physical proximity. Depending on the degree to which the professional wishes to explore family patterns (which will differ, depending on the problem presented), the genogram may yield a great deal of information on emotional responses to critical events and typical patterns of interaction as well.

Once rapport has been established, all of this can be elicited in a nonthreatening manner through the process of constructing the genogram, which allows parents to relax and focus on a topic in which they are the experts (Webster-Stratton & Herbert, 1994), and which encourages the family to see itself as a unit (Holman, 1983). Bowen (1978) has been credited with the introduction of the genogram to clinical practice, and its popularity is attested to by its frequent use in illustrating case studies in family therapy books. (See McGoldrick, Gerson, & Shellenberger, 1999, for a detailed description of genograms and their use in clinical practice.)

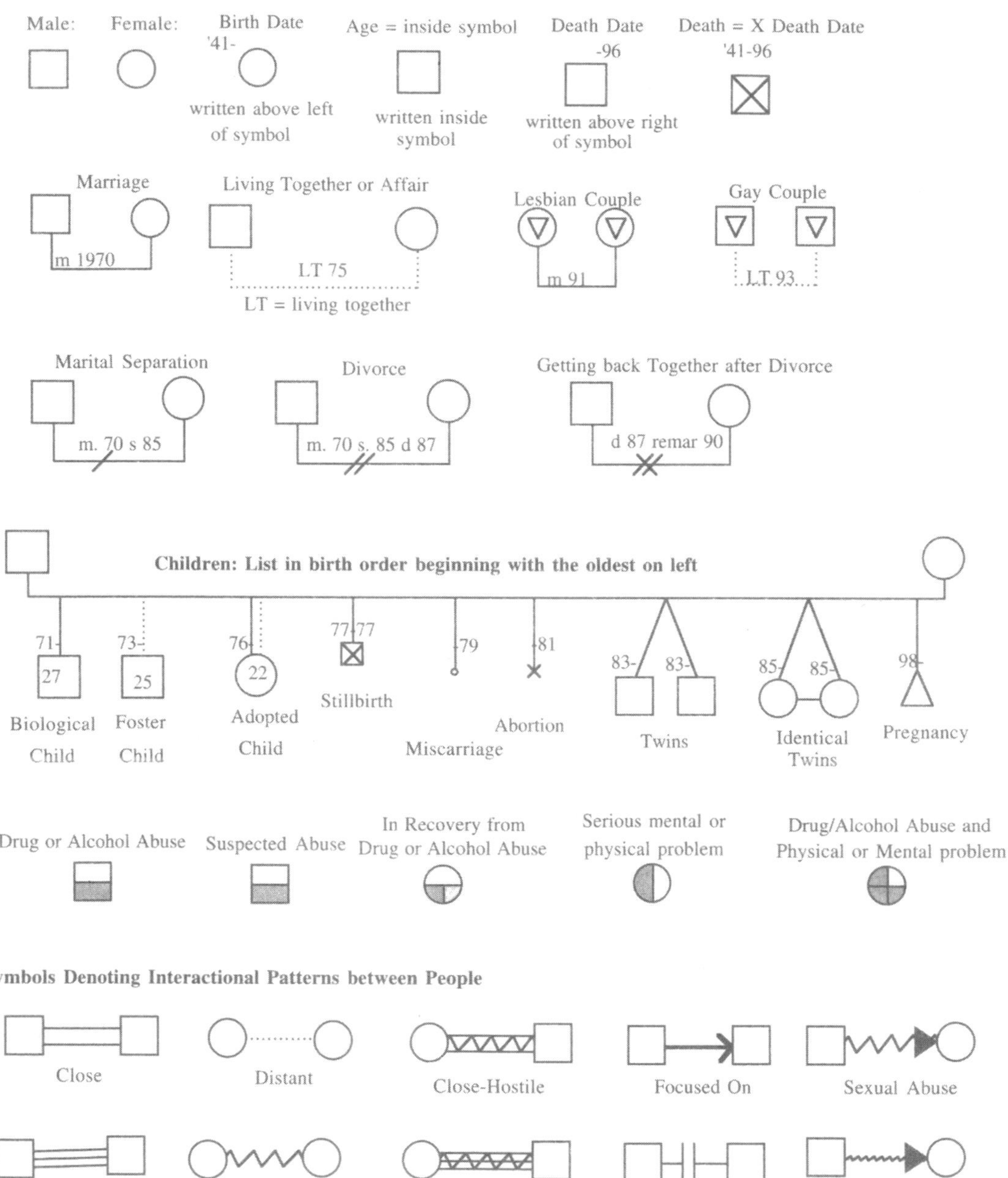

FIGURE 8.2. Symbols for constructing a multigenerational genogram. From McGoldrick, Gerson, and Shellenberger (1999). Copyright 1999 by Monica McGoldrick and Sylvia Shellenberger. Copyright 1985 by Monica McGoldrick and Randy Gerson. Used by permission of W. W. Norton & Company, Inc.

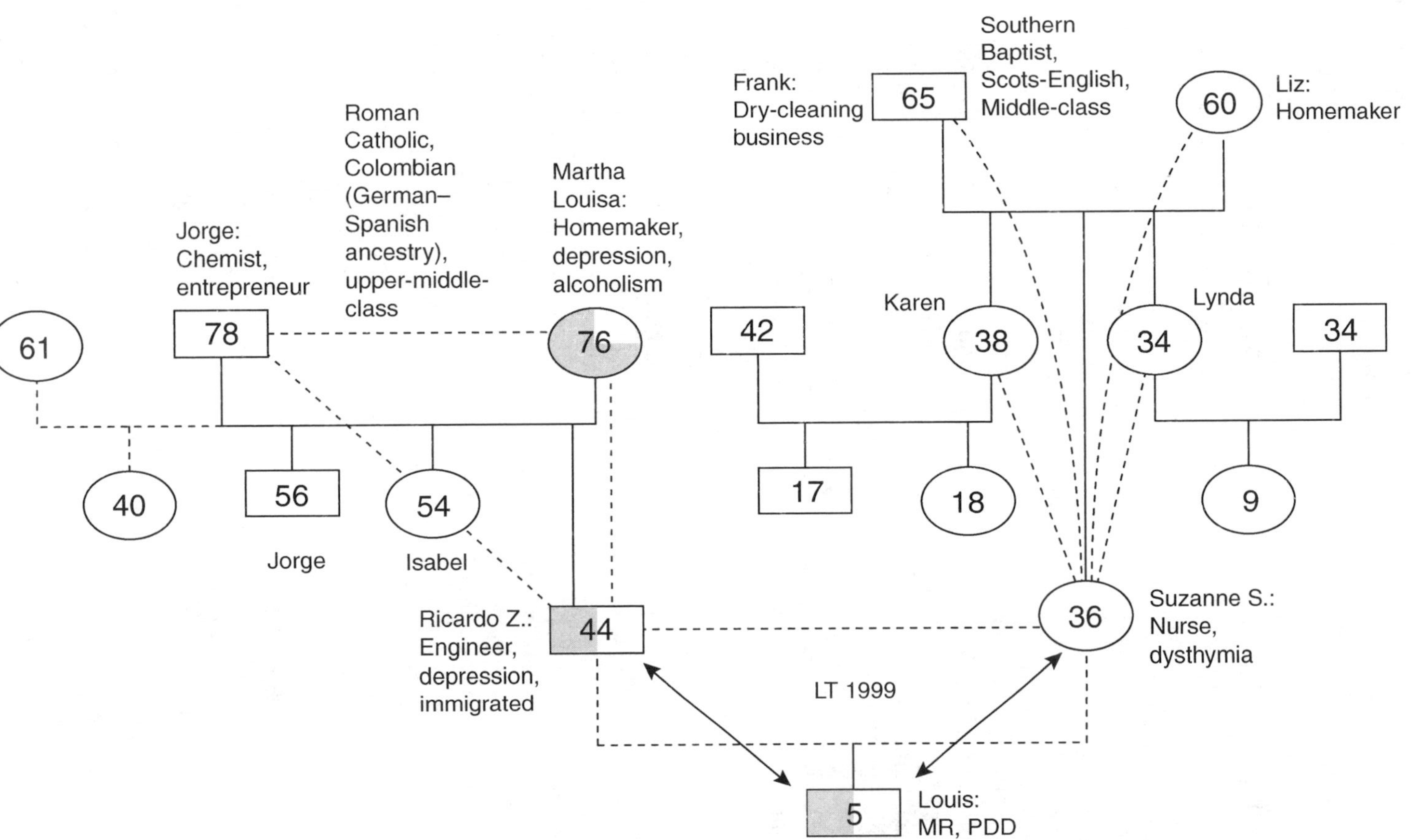

FIGURE 8.3. Genogram for Louis's family.

The genogram is a very flexible clinical tool. It can be used to quickly gather demographic information on the family, including who the members are; their relationships (both formal, in the sense of marriage, and informal, in the sense of cohabitation); their ethnic/cultural heritage; their educational, occupational, athletic, and artistic accomplishments; and their background in regard to major mental illnesses, developmental disabilities, and other health-related issues. It can also be used to gather fairly personal information about family dynamics, values, expectations for members, and general patterns of leading life.

It is our experience that families seem to enjoy constructing the genogram (in general, people like to talk about their families). When used to gather rather quick, somewhat superficial information about the family, it can be introduced fairly early in an assessment session. However, when emotional and interactional information is to be gathered as part of this procedure, it often works best after some trust has been developed between the professional and the family. A brief introduction (e.g., "This is an exercise that might help me know who is in the family and help all of us understand more about the problem") is usually sufficient to get the family involved.

With the family members gathered in a circle around the table, the professional can ask individual members specific questions. A large sheet of paper or white cardboard is used to integrate the elicited information into the genogram, while providing plenty of room to draw in an area that the entire family can see.

At a minimum, the following information should be obtained for the genogram: (1) family members (by first name); (2) dates of birth, death, marriage, divorce, separations, and major illnesses; (3) occupations; (4) education; (5) family members' health, occurrences of physical or mental illness, involvement with the legal system, suicides, learning disabilities, and hereditary degenerative diseases or common causes of death or brain injury; and (6) other important facts, such as SES, ethnicity, and religious affiliation.

In situations where a professional wishes to explore more dynamic aspects of family life, two types of additional information can be solicited. First, two-word descriptions may give some idea of family myths and individual members' role assignments. For such information, Karpel and Strauss (1983) suggest asking, "What word or two, what pictures come to mind when you think about this person?" (p. 56). Second, family members can be asked to describe the relationships between themselves, referring first to either the father or the mother, and then to other individuals on the map. This can be done for both parents, for all the children, and then for the parent's parents, siblings, and so forth, until a fairly comprehensive description of the interrelationships in the three generations of family life has been achieved.

The professional can then comment on patterns observed (e.g., inherited musical talent, or a history of marriages compelled by pregnancy across generations in the mother's family). Non-normative or unusual events (e.g., a life-threatening illness in a relatively young parent, severed relationships among family members, or the impact of historical events on family experiences [such as the impact of serving in the Iraq war on the father's occupational success and emotional adjustment]) are also identified, and their relevance to their historical family identity and current family/child difficulties is illuminated.

One of the major advantages of the genogram is that it allows family members to step back and take a look at themselves as a currently functioning, yet historically influenced, unit. Biological and cultural roots, and the important influence of past family experiences on current family life, are highlighted by this technique. The information provided is so useful that we recommend administering it as part of most parent interviews—whether on a more superficial level, as would be appropriate when a therapeutic relationship is not going to evolve out of the assessment, or at a more detailed, in-depth level, when a therapeutic relationship will follow. The genogram covers the major family bases systematically and efficiently, quickly orienting the professional to the complex and multifaceted world of any human family.

From the family genogram, the assessor can identify the current stage of the family life cycle and related issues confronted by the family. The assessment as a whole will shed light on how well the family is coping with its developmental tasks and common challenges.

Timelines are very useful in case formulation and in treatment. Duhl (1981) recommends using a chronological chart, with a column for each family member's name intersected by rows for specific family events (births, deaths, etc.). Each family member writes his or her age and reaction to the event on the form. The timeline tracks "family interactions in relations to specific events," highlights the "intrapersonal and interpersonal impact of events across time" (Deacon & Piercy, 2001, p. 364), and can help in coordinating this material with the presentation of the target child's developmental milestones and symptoms. From a history-taking perspective, timelines can be cross-checked with school/center records; family videotapes, baby books, and photo albums/discs; and past evaluations. From a treatment perspective, the assessor and family can explore the ramifications of events for family and individual functioning, help the family process feelings associated with painful events, and discover connections that may explain a child's difficulties (e.g., separation anxiety in a 4-year-old associated with postpartum maternal depression after the birth of twins). McGoldrick et al. (1999) give many clinical examples of the use of a timeline in conjunction with a genogram for family assessment.

Current Social and Physical Environment

A clear picture of the family's current living arrangements and environment can be obtained through a combination of an eco-map, interview, observation, and questionnaires about family needs and social supports.

An increasingly popular and easy tool for use in family assessment is the *eco-map* (Brassard, 1986; Hartman, 1979; Holman, 1983). Hartman developed the technique to help public welfare workers assess individual family needs, and its rationale emanates from a growing body of literature that documents the relationship between social support systems and the mental health of adults (Henderson, Byrne, & Duncan-Jones, 1981; Henderson, Duncan-Jones, Byrne, & Scott, 1980), the functioning of families with young disabled children and social support (Dunst et al., 1988), and the inverse relationship between extrafamilial contacts and child maltreatment (Salzinger, Kaplan, & Artemyeff, 1983; Wahler, 1980).

The eco-map visually portrays or maps a family's ecological system, showing the interactions of each member with outside resources (extended family, early intervention center, schools, churches, healthcare, friends, work, etc.). The eco-map identifies stresses and supports within and outside the family system by portraying the nature and flow (uni- or bidirectional) of the relationships between the family and its members and outside resources. It also portrays where individual or family needs are unmet and where untried resources might be available.

The eco-map is easily administered. Holman (1983) suggests involving as many family members as possible in its development, because this provides both the professional and the family with a comprehensive understanding of the family's perceptions of its ecological system. She recommends sitting down with the whole family or several members grouped around the eco-map protocol (which is usually a large sheet of white cardboard), with the usual environmental resources drawn in (see Figure 8.4 for symbols used in constructing and interpreting the eco-map, and Figure 8.5 for a case example). Initially, nonthreatening and nonintrusive questions should be asked, such as "Do you have much family?" or "Do you work at a job?" More specific questions can then gradually be posed, such as "Have you worked there for a while?" or "How do you get along with the family?" Family members tend to feel comfortable providing the information requested, and because of the engaging nature of the task, they may volunteer additional information that might not be typically provided (Hartman, 1979). This technique is particularly recommended for nonverbal or easily threatened family members who are reluctant to divulge information.

The household members can first be drawn in the center circle of the eco-map in the fashion of genograms, with squares for males, circles for females, and lines for generational connections (see the previous discussion of the genogram). Then the family as a whole or individual members can be connected with important extrafamilial systems.

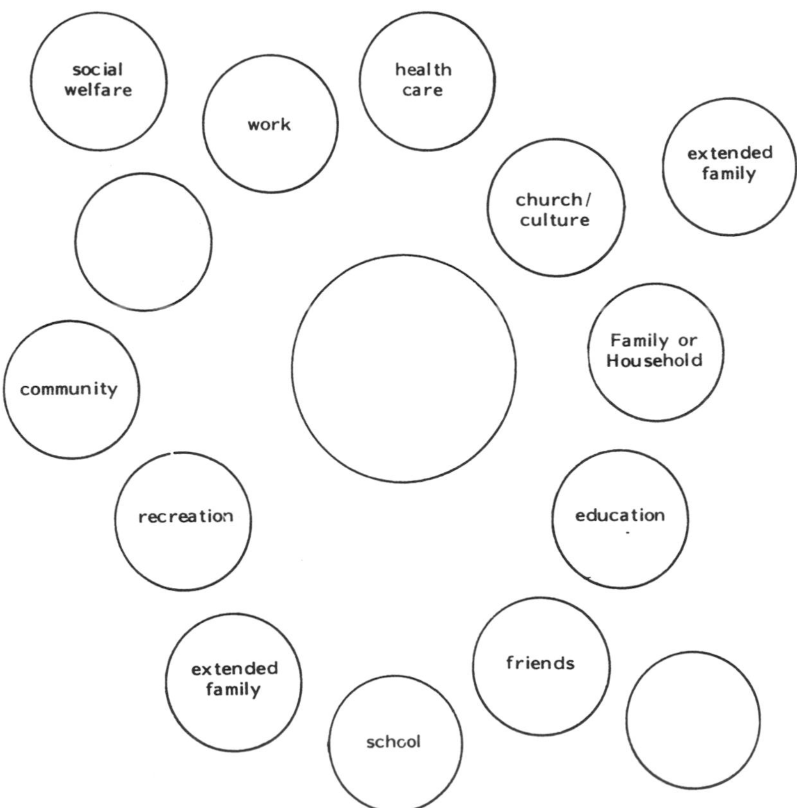

FIGURE 8.4. Symbols and form for constructing an eco-map. From Holman (1983). Copyright 1983 by Sage Publications, Inc. Reprinted by permission of Sage Publications, Inc.

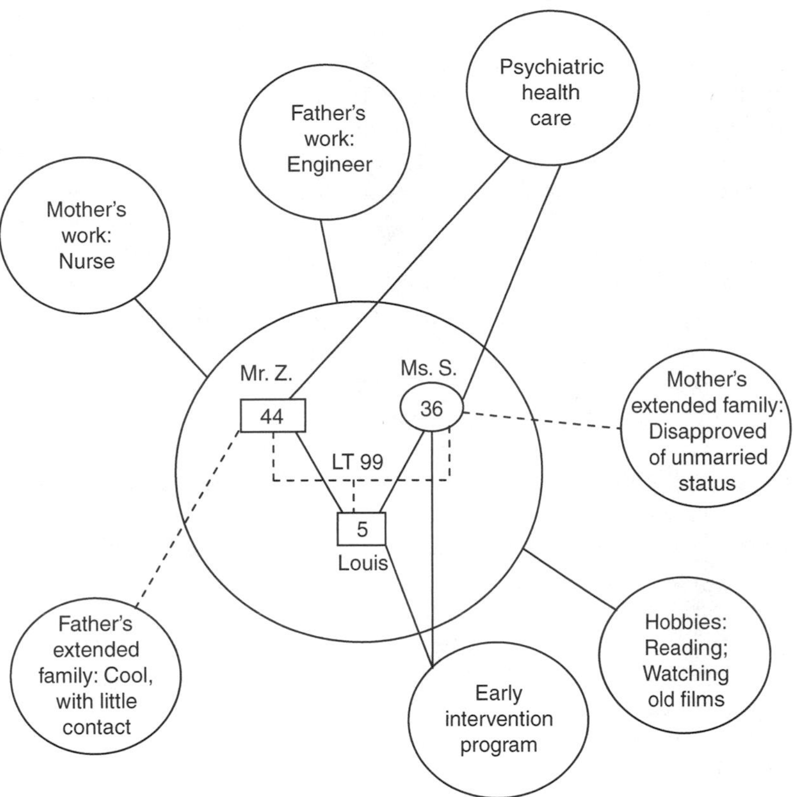

FIGURE 8.5. Eco-map for Louis's family.

Different types of lines are used to illustrate the types of relationship involved (e.g., unidirectional, tenuous, high-intensity, conflicted). For example, if one of the children has a chronic illness with heavy medical involvement, a connecting line would be a solid, heavily drawn line with arrows pointing from the hospital or medical center to the child, to indicate the amount and direction of energy expended by the medical professionals in dealing with this problem. After these system connections are drawn, empty black circles can be used to individualize the eco-map for the family. For example, a child with an autistic spectrum disorder (ASD) and mental retardation might have a strong bond with a private therapist, and this relationship may play an influential role in family routines, vacations, and financial expenditures.

The eco-map provides the professional with a great deal of information on the family's social environments, its significant sources of stress, and available used and unused resources or social support. An eco-map generates much information in a short period of time and is a very useful initial interview tool because of the engaging nature of the process and the usefulness of the information for the family. It is especially useful when more time-consuming, standardized measures of social support, family stress, or family social environment cannot be administered or are not important to the overall assessment. Finally, the eco-map's self-reported information can be verified by independent sources or by comparisons to other family-completed measures if its validity is in doubt.

As part of a family assessment, it's often useful to interview the family members about the circumstances of their daily lives and to visit their home and neighborhood. This provides the professional with salient information about environmental constraints and patterns that are useful in planning interventions. In a home description or visit, it's useful to obtain information regarding the number and types of rooms, who sleeps where, number of bathrooms and where they are located, and where the family usually spends time together (Karpel & Strauss, 1983). In a clinic setting, the family can be asked to draw a floor plan of the family home. The quality of the neighborhood is important to assess as well. What are the neighbors like? Do they have children the same ages as family members? What are the religious or ethnic influences, accessibility of recreational facilities, and safety and environmental quality (e.g., beauty, noise level, presence of crime)? The Home Observation for Measurement of the Environment (HOME; Caldwell & Bradley, 1984, 2003), an observation measure described in a later section on observing parent–child interaction, can be used to organize a home visit and to assess not only parent–child interaction, but the degree to which the home environment provides cognitive, academic, and socioemotional stimulation and support.

Another important source of information regards the family members' typical weekday and weekend routines. Descriptions of these might include weekday morning rising habits and sequences, how meals are handled, who attends them, where different individuals sit, the comings and goings of members during the day, and arrivals at home; how evenings and weekends are spent; and what family conversations and general interactions are like (e.g., warm and open, inquisitional, catch-as-catch-can). Such information can be obtained through daily/weekly schedules.

Many clinicians assessing families of children with suspected disabilities, or wishing to evaluate a program that serves these families, may wish to have more objective and specific information than the general overview provided by the eco-map. Several different types of scales have been developed by researchers from special education/early intervention programs to specifically assess such families. The scales cluster into measures that identify specific areas of family needs (including needs for support, information, financial assistance, etc.), and inventories that identify families' social, physical, and other resources. Each of these will be described next.

Family Needs

Bailey and Simeonsson (1988) and Dunst et al. (1988) have been involved in the development of family needs measures that focus specifically on the needs of families with disabled children from birth to preschool years. The scales are purposely not clinical or unduly intrusive; they provide information directly relevant to early intervention programs designed to address these children's needs and the needs of their families. Because of their brevity and focus on universal concerns and types of relationships, all of the scales could be easily translated in other languages. Appendix 8.1 contains a review of each measure and its psychometric characteristics.

FAMILY NEEDS SCALE

The Family Needs Scale, developed by Dunst, Cooper, Weeldreyer, Snyder, and Chase (1988), is used to obtain a list of family-identified needs for a variety of resources and supports, which can then be prioritized and addressed jointly by the family and the professional. The 41 items on this measure, which are rated on a 5-point scale by each parent, are organized into nine categories. The issues covered include financial resources;

adequacy of water, food, housing, plumbing, clothing, shelter, jobs, transportation, counseling, healthcare, and childcare; and recreation, educational, and intervention opportunities for the child. The authors report that adequacy of resources was significantly related to overall well-being, decision making, and internal locus of control in families with at-risk or disabled children. Reliability and validity are adequate for the scales intended purpose intervention.

FAMILY NEEDS SURVEY

Developed by Bailey and Simeonsson (1990), the Family Needs Survey is similar to the Family Needs Scale. The instrument consists of 35 items that have been organized into six categories: Needs for Information, Support, Understanding from Others, Community Services, Financial Resources, and Family Functioning. Items are responded to on a 3-point scale that ranges from "I definitely do not need help with this" to "not sure" to "I definitely need help with this." Only items marked "I definitely need help with this" are identified as targets for intervention. The items marked "not sure" may be queried during the interview.

The authors recommend that parents complete the scale separately, because they find that mothers and fathers provide different profiles of needs. The differences seem to reflect either the unique needs of each parent or different perceptions that might be usefully discussed as part of regular meetings. They recommend, in addition to using their instrument, asking parents to list their five greatest needs as a family. They found in one study that there was considerable overlap between the needs generated in that format and those identified on the Family Needs Survey, but that there were frequently surprises as well. Listing the greatest needs also serves as a framework for prioritizing goals. Garshelis and McConnell (1993) found that individual professional and early intervention team members identified only 52% and 74%, respectively, of mother-identified needs; this finding confirms the importance of surveying parents directly, followed by personal discussions. Clinically, the Family Needs Survey is a very straightforward and useful scale that should be acceptable to most families. Reliability and validity data are adequate for its use as both a research and a clinical tool to assess the unique needs of families (Sexton, Burrell, & Thompson, 1992).

Social and Other Resources

Social support has been acknowledged as the central resource for effective family functioning. It is frequently an intervention target for programs that work with young children and their families, as are physical and other resources (to a lesser extent).

The research efforts of Dunst and Trivette at the Family, Infant, and Preschool Program in western North Carolina have resulted in the development of several good measures of social support and other resources available to young children with disabilities and their families. As part of their research focus on the description of changes in child, parent, and family functioning and the identification of factors that are associated with those changes, Dunst and Trivette employed, analyzed, and developed measures specifically tailored to examining the role of these resources in promoting adaptations to the demands of rearing children with disabilities. In particular, they assessed the direct and indirect influence of social supports on parent well-being, parent–child interaction, family integrity, and child behavior and development. Dunst, Trivette, Hamby, and Pollack (1990) found that social support affects parent well-being, health, and family integrity, each of which in turn affects styles of parent–child interaction and child behavior and development. The measures of social and physical resources that they have developed include the Family Support Scale, the Family Resource Scale, and Inventory of Social Support (see Dunst et al., 1988), each of which is described below.

FAMILY SUPPORT SCALE

The Family Support Scale assesses the helpfulness of social resources to families (Dunst, Jenkins, & Trivette, 1984). The scale asks parents to indicate how helpful each source was to their family during the past 3–6 months. Parents can also indicate whether the source of help was not available to the family during that period of time with a "not available" response. Sources of support listed include such individuals as the respondent's or spouse's parents, coworkers, early child intervention program, staff members, and so on. Respondents check on a 5-point scale the degree to which these individuals have been helpful, with responses ranging from "not at all helpful" to "extremely helpful."

Although the technical data on this scale are limited, it has promising reliability and validity. In addition to the sample of 139 parents of preschool children with or at risk for developmental disabilities used by Dunst et al. (1984), two other studies have reported good construct validity and adequate internal consistency for screening measures. Taylor et al. (1993) used a sample of 900 families recruited nationwide from several early intervention studies and Hanley et al. (1998), a sample of 204 parents from low-income families in Head Start to examine the psychometric properties of the scale. The number of factors found in exploratory factor analysis has ranged from four to six but all the factor solutions are conceptually similar. The total scale is related to personal well-being of parents, integrity of the family unit, and parent perceptions of child behavior (Dunst et al., 1988). Overall, the FSS is easy to use, appears nonintrusive to families, and is an essential measure if one component of intervention will be fostering the growth of informal and formal social support.

FAMILY RESOURCE SCALE

The Family Resource Scale assesses parents' perception of the adequacy of different resources in a household (Dunst & Leet, 1987a, 1987b). Parents are asked to rate the degree to which they or their family have had adequate resources of time, money, energy, and so forth to meet the needs of the family as a whole, as well as individual family members' needs, over an unspecified period of time. Responses are again made on a 5-point scale and range from "not at all adequate" to "almost always adequate." The authors created the measure as a clinical tool for intervention with families with young children with disabilities. They found that total scores on the measure were consistently related to maternal well-being (r = .57) and predicted parental commitment to prescribed early intervention programs (r = .63).

Other researchers have found the FRS to be a much more sensitive measure of family resources than income level and SES, especially in low-income families. The FRS taps strengths, such as time to spend with family members and family help that are missed when objective but superficial external evaluations are made (e.g., Brody & Flor, 1997). Parents' perceptions of family resources on the FRS affect parenting and parents' school involvement, which in turn affects children's emotional self-control, and thus, their academic and social behavior (Brody & Flor, 1997; Brody, Flor, & Gibson, 1999).

Using very large samples of former Head Start families from 31 sites, Van Horn, Bellis, and Snyder (2001) developed a 20-item version, the FRS-R, with broader applicability than to families of young children with disabilities. This shorter version has four interpretable subscales, developed through exploratory and confirmatory factor analysis, with excellent construct validity for kindergarten and third-grade samples. The subscales are Basic Needs, Time for Self, Time for Family, and Money. As the subscales had unique relationships with variables such as distance from the poverty level, social skills, and picture vocabulary; accounted for more variance when entered separately than as a Total Scale; and provided useful information about families, the authors recommend interpreting them separately.

Overall, the FRS is a brief, clinically useful tool with good psychometric characteristics. Assessors working with families with young children with disabilities may want to use the FRS, while those working with broader populations will prefer the FRS-R.

INVENTORY OF SOCIAL SUPPORT

The Inventory of Social Support (Trivette & Dunst, 1988) asks about people or groups that may provide the family with help and assistance. Parents are first asked to respond to a list of individuals and groups with which the family may have had contact. For each source, they are asked to indicate how frequently they have been in contact with that person or group during the past month and to add any person or group that is not included on the list. Specifically, respondents are asked to note how frequently they have had contact with their spouse or partner, children, other relatives, health department staff members, and so on, ranging from "not at all" to "almost every day" on a 5-point scale.

Parents are then asked to list up to 10 needs or activities that are of concern to them, such as finding a job or paying the bills. After they have listed these needs or activities, they are asked to indicate which person or group they would go to if they needed help with any of the projects. Projects are listed down the left-hand side of the page, while across the top of the scale are listed all of the individuals and groups that the respondent has indicated having regular contact with in the first part of the scale. Finally, the same list is given to the parents, who are asked to indicate to what extent they can depend on any of the following sources of help for assistance when they need it, on a 5-point scale ranging from "not at all" to "all of the time." Trivette and Dunst's research indicated that family and personal well-being were significantly related to adequacy of support, and that lack of support placed more time demands on parents. Financial support was the only factor that was significantly related to family well-being. Emotional, child-related, and instrumental supports were significantly related to personal well-being of the parent.

Step 5: Screening Family for Parenting Stress, Marital/Couple Problems, Family Violence, and Mental Health Problems

Parenting Stress

Although every family is unique, some common challenges are faced by parents of young children with disabling conditions. Fish (2002) has organized these common challenges into the following categories:

- Increased financial hardship (e.g., unreimbursed expenses, such as remodeling a house for a child with cerebral palsy; a parent's quitting work or forgoing promotions because of high care demands).
- Daily care needs (e.g., a 4-year-old in diapers, a child with behavior problems who can't be taken to grocery stores).
- Socialization and recreational opportunities (e.g., parents' feeling isolated, finding

it hard to hire babysitters, or being unable to take the child along on family outings because of the perceived negative attitudes of the general public).

- Concerns about the future (e.g., worries about what will happen to the child, especially when the parents are gone).
- Family members' emotional reaction to the child's disability (e.g., shock, denial, depression, etc.).

Parents can be asked how each of these challenges have affected them, and/or they can be given one of two widely used measures of parenting stress to assess the stressors they are experiencing and how they are coping. The family needs measures described above also cover some aspects of the same material. The Questionnaire on Resources and Stress (QRS) has a clear focus on families of children with disabilities, while the Parenting Stress Index—Third Edition (PSI-3) is appropriate for assessing stress in all parent-younger child relationships.

QUESTIONNAIRE ON RESOURCES AND STRESS

The QRS is one of the oldest and most frequently used measures for families with a disabled or chronically ill child or other family member (Holroyd, 1974, 1987). Consisting of 285 items (66 items for the short form) written at a sixth-grade reading level, it has 15 subscales that are organized into three general domains. The Personal Problems domain consists of subscales assessing poor health or mood, excessive time demands, pessimism, lack of social support, negative attitude, overprotection/dependency, and overcommitment/martyrdom. The Family Problems domain consists of subscales assessing lack of family integration, financial problems, and limits on family opportunity. The third domain, Problems of Index Case, consists of subscales assessing physical incapacitation, lack of activities for index case, occupational limitations, difficult personality characteristics, and social obtrusiveness.

Items are scored true or false, and the instrument takes about 1 hour to complete for the long form, 20 minutes for the short form. Problem areas are identified as all areas with *T*-scores above 70, which suggest a significant problem. The manual suggests that clinicians identify family problem areas of concern and then assist families in prioritizing the issues of most concern.

Validity data suggests that the QRS can differentiate between married and single mothers, between mothers and fathers, and between mothers of children with mental retardation and mothers of children with emotional problems (Holroyd, 1974). It has also been used to compare stress levels between parents of children with autism and children with Down syndrome (Holroyd & McArthur, 1976), and between families of institutionalized and noninstitutionalized children with autism (Holroyd et al., 1975). There is a relationship between stress levels as measured by the QRS and a child's level of functioning (Beckman, 1983; Holroyd & Guthrie, 1979), as well as interview-based rating of stress (Holroyd, Brown, Wilker, & Simmons, 1975). Norms are available for families with members who have four major types of disabilities: psychiatric, developmental disabilities, chronic medical illness, and neuromuscular disease.

Friedrich, Greenberg, and Crnic (1983) developed a shortened version based on 289 parents of children of all ages diagnosed with autism, cerebral palsy, cystic fibrosis, Down syndrome, hematological disorders, neuromuscular disease, psychiatric disorders, renal disease, and mixed developmental and/or retardation disorders. The factor-analytic techniques they used yielded four distinct factors based on 52 items: Parent and Family Problems, Pessimism, Child Characteristics, and Physical Incapacitation. The correlation between the full QRS and this version of the short form was .99. As Friedrich et al. note, if the total score is what is of most interest, the short form is faster and equally effective at assessing total stress. Holroyd (1987) states that the longer form provides more detailed information about particular sources of stress, making it potentially more useful clinically, while the short form serves as a screening tool.

The clinical usefulness of the QRS, its ease of administration, and its appropriateness for a multitude of disabling conditions makes it popular with programs serving disabled children of all ages. Additional advantages are its psychometric characteristics, sixth-grade reading level, and the flexibility offered by four versions—one long form, two short forms, and a form for young siblings of disabled children (Crnic & Leconte, 1986). A weakness of the QRS is one of its strengths: Its age breadth means that a number of items are not relevant for preschool children. This is particularly so for Friedrich et al.'s Physical Incapacitation factor. Items such as "__________ can ride a bus," "__________ knows his own address," and "__________ is able to take part in games or sports" are certainly related to a child's dependence on parents, but are not developmentally appropriate and may not be related to stress above and beyond that experienced by any parent of a young child.

PARENTING STRESS INDEX—THIRD EDITION

The PSI-3 (Abidin, PAR staff, & Noriel, 1995) assesses parents' perception of stress and is designed for screening parents of children under the age of 12 (with a particular focus on birth to age 3) for high levels of stress between parent and child and within the parent or the situation. In addition to screening, it can also be used as part of an individual diagnostic assessment, as a pre- or posttreatment measure of intervention effectiveness, and has been used for research on the effects of stress. There is both a long form and a short form.

The PSI-3 long form contains 120 items, each of which is rated by a parent from 1 (lowest level of stress) to 5 (highest level of stress) The scale is divided into two major domains:

Parent Domain
(Related to Parent Motivation)
- Depression
- Attachment
- Restrictions of Role
- Sense of Competence
- Social Isolation
- Relationship with Spouse
- Parental Health

Child Domain
(Related to Child Temperament)
- Adaptability
- Acceptability
- Demandingness
- Mood
- Hyperactivity and Distractibility
- Reinforces Parent

The PSI-3 short form consists of 36 items derived from the long form that are organized into three scales: Parental Distress with items drawn from the long form's Parent Domain; Parent–Child Dysfunctional Interaction with items from the Parent and the Child Domains; and Difficult Child with items drawn from the Child Domain. The Total Stress Scores on the long and short forms correlate .94 and there are high correlations as well between the Parental Distress and the Parent Domain (r = .92) and between the Difficult Child and the Child Domain (r = .87).

The excellent manual includes a detailed description of the standardization sample and norms. The normative sample was drawn primarily from pediatric clinics in central Virginia and included children with and without problems, was predominantly white, and had a range of SES levels and parental age levels. The Spanish version was normed on 223 Hispanic parents. The manual provides percentile ranks for scaled scores and information about possible clinical interpretations. Clinical interpretation of the PSI-3 should be based on the measure's status as a screening instrument. Thus, Lloyd and Abidin (1985), discussing an earlier version of the PSI, recommended that a tentative hypothesis should be generated based on extremely high or low total scores (see manual for cutoff) and domain differences, which should then be explored through interview and other assessments with the family. Scores on subscales are used to generate a more refined hypothesis, and suggestions are offered on how best to approach intervention, given a particular profile.

The PSI-3 has strong psychometric characteristics, and the manual presents a wealth of data supporting the content, criterion-related, and predictive validity of the instrument in screening and assessing intervention effectiveness (Abidin, 1995; Grotevant & Carlson, 1989), although it is more effective as a measure of child and/or parent maladjustment than as a measure of stress per se. Reviewers note that the large normative sample was not random or stratified to be representative of the U.S. population. It had an East Coast geographic bias and consisted almost entirely of mothers, with only a small sample of fathers (who report lower stress than mothers) (Allison, Barnes, & Oehler-Stinnett, 1998). Bailey (1988) criticized an earlier version of the PSI as a tool for early interventionists because of its length, the clinical training needed for interpretation and intervention, the ambiguity of item content (acknowledging that an event is stressful does not necessarily mean that a family wants help dealing with the stressful event), and the use of the PSI in program evaluation (because he questions whether stress can ever be significantly reduced in families of children with disabilities). If a professional has sufficient time and appropriate training, however, the PSI-3 is a valuable clinical tool.

Marital/Couple Functioning

The parents' couple relationship has an important causative role in the emotional health and general development of children (Belsky & Vondra, 1989; Christensen & Margolin, 1988; Easterbrooks & Emde, 1988; Engfer, 1988; Gottman et al., 1997). In addition, several family therapists have asserted on the basis of their clinical experience that covert marital/couple discord is frequently evident in the emotional and behavioral symptoms of children and adolescents (Ackerman, 1987; Alexander & Parsons, 1982), and that poor child management skills may be causally related to increased marital/couple distress (Fleischman, Horne, & Arthur, 1983). Thus there are critical reasons to assess the quality of the parents' relationship as part of the family assessment. Although school-based professionals do not view marital/couple assessment and intervention as a legitimate school role, it is often appropriate in a clinical or community agency setting. The two instruments that we have used to screen for marital/couple satisfaction are the widely used Marital Adjustment Test (Locke & Wallace, 1959) and the Dyadic Adjustment Scale (Spanier, 1976). In any setting, the issue of marital/couple functioning must be addressed tactfully. For example, an assessor might say, "Many families find parenting preschoolers stressful. How are you dealing with it personally? As a couple? What do you do to get away and renew yourselves and your relationship?"

Family Violence

Family violence, in the form of intimate partner violence and parental psychological and physical abuse of children, is surprisingly common (Straus & Field, 2003; Straus & Kurz, 1997). Families of young children presenting with emotional or behavior problems have particularly high rates of family violence (Patterson, Reid, & Dishion, 1992). The Conflict Tactics Scales (Straus, 1979) is a brief set of scales that can be used to screen for intimate partner violence, and its parent–child version can be used to screen for psychological and physical child abuse (Straus & Hamby, 1997). It has adequate internal consistency and validity for screening. We do not give this measure to every family in our setting. High levels of anger, aggressiveness, and hostility in family or parent–child interaction, or signs of fear on the part of family members, are signals to us that this area should be assessed (see Brassard & Rivelis, 2006). Barkley's (1997a) Clinical Interview—Parent Report Form, which we use routinely also, asks whether a child has a history of physical or sexual abuse. If a parent/caregiver answers in the affirmative, follow-up questions in regard to the abuse should be as concrete as possible, since different cultures and individuals may define abuse in various ways.

Parental Mental Health

It is important to note any signs of distress or impairment in a family member during an assessment. Of particular concern are depression, tangential or loose thinking, intense anxiety, suicidal ideation, paranoid-sounding expressions, or any other signs that indicate distress in a family member; these should be evaluated in an individual meeting with the person or a conjoint meeting with the person and the spouse/partner. Because of high rates of depression and stress in parents (particularly mothers) of children with disabling conditions, many clinics routinely administer the Beck Depression Inventory–II (Beck, Steer, & Brown, 1996) or the PSI-3, which has a depression scale. High scores would then prompt a screening for depression, suicidality, and receptivity to a referral for mental health services, if warranted. Barkley's (1997a) Clinical Interview—Parent Report Form asks for a family psychiatric and learning history, which may reveal past and/or current problems in the parents or other family caregivers. Follow-up questions on the status of the problem and its impact on family and child functioning are appropriate.

Step 6: Reviewing Symptoms and Severity for Diagnoses Being Considered

If a specific diagnosis (e.g., ODD or an ASD) is being considered, then specific symptoms and their degree of severity need to be reviewed with parents. Depending on the diagnosis being considered, there are disorder-specific measures that can be used for parental ratings and structured interviews for diagnosis. (See Chapters 13 and 14 for details.)

Step 7: Assessing Child Adaptive Behavior across Developmental Domains

We also administer a measure of adaptive behavior, such as the Vineland Adaptive Behavior Scales, Second Edition (Vineland-II; Sparrow, Cicchetti, & Balla, 2005). The Vineland-II (reviewed in Chapters 12 and 13) is widely used for developmental assessments in referred children ages 0–5, as well as individuals of all ages with suspected mental retardation, ASD, dementia, or other cognitive impairments. The Socialization domain assesses the development of interest in others, emotional responsivity, emotional expression, emotional understanding, and success in making friends. The absence of these skills, when they would be expected based on either chronological age or mental age, should alert the evaluator that a more extensive assessment of emotional and social functioning may be appropriate. This subscale is particularly sensitive in identifying children with ASD. If adaptive behavior is low across the board or for the domains of Communication or Daily Living Skills, administration of an individually administered intelligence test by the psychologist and consultation with a speech and language pathologist would be in order. If the Motor Skills score is low, assessment by a physical or occupational therapist would be desirable.

Step 8: Observing Parent–Child Interaction in the Clinic and/or the Home

Direct observations of parent–child interaction are very useful for both diagnosis and treatment planning. Because of the training involved in mastering structured systems and maintaining interrater agreement, many examiners either omit direct observation or do it informally (see Chapters 4 and 5). There are three observation measures that may be worth spending the time to master, depending on the types and numbers of clients seen. If a child is referred for disruptive, noncompliant behavior, or if the assessor simply wishes to make a quick appraisal of the ability of a parent and child to cooperate and relate to one another, we recommend the Parent–Child Game developed by McMahon and Forehand (2003) (see Chapter 14 for a description and review). If the child is referred for delays in emotional milestones, we recommend the Functional Emotional Assessment Scale (again, see Chapter 14). The HOME (Caldwell & Bradley, 2003), which assesses the child's home environment and the degree to which it supports cognitive and emotional development, is useful in the assessment of any child referred for learning or behavior concerns.

The purpose of the HOME is to serve as a screening device to describe the "stimulation potential of the early developmental environment" (Caldwell & Bradley, 1984, p. 2), which might impede or foster cognitive development and to identify high-risk home environments. In developing the HOME, its authors identified the following features of home environments that show a relatively consistent relation to development:

1. Environment that ensures gratification of basic physical needs, health, and safety.
2. Relatively high frequency of contact with a small number of adults.
3. Positive emotional climate.
4. Optimum level of need gratification.
5. Varied sensory input that does not overload the child.
6. A physically, verbally, and emotionally responsive environment that reinforces valued behaviors.
7. A minimum of social restrictions on exploratory and motor behavior.
8. Organization of the physical and temporal environment.
9. Provision of rich varied and shared cultural experiences.
10. Availability of play materials that facilitate coordination of sensory–motor processes.
11. Contact with adults who value and foster achievement.
12. Cumulative provision of experiences that match the level of the child's cognitive, social, and emotional development.

The list above was used as a guide in scale development. Items developed were selected first empirically and then validated by their usefulness in practice.

The Infant–Toddler HOME (ages 0–3 years) was developed in the 1960s to study longitudinally the effects of daycare, home environments, and the children's development (Elardo, Bradley, & Caldwell, 1975). It has provided to be a remarkably effective instrument for describing critical aspects of children's homes that appear to play a causal role in development. The Early Childhood HOME (ages 3–6 years) was developed in the late 1970s as a screening instrument for children at risk of developmental problems. The Middle Childhood HOME (ages 6–10 years) and Early Adolescent HOME (ages 10–15 years) were added in the 1990s. The original items of the Infant-Toddler and Early Childhood forms have not changed, but their location on scales and scale names have changed over time, which is reflected in the versions of the manual (Caldwell & Bradley, 1984, 2003).

The HOME procedure involves both observation in the home and interviewing the family caregivers. The appropriate inventory is administered during a home visit while the child is awake. This procedure ensures that the observer/interviewer can observe the interaction between the child and mother (or primary caregiver). Administration takes about 1 hour. The interview is presented in a nonstandard format to put the caregiver at ease. Useful and extensive suggestions are presented for conducting the interview. Responses to items are coded and scored before the interviewer leaves the home. Interpretation is based on looking at scores that fall in the top, middle two, and bottom quartiles, with those in the bottom indicating an environment that places a child at risk for problems in one or more areas of development, identified by examining the patterns of subscale scores.

The 55-item Early Childhood HOME has eight subscales, established through factor analysis:

1. Learning Stimulation
2. Language Stimulation
3. Physical Environment
4. Warmth and Acceptance
5. Academic Stimulation
6. Modeling
7. Variety in Experience
8. Acceptance

There is a considerable body of evidence supporting the validity of the HOME. As early as 6 months of age, it correlates well with intelligence scores obtained at 3, 4, and 4-6 years of age (Bradley & Caldwell, 1976; Elardo, Bradley, & Caldwell, 1975), and it was sensitive to home environments associated with low IQs. Low scores on the HOME in the first few years of life were also found in separate studies to predict later problems, such as malnutrition and language delay (Cravioto & DiLicardie, 1972; Wulbert, Inglis, Kriegsman, & Mills, 1975). Across the different samples, there was a clear indication that SES and most HOME subscale scores were significantly related at each age level.

In a large national data set the Learning Stimulation subtest on the HOME short form was associated with early motor, language, and social development and academic achievement in poor and nonpoor white, black, and Hispanic children (ages 0–13 years). This subscale was also inversely related to behavior problems after controlling for other demographic factors and other HOME subscales (Bradley, Corwyn, McAdoo, & García-Coll, 2001b). This study conclusively demonstrated that home environments are significantly different for poor and nonpoor children (ages 0–13 years) in the three main ethnic groups in the United States. Poverty accounts for more of the differences than ethnicity (Bradley, Corwyn, Burchinal, McAdoo, & García-Coll, 2001a). The relationship between cognitive functioning and the HOME is stronger in white and black families and for those in higher social classes but it is still significantly related to children's development in other ethnic groups. The HOME can discriminate between poor mothers and poor mothers with mental retardation, the quality of rearing environment provided by mothers with different psychiatric diagnoses, and later attachment style of a child, to name just a few of the studies that support its validity (see Totsika & Sylva, 2004 for a recent review).

In general, the HOME is recommended as a useful screening instrument that provides a more objective and accurate view than self-report checklists do of supports in the home for child development and parent–child interaction. As such, it offers information useful for designing interventions that help parents provide a more intellectually stimulating environment, and/or a more positive and less punitive approach to discipline and guidance. It is easy to use and has demonstrated good construct and criterion-related validity in many studies with diverse samples within the United States and countries throughout the world. As with all observation measures, careful training and regular conferences between raters are necessary in order to maintain interrater agreement. Its one drawback is that assessors often do not have the time to make a home visit.

Step 9: Assessing the Child's Perception of the Family

Very few instruments are available to assess parent–child and child–sibling relationships from the perspective of the preschool child. The MacArthur Story Stem Battery (MSSB; Bretherton, Oppenheim, Buchsbaum, Emde, & MacArthur Narrative Working Group, 1990; Emde, Wolf, & Oppenheim, 2003) is a clinical tool developed by researchers to gain access to young children's "representational worlds, to what they understand, to their inner feelings" (Emde, 2003, p. 3). It uses a story stem technique, along with human and animal figures, to set a stage that encourages a child to complete a story drawing from his or her personal experience and internal representation of the social environment. Designed to be used with verbal children from age 3 or 4 up to age 7 (age 3 is the lower limit for middle-class children, 4 for high-risk samples), the MSSB has been used to assess attachment, moral development, family relationship conflict, empathy, prosocial orientation, dissociation in maltreated children, and propensity for behavioral problems and emotional stress. It is reviewed in detail in Chapter 14.

Step 10: Developing a Case Formulation from a Family Perspective

A comprehensive psychoeducational assessment of a child suspected of having a disability produces a wealth of information, which must be organized into a coherent framework that explains the problem to the referral source and guides intervention (see Chapter 14 for a detailed discussion of case formulations for the diagnosis of a child). The family assessment component of this evaluation may have a central role in the case formulation (e.g., child neglect as the result of substance abuse and depression in a parent; anxiety and inattentiveness in a child whose family is homeless), or may be largely irrelevant for diagnosis but critical for effective intervention (e.g., stress in the family of a child with an ASD).

Each child's family is unique and needs to be addressed with that uniqueness in mind. Families differ greatly in what they identify as their needs and priorities, their social and financial resources, the other demands on their energy and time, the particular challenges faced by individual families (e.g., second-language background), and the specific challenges involved in parenting a child with a disability. Nonetheless, all families should be assessed for their needs in four areas and offered help as indicated:

- Information (e.g., about the particular disability or condition, special education regulations, community support groups).
- Stress reduction and/or support to help them cope with the pressures and/or disappointments of raising a child with a disability, including its impact on marital/couple and sibling relationships (e.g., need for respite care, appropriate schools, transportation, or other services).
- Social and financial resources to help them meet their other needs, particularly those they prioritize as most important.
- Parents' interest and ability to participate effectively in a home-based intervention, if such an intervention is relevant.

Families' need for or interest in stress reduction or mental health support can be addressed directly with parents. We always ask them about the effect of their child on couple and family functioning. It is not uncommon for parents to acknowledge the loss of time for intimacy in the couple relationship as a result of the demands of having a special-needs child. Conflict also arises because of different approaches to the problem. For example, a father, while recognizing that something is clearly wrong with his son, may resist an evaluation or any type of labeling for fear of "pigeonholing" his child in special education for life. An equally concerned mother may want whatever early intervention is available, even if it comes with a label, in order to ensure that everything possible is being done to promote her son's optimal development. Exploration of these issues in the interview can be very helpful for parents.

A common situation that we see clinically is a father's talking with real sadness about how intimacy, closeness, and time alone as a couple have completely disappeared since the birth of the child with a disability, and what a loss that has been. His wife, having immersed herself in seeking the best possible educational placement and running an extensive home program, may have pushed aside her own needs for closeness; her husband's comments may leave her first taken aback and then willing to acknowledge what a loss it has been for them as a couple to have made their disabled child the unchallenged priority in their life. Bringing these issues out into the open helps the parents think about how their family life is and how they would like it to be. This gives them an opportunity to reevaluate how they've been functioning and to create some alternatives that may be more satisfactory to them. We follow up on these issues with parents and may ask whether they would find a parent support group helpful. If the couple seems hostile or disengaged, or if one or both partners seem in distress, we explore these issues enough to see whether a referral is in order and what type of referral might be helpful. For example, depression might involve an assessment of its severity (including risk of suicide) and referral to a crisis center, mental health professional, or psychiatrist. Treatment might also involve couple or family therapy to improve the social environment at home and make family life more balanced and enjoyable for everyone.

The impact of having a disabled child in the family care be very strong for siblings as well. When a normally functioning sibling is older, the parents may be relieved that this sibling needs relatively little attention, allowing them to focus more on the needy younger child with a disability. They may be unaware of how this has affected the older child who may have felt abandoned by the parents after the birth of the disabled sibling. Therefore, it is important to get both parents' perceptions of how the older sibling is functioning, as well as to talk with the older sibling him- or herself. Perceptions of the younger child's disabling condition, beliefs about what it means to have the particular disability, feelings about family organization, and so forth can all be assessed and explored. When the nondisabled sibling is younger than the child with a disability, other issues can arise. Sometimes parents are shocked at how competent the younger sibling is, and they may become quite concerned that the younger child is going to "show up" and possibly embarrass the disabled older child. Consciously or unconsciously, they may try to hold this child back and limit his or her opportunities for development. In other situations, they may be delighted with the younger child's competence and actually push him or her toward earlier independence, because it lightens their parenting load. Some parents, in hopes that the younger child's competence (particularly in social areas) might rub off on the older child with a disability, may insist that the disabled child accompany the nondisabled sibling on all social outings with friends. Although this provides the disabled child with more opportunities for normal social contact, the nondisabled sibling may experience it as a burden. Each sibling's response to a brother or sister with a disability is unique. One cannot know how siblings feel without asking them. Some siblings report as adults that having a sister or brother with a disability was a wonderful experience, promoting a deep empathy for such individuals. We have educated many school psychologists and special educators who have gone into these fields because of their desire to help children with problems similar to those of their disabled siblings.

In addition to seeking a diagnosis, coping with complex emotions, finding an appropriate treatment program, and making a decision about whether to participate in a home-based treatment component, parents are also expected to be full members of the IEP team. This can be a very demanding role for parents, particularly if they have a child in a district with limited services for children with disabilities in general or for youngsters with their child's specific condition. Some parents, once they find an appropriate educational program, are offered the opportunity to be trained in techniques that will help their child master behaviors in the home and in the community. Some parents are very active in parent training and implementation of techniques at home, while others are not. An assessment, if the point is relevant, should explore parents' interest and ability to participate in parent training, as it may influence which programs will accept a child. Parent training has the advantage of offering a child round-the-clock treatment, but the drawback of increasing family stress to a point that functioning deteriorates (Schreibman et al., 1984). Training parents who will not continue to apply the intervention after the program ends wastes valuable professional and family time. Kozloff (1984) found that one-third of the families he trained had not changed following a yearlong program designed to improve their interactions with their disabled children. Kozloff offers advice on assessing parents' readiness to change (e.g., acceptance of the program's philosophy, a willingness to change in order to change a child's behavior), but such assessment is still subjective (Newsom & Hovanitz, 1997).

Based on family members' response to the procedures and measures described in this chapter, we develop a case conceptualization, share it with the family, work toward a shared understanding of the problem, and then draw on our collective knowledge of appropriate and accessible interventions to address the concerns that have motivated the referral and other issues that have arisen during the assessment.

Step 11: Making a Therapeutic Presentation of the Findings

Parenting a preschool child is demanding. Parenting a preschool child with learning or behavior problems is even more so. Parents are usually the first to realize that there is something unusual or wrong with their child, and yet it may take some time and considerable persistence on their part before they obtain a confirmed diagnosis that seems to make sense. Even when they have wanted to understand what is wrong with their child, it still may be very difficult to accept a diagnosis—especially if it implies lifelong developmental disabilities or if family factors are implicated in the origins of the problem. This situation can create a very complex set of emotions in parents, including tremendous sadness and disappointment that their child has such a significant problem; shame that they have contributed "bad genes" or are incompetent in parenting; despair over the future of their child or the family; frustration over the differing diagnostic opinions they may receive; frustration over the difficulty of finding appropriate services for their child; anger at professionals who may be insisting that their child has a diagnosable problem when they're not yet ready to accept that diagnosis; or professionals who say "Wait and see" when the parents believe there's clearly something wrong.

Many parents accept a diagnosis, but struggle with what it means. They ask, "Why did it happen?" or "What did I do wrong for my child to have this?" We often see both self-blame and blaming of others; the latter may take the form of displacing anger on a spouse/partner, therapists, teachers, other professionals, the theoretical approach of the child's program, and so on. Feeling ashamed and stigmatized is another common reaction.

Judging from the copies of previous evaluations that we have received for children who are evaluated by our clinic, and our past experiences on preschool committees for disabled children, many schools and clinics delay giving firm diagnoses until children enter elementary school and parents "figure it out for themselves," as one preschool speech pathologist put it. This is particularly the case if a child has mental retardation, even when schools and clinics have compelling evidence to support their opinion. We believe that much of this is driven by the very real unpleasantness of giving parents information that they often find difficult to accept.

Our philosophy in reporting diagnoses to parents is to be cautious and give a provisional diagnosis, with suggested retesting a year later, if we are uncertain. When we are confident of our diagnosis, then we state it clearly in the belief that our clients are entitled to our professional opinion, even if our findings are disappointing to them at the time. Just as an oncologist would not obscure a finding of cancer, we believe that we cannot hide a finding of a disability—especially one that may have an improved outcome with appropriate diagnosis and early intervention.

The strong emotional reaction of some parents has taught us to role-play feedback sessions we think will be difficult, so that we can be confident that our message is clear and respectful, and that it emphasizes strengths possessed by the child and the family. We sometimes present findings in dyads, so that one member of the team can focus on the presentation of findings and the other on monitoring the parents' understanding of the information and emotional state. We try hard to be nondefensive, focusing empathetically on parents' distress over their child's disability, while still making it clear that we are offering our well-considered professional opinion. We accept the fact that we have limited control over how parents will respond to our findings, and that many parents find denial and minimization of their child's problems helpful in coping with the day-to-day burden of rearing a child with a disability. We acknowledge that all children are unique and that some children referred for evaluation fit poorly into current diagnostic categories, increasing the potential for diagnostic error. Similarly, we acknowledge that we are not infallible as diagnosticians. To minimize diagnostic error, we consult frequently with colleagues; work as a multidisciplinary team; listen closely to parents (some of whom are very well read on the most current theories and research findings related to their child's problem, attend most research conferences, and network with other parents); and work hard at keeping up with the literature on emotional, behavioral, and learning problems in young children and their families.

Step 12: Co-Constructing Recommendations and Interventions

If a child has been previously assessed, or if the family is able to accept the assessment findings easily, we may be able to move quickly in the feedback session to a discussion of recommendations and possible interventions for the family and the child. We focus first on the child in terms of school and then home recommendations, offering suggestions to address problems that the family and possibly the center/school have identified. We discuss options with the recognition that in our setting (a university clinic), we are consulting with them. It is their prerogative to take what they find useful from the assessment process and to leave the rest. After we have focused on the problems that they have identified, we often have suggestions for problems we may have identified.

In order to make our evaluations more helpful for parents, we schedule a follow-up telephone call or a face-to-face meeting a week after they have had time to review the report carefully. We ask them whether they have any questions or concerns, whether we made any factual errors, and whether our conceptualization of the case makes sense. We have learned from this how sensitive many parents are about language used to describe their child and family functioning. Parents are highly attuned to words that seem pathologizing to them (e.g., "peculiar," a word used on an autism subtest); are quick to pick up professional disapproval of perceived parental denial of a child's disability (one mother was very hurt when a report described as "unrealistic" her hope that her son, who had mild mental retardation and autism, would attend college—she continued to have this hope, despite her awareness of its improbability); and find behavioral descriptions of sometimes very difficult living situations painful. They are also grateful for strengths that we identify in the family and child, and statements that reinforce what they see that their child is able to do. They let us know which recommendations are helpful and which are not. We use their feedback to maximize the therapeutic value of our future reports.

CASE STUDY

Louis, a 5-year-old boy, diagnosed at age 2-6 years as having a pervasive developmental disorder (PDD) and at age 3-6 years with mild mental retardation, was referred by his parents to obtain another perspective of their son's functioning and to get help with behavior problems at home. Louis was the only child of Ms. S., age 36, a registered nurse, and Mr. Z., age 44, an engineer. They were an unmarried couple, no longer involved romantically, living together in a small two-bedroom city house owned by Mr. Z.

Ms. S. contacted the university clinic for an evaluation. The brief telephone intake—designed to get an overview of the problem, obtain consent to visit Louis's early childhood program, and arrange to send out behavior rating scales—turned into three long conversations over the course of a week about the mother's intense psychological distress over her son's difficulties and her tenuous relationship with Mr. Z. It was very difficult to establish boundaries with her. She shared suicidal–homicidal fantasies that created great concern and elicited a suicide and harm risk assessment. Even though she did not seem to be actively suicidal or have any intention to harm her child, permission to talk with her therapist was requested and granted.

Mr. Z., on the other hand, was very difficult to engage. He saw the referral as driven by Ms. S.'s need to manage Louis's tantrums at home—a problem he did not experience. Only when staff members insisted that his participation was essential did he agree to participate by conference call. However, on the day of the assessment he appeared in person. He sat at a distance, kept his emotions tightly in check, and gave precise answers to questions. Ms. S. sat close to the assessor, articulately shared painful emotions and experiences, wept frequently, and gave long and highly detailed answers to questions.

The parents presented with three primary concerns. First, Louis did not have behavioral problems in his special education program at school, but at home he often had tantrums and sometimes screamed for up to 3 hours. According to his mother, the tantrums were brought on when he was not given what he wanted or when restrictions were placed on him. At other times, however, there did not appear to be a clear antecedent to the behavior. Louis's tantrums occurred more frequently when he was with Ms. S. Both parents agreed on using disciplinary techniques, but they responded differently to Louis's behavior. Mr. Z. usually ignored the behavior or placed Louis in time out. Ms. S., who spent more time with Louis, did not have a systematic way of responding; sometimes she ignored his behavior until she could take it no longer, sometimes she screamed back at him, and sometimes she bribed him with food. It was very hard to get a clear picture during the interview of the exact context in which the tantrums occurred. Second, the parents were concerned about Louis's weight. He was obese, and the school was complaining that his weight was interfering with physical activities. Third, they wanted to know whether Louis was in the best possible placement. He was currently attending an early intervention center for students with PDD. The teaching approaches used in the classroom consisted of discrete-trial teaching (applied behavior analysis), with group activities focused on socialization, communication, and daily living skills. Louis also received occupational therapy, physical therapy, and speech and language therapy twice a week for 30 minutes. The parents liked the program, but wondered whether he would do even better if he had regular contact with typically developing children.

Ms. S. reported a full-term pregnancy with a birth weight of 10 pounds. Louis's developmental milestones were delayed in all areas, however. He never crawled, yet took his first steps alone at 15 months. He spoke his first word at 1 years, his first phrase at 3 years, and his first sentence at 4 years. His vision and hearing were normal, but his speech was difficult to understand. Prior psychological evaluations had concluded that Louis had a PDD (age 2-6 years) and that he had mental retardation (age 3-6 years; IQ = 57). Testing was negative for Prader–Willi, fragile X, ataxia, and dysmetria. He had had two seizures, one at age 20 months and the other at age 4 years. Subsequent EEGs were normal. His parents reported normal social interaction and age-appropriate behavior prior to the first seizure.

Previous occupational and physical evaluations had assessed Louis's gross motor development to be at the level of a 2-7-year-old. His fine motor skills and visual perception were determined to be at a 3-9 to 4-3-year-old level. Louis's overall gross motor abilities were hindered by his weight. He had difficulty in standing up from a sitting position on the floor, as well as seating himself on the floor. Louis could run on the playground and could kick, catch, and throw a ball, but was unable to jump or balance himself on one leg. In the area of fine motor skills, he was able to string small beads and manipulate small toys. Due to weakness in his hands and fingers, however, he was sometimes unable to push large or small Legos together and was often unable to lift large wooden blocks without losing his grip. Louis could hold crayons and pencils in a weak tripod grasp, but was unable to apply much pressure when doing so.

The family genogram is shown in Figure 8.3. Mr. Z. came from an educated upper-middle-class Colombian family. He was the only family member to immigrate, having done so for graduate school. He reported a distant relationship with his family of origin, whose members he described as emotionally cold. There was a history of depression and alcoholism on his mother's side of the family and he reported lifelong problems with depression as well (see below). Because he had never married Ms. S., he reported that his family refused to acknowledge her or Louis. He thought this was related to the fact that his father had a daughter with a long-time mistress who was never formally acknowledged by the family. Similarly, Ms. S.'s middle-class Southern Baptist family in the American South disapproved of her living with a man who was unwilling to make her his wife. They were also uncomfortable with his Hispanic and Roman Catholic background. The birth of a grandson with developmental disabilities, Ms. S. believed, only strengthened her family's view of her as the "unsuccessful child."

An eco-map of the family is shown in Figure 8.5. The most notable feature was the degree of isolation experienced by the family. Except for each parent's psychotherapist and the early childhood program staff, there were no other social supports. Each parent's relationship with Louis was the most positive and least ambivalent relationship each had with anyone. This was confirmed by the social support measures. The family needs measures showed Ms. S. as wanting time for herself. She also reported being intensely lonely. She and Mr. Z. had an ambivalent relationship that left her feeling insecure. She had made repeated efforts to develop friendships with coworkers, and with other parents of children like Louis in a support group, but had always been rebuffed. Her hypothesis was that she presented herself as too intense and needy. She also said that she would like more money to pay bills, as well as help with managing her son at home. Mr. Z wanted help in planning for his son's future and time to keep in shape.

Both parents reported mental health problems. Mr. Z. had had chronic dysthymia and repeated episodes of major depressive disorder since his teenage years, for which he took antidepressants and sleeping pills. Ms. S. reported high levels of parent-related and child-related stress on the PSI-3 (depression, low sense of competence, social isolation, relationship with spouse, demandingness, adaptability, mood, dysthymia, and chronic low self-esteem). In regard to their partnership, they reported cooperating on parenting tasks, but Ms. S. felt very insecure in the relationship and Mr. Z. very ambivalent. Mr. Z. owned the house, but he was distant and gave her no reason to believe that he wanted her to stay. Neither parent had made efforts to meet other people romantically.

At home Louis followed a routine in some respects, such as waking at the same time every day, being dressed by his mother, and waiting with his father for the school bus. When he returned home from school, Louis had a snack and played on his own while his father did his work. He had no set bedtime and usually went to sleep late. There was also no routine for mealtimes, and Louis ate at various times throughout the day.

When observed at home, Louis was dressed comfortably in a long-sleeved T-shirt, pants, and sneakers. He had dark curly hair and big brown eyes with long lashes; he was of average height for his age, but was very overweight. Louis appeared to spend much of his time at home eating, but he also seemed to be reasonably self-sufficient and independent in feeding himself, as he was observed retrieving his own food and drink from the kitchen and attempting to use a knife to cut a pastry. When his attempt failed, he looked at his mother for help and said, "Mommy, please." Ms. S. stated that Louis had a limited vocabulary and spoke in short phrases. The small house in which the family resided was tightly packed with furniture, books, stacks of magazines, and art, with little room for Louis to move about actively. The small yard was landscaped as an urban garden, which also limited movement. Although Louis showed some interest in the observers by looking curiously at them and playing near them, he interacted little with them. He enjoyed rolling on a large ball, as well as appropriately playing with a train set and a puzzle with his mother. However, these activities did not hold his attention for a long period of time. He displayed much affection toward his parents, such as giving them hugs and kisses. The family obtained high scores on the HOME, because the parents provided a warm and intellectually stimulating environment with age-appropriate toys, verbal interaction, promotion of maturity, and many opportunities to get out and explore the community.

Louis was also observed during group time, recess, lunch, and art (painting) in his early learning center class one morning. He was in a class consisting of 11 students with PDD, as well as one teacher and two aides. During group time, Louis pointed to his nose, ears, and eyes when asked to do so by Mr. X., his teacher. He cooperatively followed directions and was polite, as indicated by saying "please." He sat passively during a song that involved hand clapping and foot stomping. Although he did not sing, Louis was attentive throughout the activity. Louis had to be helped by an aide when the children were instructed to stand up and shout "hooray." When instructed, through the modeling of the teacher, to put his head on his hands, Louis correctly copied the behavior.

During recess, Louis spent the majority of the time by himself. At this time, Mr. X. suggested to Louis that he go down the slide. Louis ran toward the slide, bypassed it, and kept on running. When he was told that recess was over, he cooperated and went inside. During lunch, Louis sat quietly and waited patiently for his hamburger, French fries, and milk. He politely accepted the meal when it arrived, and he diligently and neatly put ketchup on his plate. During his meal, Louis was generally quiet and focused upon eating his lunch, chewing with his mouth closed. Mr. X. mentioned that if Louis was not closely monitored, he would eat from the plates of his classmates. Louis was observed using some two-word phrases during lunch; for instance, without a prompt, he said, "More milk." Holding the carton in both hands, Louis poured the milk into his cup without spilling anything. When the milk carton was empty, he proceeded to lick it. Although Louis still had fries on his plate, he took some from the child sitting next to him. Louis finished his lunch and put his garbage in the trash without being told to do so. Louis then returned to the table and waited quietly and patiently for the art activity to begin. The children were given paint, paper, and paintbrushes to work with during this activity. Louis worked intently on the task, but he used only one paint color on each page. He then got ready to go home and left the classroom with the aides and the other children.

His teacher reported that Louis exhibited significant delays in all areas of development—including cognitive skills, expressive and receptive speech and language, motor skills, and socioemotional skills—but he continued to make slow and steady progress in his current classroom setting. Louis was cooperative, worked well in a group setting, and was able to follow routines. Louis also had some preacademic skills, including the ability to identify colors, shapes, and numbers. Mr. X. reported frequent contact with Ms. S. via phone calls and a daily online journal.

Consistent with past testing, Louis earned an IQ of 61 with an adaptive behavior composite of 50. Age scores ranged from a 1-3 on socialization to a high of 2-7 on motor skills. Trial teaching on portions of the Hawaii Early Learning Profile, Assessment Strands: Ages 3–6 Years indicated delays in both cognition and language, with a pronounced delay in expressive language. He required redirection numerous times in order to attend to the tasks and was reinforced with cookies and verbal praise. Results of the assessment indicated relative strengths in interacting and cooperating with adults, adapting to change, nonverbal communication, receptive language, and emotional response. He showed particular weaknesses in expressive language, cognitive functioning, attention, and gross motor skills. During the administration of the Hawaii Early Learning Profile, Louis repeated the last word of the directions given to him and imitated several of the examiner's behaviors and sounds. He was easy to redirect with a verbal prompt. He responded to both social and edible reinforcement from the examiners; the social reinforcement included high-fives, handshakes, and verbal praise.

Although a prior assessment had indicated a diagnosis of PDD, the present evaluation found him just missing meeting criteria for autism or other ASD/PDD. Louis did demonstrate some autistic features, such as failure to develop peer relationships appropriate to his developmental level, delay in the development of spoken language, and stereotyped and repetitive motor mannerisms. However, Louis displayed multiple nonverbal behaviors, engaged in social and emotional reciprocity, was flexible with changes in routines, and exhibited other behaviors that are not characteristic of autism. It seemed likely that he was responding well to the early intensive intervention he was receiving, and it is not uncommon for children with mild cases of ASD to move in and out of the diagnosis over time.

The S./Z. family had many strengths. Both parents were well educated, had adequate financial resources, and were devoted to Louis. They were completing all of the tasks of raising preschool children adequately (see Table 8.1), with the exceptions of providing a structured environment with eating and sleeping routines, contingent reinforcement of rules (by the mother), and supporting the development of peer relationships by modeling and providing opportunities to interact with peers outside structured school settings. The parents were severely lacking in social support, and they struggled with a sense of shame over their relationship with each other and Louis's disability, stemming in part from their families' rejection of their unmarried status.

In response to the first referral question (Louis's tantrums at home), we told the parents that we were confident that a behavioral family therapist working with them in the home could quickly help them identify exactly what was triggering the tantrums and find alternative responses for both Louis and his mother. Louis's early childhood center reported that they had repeatedly offered such help and Ms. S. had not accepted it, and we wondered why. Ms. S. replied that she was very conflicted about putting constraints on Louis at home. She wanted home to be a retreat where Louis could relax and be a "normal kid," not a "special-needs child" who required a behavior plan with reinforcers and time out. Setting and maintaining regularly scheduled, calorie-controlled meals as a way of addressing the second referral question met with the same objections. Louis liked to eat; it was his main pleasure in life. Restricting his food meant taking away the one thing that mattered most to him.

Acknowledging the worthiness of her goal of wanting home to be a place of comfort and enjoyment for Louis and for his parents, we explored other ways of framing the situation. Perhaps seeing Louis's tantrums as his way of communicating his dissatisfaction with things—a means of communication that was painful and frustrating to all—might enable her to work with the therapist to find more satisfying ways for them to communicate and negotiate with one another. We also explored other metaphors for dieting. Instead of framing it as restricting pleasure, couldn't the family view healthful eating as an expression of love and nurturance? Working with a nutritionist to plan meals for the family could result in delicious, nutritious, and calorie-controlled meals. Ms. S. and Mr. Z. were open to our suggestions but said that they needed time to think about them. Because Mr. Z. had mentioned that he would like more time to keep in shape, we wondered whether he might turn his daily outing to the bus stop with Louis into a longer walk that would provide exercise for both of them, or whether he might find some other physical exercise for them both, separately or together. We encouraged Ms. S. to exercise as well, given its effectiveness in improving moods.

The most difficult part of the session was talking about the parents' loneliness and insecurity in their couple relationship, and the isolation of the family as a whole. We felt that the cutoffs both parents felt from their families of origin because of their unmarried status might be playing a role in keeping them stuck in their relationship—feeling too needy to move closer together or to move on romantically. In addition, there were issues of intense, unresolved shame about their child and their mental health problems. Ms. S. also felt like a social reject as an adult, despite having had friends as a child and adolescent. We recommended that they continue their individual therapies, but also consider working with a family therapist so that they could find a way to have more satisfying, secure lives—perhaps reconnecting with their families and sharing with them the wonderful Louis, who, while intellectually limited, was also loving and fun to be with. We suggested that having family support, should that transpire, might help Ms. S. feel less needy and thus make her more attractive as a friend. To Mr. Z., we noted that family members change over time, and that it might be worth an overture to see whether this was true of his family.

In regard to the third referral question (the quality of Louis's educational placement), Louis was enrolled in an excellent preschool program that was well tailored to his educational needs. He liked going to school and was making steady but slow progress. Unfortunately, the lack of typically developing peers in his program meant that he had no models or experience with normal peer relationships. Being an only child in a socially isolated family further limited his social development. We explored with the parents the pros and cons of alternative placements with typical peers. Because of her own social problems, Ms. S. was reluctant to leave a program that had been so supportive of her personally. She felt overwhelmed at the thought of negotiating with the school district to get a satisfactory placement for her son and work out a comfortable relationship with his teacher. Mr. Z. volunteered to help her explore options.

We called the family a week later to solicit feedback on the report and the assessment process, answer questions, and see how we could help. Ms. S. had called her parents and sisters and was planning a visit to the South with Louis. Mr. Z. had set up two visits to inclusion programs for typically developing children and children with PDD. Mr. Z. had also expanded his walk to the bus with Louis. The couple was not yet ready to see a family therapist, invite a behavioral consultant into the home, or modify Louis's diet. They wanted a report for the school that kept family information to a minimum. We offered to attend an IEP meeting in the future if they thought it would help them get the services they wanted for Louis, and we wished them well.

SUMMARY

This chapter describes family assessment and consultation as one component of a comprehensive psychoeducational evaluation of a preschool child suspected of having a disability. Procedures and measures are described for identifying family factors that enhance a child's competence; factors that might contribute to the child's emotional or educational problems; and needs that, if met, might enhance the family's ability to function more effectively. Healthy families produce healthy children. Professionals should make every effort to understand and offer nonjudgmental support and concrete assistance to parents as they carry out their challenging mission of raising a child with a disability.

APPENDIX 8.1. Review of Measures

Measure	**Family Environment Scale—Third Edition (FES-3). Moos and Moos (1994).**
Purpose	Measuring individuals' perceptions of the social and environmental characteristics of their families.
Areas	Family Relationships, Personal Growth, and System Maintenance.
Format	Questionnaire. Four forms: the Real form (R), the Ideal form (I), and the Expectations form (E) for adults, as well as a children's version (ages 5–12).
Scores	Standard scores.
Age group	Parents and adolescents.
Time	15–20 minutes.
Users	Professionals.
Norms	Form R, based on 1,125 normal and 500 distressed families from a variety of sources; Form I, based on 281 families.
Reliability	Internal consistency, .61–.78; test–retest (2, 3, and 12 months), .52–.91.
Validity	Construct, discriminant, and content, all supported.
Comments	Easy to administer and score. Assessors should use caution when interpreting for nontraditional families or families from nonmajority cultures. More useful for research than for clinical practice.
References consulted	Mancini (2001); Sporakowski (2001). See book's References list.

Measure	**Family Needs Scale. Dunst, Cooper, Weeldreyer, Snyder, and Chase (1985).**
Purpose	Assessing the family's needs for a variety of resources and supports, which can then be prioritized and addressed jointly by family and professionals.
Areas	Basic Resources; Specialized Child Care; Personal/Family Growth; Financial and Medical Resources; Child Education/Therapy; Meal Preparation and Adapted Equipment; Future Child Care; Financial Budgeting; Household Support.
Format	41 items, 5-point rating scale.
Scores	Total and subscale raw scores.
Age group	Parents of young children with disabilities.
Time	5 minutes.
Users	Professionals.
Norms	Data collected on 54 parents of preschoolers with mental retardation, other disabilities, or developmental risk.
Reliability	Internal consistency, .95; split-half, .96.
Validity	Construct, supported for the nine components; criterion-related, .28–.42 (subareas, .35–.57).
Comments	The measure has adequate reliability and validity for its intended purpose, intervention.
References consulted	Dunst, Trivette, and Deal (1988). See book's References list.

Measure	Family Needs Survey. Bailey and Simeonsson (1990).
Purpose	Assessing parental perception of the needs of families of children with disabilities.
Areas	Need for Information, Support, Understanding from Others, Community Services, Financial Resources, and Family Functioning.
Format	35 items, rated on 3-point scale.
Scores	Raw scores.
Age group	Parents of young children with disabilities.
Time	5 minutes.
Users	Professionals.
Norms	Local norms should be collected.
Reliability	Internal consistency, .91; test–retest (6 months), .67.
Validity	Criterion-related, .47–.52 (range for subareas, .28–.68).
Comments	Authors recommend that mothers and fathers complete the scale separately because of a tendency to report different profiles of need. Useful for designing and assessing intervention.
References consulted	Sexton, Burrell, and Thompson (1992). See book's References list.

Measure	Family Resource Scale. Dunst and Leet (1987a).
Purpose	Measuring parent perceptions of the adequacy of various resources in families with young children.
Areas	FRS: Growth and Financial Support; Health and Necessities; Nutrition and Communication; Physical Shelter; Intrafamily Support; Communication and Employment; Child Care; Independent Source of Income. FRS-R: Time for Self; Time for Family; Money; Basic Needs.
Format	FRS: 31 items, 5-point rating scale. FRS-R: 20 items. Can be administered as an interview or rating scale.
Scores	Total and subscale raw scores.
Age group	Parents of young children.
Time	5 minutes.
Users	Professionals.
Norms	FRS: Data collected on 45 mothers of preschoolers with mental retardation, other disabilities, or developmental risks. FRS-R: Data collected on 2,441 kindergarten and 1961 third-grade former Head Start families from 31 sites in all regions of the United States for the exploratory factor analyses, and 1 year later, an additional 2,688 kindergarten and 2,101 third-grade families for the confirmatory factor analyses. Families were 47% white, family income was below the federal poverty line, and median educational level of parents was a high-school diploma.
Reliability	FRS: Internal consistency, .92; test–retest (2 months), .52; split-half, .95. FRS-R: Internal consistency, .72–.84 for the four subscales.

Validity	The FRS taps strengths that are missed when objective but superficial external evaluations of resources are made (e.g., Brody & Flor, 1997). Parents' perceptions of family resources on the FRS affect parenting and parents' school involvement, which in turn affects children's emotional self-control, and thus, their academic and social behavior (Brody & Flor, 1997; Brody, Flor, & Gibson, 1998). Total scores are related to maternal well-being and commitment to prescribed early intervention programs (Dunst & Leet, 1987a). On the FRS-R, subscale Time for Self uniquely predicts variance on the SSRS; subscale Basic Needs, kindergarten PPVT-R scores; and subscales Money, Time for Self, and Basic Needs are significantly and positively correlated with distance from the federal poverty level.
Comments	Overall, the FRS/FRS-R is a brief, clinically useful tool with good psychometric characteristics. Research shows that family resources are more than income level and parents' perceptions of family resources are more predictive of quality of parenting and child outcomes than external measures. Assessors working with families with young children with disabilities may want to use the FRS while those working with broader populations will prefer the FRS-R. Test–retest correlations are moderate at best.
References consulted	Dunst, Trivette, and Deal (1988); Van Horn, Bellis, and Snyder (2001). See book's References list.

Measure	**Family Support Scale. Dunst, Trivette, and Jenkins (1984).**
Purpose	Measuring the helpfulness of sources of support to those raising young children.
Areas	Informal Kinship; Social Organization; Formal Kinship; Immediate Family; Specialized Professional Services; Generic Professionalized Services. Taylor, Crowley, and White (1993) identified 4 factors, labeling their scales Familial, Spousal, Social, and Professional Support. Hanley, Tassé, Aman, and Pace (1998) obtained a 5-factor solution with subscales labeled Community, Spouse and In-laws, Friends, Specialized/Professional, and Own Parents and Extended Family.
Format	18 items, listing sources of support (e.g., other parents) rated on a 5-point scale as to how helpful the source is to the respondent. Two blank items allow the respondent to list additional sources of support.
Scores	Total and subscale raw scores.
Age group	Parents of young children.
Time	5 minutes.
Users	Professionals.
Norms	Data collected on 139 parents of preschoolers with mental retardation, other disabilities, or developmental risks. Taylor et al. (1993) collected data on 900 families recruited nationwide from several early intervention studies that were mostly white, married, and of middle-class income. The sample of Hanley et al. (2001) was 204 low-income, mostly minority and single-parent families with children in Head Start.
Reliability	Internal consistency, .77; test–retest (1 month), .91; test–retest (18 months), .47; split-half, .75. Taylor et al. (1993) reported a Cronbach's alpha of .80, total scale and .35–.76 for subscales. Hanley et al. (1998) reported Cronbach's alpha of .85, total scale; split-half, .72; and subscale alphas of .60–.78. Test–retest over an unspecified time was .73 for the total scale and .60–.78 for subscales.

Validity	Criterion-related, supported. The total scale is related significantly to personal well-being of parents, integrity of the family unit, and parent perceptions of child behavior (Dunst et al., 1988). Construct validity somewhat supported by exploratory factor analysis on three samples showing conceptual similarity in factors obtained although number of factors and assignment of items to scale varied.
Comments	It is reliable and has criterion and construct validity in families with young children at risk for or diagnosed with disabilities. It is easy to use, appears nonintrusive to families, and is an essential measure if one component of intervention will be fostering the growth of informal and formal social support.
References consulted	Dunst, Trivette, and Deal (1988); Hanley et al. (1998); Taylor, Crowley, and White (1993). See book's References list.

Measure	**Home Observation for Measurement of the Environment (HOME). Caldwell and Bradley (2003).**
Purpose	Describing the quality and quantity of stimulation and support available to the child in the home environment and identifying high-risk home environments.
Areas	Early Childhood HOME: Learning Stimulation; Language Stimulation; Physical Environment; Warmth and Acceptance; Academic Stimulation; Modeling; Variety in Experience; Acceptance.
Format	Semistructured observation and parent/caregiver interview in the home. Four levels (for infants, preschoolers, middle childhood, and early adolescent).
Scores	Means, SDs for subscales and total score. Items scored yes or no.
Age group	Infant–Toddler HOME, 0–3 years; Early Childhood HOME, 3–6 years; Middle Childhood HOME, 6–10 years; Early Adolescent HOME, 10–15 years.
Time	1 hour.
Users	Professionals.
Norms	Original data collected in the mid-1960s 174 families from Little Rock, Arkansas, both receiving and not receiving welfare; overrepresentation of black and single-parent families; not representative of national population. Since then the HOME has been used in an enormous number of published studies within the United States and around the world, among all SES groups and with families with children with different disabilities, illnesses, and adverse experiences.
Reliability	Internal consistency for the Early Childhood HOME: The authors no longer calculate this because the HOME is presumed to be a causal variable with no assumed covariance structure, and not a dependent variable for which Cronbach's alphas are appropriate. They argue that coefficients of internal consistency do not provide good estimate of reliability for causal measures. Past reports show total scores to be .93 using split-half reliability (KR-20) and subscales from .53–.83. Test–retest for subscales and total score was .05 to .70 over a period of 18 months. More recent studies with the IT-HOME have shown much higher test–retest reliability and stability. Interobserver agreement with training is at least 90%.

Validity	Construct, strong, predictive, strong. It is best as a broad measure of the home environment and at discriminating poor from adequate environments. The HOME has been validated as a measure of home environment factors that promote cognitive development as early as 6 months but with higher correlations after 2 years of age. The Learning Stimulation subtest on the HOME short form was associated with early motor, language, and social development and academic achievement in poor and nonpoor white, black, and Hispanic children ages 0–13 years. The HOME can discriminate between poor mothers and poor mothers with mental retardation, the quality of rearing environment provided by mothers with different psychiatric diagnoses, and later attachment style of a child, to name just a few of the studies that support its validity.
Comments	Useful as a screening instrument. Thorough manual. Extensive validity studies with diverse and international samples suggest that the HOME correlates well with early measures of cognitive development and moderately with SES (as intended by the authors). HOME scores as early as 6 months of age have been shown to predict Stanford–Binet IQ scores at ages 3, 4, and 4-6 years. Offers information useful for designing interventions to help parents provide a more intellectually stimulating environment and/or a more positive and less punitive approach to discipline and guidance.
References consulted	Bradley (1994); Bradley, Corwyn, Burchinal, McAdoo, and García-Coll (2001a, 2001b); Linver, Brooks-Gunn, and Cabrera (2004); Totsika and Sylva (2004). See book's References list.

Measure	**Inventory of Social Support. Trivette and Dunst (1988).**
Purpose	Provides a map of a parent's social network and assesses the extent to which identified needs are being met by the members of the social network. Particularly suitable for low-income families with developmental disabilities or problems. Used in conjunction with the Support Functions Scale.
Areas	There are 12 different types of help and assistance identified and 19 potential sources of support ranging from intrafamily to informal to formal support sources. Respondents first indicate frequency of contact with each source and then whom he or she goes to for support or to receive help for different types of needs.
Format	Either self-report or interview-format questionnaire.
Scores	A completed questionnaire provides a graphic display of the individual's personal social network in terms of both source and type of support.
Age group	Parents of young children with developmental problems or disabilities.
Time	5–10 minutes.
Users	Professionals.
Norms	Data collected on 120 parents of preschool children with developmental disabilities or at risk for them.
Reliability	Not reported.
Validity	There were significant differences in the number of types of help provided by different sources of support, with spouse/partner the most frequent, followed by respondent's parents, then friends, then the respondent's brothers and sisters, and then the early intervention program the child was enrolled in. An exploratory principal components factor analysis produced a 5-factor solution that accounted for 58% of the variance and demonstrated that different types

	of help are provided by different sources of social support. These factors were Formal Kinship I (spouse or respondents' parents, spouse or partner, and spouse or partner's siblings); Formal Kinship II (respondent's parents, siblings, and other relatives); Individual Source of Support (included early childhood program, private therapist, friends); Medical (child or family's physician); and Respondent's Children. All of these factors were related to personal well-being except for Formal Kinship II. Formal Kinship I and Medical were related to family well-being.
Comments	Used as an informal clinical tool to provide insight into respondent's sources of support and types of support as part of an intervention to empower parents to meet family needs through their own networks.
References consulted	Brassard review. See book's References list.

Measure	**Parenting Stress Index—Third Edition (PSI-3). Abidin, PAR staff, and Noriel (1995).**
Purpose	Identifying potentially dysfunctional parent–child relationships that may place a child at risk for emotional disturbance.
Areas	Long form: Child domain (Adaptability, Acceptability, Demandingness, Mood, Hyperactivity and Distractibility, Reinforces Parent); Parent domain (Depression, Attachment, Restrictions of Role, Sense of Competence, Social Isolation, Relationship with Spouse, Parental Health); Life Stress. Short form: Parental Distress; Parent–Child Dysfunctional Interaction; Difficult Child.
Format	Long form: 120-item, 5-point scale self-report questionnaire. Short form: 36 items derived from long form.
Scores	Percentile ranks.
Age group	Parents of children ages 1 month–12 years.
Time	Long form: 20–30 minutes. Short form: 10 minutes.
Users	Professionals.
Norms	Data collected on 2,633 mothers (ages 16–61) of children ages 1 month–12 years, 200 fathers (ages 18–65) of children ages 6–12 years; 223 Hispanic parents used as norming sample for Spanish version; sample not random or stratified.
Reliability	Long form: Internal consistency, .95; test–retest (1 year), .65; test–retest (1–3 months), .96. Short form: Alpha reliabilities, .87 for Parental Distress; .80 for Parent–Child Dysfunctional Interaction; and .85 for Difficult Child.
Validity	Research indicates strong validity, especially cross-culturally. May have questionable factor structure. PSI-3 long form and short form correlate .94 for Total Stress.
Comments	Has a short form, long form, Spanish-version, and Swedish version. Useful for screening purposes. Easy to score. Nonrepresentative norming sample. Good psychometric characteristics.
References consulted	Allison (1998); Barnes (1998); Oehler-Stinnett (1998); Grotevant and Carlson (1989). See book's References list.

Measure	**Questionnaire on Resources and Stress (QRS). Holroyd (1987).**
Purpose	Measuring stress in families caring for ill or disabled relatives.
Areas	Short form: Parent and Family Problems, Pessimism, Child Characteristics, and Physical Incapacitation. Long form: Personal Problems, Family Problems, and Problems of Index Care.
Format	Two forms. Short form, 66-item self-administered true–false checklist; long form, 285-item self-administered true–false checklist. Short form and long form correlate .99.
Scores	*T*-scores for total and subscale scores.
Age group	Parents with at least sixth-grade education.
Time	1 hour for long form; 20 minutes for short form.
Users	Professionals.
Norms	Long form: 107 cases from California, Georgia, and New Zealand; sampling not random. More recently, norms have been developed for families with a member who has 1 of 4 disability categories: psychiatric; developmental disabilities; chronic medical illness (renal disease, leukemia, cystic fibrosis); and neuromuscular diseases (cerebral palsy, Duchene's dystrophy), based on 329 cases. Of these, 98 had psychiatric problems, 145 had developmental disabilities, 49 had medical illnesses, and 37 had neuromuscular disease. Short form, Friedrich, Greenberg, and Crnic (1983): 289 parents of children with a wide variety of developmental disabilities, diseases, and psychiatric problems.
Reliability	Internal consistency, .96 (long form), .79–.85 (short form); test–retest, not available.
Validity	Content, established; criterion-related, weak; construct, not established.
Comments	Short form is designed for screening purposes. Useful for initiating conversations with families about stress. Small norming sample and absence of test–retest and alternate-form reliability information limit the general usefulness of this instrument.
References consulted	Erickson (1992). See book's References list. www.assessmentpsychology.com

Chapter 9

Assessment of Linguistically and Culturally Diverse Preschoolers

INCREASING CULTURALLY SENSITIVE PRACTICES

Assessing children from linguistically and culturally diverse backgrounds in a valid and fair manner presents a complex challenge for all assessors. Schools and agencies need to make decisions about children who need special services, as well as to engage in appropriate curriculum planning (including placement in mainstream or bilingual programs). Public Law 99-457 requires that all preschoolers be assessed for potential disabilities in learning. The original IDEA and IDEA 2004 furthermore mandate that children be assessed in the language(s) that they understand and use, if this is at all feasible, and that tests and other procedures be selected and administered in a nondiscriminatory fashion. IDEA 2004 takes note of the fact that the population with *limited English proficiency* (LEP) is the fastest-growing in the nation, and that children with LEP are disproportionately referred to and placed in special education. It requires states to have policies and procedures in place to prevent this overidentification.

Differentiating children with LEP, who are now more commonly referred to as *English-language learners* (ELLs), from those with language disorders and learning delays is not a new challenge. However, steadily increasing immigration in North America and the availability of reliable and valid tests only in English (and, in some cases, Spanish) has created an ongoing educational crisis. For example, one New York City district has more than 140 dialects and languages represented within the school population. Meeting the needs of children who are ELLs was a challenge only in urban areas at first, but it is increasingly a suburban and rural challenge as well. Furthermore, some children who speak English come from other cultures, such as the Caribbean (e.g., Antigua, Trinidad), where dialects other than standard American English are used. Assessment tools do not exist for most of this group. Fortunately, more often a single language or dialect (e.g.,

Russian, Cantonese) predominates among the local population of children who are ELLs, allowing assessors to focus their efforts on developing competence in the assessment of one or two groups.

Assessment practices are closely connected to community values, school practices and priorities, and teacher/assessor/interviewer attitudes. As IDEA 2004 notes, in some cases this has resulted in disproportionate numbers of minority children and children who are ELLs being "misdiagnosed as having language disorders—or remain[ing] undiagnosed" (Schiff-Myers, Djukic, McGovern-Lawler, & Perez, 1993, p. 237). As a result, such children are often either placed in special education, or deemed not ready for kindergarten or first-grade entrance and placed in transition or bilingual classes, often with watered-down or skill-oriented curricula. These interconnected factors are summarized in Figure 9.1.

The purpose of this chapter is to provide a guide to screening and assessing linguistically and culturally diverse preschoolers in a manner that, although it cannot eliminate bias, attempts to reduce it. Our intent is simply to raise issues and suggest solutions to commonly encountered problems; because of the complexities involved, no attempt is made to present a best-practices approach that can or should be universally adopted. The first section of the chapter focuses on assessors' exploring their own attitudes toward diversity and ways in which these attitudes might affect the assessment process. The second section focuses on general characteristics of various cultures and their implications for assessment and intervention with young children and their families. The third section addresses misconceptions about bilingualism and presents a variety of strategies for reducing cultural bias throughout the assessment process. Particular emphasis is placed in this section on efforts to gather local language/cultural/demographic information; recruit and train staff members for diversity; create a culturally friendly screening environment;

Community

- Political climate
- Prevailing belief systems and attitudes toward diversity
- Financial resources
- Extent of diversity represented
- Local issues

School

- Teachers' belief systems and prior experiences with diversity
- Level of in-service training related to diversity
- Availability of alternative programs
- Flexibility for movement within and across programs
- Nature of curriculum of the bilingual program vs. the mainstream program

Assessor

- Belief systems
- Awareness of and sensitivity to diversity-related issues
- Familiarity and comfort with cultural and linguistic diversity
- Training
- Familiarity with limitations of traditional assessment approaches
- Familiarity with alternative assessment approaches and new instruments
- Willingness to confront dilemmas and advocate for children

Families and children

- Length of time in this country; history
- Languages spoken
- Child-rearing beliefs and practices
- Beliefs regarding learning/disability/help seeking
- Attitudes regarding assessment and intervention
- Degree of assimilation to European American attitudes

FIGURE 9.1. Influences on assessment practices and outcomes.

and select, use, and modify measures in ways that reduce bias. The final section presents selected strategies and tools for screening and assessing linguistically and culturally diverse preschoolers and making educational recommendations.

EXPLORING ATTITUDES TOWARD DIVERSITY

Rogoff (2003) argues that humans are biologically cultural: "People develop as participants in cultural communities. Their development can be understood only in light of the cultural practices and circumstances of their communities—which also change" (pp. 3–4). Anderson and Fenichel (1989) define a *culture* "as the specific framework of meanings within which a population, individually and as a group, shapes its lifeways. A cultural framework is neither static nor absolute. It is, in a sense, an ongoing process, within which individuals are constantly reworking or trying out new ideas and behaviors" (p. 8).

All of us grow up within a cultural group (or groups) that passes along its ways of living, language, and values. These in turn influence caregiving practices, values, and expectations (Polk, 1994), including feeding, sleeping, toilet training, the amount of independence a child is allowed, use of discipline, quality and type of play, and literacy-related experiences. Within as well as between cultural groups, there are wide differences regarding child-rearing practices, belief systems, and family lifestyles. Early childhood specialists need to "discern where on the continuum of assimilation into the majority culture a family functions, and recognize that this may change" (Vincent, Salisbury, Strain, McCormick, & Terrier, 1990, p. 178). Green's (1982) description of four categories of cultural integration as a means of understanding the continuum is useful here. These categories, as applied to families, would range from (1) mainstream, fully integrated families; (2) bicultural families who maintain a commitment to both cultures, such as Crystal and Jack's family described later; (3) culturally different families who adhere to their culture of origin, often in minority enclaves, such as Maria's family described later; to (4) culturally marginal families who don't seem to have connections or commitments to any cultural group (see also Lynch, 2004a). Interview is the best way to assess acculturation and Rhodes, Ochoa, and Ortiz (2005, p. 132) provide sample questions for such an interview. To the degree possible, educational personnel want to ensure continuity with the activities and procedures used in their setting and those used in the home to facilitate children's development.

Forms of Cultural Bias

Cultural bias takes many forms that assessors need to consider. As a first step, assessors need to reflect on their own attitudes and beliefs. Next, they need to consider the multiple ways bias can enter the assessment process. They must recognize that all tests are culturally loaded, in that they assess culturally valued aptitudes or skills and tap these aptitudes and skills through items containing material familiar to most individuals within the mainstream culture in which they were developed. Thus children from other cultures are likely to be assessed *unfairly* by tests developed and normed on mainstream groups in the United States and Canada, for a variety of reasons:

1. Children who are ELLs generally have nonexistent or emerging English-language skills, by definition. Thus any test given in English may be, to an unknown degree, simply a test of such a child's English-language skills.

2. Each culture has very different ideas about what are important things for preschool children to know. For example, in some Malaysian coastal communities, 5-year-olds are expected to be highly competent at rowing large boats through choppy waters and docking them underneath their homes, which are on stilts. Assessors need to take into account that adaptive, motor, language, and cognitive behaviors are culturally defined. What is valued in one culture may not be fostered in another culture, and what is viewed as an impairment or deficit in one culture may not be so considered in another. These facts contrast sharply with the yardsticks for making referral decisions—generally norms based on Western and largely middle-class populations.

3. Children's past experiences influence their responses in a testing session. Lynch and Hanson (2004b) give the example of a young child who had recently moved with his family to California from Samoa. During testing, the boy appeared to show delayed motor development; in a later home visit, however, the child appeared to have age-appropriate motor skills. The authors noted that his home had mats and very low furniture, not the furniture and large obstacles found in most American homes or in the testing situation. They concluded that his cultural experiences interfered with his successful performance upon what many consider to be culturally invariant measures (test of motor skills). The screening or assessment situation thus may require the use of measures that *do not* involve culture-specific materials or tasks, or that are relevant to a child's own culture rather than the mainstream culture.

4. Even if a child has relatively good English skills, mental processing in his or her second language may be slower and less efficient (American Educational Research Association [AERA], American Psychological Association, & National Council on Measurement in Education, 1999; Cummins, 1980; Schiff-Myers et al., 1993).

5. An assessor's lack of in-depth knowledge about culturally relevant practices may result in misinterpretation of behavior and misclassification. The assessor, for example, may interpret the profile of a child who is an ELL as if he or she was from a monolingual English background (Cummins, 1980), which would grossly underestimate the child's vocabulary development, or conclude that the child needs speech therapy because his or her English pronunciation is influenced by another language (Fantini, 1985).

These are just a few of the culture-related issues that can lead to invalid results in assessment situations. For a more detailed analysis of some of the complexities and problems in assessing culturally and linguistically diverse groups, see Bialystok (2001), Collier (1988), Figueroa (1990), Garcia (1993), Genesee, Paradis, and Crago (2004), Green (1982), Lynch and Hanson (2004a), Ortiz (2002), Paredes Scribner (2002), Rhodes, Ochoa, and Ortiz (2005), and the *Standards for Educational and Psychological Testing* (AERA et al., 1999).

In addition to the diversity of languages and dialects in which children need to be assessed, and the lack of valid instruments for doing this, there is a scarcity of bilingual personnel—a problem that is likely to continue (Lopez, 2002). As a result, early childhood teachers and specialists tend to be from the majority European American culture and have been socialized into that culture; at worst, their practices may reflect institutional racism and classism. Some of these insensitivities are unintended and subtle, such as feeling stigmatized by working with poor minority or immigrant children. Others are overt, as in an attitude of "If you don't like it here, go back to where you came from." Therefore, attention needs to be focused on increasing cultural and linguistic sensitivity, and empathy toward diverse cultural values, among all those involved in the assessment process. To achieve this goal, assessors need heightened awareness of (1) possible cultural and linguistic barriers to communicating with families that make it difficult to get good information on children and their development, or to design intervention programs that might be successful; and (2) professional habits or accepted practices that may result in strained communication with linguistically and culturally different families and children. Professionals thus need to move past a focus solely on assessment instruments and their interpretation, and to examine their own attitudes, stereotypes, and awareness of cultural values and goals.

Increasing Cultural Sensitivity through Self-Assessment

Cultural competence includes an awareness of one's own cultural frameworks, an openness to and respect for cultural differences, a view of intercultural interactions as opportunities to learn about other world views, a willingness to use cultural resources in intervention, and a recognition of the integrity and worth of all cultures (Green, 1982). Becoming culturally competent is important for all professionals, regardless of their race or ethnicity. This is almost impossible to do without certain experiences, such as participating or living in another culture or spending time with bicultural people. Cultural competence requires at least four critical steps:

1. An exploration of one's own cultural heritage, including such information as place of origin prior to coming to the United States or Canada, time of immigration, languages spoken prior to immigration, religious background, and place of the family's first settlement in North America.
2. An examination of the values, beliefs, behaviors, and typical customs associated with one's own cultural background, bearing in mind the tremendous diversity within each cultural group and the influence of such factors as time in country, community experiences, education, and SES on one's values and beliefs. Lynch (2004b) provides a values clarification exercise ("a cultural journey") that guides professionals through an exploration of this process. Preschool assessors in particular need to focus on their own beliefs about "appropriate" child-rearing practices (including fostering independence, discipline, sleeping patterns, etc.), approaches to disability, and interactions with help providers.
3. Becoming aware of other cultures represented in the population to be assessed and how their values and beliefs differ from those of one's own culture and background, with the goal of becoming more able to look at behavior through the lenses of individuals from these other cultures. This can be accomplished through participating and/or living in other cultures, through ongoing in-service training with consultants representing cultural/linguistic groups of interest, through viewing films, through attending multicultural workshops, and through reading books.[1] Lynch and Hanson (2004a) provide an anno-

[1] Books that we have found particularly helpful include Lynch and Hanson's (2004a) *Developing Cross-Cultural Competence: A Guide for Working with Children and Their Families* (3rd ed.); Whiting and Edwards's (1988) *Children of Different Worlds: The Formation of Social Behavior*; Korbin's (1981) *Child Abuse and Neglect: Cross-Cultural Perspectives*; Ramsey's (1998) *Teaching and Learning in a Diverse World: Multicultural Education for Young Children*; Waxler-Morrison, Anderson, and Richardson's (1990) *Cross-Cultural Caring: A Guide for Health Professionals in Western Canada*; and Rogoff's (2003) *The Cultural Nature of Human Development*; and Hanson and Lynch's (2004) *Understanding Families: Approaches to Diversity, Disability, and Risk.*

tated bibliography of popular books and films depicting the cultural experiences of various ethnic groups.

4. Developing skills in interviewing the caregivers of culturally and linguistically diverse children. Such skills, according to Collier (1988), include (a) *nonverbal reflection*, which involves adjusting to and using the body language and gestures of the person who is being interviewed (e.g., avoiding eye contact as a sign of respect or using gestures); (2) *verbal reflection*, such as adapting to the interviewee's tone, intonation, latency, and rate of speech, which have different meanings across cultures; and (c) *culture comfort zone*, or awareness of one's own cultural practices in relation to the cultural practices of the person interviewed, which may be reflected in such behaviors as touching the person and responding to discomfort.

Potential sources of misunderstanding between cultural minority groups and mainstream American professional groups, which are relevant to the assessment of preschool children, have been identified by Harry (1992) in an influential paper. These include (1) the meanings of disability; (2) family structure and identity; (3) parenting styles; (4) goals of early intervention; (5) communication styles; and (6) professional roles. Contrasts between mainstream views and culturally different views of these issues are presented in Table 9.1. Harry urges professionals to become aware of the values and parental goals of cultural minority families with young children, as well as the cultural assumptions on which special education law and much professional training are based.

In addition, it is important for assessors to review studies of cross-cultural differences in child development, in order to understand which factors are universal across cultures (e.g., timing of some developmental milestones, such as walking and talking) and which are open to great variation (e.g., ages at which children are considered competent child caregivers, can use sharp knives, are free to roam the community). Dreher, Nugent, and Hudgins (1994) point out how important knowledge of this research is, to challenge our current assumptions about human behavior and to free us from our own ethnocentrism.

Teachers' beliefs may influence who is referred for assessment. This may result from a lack of familiarity with a particular culture or language, or from the teachers' own feelings of not being able to cope (Gersten & Woodward, 1994). Therefore, assessors must be concerned about setting the stage for others to reflect on these issues, and must create opportunities for staff members to share their concerns and areas of expertise.

GENERAL CHARACTERISTICS OF CULTURES AND THEIR IMPLICATIONS FOR ASSESSMENT AND INTERVENTION

Professionals' first interactions with families of different cultures are critical in that they may determine success of a long-term relationship. Because cultural and linguistic gaps can be so large, it is imperative that assessors become as familiar as possible with each cultural group with which they work, and in particular become aware of their customs and social manners. In this section of the chapter, we briefly describe some of the beliefs, values, and practices of the cultural groups most frequently encountered in the North American educational system; we draw heavily on Lynch and Hanson (2004a) and our own experiences over many years of supervising culturally diverse graduate students assessing culturally diverse children. Table 9.2 summarizes important cultural customs

TABLE 9.1. Developing Cultural Self-Awareness: Mainstream Views That May Clash with Culturally Different Views

Source of bias	Mainstream view	Culturally different view
Meanings of disability	• Disability is an intrinsic deficit.	• Disability is within the normal range (low-income Puerto Rican and some Native American) or has spiritual causes (some Hispanic, Native American, and Southeast Asian groups).
	• Education and/or medical treatment is needed.	• No need for treatment may be perceived, or spiritual treatment may be preferred.
	• Biological abnormalities should be corrected.	• Biological abnormalities may be seen as rewards or blessings (e.g., Hmong).
Family structure and identity	• *Family* refers to biological family.	• Extended or informally adopted family members care for children in many cultures. Many immigrants leave children in homeland in such care; this is not seen as parental neglect or lack of interest.
	• Parents are main authorities.	• Grandparents, other family/clan members may be authorities.
	• Collective sense of identity is seen as enmeshment.	• Collective sense of identity is normal in many Hispanic and Asian American families.
Parenting styles	• Verbally rich environment is a sign of good parenting.	• Nonverbal style, related to greater attention to visual detail, is seen in Native American parents. • High levels of nonverbal and physical attention are seen in rural African American parents.
	• Democratic child rearing is superior to authoritarian styles.	• Corporal punishment is considered appropriate by some African Americans/ Asian Americans. • Shaming is practiced by some Asian groups.
Goals of early intervention	• Verbal development is given high priority.	• Families in many cultures (see above) show less concern and have fewer expectations for early achievement of verbal milestones.
	• Independence at earliest possible age is promoted; close supervision for age is seen as "overprotective."	• Families in many cultures show less concern for independence, provide closer supervision.
	• Individual orientation; best interests of the child are seen as most important.	• Collectivist orientation; best interests of the group are seen as most important.

(continued)

TABLE 9.1. *(continued)*

Source of bias	Mainstream view	Culturally different view
Communication styles	• Professional self is different from personal self, and it is important to maintain distinction.	• Sharing of personal self is important in developing trust with many minority clients.
	• Coming directly to the point is appropriate.	• Abrupt introduction of topic is offensive and leads to resistance and opposition in many Hispanic, Asian, and Native American groups.
Professional roles	• Collaborationist role is currently popular.	• Expert role is expected by many Asian, Native American, Hispanic, and low-income groups.
	• Families should openly convey doubts and disagreements with professionals.	• Families should show respect and defer to professionals, regardless of professionals' views or recommendations.

Note. Adapted from Harry (1992). Copyright 1992 by PRO-ED. Adapted by permission.

TABLE 9.2. Culturally Appropriate Manners for Professionals Working with Diverse Ethnic Groups: Some Representative Examples

European Americans

- Be on time for appointments.
- Give equal respect to everyone, regardless of sex, age, or position.
- Greet everyone directly and warmly.
- Get to the point of the interview or meeting.
- Keep a physical distance of about 3 feet.
- Do little or no physical touching, except by shaking hands.
- Make direct eye contact with each person, regardless of age or sex.
- Avoid any behavior that suggests patronization on the basis of class (e.g., offering toys or used clothing to poor children).

Native Americans

- Take time to develop a trusting relationship.
- Be reserved, and be tolerant of periods of silence.
- If making a home visit to a family without a telephone, honk the horn when you arrive, and then wait for someone to come and greet you. If no one does, assume that your visit was inconvenient and try again.
- Accept offered food and drink.
- Discuss family roles, as grandparents may be responsible for making decisions about the child, and other relatives may have the disciplinarian role.
- Consult with the family to see whether toys or pictures used in tests or intervention are acceptable (some may be considered bad luck).
- Treat any ceremonial markings or objects a child bears or wears with respect, and ask permission before removing any of them.

(continued)

TABLE 9.2. *(continued)*

African Americans

- Convey competence through a professional manner.
- Greet adults formally, using Mr. or Ms. to show respect, unless given permission to use first names.
- Follow the clients' lead in any discussion of racial issues, and do not minimize their concerns.
- Make no assumptions about family functioning based on poverty or single parenthood.

Hispanic Americans

- Allow for a flexible interpretation of when the appointment will start.
- Greet husbands first, then wives, when both are present.
- Present a professional appearance and use your title.
- Engage in relaxed social conversation before addressing the purpose of the meeting.
- Do not rush through the meeting, as being in a hurry indicates disrespect.
- Always solicit the father's views on any treatment plan, even if he is not present.
- Expect warm physical touching and decreased spatial distance between conversational partners.
- Accept any food or drink offered.

Asian Americans

- Respect the family hierarchy by greeting the oldest (and usually male) family members first, and seeking their opinions in this order as well.
- Avoid physical contact, particularly between men and women; men may shake hands, but the younger man should wait for the older man to initiate.
- Do not make or expect extended eye contact.
- Be formal, reserved, and polite.
- Treat business cards with great respect; inspect them closely before putting them away.
- Remove shoes before entering a private home.
- Accept any food or drinks offered.
- If a gift is given, accept it with both hands and open it later.

Note. Some data from Lynch and Hanson (2004a).

and polite behavior relevant to developing rapport with families within the most common ethnic groups in North America. Lynch and Hanson cover each of these groups in detail, as well as families with Pacific Islander (e.g., Filipino, Native Hawaiian, Samoan) and Middle Eastern roots.

An essential principle in working with all families is *not to make any assumptions* about their priorities, concerns, or resources. This principle is even more important in working with families of cultural backgrounds different from one's own. Once again, assessors must acknowledge the many and wide variations that exist within cultural groups, and must take care not to perpetuate stereotypes (Vincent et al., 1990). As noted earlier, families function on a continuum of assimilation into the majority culture. Furthermore, cultures are dynamic and ever-changing; the cultural practices that families remember and practice from their home countries are often different from the practices that are occurring in those countries today. In addition, not only culture, language, ethnicity, and race, but SES, educational level, occupation, past experience, and personality all exert a powerful influence over how individuals and families define themselves and function. Thus there is wide variation among children coming from a particular language background, such as Spanish, in tradition and cultural practice. The brief descriptions of cultural stances and manners that follow are meant to serve only as a rough guide to cross-cultural interactions with families.

European American Families

European Americans have been described as valuing individualism, privacy, informality in interactions with others, timeliness and punctuality, high achievement, action, hard work, materialism, and interactional styles that are direct and assertive. In addition, they believe in the general goodness of humanity and the quality of all individuals (Althen, 1988). Again, cultural courtesies that are valued by this group and the others described here are listed in Table 9.2.

Native American Families

Native American tribes (or First Nations, as they are known in Canada) represent tremendously diverse cultural and language groups. There are about 550 federally recognized tribes in the United States (Dauphinais & King, 1992). Some tribes have a matriarchal family structure, others have a patriarchal structure, and still others have a combination structure. Some tribes have been polygamous while others have been monogamous in the past (McAdoo, 1978). The few generalizations that can be made are that there is an emphasis on group life; on respect for elders, experts, and spiritual leaders; on harmony; and on observable behaviors rather than verbal statements. In addition, supportive nonfamily members are incorporated into the family network, and there is a general tendency to accept situations as they are without focusing on how to change them. Many families have developed great distrust for public institutions because of past racism and cultural insensitivity; respectful interaction is thus especially important if a good relationship is to be developed (Joe & Malach, 2004). English is the most common second (and often first) language.

Families of African Descent

Families of African descent also come from a great variety of backgrounds; some families' ancestors were forcibly brought to the United States as slaves, and other families have immigrated voluntarily from the Caribbean or from African countries. Racism and oppression have been common experiences regardless of country of origin or time of arrival. On the whole, Americans of African descent tend to have a collective orientation; are more oriented to a situation than to time; have great respect for elderly persons and give them major family roles; have more authoritarian child-rearing practices than mainstream families; tend to have strong religious and spiritual orientations; place importance on kinship and extended family bonds; and engage in what is called "high-context" communication, in that they are likely to use a great deal of gesture and nonverbal communication that is meaningful in context, as opposed to the greater emphasis on precise use of language emphasized by mainstream culture (Willis, 2004). These families are also notable relative to other groups in the degree to which their family organization is represented by single-parent homes. Although this may be the case for economic reasons, this type of family organization seems to have strong cultural roots as well (see Whiting & Edwards, 1988). This does not mean that fathers are not involved in families, but that mothers often have the primary responsibility (and resultant credit) for raising their children.

Hispanic Families

Hispanic families in the United States come from many different places; the largest groups are from Mexico, Puerto Rico, and Cuba, but increasing numbers of families are immigrating from the Dominican Republic and from South and Central America as well. Within the Hispanic community, there are clear status distinctions among countries of origin and class distinctions within each country. Class standing has a strong influence on the behavior of individuals within a group and on intragroup relationships. On the whole, those of Hispanic descent (who are also often known as Latinos or Latinas, depending on gender) place a very strong emphasis on the importance of the family, regardless of class, background, or country of origin. The emphasis on collective identity and socialization means that interdependence and good interpersonal relationships are often valued more highly than independent achievement. Hispanic families tend to have relaxed standards about the age at which children will achieve certain milestones, and they show a great deal of respect for elders (Zuniga, 2004). Family structure tends to place a great deal of authority and responsibility in the hands of fathers in middle-class families; families from impoverished backgrounds, in our experience, often have little father involvement. The mothers in these families are often passive and deferential when interacting with educational, mental health, and health professionals. Catholicism, evangelical Protestantism, or other forms of spirituality are often important in family life.

Asian American Families

Asian Americans also come from a tremendous variety of traditions and unique cultures that have arisen from ancient civilizations (e.g., Chinese, Korean, Vietnamese, Japanese, and Indian). Across these various cultural groups, however, there are some transcending Asian values. As with most of the other cultures we have briefly reviewed, the family is the basic societal unit and the center around which most individuals' lives revolve. Academic achievement is highly valued and considered an honor bestowed in gratitude to one's parents and one's family. Culturally valued are the virtues of patience, perseverance, social harmony, humility, stoicism, hard work, and self-sacrifice. Asian families are hierarchically structured, with particular respect paid to elders (particularly male elders). Children are expected to respond with unquestioning obedience and loyalty to their parents, who have a great deal of authority over them. Children are also expected to respect their school teachers and other authority figures. They are expected to work hard and do things over and over until these are mastered, and not to ask questions. The orientation is toward group welfare and mutual interdependence (Chan & Lee, 2004). Asians tend to be subtle and indirect in their communication, using a lot of implicit and nonverbal cues to communicate feelings and opinions. It is not uncommon for nonverbal behavior to contradict verbal behavior (Chan & Lee, 2004). In their religious lives, Asians tend to be polytheistic, blending Buddhism, Taoism, Confucianism, and ancestor worship into a mixture of beliefs and religious practice; however, many from the People's Republic of China are atheists, and many Asians immigrating to the United States (particularly Koreans) are Christians.

ISSUES IN BILINGUALISM AND SECOND-LANGUAGE ACQUISITION

Most individuals in the world are regularly exposed to and have some proficiency in more than one language (Duncan, 1989; Grosjean, 1982); in other words, bilingualism, rather than monolingualism, is the more common pattern. However, monolingualism has been the predominant pattern among members of the mainstream culture in the United States, and to a lesser extent in Canada. Bilingualism, though common, is not generally valued or supported by public schools in the United States (Bialystok, 2001; Ovando, 2003). The focus is on proficiency in English as soon as possible, with transitional bilingual education—in effect, a move from monolingualism in the native language to monolingualism in English (Snow & Hakuta, 1992)—the predominant mode of education for Spanish-speaking students, who constitute by far the largest group of students who are ELLs in the United States (Paredes Scribner, 2002). Non-Spanish-speaking children who are ELLs are generally placed in English immersion (called *submersion* by critics) or English as a second language (ESL) programs, with little or no instruction in their first language (Paredes Scribner, 2002). This is unfortunate, as a large body of international and domestic research, much of it conducted in Canada, strongly supports high-quality bilingual education (i.e., continued instruction in both languages) for children learning a second language (for reviews, see Cummins, 1984, 2000; Duncan, 1989; Genesee, Paradis, & Crago, 2004; Rhodes, Ochoa, & Ortiz, 2005; Thomas & Collier, 1997, 2002; U.S. General Accounting Office, 1987; and Willig, 1985). Transitional bilingual education is associated with lower levels of proficiency in the second language, lower academic achievement, and psychosocial problems (Hakuta & Feldman Mostafapour, 1996).

In the United States, the NCLB Act of 2001 has mastery of the English language by all children in America's schools as one of its major priorities. Annual assessment of English proficiency in oral language, reading, and writing skills are mandated for all children who are ELLs and have been in U.S. schools for 3 consecutive years. Under the NCLB legislation, each state is free to devise its own approach to ensuring proficiency in English, as long as the curriculum used is based on scientific research and has been demonstrated to be effective. We hope that the emphasis on curricular effectiveness in the NCLB Act triumphs over hostility to bilingual education, some of it based on common myths about bilingualism described below, as states experiment with ELL/ESL programs.

In addition to the many children who are bilingual, some children speak only or primarily English but are exposed to one or more languages through contact with parents, other relatives, or caregivers. According to the U.S. Bureau of the Census (2003) about 18% of individuals age 5 and over speak a language other than English at home. In the states of Hawaii, California, New Mexico, Arizona, Texas, New Jersey, and New York, from 25.5% to 39.5% of the state populations do so. Of nursery and kindergarten children in the United States in October 2003, 20.1% had at least one foreign-born parent. This was true for 62.2% of Hispanic children and 88.8% of Asian children in this age group (U.S. Bureau of the Census, 2003), suggesting high levels of exposure to other languages. In Canada—a country with two official languages, English and French—9.53% of 5- to 9-year-olds in 2001 spoke a nonofficial language at home. The distribution of foreign-born (and thus nonofficial-language-speaking) populations was highly concentrated in a few metropolitan areas; Toronto's population, for example, was 43.7% foreign-born, and Vancouver's was 37.5% foreign-born. (*Canada's Census Information*, n.d.). However, the total figures for children not speaking an official language at home also included some First Nations children.

Levels of proficiency range from a high degree of competence in two languages (the most common meaning of the term *bilingualism*) to limited competence in either (known as *semilingualism*; Duncan, 1989). Bilingual competence is most likely to occur when a child comes from a literate home that values both languages and provides a linguistically rich environment, with some community support for the nondominant language (Cummins, 1984, 2000; Romaine, 1995). Semilingualism is most likely to occur when a child is exposed to two languages at once, or first one and then another, in a linguistically impoverished environment and masters neither. Or a child may be proficient in one language and then be exposed to another; in time, the second language becomes dominant and the first language begins to atrophy. This happens to many children from non-English-speaking backgrounds once they begin attending North American schools, unless they are part of a large immigrant group with many opportunities to use their first language or they attend a school that respects and explicitly fosters their language and culture. Moreover, the form of a particular language used locally may change as the population using it is exposed over time to English; this unique form of a language is called a *contact dialect* (Haugen, 1977).

Misconceptions about Bilingualism

Many misconceptions about bilingualism continue to influence educational policy and professional practice. Four of these misconceptions are summarized below.

1. *Knowledge and use of another language endangers the development of English proficiency.* This is the view that bilingualism is subtractive rather than additive. *Subtractive* refers to any negative effects on the first language as a result of learning the second language. *Additive* refers to any positive benefits occurring to the first language from learning the second. These two outcomes, however, are related to environmental circumstances, not to learning a second language itself.

Reviews of studies examining the conditions under which each form of bilingualism arises suggest that subtractive bilingualism is most often found among disadvantaged immigrant or minority populations where the first language is gradually supplanted by the higher-status majority language. Since the first language is likely to atrophy faster than the second language develops, a child may experience academic difficulties and end up less proficient in both languages than a monolingual speaker of either language (Cummins, 1984, 2000; Ovando & Collier, 1998).

Additive bilingualism is most likely to occur in children who speak the higher-status majority language, which is not in danger of being replaced by the second language. Anglophone Canadian children educated in a French-language school are a good example. Children from minority language backgrounds may achieve additive bilingualism if their first language is strongly supported in school (Cummins, 1984, 2000) or at home and in the community, as seen in children whose parents speak a minority language at home and send their children to language/cultural classes on the weekends.

Because of the fear of subtractive bilingualism, some parents have been told to speak to their preschool children in English even if they are not fluent in it, so that their children will be better able to master the English they are learning at school. This practice is to be avoided, since it reduces the children's exposure to the sort of linguistically rich environment that most parents of non-English backgrounds cannot provide in English. It also degrades the culture and language of the home. Most importantly, dual-language exposure does not appear to be a risk factor in language development. The little evidence that exists suggests that simultaneous bilingual children with language impairments acquire language at the same rate as monolingual children with language impairments (Paradis, Crago, Genesee, & Rice, 2003).

2. *Bilingualism impedes cognitive development.* This misconception is countered by the work of Cummins (1976, 2000), who proposed the *threshold hypothesis*, which has since been supported by a number of studies (see Bialystok, 2001, for a recent review). According to this hypothesis, the positive effects of bilingualism on cognitive development do not come into play until a minimum level of proficiency is achieved in the first language. This first threshold prevents any negative effects from learning the second language, and the achievement of a higher level of proficiency leads to accelerated cognitive growth. The research shows that additive bilingualism is related to more rapid development of selective attention—an important component of many forms of problem solving—than is monolingualism (Bialystok, 2001). Other benefits of bilingualism include competence in two languages, participation in two cultures, and the ability to interpret from one language to the other. For subtractive bilingual children, it is not bilingualism per se that accounts for the children's academic difficulties. Rather, it appears to be the lack of adequate conceptual development in the first language that leads to the cognitive confusion seen in these children. For children of lower intellectual ability, placement in a dual-language program that begins with a focus on the second language, is not related to lower native-language development or to lower academic development if children are regularly exposed to a rich language environment in both languages. They do as well in each of these areas as monolingual peers of lower intellectual ability (Genesee, 1976, 1987).

3. *Oral proficiency in conversation with others is representative of a child's total competence in English, including his or her ability to use cognitive and academic language.* Second-language learning seems to develop in a very similar pattern to first-language learning of English. This assumption presents no major problems for preschoolers, who have not generally developed reading and writing skills, but older students' bilingual competence is frequently judged on the basis of their skill in communicating orally, face to face in a particular context. Although they may appear highly fluent, their ability to communicate out of context and their literacy (reading and writing) are other matters.

Proficiency with literacy in a new language takes considerable time. Gifted individuals, and those from highly academically oriented environments, may become quite competent in a language after 2 years. Most children coming from educated and literate homes (and who are also at least 8 years of age, have acquired some literacy skills in another language, and have suffered no traumatic or major economic dislocation) take 4 years on the average to reach the 50th percentile on English competency tests such as the verbal sections of the California Achievement Test. The average child with LEP coming into the North American school system takes 5–7 years to reach an average level of academic competence (Cummins, 1980, 1984). Although Cummins's discussion is focused on school-age children, many of the issues are also relevant to early childhood populations. For example, readiness testing in English for entrance into kindergarten or first grade, the results of which may be used to exclude children, is a poor practice to begin with and is particularly inappropriate for bilingual children.

Bilingual preschool-age children, once they are *regularly* exposed to English as a second language through nursery school, preschool, or childcare, typically become orally proficient in conversation within 18–36 months (Duncan, 1989); for many preschoolers, this is most of their lives. This is a key point for assessors, because if such proficiency does not develop, it could signal some language or cognitive difficulties, or possibly some emotional problems or some cultural inhibition against learning ESL. It is essential for an assessor, therefore, to determine how long a child has been exposed to English and under what circumstances before presenting assessment measures and interpreting outcomes. If a child has strong cognitive, linguistic, and emergent literacy support for one language at home, a strong preschool and kindergarten program in English should provide enough knowledge of the language for the child to be competent in first-grade reading in English (Bialystok, 2001). If a preschool child does not have such support at home, and the school provides only instruction in English, the child may lack the conceptual knowledge and the emergent literacy background to respond successfully.

4. *Communicative differences are indications of communication disorders.* According to Mattes and Omark (1984), communicative differences, such as frequent requests for repetitions when communicating in English, pauses before speaking, articulation difficulties, and word-finding problems, are typical of children learning a second language. Assessors should note that these problems do not necessarily occur when a child speaks his or her native language. Communication disorders are present when spoken language is so poor that communication with partners who speak the same language and dialect is impaired. If these problems do occur in a child's first language, as well as in the second language, then the child is considered to have a communication disorder.

How can professionals distinguish between communicative differences and communication disorders? To determine whether or not a child has a language disorder requires not only taking a careful family history, but also comparing the child's language behavior with that of other bilingual speakers who have had similar language and cultural experiences.

Research has shown that children who are identified as having language problems on the basis of *pragmatic* dysfunctions (problems in using language to convey needs and wants) are much more likely to have serious language problems than those identified for grammatical dysfunctions. In particular, Damico and Oller (1980) have shown that teachers can be trained to be highly effective assessors of pragmatic language competence. When trained to refer children on the basis of pragmatic problems, they have much higher rates of identifying children with language dysfunctions than when problems with the structural features of language are used as the referral basis. These pragmatic criteria are also effective in separating out bilingual children with language disorders from those who are simply in the process of acquiring a second language (Damico, Oller, & Storey, 1983). Pragmatic problems described by Damico and Oller (1980) include the following:

- *Linguistic nonfluency*—the child's speech is disrupted by an excessive number of repetitions, unusual pauses, and hesitations or "uh's."
- *Revisions*—the child's speech is broken up by many false starts or self-interruptions, in which he or she revises what has already been said.
- *Delays before responding*—when others attempt to initiate conversation, these efforts are met with long pauses by the child.
- *Nonspecific vocabulary*—the child says "this," "that," "then," "he," "over there," "thing," "stuff," "these," and "those" when the conversational context makes the referents unclear and a typically developing child would probably have used specific names or somehow made the referents clear.
- *Inappropriate responses*—the child's conversational responses seem only tangentially or not at all related to the prompts or probes of an adult or peer partner. These are easy to identify, even though they are harder to describe.

- *Poor topic maintenance*—the child makes rapid and inappropriate changes in topic without providing conversational clues to the listener.
- *Need for repetition*—the child requests many repetitions, but they do not seem to help comprehension.

Speakers of a child's first language can observe pragmatic difficulties as a child converses in a natural context. Family members may report spontaneously, or in response to questioning, that a child has language delays or deviancies relative to an older sibling or cousin. In addition to getting a history of language development, an assessor can use the pragmatic problems described above to guide follow-up questions. If a language problem is suspected, then an observation and language sample should be obtained and analyzed, as described later in this chapter and in Chapter 10. It is important to remember that a child has a true language disorder *only* if problems are present in the child's first language; he or she cannot have a language disorder in English as a second language and function normally in the first language.

One of the fundamental findings of linguistic studies is that early-emerging morphology and syntax in English seem to develop in a highly similar pattern in first- and second-language English in early childhood (Dulay, Hernandez-Chavez, & Burt, 1978; Duncan, 1989; Kessler, 1984). As a result, descriptive developmental profiles of the structure of first-language English can be used to chart the *morphosyntactic development* (the different grammatical uses of *morphemes*, or word endings that affect number, tense, location, etc., and the rules governing their use) of children who are ELLs (see Duncan, 1989, for a detailed demonstration).

It is also helpful to keep the following descriptions of second-language learning in mind (see Mattes & Omark, 1984, for more details). First, children learning a second language make grammatical errors similar to those of children learning their first language. One only has to think of having oneself judged as communicatively competent or incompetent based on proficiency in an unmastered second language to understand this. Second, when children have few opportunities to learn and use their first language, they lose fluency. Third, another frequent pattern involves code mixing and/or code switching. Borrowing terms from another language (particularly terms with no counterpart in the first language) is called *code mixing*. Code mixing and *code switching* (moving back and forth from one language to another within a sentence) are both normal phenomena in many bilingual populations and not necessarily signs of language disorder. Assessors need to be aware of local norms for code mixing. As Genesee, Paradis, and Crago (2004) point out, some communities frequently code mix, like Miami, and some almost never do, like Montreal. Violations of local norms for language behavior, if a child has had time to become familiar with them, may indicate a need for assessment and intervention. The use of contact dialect is also normal, as noted earlier.

Points to Consider Prior to Screening Children from Linguistically Diverse Backgrounds

Preschool screening programs are designed for a variety of purposes, one of which is to identify very quickly (in no more than 20–30 minutes) children who need to be more thoroughly evaluated for potential learning or behavioral problems. This is a problematic process even with monolingual English-speaking children from mainstream cultural backgrounds, because most such measures have limited reliability and validity, due to their brevity and to the developmental fluidity of preschoolers (see Chapters 6 and 7).

When children from non-English or ELL backgrounds are screened, the time and staffing demands and the psychometric challenges can seem insurmountable, as the children must first be assessed for language proficiency in English and their primary language(s) and then screened for potential learning problems. Here is the dilemma: In many cases there are no adequate measures of language proficiency, and even when language proficiency and dominance are clear, no appropriate screening measures in children's primary language exists. In what follows, we cover major points that screeners and assessors need to take into account.

Establishing a Child's Linguistic Background

Prior to screening for cognitive, language, emotional, behavioral, sensory, or physical problems, consideration of a child's linguistic background is essential. It is necessary to determine (1) which languages a child speaks and/or understands, and (2) how proficient a child is in English *and* in the other language(s) that a child may have been exposed to or uses. Thus it is important to assess *all* of a child's languages even when one is dominant, in order to determine a child's communicational competence and develop educational plans.

Linguistic background has to do with the languages a child understands or speaks because of regular exposure. Language proficiency has to do with the level of competence a child has in each of several languages which can range from negligible to very limited to limited to fluent to advanced if one used the cognitive academic language proficient (CALP) terms developed by Cummins (1984). Language dominance is "a measure of the relative proficiency between two languages that the child is learning" (Genesee, Paradis, & Crago, 2004, p. 80). The dominant language usually has a longer mean length of utterance, more advanced grammar, greater vocabulary, more verb types, fewer pauses and hesitations, and greater fluency. Most bilingual children are dominant in one of their two (or three) languages, as illustrated in the following example.

> Crystal, age 4-7, and Jack, age 2-5, have lived in the United States since birth. They have a mother who is from Shanghai, China and a father who is European American. They spend several mornings a week with their American grandmother who lives several miles away. Their mother, a native speaker of the Shanghai dialect, is fluent in English but speaks to the children in Mandarin because the parents want them to be bilingual in Mandarin and English. Their father speaks to them in English (although he is fluent in Mandarin), and they are exposed to their mother conversing with her parents in the Shanghai dialect during the grandparents' annual 3- to 5-month visits. Crystal understood but refused to speak Mandarin until she was 4 years old, when her family moved to Taiwan for 4 months and enrolled her in a Chinese preschool. Living in an all-Chinese environment, she became sufficiently fluent in Mandarin, which she speaks with a slight American accent, to do well in the preschool and is now able to translate simple language for her English-speaking grandmother when both sides of the family get together. Crystal is English-dominant, converses well in Mandarin, and understands but does not speak the Shanghai dialect. Jack, on the other hand, is dominant in Mandarin, understands and speaks at a beginning level in the Shanghai dialect, and understands and speaks a little English. His Chinese grandparents have lived in his family's house for 12 of the 27 months of his life, the family lived in Taiwan for an additional 4 months, and the family has had a nanny, who speaks only Mandarin, since he was one and a half years old. His only English exposure is from his father and his paternal grandmother. By age 2 he

knew to speak to them in English, but his vocabulary was so limited that he frequently interjected words from Mandarin. Recently, he has started to attend Mommy and Me classes in his American community twice a week and his American grandmother has noticed a marked improvement in his English.

When learning two languages, young children focus on giving priority to new words over learning the equivalent word in each language (Taeschner, 1983). Children have different experiences in each language (e.g., daycare in English, home and church in Russian) that result in different vocabularies in both languages. A study of English–Spanish bilingual toddlers in Miami found that they had an average of 30% of words that were translation equivalents, a figure that had increased to 50% by age 6 (Pearson, 1998). Thus bilingual individuals, even those who are equally proficient in both languages, generally know fewer words in any one of the two languages than a monolingual individual does. The result of this process is illustrated by Erickson and Iglesias (1986) in their example of a Spanish-dominant child who was administered the Spanish and English versions of the original Boehm Test of Basic Concepts. The authors noted that her performance on each version was 3 *SD* below the mean. However, when the number of concepts she knew across both measures was tabulated, her performance was slightly above the mean—a very different picture of the child. Bilingual children know many more concepts when both languages are examined than when each language is examined individually; this point has important implications for curriculum planning.

Children's use of language and choice of language also vary, depending on the topic, the context, the conversational partner, and the emotional tone of the language. Therefore, professionals should take a child's *total* language experience and knowledge into consideration when judging his or her communicative competence. In particular, assessors need to review the content of brief screening measures and the extent to which they tap a child's background, knowledge, and understanding.

Related issues that merit consideration include how long a child's family members have been in this country (i.e., recent immigrants vs. second- or third-generation residents); the extent to which the family embraces English as a second language; the child's attitude toward the native language and English (a child with only one parent who speaks a foreign language, and with no community support for that language, often understands but refuses to speak that language, as was the case with Crystal before the family moved to Taiwan); educational background; and other factors affecting a family's status (e.g., being refugees from war, being discriminated against for the first time). After a child's linguistic background is established, the child can then be assessed more accurately.

Assessment of potential disabilities is further complicated by three critical factors: a lack of research regarding typical patterns of language development for many languages (Stokes & Duncan, 1989); a lack of appropriate instrumentation and norms for expected levels of development across all developmental domains for different cultural groups and for bilingual children in particular; and a lack of trained staff members to conduct these assessments. These difficulties compound the fact that even the best general screening measures have only moderate reliability and validity (see Chapter 6).

Routine Language/Cultural/Demographic Survey of District Families

In order to prepare for efficient, valid screening and in-depth assessment of culturally and linguistically diverse children, districts need up-to-date information on the language/cultural backgrounds and demographic status of families living in the district. Such information could be very helpful to administrators in planning for screening as well as programming needs (Braden, 1989). Figure 9.2 illustrates the type of form suggested.

As a first step, this type of information could be collected as part of a door-to-door census, which many districts conduct every year. It could also be done as part of a telephone survey (families without telephones would need home visits), or it could be completed when parents enroll their children for kindergarten. Many families do not have any adult members who are fluent in English, so mail queries will not elicit adequate

Child's name:

Child's birth date:

Age (clarify; some cultures do not record birth dates or start counting the first year at birth):

Gender: Male Female

Address:

Telephone number:

Language/dialect child speaks at home:

Child's primary language:

Child's first language (if different):

Does the child speak English? Yes No

Does the child understand English? Yes No

Parent/guardian name:

Address (if different from child's):

Telephone number(s):

Please list all of the people who live at home with your child:

Name	Relation to child	Primary language/other languages used or understood
Adults:		
Children (ages):		

How long (months or years) have you been in the U.S./Canada (or off the reservation)? Your children?

How long (months or years) have you lived in this community?

Who takes care of the child after school? What language does this person (or persons) use with the child?

Name, address, and telephone number of person in the family or community who might serve as an interpreter (if applicable)?

FIGURE 9.2. Family/child language, cultural, and demographic survey.

information unless forms are translated; even then, some parents may not be fluent readers of their own language, or they may fail to return the forms. Because of the risk for educational difficulties that many children from these families have, Braden (1989) recommends that parents or guardians be required to fill out a survey form at the time the students are enrolled (with translated forms available). Another approach is to contact community agencies that are involved with non-English-background groups and ask them to encourage their members to make sure that all of this information is on file with the local school district. Listing the name and address of a cultural community member who is willing to serve as an initial contact, and prominently advertising the availability of trained interpreters (if available), are effective strategies as well (Anderson & Fenichel, 1989). If the local population includes many undocumented immigrants, school personnel may want to emphasize that they do not report families to the federal Immigration and Naturalization Service. Demographic information collected in this fashion can be used for instructional planning and to evaluate the effectiveness of outreach programs and intervention programs by identifying particular groups that are either not being served or are having particular difficulties in their programs (Braden, 1989). A group in need of special outreach consists of migrant worker families and their children, many of whom are ELLs. Districts that serve this population will also need to reach out to other districts that educate these children, in order to ensure a timely exchange of educational records (as is required by the NCLB Act of 2001).

As much information as possible about a particular language community should be gathered, particularly information about degree of literacy, attitudes toward disability, expectations of professionals, and cultural courtesies and customs. The National Center for Clinical Infant Programs recommends that states employ professionals skilled in survey data collection and ethnographic fieldwork to gather this data continuously (Anderson & Fenichel, 1989). Knowledge of the historical and cultural context of various groups; their patterns of migration; their practices or preferences regarding child rearing and family roles; their SES level(s), religion, age distribution, employment patterns, housing conditions (location and stability), educational facilities, and degree of isolation; health problems/disabling conditions prevalent in their group; and the effects of racism on the population are all very helpful in preparing staff members to reach out in a culturally friendly manner (Anderson & Fenichel, 1989; Vasquez-Nuttall, De Leon, & Del Valle, 1990). Refugee groups that may have experienced war or other traumatic circumstances prior to immigrating will have a different set of problems and living conditions from that of a middle-class elite motivated to immigrate because of economic circumstances and welcomed into the country because of their vocational skills.

Hiring and Training Staff Members for Linguistic and Cultural Diversity

The language/cultural/demographic survey will give a district information on the size and diversity of its language populations—information that is useful in deciding what language and cultural groups will need representation on the screening and assessment team. This survey needs to be supplemented by follow-up contacts with leaders of cultural groups and community agencies that regularly serve immigrant or minority families, to ascertain whether there is a greater prevalence of particular health problems (e.g., otitis media in Navajo children) or mental health needs (e.g., psychological trauma in Afghani refugees) among these families. If so, augmentation of the staff may be required.

The issues raised thus far are further complicated by the lack of bilingual professionals who are sufficiently knowledgeable about early childhood to carry out in-depth assessment. The sheer diversity of languages represented in the North American school system means that even if there were enough bilingual early childhood specialists in the more common languages, there would still be a need for interpreters and translators of written material (e.g., consent forms for evaluation, IEPs, and special education guidelines) in less commonly represented languages. This shortage represents a tremendous challenge at the early childhood level, where many children do not have well-developed verbal skills to begin with. The assessor confronted with understanding the extent and nature of a problem, along with the child's strengths and learning strategies, may find it necessary to use an interpreter to conduct a family interview, administer a language proficiency exam, or elicit a language sample. Although this practice may be unavoidable, it often introduces error, and conclusions need to be drawn with caution.

As pointed out by Ohtake, Santos, and Fowler (2000), "Interpretation is a process in which interpreters convey information, thoughts, and feelings attached to sentences, actions, and gestures by the speaker, considering contexts in which both the particular sentence is conveyed and the cultures in which the speaker and listener lives" (p. 13). This activity requires training and practice. Plata (1993) details guidelines for the selection of interpreters in special education, along with the limits of their responsibilities and ethical issues. Desirable characteristics include the following:

1. Proficiency in a child's first language, including the nuances and pragmatics of that language.
2. Sufficient familiarity with the culture to pick up nonverbal cues and to understand child and family needs.
3. Knowledge of special education concerns, terminology, and procedures.
4. Ability to relay information accurately and to take a secondary role in the referral and placement process.
5. Ability to read and write English.
6. Ability to interact appropriately with individuals from varying cultures and educational backgrounds.
7. Ability to be trusted, abide by school rules, maintain confidentiality, and respect the rights of others.

Plata also details potential problems in using interpreters or translators of English-language tests, including the stress of on-the-spot interpretation, loss of meaning in the translation process, geographical variations in how terms are used, and possible resentment toward monolingual colleagues or more highly paid professionals. Some interpreters may want to help the child earn a higher score and thus augment an answer. All of these issues are highlighted when interpreters are used during the administration of intelligence tests, where it is essential to pick up shades of meaning, nonverbal cues, and indicators of emerging knowledge. This is poor assessment practice and should not be used.

Barnett (1989) details steps for interacting with interpreters during speech therapy sessions that are important considerations for assessors in general. Barnett makes several specific suggestions:

1. Presession planning and discussion, including the purpose of the session, seating arrangements, type of translation to be used (word-for-word vs. sentence-by-sentence), use of eye contact, and the interpreter's role in assessment (such as eliciting a language sample).
2. Using clear, unambiguous messages to facilitate the interpretation task.

3. Providing the interpreter the opportunity to seek clarification, if needed, from the assessor.
4. Postsession debriefing to clarify misunderstandings, discuss procedures, and close up possible communication gaps.

Lopez (2002) and Rhodes, Ochoa, and Ortiz (2005) cover the same points, but in much more detail, for school psychologists working with interpreters.

If bilingual professionals and paraprofessionals are not available locally for translation and assessment, they might be borrowed from neighboring school districts, the courts, community agencies, embassies, or university training programs in school psychology, special education, bilingual education, and/or speech pathology. The National Association of School Psychologists (NASP, 2000) has published the Directory of Bilingual School Psychologists to facilitate this process for one professional group. Alternatively, the district might consider recruiting and training paraprofessionals from the local communities. In addition, representatives of local cultural groups might also be asked to consult with or serve on the screening and diagnostic team, in order to increase the team's sensitivity to each group's cultural norms and values, and to assist in the modification of existing tests or eventual development of new instruments. Table 9.3 contains guidelines for such selection and training. Because ethical standards require professionals to be fully responsible for the supportive personnel who offer clinical services under their supervision, it is imperative that supervising professionals take great care in selecting and training their assistants. Paraprofessionals should only engage in activities in which they have been trained; they must be closely supervised; and they should not be responsible for making educational or psychological decisions. To ensure quality, confidentiality, and consistency of services, bilingual paraprofessionals should be paid and treated as valued staff members (Mattes & Omark, 1984).

Regardless of who does the interpreting, Figure 9.3 is a checklist that can be used by a professional and an interpreter to evaluate their joint effectiveness in a conference or interview with parents. Plata (1993), Lynch (2004b), the Los Angeles Unified School District (1988), and Ohtake et al. (2000) are additional sources of useful information on this topic.

Strategies for Community Outreach and Creating a Culturally Friendly Screening Environment

If a screening is held at one time for all children, then an open house for community agencies and volunteer groups could be held at the same time. This would require considerable advance planning the first time it is done. However, it would facilitate community adjustment for new residents by introducing them to representatives of institutions (legal, healthcare, social service, adult educational, and religious) in which they might have an interest. It would also familiarize staff members with relevant local services and their bilingual personnel, foster community coordination, and possibly facilitate program development in conjunction with the cultures served. If screenings are scheduled individually, the school social worker or psychologist could ensure that family members are aware of local services and could provide assistance in contacting them as needed.

Since screening is often a school staff's first opportunity to interact with a family, it is essential to take this opportunity to prove a positive sense of what a home–school relationship might become, and to establish a strong beginning for what may become an important long-term relationship if the family has a child with a disability. Figure 9.4 is a

TABLE 9.3. Guidelines for Selection and Training of Bilingual Paraprofessionals and Professionals

Guidelines for selection

- Oral fluency in both English and the second language (ensure by interviewing in both languages).
- Adequate reading/writing literacy in second language (ensure by having test stimuli read orally and dictated material recorded in second language).
- Skill in relating to children and families of the cultural group to be assessed (check experience and references).
- Discretion and respect for parental and school authority (neutrality) (check references and assess by interview).
- Availability (assess priorities and potential time conflicts).
- Personal characteristics (such as age, gender, class/caste, and religion) that may make certain interpreters more or less effective with certain cultural groups (check with community leaders).

Training content

- Characteristics of the preschool child, and levels and range of development expected in the domains of cognitive, language, motor, socioemotional, and adaptive behavior.
- First- and second-language acquisition, and the differences between communicative differences and communication disorders.
- Psychological and special education terminology, and the meanings of testing practices, test results, and placements, so that they can be explained to family members.
- Goals of screening and diagnostic evaluation, and use of results in educational decision making.
- Role of the paraprofessional on an assessment team.
- Cultural differences that may affect performance, and thus test administration and interpretation.
- Procedures and observed practice in administering, scoring, and interpreting specific instruments.
- Relating effectively to parents and children of the language/cultural group to be assessed.
- Ethics and laws related to psychoeducational screening and assessment.
- Adaptations of interviewing skills for the cultural group assessed.
- Practice in role-played or actual situations, to improve the skills of both the paraprofessionals and the professionals.

Note. Data from Mattes and Omark (1984) and Barnett (1989).

checklist of things screening committees can do to establish a culturally friendly screening environment. If the language/cultural/demographic survey of the district has been conducted and cultural groups researched, the staff knows which languages and cultures are represented in their district and what needs are represented within these groups.

Assessing Language Proficiency

Language proficiency is difficult to determine in the most thorough of assessments, as it reflects so many concepts—receptive understanding, oral production, pragmatic usage, accent, reading, and writing (Bialystok, 2001). One of the best-regarded proficiency measures is the Bilingual Verbal Ability Test (BVAT-NU; Muñoz-Sandoval, Cummins, Alvarado, Ruef, & Schrank, 2005). It assesses English proficiency for ages 5 to adult-

Preconference planning

Did you:

____ Review issues of confidentiality/neutrality?

____ Discuss purpose/goals of meeting?

____ Plan the format?

____ Review and practice questions to be asked and critical content to be covered?

____ Arrange meeting space to be welcoming, comfortable, and intimate?

Considerations for a successful interview

Did you:

____ Greet parents using culturally appropriate forms of address, and obtain preferred names and correct pronunciation?

____ Ensure that the parents could see both of you (the professional and the interpreter)?

____ Introduce both yourselves (the professional through the interpreter) to the parents, including name, position, and current or future relationship to child (if any)?

____ Present yourselves as a unified team?

____ State the purpose of the meeting and its estimated length (the professional through the interpreter)?

____ (The professional) Stick to only a few topics, and pause for interpretation after several sentences?

____ (The interpreter) Clearly and precisely interpret all comments made, ask for clarification when necessary, and use language that parents could understand?

____ (The professional, through the interpreter) Summarize the meeting, ask for questions, provide answers as far as possible, and describe follow-up (if appropriate)?

____ Try not to rush parents?

Postinterview review

____ Did you review information gathered to ensure accuracy, any problems that arose during the meeting, and any problems in the interpretation process? Did you reinforce the confidentiality of the information?

____ Did either of you (interpreter or professional) experience any discomfort during this meeting?

____ Will the interpreter have further contact with the family (e.g., at the IEP meeting)?

Case notes or reports

____ (The professional) Did you indicate that an interpreter was used, the extent to which his or her services were needed, and your assessment of the effectiveness of the communication with the family?

FIGURE 9.3. Checklist for assessing interpreter's and professional's effectiveness in a parent interview.

hood, using three subtests (Oral Vocabulary, Picture Vocabulary and Verbal Analogies) from the Woodcock–Johnson Psycho-Educational Battery—Revised Tests of Cognitive Ability (Woodcock & Johnson, 1989), as well as providing translated subtests in 18 other languages (e.g., Spanish, Navajo, Arabic, Hmong). Individuals are administered the subtests in English first, and then are given those items that were missed in their native language. The score on each subtest includes the total number of items correct in both languages. The BVAT-NU uses a reasonable and efficient procedure, given the number of languages that may need to be assessed. However, assessors need to be aware that the test is an English-language measure that assesses receptive and expressive vocabulary and verbal reasoning. The verbal concepts assessed are those selected to reflect the content and order in which vocabulary develops in American children, not in children from the diverse cultures represented in the translated versions. Directions may be difficult, confounding cognitive factors with language proficiency. It also starts at age 5 or kindergarten and thus has insufficient floor (or number of easy items) for many children referred for suspected learning difficulties.

If a child is bilingual in Spanish and English, than oral-language proficiency can also be assessed with the Batería III Woodcock–Muñoz (Muñoz-Sandoval, Woodcock, McGrew, & Mather, 2005). This carefully constructed Spanish version of the Woodcock–Johnson III (WJ III; Woodcock, McGrew, & Mather, 2001a) has an extended oral-language cluster that can be useful in assessing a child's oral-language competence in both languages starting at age 2. A Comparative Language Index (CLI), consisting of the ratio between the child's Relative Proficiency Index (RPI) in Spanish on the Batería divided by the child's RPI in English on the WJ III, provides a standardized way of comparing proficiency in each language, relative to age or grade peers. For example, a Spanish/English ratio of 82/90 in Spanish and 20/90 in English would be expressed as S/E CLI = 82/20, indicating 82% proficiency in Spanish on those language tasks performed with 90% proficiency by average 5-year-olds in the Spanish normative group and a 20% proficiency on those language tasks performed with 90% proficiency by 5-year-olds in the United States.

The BVAT-NU and the Batería are problematic in that: (1) they are normed on predominantly monolingual populations, not simultaneous or sequential bilingual populations as is the norm in North America; (2) the Woodcock–Johnson, on which both are

____ Have multicultural, bilingual professionals or trained paraprofessionals available to welcome parents and answer questions.

____ Ensure that the bilingual professionals can give parents as much time as they need to understand an assessment process that may be confusing and threatening.

____ Use posters and art to indicate an appreciation of local ethnic groups.

____ Attend to literacy issues when giving written materials (i.e., adjust the reading level in English or the translated forms to the educational level of the parents; provide definitions for special education or psychological/psychiatric terms).

____ Translate all materials for parents into the major local language and dialects; both the language itself and its manner of usage and presentation are important.

____ Use videos with presentations on screening for nonreading parents of all language groups; attend to cultural issues in presentation.

____ Offer snacks and beverages that are culturally appropriate (e.g., *café con leche*, green tea).

____ Provide pamphlets on other services for children and families in the community.

____ Provide time for face-to-face feedback, and the name of a person to contact who speaks the same language if later questions arise.

____ Consider holding the screening at a site that is familiar to or owned by the cultural/language group being assessed (e.g., a building owned by a Native American tribal corporation).

____ Use warm-up activities to help the child feel comfortable and know what is expected.

____ Screen child for vision and hearing problems.

____ Take time for social interaction prior to direct interview; be willing to be either more personal and self-revealing or more formal, depending on what is appropriate for the particular culture.

____ Learn how to greet and say goodbye to family members in their native language and with culturally appropriate gestures (e.g., hand shaking, bowing, or greeting oldest male family member first).

FIGURE 9.4. Checklist for making the screening environment culturally friendly.

based, is not an appealing test for preschoolers and it can be a challenge to keep them engaged in testing and thus obtain valid results; and (3) they assess a limited array of language skills in an artificial context, which is characteristic of every formal language measure.

How can screening for language proficiency be done fairly, using nondiscriminatory practices? We offer some suggestions below.

- *Step 1*. For children of non-English backgrounds, an examination of language proficiency in both their mother tongue and English is an essential first step prior to screening for any potential disabilities or developmental delays (see Figure 9.5). Several procedures are used to obtain this information: the district language/cultural/demographic survey, or a family interview; a language proficiency measure (if available); and, preferably, observation of the children using language in a natural context (e.g., playtime, snacktime). To compile this information systematically, we have developed the form presented in Figure 9.6. All of these options have attendant problems: The district survey gives no information on language competence; the family interview is dependent on the

- **Step 1:** Determining language proficiency in English and first or primary language through language/cultural/demographic survey, proficiency test, or observation of language use in a natural context (good measures do not exist at the preschool level). What is the child's:
  Level of oral proficiency in English?
  Level of oral proficiency in first or primary language?

- **Step 2:** Screening for learning and behavior problems.

If child speaks good English, administer standard preschool screening tool in English *and* (if one exists) in first or primary language.	If child speaks some or no English, administer locally normed screening tool in first or primary language (if one exists).	If no locally normed test exists, use family interview and natural language sample to determine risk; if district has large language population, consider translating and restandardizing English test. Because of their ease of administration and psychometric properties we would recommend using Ages and Stages as a parent measure and the Early Screening Inventory—Revised for developmental screening.

- **Step 3:** Decision making or further assessment.

If child passes test in English, confer with parents and teachers regarding bilingual background and whether or not to provide support for first language. If child does not pass test in English, but passes in first/primary language, see middle column.	If child passes test in first/primary language, or if alternative methods described above indicate normal functioning, refer to bilingual education for language enrichment or dual-language program.	If child does not pass test in first/primary language, or if alternative methods described above suggest developmental delays, refer for diagnostic observation and/or special education/bilingual education evaluation. Conduct Transdisciplinary Play-Based Assessment of language and other developmental areas.

FIGURE 9.5. The screening and decision process with linguistically diverse preschoolers.

1. What language(s) does the child speak? (if more than one, circle the one that is dominant.)
2. What language(s) are spoken in the home? (If more than one, circle the one that is dominant.)
3. What language(s) do parents use to speak to each other? To the child?
4. What language(s) do siblings use to speak to each other? To the parents? To peers? To other adults in the family or to regular caregivers?
5. How long has the child's family been in this country?

Estimate how many months the child has been exposed to English:

0	3	6	9	12	15	18	21	24	27	30
					Should begin to be proficient in conversation; if not, observe carefully.				If not proficient, refer.	

Describe child's language use in everyday, natural contexts:

First or primary language:
  Family report:
  Teacher observation:

Direct observation:
  To elicit language proficiency, ask a child to:
  Retell a story,
  Play a copycat game,
  Follow your directions,
  Ask you questions,
  Talk with peers or siblings.

English:
  Family report:
  Teacher observation:
  Direct observation (see above):

In first or primary language, does the child use language to convey needs/wants?

Are any signs of language problems present in the child's first or primary language?
____ Frequent repetitions/hesitations
____ Many false starts; self-interruptions
____ Delays before responding _____ Long delays
____ Nonspecific vocabulary/word-finding difficulty
____ Requests for repetition: _____ Frequent _____ Seldom
____ Grammatical errors
____ Articulation difficulties
____ Moving back and forth between languages

Overall, estimate competence in English and first or primary language (indicate basis for your estimate):
  In English:
  In first or primary language:
  Refer if both ratings are "poor" or "very poor," based on *reliable* sources of information.

How would you describe the child's progress in other areas?

	Like most children	Have some concerns
Physical and motor skills		
Learning skills		
Getting along with others		

Comments:

FIGURE 9.6. Proficiency checklist for the first (or primary) and second languages of young children.

skill of the interviewer and the quality of the information provided by the respondents, which can range from excellent (for observant, experienced parents) to vague (for survival-focused parents) to misleading (for families from cultures where flaws in children are not shared with nonrelatives); language proficiency measures are limited by age and language, and the degree to which they sample key syntactic features is questionable; and obtaining a good language sample through observation requires a trained observer and time.

We think that the best practice is to engage in intense outreach in the cultural/language community through interviews, to identify children with possible developmental delays as early as possible (as is required by IDEA 2004). Children, who are not identified through outreach should be screened prior to kindergarten entry for sight, hearing, and health problems, and their parents should be interviewed to see if they have any concerns (as noted earlier, the assessor needs to be mindful that for some parents, such an interview is highly stressful and clashes with cultural practices). Some children will be referred for further assessment through this process. If enough such children of one language group are identified, a bilingual classroom with a qualified teacher might be the best option; if such a classroom is not available, a child might be placed in a kindergarten, with a tutor. *Instead of spending screening funds on invalid assessment tools for this population, the money could be used for training all teachers to work effectively with children who are ELLs, and to provide ongoing consultation and observation with specialists to identify children over the course of the year who may need further evaluation.* Kindergarten and first-grade teachers are more accurate than brief screening measures in identifying monolingual children with learning problems. We think that with training and the opportunity to consult with specialists, teachers could become equally good at differentiating between cultural differences and second-language acquisition on the one hand, and genuine language and learning disorders on the other.

• *Step 2*. If the language survey, family interview, or language proficiency exam suggests that a child is competent in English, he or she should be given the standard developmental screening measure in English and in his or her first language (if such a measure exists). If the child passes the test in English, it should be clearly noted on the test protocol that the child is bilingual, and the results should be interpreted cautiously with this in mind; the child may still need extra support in the classroom. It should be noted, however, that the criterion level for "pass" varies by school district. For example, what is considered within the "average" range is generally at least the 16th–26th percentile or better. This decision must be backed up by information from the family interview and discussion with the family, to decide whether or not tutorial support or a bilingual program (if one is available) will be recommended when the child starts school. Areas of potential strength or limitation can be noted as well. An English proficiency measure should not be used in isolation.

If the child is not competent in English, the family interview, a language proficiency exam in the native language, and possibly a native-language developmental screening measure (if one exists) may suggest normal development. Bilingual education or other supports should be recommended as appropriate.

• *Step 3*. If on the other hand, the family interview or scores on the native-language proficiency or developmental screening measure suggest developmental delays, a referral to determine eligibility for bilingual special education may or may not be appropriate. We recommend a more detailed family interview, an examination of test responses, and a naturalistic language sample before a referral decision is made. The family may speak a dialect that is different from the form of the language used on the screening test, or the testing materials may be culturally irrelevant even though the child speaks the language (e.g., an East Asian parent may be asked if her child uses a knife or fork). We recommend that a natural language sample be obtained by a speech pathologist (preferably a native speaker of the child's language) and reviewed by either the speech–language specialist or a native speaker of the language who can judge the age-appropriateness of the child's speech and language. Videotaping the language sample is quite useful if the sample is not obtained by the person doing the evaluating. Clearly, this procedure is not feasible for all children; it is, however, a necessary step for children for whom there is concern that special education services might be needed. The natural language sample needs to be supplemented, where possible, by observational data obtained by the parent and teacher. If a problem is identified either by family report or from the language sample, Transdisciplinary Play-Based Assessment (TPBA) might be used for further evaluation (see Chapter 4) if culturally sensitive assessors are available. These procedures may result in a more representative sample of behaviors.

Another caution in this area is to avoid making premature assumptions about language preference or dominance based on the child's last name, language spoken in the home, or country of origin. For example, in our experience, it is not uncommon to find a Mayan from Guatemala placed in a Spanish bilingual program, even though the child knows no Spanish; placement in such a case is (wrongly) based on country of origin. (One Mayan father reported, through an interpreter, that he was pleased that in the United States his children could finally learn to speak Spanish—a language that would assist them economically if they were still living in Guatemala.)

Modifying and Restandardizing English-Language Tests

If an appropriate second-language developmental screening measure does not exist, a district or community might consider thoroughly revising an English-language test so that it accurately reflects the linguistic structure and cultural relevance in item content of the second language. This could also be done with English-language preschool screening tests or curriculum-based assessment (CBA) (see Dayan, 1993). This step is labor-intensive and only worth doing if one or two large, stable language groups are present in a district, and if the information yielded leads to curriculum planning. Chapter 3 describes this process in detail. Otherwise, the choice is use of an inappropriate test (which should be avoided) or the use of alternative assessment procedures (which are described below).

SCREENING AND ASSESSMENT OF LEARNING AND BEHAVIOR PROBLEMS

Use of Family Interview

The language survey and the information obtained from interviewing the parents or other relatives in attendance at the screening or assessment session should provide a good indication of the degree to which a child is competent in various languages, as well as any concerns that the family may have about the child's development. In addition to the questions listed earlier in Figure 9.2 for the language survey, the following questions are useful: What language(s) do the parents speak to each other? To the child? What languages do the siblings use with each other? With peers? Have the parents or other relatives noticed any problems with language development, behavior, thinking, self-help skills, or motor skills? Have any other family members had any problems in any of these areas? In asking these last two questions, it is helpful to know (1) whether the family is from a culture that feels comfortable acknowledging problems on the part of family members; (2) what expectations the culture has for children's achievement of developmental milestones; and (3) what behaviors and skills it values and fosters in preschool children. If the family reports a concern, further evaluation is indicated.

Non-English Versions of Early Childhood Measures

Of the widely used screening and diagnostic measures used in early childhood assessment, a number are now available and normed in Spanish. Some examples of such screening measures include the Boehm Test of Basic Concepts—Third Edition and its preschool version (Boehm-3 and Boehm-3: Preschool; Boehm, 2000a, 2001); the Preschool Language Scale—Fourth Edition, Spanish Version (PLS-4; Zimmerman, Steiner, & Pond, 2002); the Early Screening Inventory—Revised (ESI-R; Meisels et al., 1997); the Developmental Indicators for the Assessment of Learning—Third Edition (DIAL-3; Mardell-Czudnowski & Goldberg, 1998); and the Ages and Stages Questionnaires—Second Edition (ASQ; Bricker & Squires, 1999). Some examples of such diagnostic measures include the Batería III Woodcock–Muñoz (Woodcock, Muñoz-Sandoval, McGrew, Mather, & Schrank, 2005) and the Wechsler Intelligence Scale for Children—Fourth Edition (WISC-IV) Spanish (Wechsler, 2004). In addition to normed tests, numerous translations of measures exist. For example, the original version of the Child Behavior Checklist (Achenbach & Edelbrock, 1983) was translated into many languages, but the norms used in the past were based on the mainstream U.S. population. Publishers and test authors are the best sources of information, although they do not necessarily know of work that has been done across North America or abroad. R. Paul (2001) is a good source of information on early childhood measures available in languages other than English. Presently, as major tests are being revised or developed, they are being made available, normed, and validated in Spanish.

Developing CBA instruments in other languages for kindergarten and first-grade students is another option (Dayan, 1992). However, this approach has been criticized as highly susceptible to bias if students are in bilingual programs that do not provide enough instructional support for their first language. Without such support, they will not be able to make adequate progress relative to the test's grade equivalents (Figueroa, 1990; see also Gersten & Woodward, 1994). This is less of a concern with preschool and kindergarten children in initial screening and assessment, but the criticism might apply to reevaluations using CBA. If support for the first language is provided, the CBA approach has much promise because of its built-in evaluation of student progress.

Reducing Bias When English-Language Tests Are Used

If a child has sufficient English to be given the standard instruments in English, several modifications can be made to reduce bias. These suggestions are derived from Erickson and Iglesias (1986).

1. Before using a test, examine each item to evaluate whether the child will have had access to the information being tested.
2. Administer the test in a standardized form, followed by testing of the limits, which should include the following:
   a. Rewording instructions.
   b. Providing additional time for the child to respond.

c. Continuing testing beyond the ceiling.
d. Developing warm-up practice items if the test does not have any, so that the process of "taking the test" is established.
e. Having the child name an item in addition to pointing on picture vocabulary tests, in order to ascertain what word the child uses and to tell what the child thinks he or she is seeing.
f. Having the child explain why the "incorrect" answer was selected.
g. Having the child identify actual objects, body parts, actions (in photographs), and so forth, particularly if he or she has had limited experience with books, line drawings, or the testing process.

3. Record all responses, particularly when the child changes an answer, explains, comments, or demonstrates.
4. Consider the influence of dialect and learning a new language when evaluating responses. Rescore articulation and expressive language samples as necessary, giving credit for variation or differences.

Observing Communication and Developmental Achievements in Natural Settings

Probably the most valid assessment method for a young child is observation of the child interacting with his or her caregiver in a familiar setting, such as a classroom or home environment. A clinic playroom is the next best alternative, since play is a natural activity for children. Observations in the familiar setting are typically used as a last resort because of professional time constraints, unless a child is suspected of having a disability (see Linder, 1996, for a model of assessing children while at play). If this powerful assessment approach cannot be employed, assessment should involve collecting a language sample, possibly with the mother or other caregiver present, that can be tape-recorded by a staff member or the caregiver at home and analyzed later by a staff member, professional, or paraprofessional with knowledge of that particular language (see Miller, 1981, and Chapter 10 on obtaining language samples). If an appropriate interpreter is available, the mother can be interviewed about language and adaptive behavior; of course, the interviewer must bear in mind that each culture has different norms and expectations for children in terms of communication and social behavior.

Regardless of the approach or methods used in screening for potential learning or behavioral problems, the ethics of the American Psychological Association (2002) require psychologists to note any reservations they may have about assessment results because of the assessment circumstances or because of questions about the appropriateness of norms for the person tested.

In-Depth Assessment Considerations

Assessment Decisions

WHEN TO RECOMMEND NO SPECIAL SERVICES

Bilingual children need no special services when they can perform at a level comparable to that of the average monolingual English-speaking child. This usually means performance at the 16th–25th percentile or better on either nationally or locally normed tests of academic preparedness/progress and language development. Regardless of whether a child needs to be referred for a possible learning problem, a child who is bilingual also needs to be thoroughly assessed in his or her first language, so that an appropriate educational program can be developed. The research of Ellis (1981) showed us that teaching English or another second languages to a child who is still developing in his or her first language may have adverse consequences for the development of both languages, if the structured form of input is not in line with the child's acquisition level. Thus formal instruction should be preceded by careful assessment in all areas of both languages, so that appropriate stimulation programs for developing normal language patterns, and possibly for remediating deviant or delayed language patterns, can be devised (Duncan, 1989). Furthermore, a delay in both languages does not necessarily mean that a child has a learning disability. Schiff-Myers et al. (1993) underscore the fact that many children with LEP learn language normally; they do not have disabilities. They caution assessors to (1) recognize that a child's learning of a second language may result in loss of proficiency or arrested development in the child's first language; (2) consider the types of errors the child makes and the possible reasons for these errors (including limited vocabulary, syntactic or pragmatic errors, receptive and productive skills, comprehension, content, and the use of language); and (3) consider interventions that might take place in regular education contexts, such as language tutoring, so that the child will not be classified as having a language disorder.

> Ricardo, age 5-5 and in kindergarten, was referred by his mother for an evaluation because of concerns about his expressive-language skills (he would get frustrated when he couldn't find the right word) and separation anxiety. English and Spanish are spoken in his home by both of his parents and he is cared for by his grandmother who speaks only Spanish. He had received early intervention for language in English from ages 2-5–4. He attends an English-only kindergarten which he enjoys and where he has many friends. On the Extended Oral Language cluster of the Batería and the WJ III he had a Spanish/English CLI of 2/89, indicating that he was monolingual and competent in English. All of his readiness skills on the Brigance Inventory of Early Development—II were age appropriate or above, indicating good preparation for first grade. On the Boehm Test of Basics Concepts—Third Edition in English his score fell at the 70th percentile, indicating an adequate mastery of concepts important for following teacher directions. Because of his good oral language, competence in readiness tasks, reports by his teacher that he is one of the best beginning readers in the class, his knowledge of basics concepts, and his good social and behavioral adjustment at school, there was no educational reason for him to be in a bilingual program unless his parents wanted to have him educated in both languages. As this was not a priority for them, bilingual education was not recommended.

WHEN TO RECOMMEND BILINGUAL EDUCATION

Children who are ELLs are entitled to a free, appropriate education, which should include instructional services in their primary language if it is not English. If the results of the screening and the information furnished by the family and other service providers suggest that the child's primary language is not English, then bilingual education might be considered for the child when he or she enters school. The specific form of bilingual service will vary and is usually determined by the types of bilingual programs available in a particular school district, the preferences of parents, and the needs of the child. If a large number of students (22 or more) of the same language background (almost always Spanish) need services, then a bilingual class is sometimes provided. If fewer students are involved, then a tutor may be provided or the child may be placed in a multilingual ESL class. However, regardless of what programs are available, they should involve appreciation of, and development and/or maintenance of, the child's native language while also providing opportunities to learn English (see Duncan, 1989; Genesee, Paradis, & Crago, 2004).

> Martha, age 5-1, the daughter of recent immigrants from the Dominican Republic, was referred by her parents who were concerned about whether she should stay an extra year in her prekindergarten/kindergarten program or move to a different program for first grade. Martha had a history of separation anxiety and her parents were concerned about how she would do if moved but they were also concerned that she did not seem to be learning as much as they had hoped. Although most of the students and the teacher in her prekindergarten class were Hispanic, English was the language of instruction. Observation in the classroom indicated that Martha was well adjusted and happy in her well-managed classroom. The classroom curriculum was clearly at a preschool level with limited time spent on emergent literacy or math activities. On the WJ III and the Batería Extended Oral Language Cluster Martha had a Spanish/English CLI of 2/81, indicating that she was monolingual but below average in her mastery of English. This was believed to be an underestimate of Martha's knowledge of Spanish because she spoke fluently with her mother in Spanish between subtests, even though she preferred English with the examiner for both casual conversation and on her response to Spanish language tasks. On the Spanish version of the Vineland Adaptive Behavior Scale—II her mother's responses placed her at the 82nd percentile, high average on the Communication domain, and her teacher's ratings on the BASC-2 Functional Communication subscale placed her at the 86th percentile. On the BTBC-3 in English she was at the 5th percentile, low average, and in Spanish at the 25th percentile, low average. When given credit for all the concepts she knew in either language she was at the 53rd percentile, average. Concepts known in one language can be easily taught in the other language. Her readiness skills on the Brigance Inventory of Early Development—II suggested that she had mastered many readiness skills in math and writing and some in reading. A well-regarded dual-language program in another school for first grade was recommended because Martha appeared to be a mixed bilingual, and education in Spanish as well as English would not only allow her to maintain the language of her family and community, but it would offer her the best chance of mastering English and doing well academically over the course of her education.

WHEN TO RECOMMEND FURTHER ASSESSMENT FOR POSSIBLE PLACEMENT IN BILINGUAL SPECIAL EDUCATION

Before a child is recommended for services as in need of both special education and ESL instruction, a fair, nondiscriminatory screening must be conducted in the child's primary language (we recommend conducting it in both or all languages, for reasons described previously). If the results of the screening indicate that he or she exhibits developmental delays in one or more areas, there are two options. The first is a referral for a formal assessment by the school's or district's committee on special education, in conjunction with the bilingual education staff (see Fradd & Weismantel, 1989, for a description of process and content). During this formal diagnostic process, assessors need to be cautious about interpreting outcomes, to avoid bias with far-reaching implications—for example, labeling a child as "deficient" on a test administered in his or her weaker language (Cummins, 1980, 2000; Genesee, Paradis, & Crago, 2004). Such a label poses a challenge for assessors, who need to determine whether (2) learning problem or an English-language proficiency problem exists. Alternative assessment procedures, such as dynamic assessment, probes, and play assessment, need to be used to understand the basis of the difficulty.

Even more desirable is the second option. Some states allow for a *diagnostic placement* (a limited period of close observation by a teacher and other professionals, to determine whether a special education referral is necessary or to provide more information to a special education team prior to final diagnosis and placement). This seems particularly appropriate for children who are both culturally and linguistically different, and we highly recommend the practice in general. Figure 9.5 has summarized the screening and assessment process.

Feedback to Families

School personnel in the United States have a habit of interacting primarily with a child's mother. In other cultures, the mother may be in charge of all caregiving, but other individuals may be more influential in making decisions about a child—including decisions about education and the receipt of special services. Grandparents, fathers, and influential uncles and aunts may have a predominant role; if the school does not seek contact with such persons, the home–school relationship may go awry. Even if the involvement of the extended family at the initial screening is minimal, if a child is being referred for further assessment it is important that other influential family members be identified at the time of feedback and that efforts be made to involve them in all further assessment and educational planning decisions.

Trust in professional judgment, even when culturally prescribed, may be easily undermined when parents discover the discrepancy between their beliefs about children and child rearing and those of school professionals (e.g., the degree to which children should be involved in making choices). Harry (1992) recommends examining one's own professional views from the context of cultural relativity, treating parents' "most un-American beliefs" (p. 346) with respect, and explicitly discussing with parents different cultural values and practices, in order to find a way to discover and address common goals that will offer real assistance to families and their children. This respect and open dialogue may then increase parents' willingness to consider professional evaluations and recommendations, and to proffer their own wishes and concerns.

SUMMARY

This chapter attempts to provide practical suggestions for accomplishing a professionally difficult and time-consuming task: screening and assessing culturally and linguistically diverse preschoolers for potential learning problems in a less biased manner than has previously been the case. The task requires an interest in and respect for bilingualism and cultural diversity, a willingness to reflect on cultural relativism, and the energy to work at achieving best practices at a local level. To highlight the key points of this chapter and provide an opportunity for self-assessment, we have listed below some major questions assessors need to be raising when they work with linguistically and culturally diverse families and their children. Table 9.4 provides a parallel list of questions for districts and agencies.

- Have you examined your own culture from a relativistic perspective?
- Do you know enough about second-language (and first-language) acquisition to make decisions about the developmental progress of bilingual children?

TABLE 9.4. Self-Evaluation of District/Agency Support and Assessment Practices for Children Who Are ELLs

Education practices/beliefs

1. Are children's first languages supported by the agency/school?
2. What is the local philosophy about bilingual instruction?
3. What are the early childhood teachers' belief systems about bilingualism?
   - Does it impede cognitive level?
   - Does it have cognitive benefits?
   - Should parents be encouraged to speak only English to their children (even if they are not fluent in it)?
   - Is African American English respected, or viewed as "inferior"?
4. What are the beliefs of mainstream parents? Of culturally different parents?

District/agency assessors' practices/beliefs

1. Have assessors examined their own cultural attitudes/feelings?
2. What are their beliefs about bilingualism?
3. Do they know enough about both first- and second-language acquisition to make sound decisions?
4. Do they know enough about the specific language groups in your district?
5. To what extent are assessment results used to formulate intervention carried out in classrooms or by specialists?

Typical assessment situation

1. Is instrument, rating scale, etc., translated and normed?
   - Translated only?
   - Spontaneously translated?
   - Norms appropriate to the child's particular cultural subgroup?
2. Is child's performance on English version *and* translated version (if one exists) of a test considered?
3. Is child's knowledge base (correct response to different items) assessed *across* test versions?
4. Are instrument/materials/procedures/items relevant to child's culture?
5. Has the test been administered in a standardized form?
6. Is standardized testing followed by testing of the limits?
7. Have observations of language use and learning been made in natural contexts?
8. Are outcomes compared across measures?
9. Have performance-based measures been used?

Ongoing evaluation of procedures

1. Do culturally different families feel welcome?
2. Are children who are ELLs being disproportionately referred for special education evaluations?
3. Is input on district/agency practices routinely sought from the culturally different community?
4. Is there outreach to culturally different families?
5. Are bilingual assessors adequately trained?
6. Are bilingual interpreters trained in interviewing, their role during test administration, confidentiality, special education/testing terminology, and their role as members of a team?
7. What questions and concerns do interpreters have? What advice can they give?

- Have you surveyed your district to ascertain the language groups your district or catchment area includes and the range of cultures represented (e.g., are there numerous Spanish-speaking cultural groups)?
- Do you and your staff members (all who meet the public) know enough about the cultures you are serving to interact in a manner that communicates respect and may lead to the development of trusting relationships?
- Have you checked to see whether any extant language dominance or screening measures could be appropriately used in your setting?
- If no extant measures are appropriate, and the district and/or setting has a sufficient and stable population of speakers of one or more languages, have you formed a team to modify and restandardize one or more English-language tests or develop comprehensive alternative assessment approaches?
- Do you know all of the bilingual psychologists, speech pathologists, special educators, and other educators available for evaluations, interpretation, or translations in your community? Do you know their language/dialect background, SES, age, and religion, so that you can best match a particular bilingual professional with a particular family?
- If appropriate bilingual professionals are not available, have you pursued the selection and training of paraprofessional interpreters or bilingual facilitators, perhaps in conjunction with other agencies and institutions?
- If you use interpreters, have you role-played various situations with them to improve your skills in communicating with their assistance?
- Do you know how to conduct an effective observational assessment (e.g., TPBA) for those children who cannot be efficiently screened as part of the traditional process and who appear to have significant problems? Are you able to adapt this for families of different cultures (e.g., for those who are not comfortable with playing on the floor or with their children, or for mothers who are comfortable playing only without their husbands watching)?
- Do you have a flexible and sensitive plan to provide all families—and culturally different families in particular—with feedback on their children's developmental status, and to work with them on decision making as needed?

Chapter 10

Assessment of Language Development

This chapter is presented to help individuals involved in preschool assessment understand the complexity of language, appreciate the important role of the speech–language specialist, and be prepared to contribute their observations to language assessment as team members or through their own reports and recommendations. (This chapter does *not* cover speech disorders per se, including problems with production, articulation, voicing, or syllable structure.) The chapter is divided into two major sections. The first section provides the foundations for the assessment practices detailed in the second section and covers (1) the development of language among preschool children; (2) the interacting components of language; (3) sources of variability in the language behaviors of young children; and (4) forms of disability that affect language development. The second section covers procedures assessors can use to gain a representative sample of children's language abilities, and provides suggestions for linking assessment outcomes to intervention. The works of Bloom (1970, 1974, 1991), Bloom and Lahey (1978), Hart and Risley (1995, 1999), Lahey (1988), Miller (1981), McLean (1990), Olswang and Bain (1988), Owens (1995, 2004), R. Paul (2001), Prizant, Wetherby, and Roberts (1993), and Wells (1985) have been particularly influential in the preparation of this chapter.

FACTORS TO BE CONSIDERED IN THE ASSESSMENT OF LANGUAGE DEVELOPMENT

Communicative skill is a broad concept that involves multiple behaviors on the part of young children—including signs, gestures, facial expressions, and sounds, as well as speech and language. The focus of this chapter is on verbal language, as opposed to communication through gesture. As communicative skill develops, however, it becomes a means of social and emotional interaction that builds on both verbal and nonverbal behaviors; it thus involves not only the content of what is said, but also the attitudes that people convey with their faces, voices, and body actions. The development of language is closely linked to all other developmental domains: the socioemotional exchanges of the child with caretakers and peers, the child's sensory–motor development, and the child's cognitive capacities (see Figure 10.1). Since the child's daily experiences are key to language development, the nature and quality of the interactions between parents (or other caregivers) and the child need to be integral components of the assessment process. Assumptions that underlie this chapter include the following:

1. Language is a complex, rule-governed symbol system that is used for the purposes of communication (Lahey, 1988).
2. Language development influences cognitive development, and the cognitive concepts a child develops influence language.
3. Socialization depends on the acquisition of language, and language "bears the marks of socialization" (McNeill, 1970, p. 1061). Parents and children are partners in the interaction ("social dance") that serves as the basis for language development (Hart & Risley, 1999).
4. Language serves many purposes, including sharing experiences and communicating with others (both present and absent); communicating desires, thoughts, and feelings; gaining information; making requests or responding to the requests of others; understanding the feelings and thoughts of others; and establishing and maintaining social interaction.

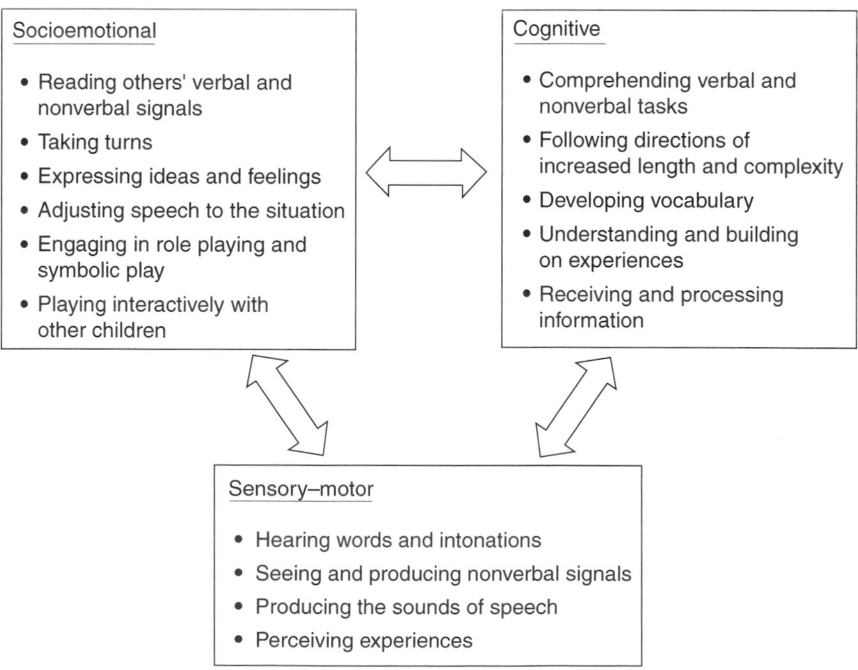

FIGURE 10.1. Interaction of language with major developmental domains.

5. A child's perceptual and motor functioning influences what he or she can perceive and do. A child with a hearing impairment will have considerable difficulty acquiring verbal language, but not nonverbal language such as American Sign Language (ASL); a child with a cleft palate will have considerable difficulty in producing sounds.
6. Many environmental factors, including culture, modeling, opportunities for communication, feedback, and range of experiences, influence language development.
7. Spoken language is one component of the child's larger communication system, which includes gestures, eye contact, and (later on) reading and writing.
8. Assessing language involves multiple steps that need to be linked with intervention.

The Development of Language among Preschool Children

The Sequence of Typical Language Development

The ages 3–5 years are a time of great development in a child's learning and use of language. According to Bloom (1991), children learn the basics of language in the year from 2 to 3, and during this year "most children will have acquired much of what they need to know for forming sentences and making conversation" (p. 1). Thus, in the course of normal development, children by age 3 will have acquired the basics of the sound system, will be using sentences, and will be carrying out conversations. Children's vocabulary is expanding rapidly and grows to more than 2,000 words between the ages of 3 and 5. By the time children are 6 years of age, they will have an expressive vocabulary of more than 2,500 words (Sweeting, 1981) and a receptive vocabulary of 14,000 words (Goswami, 2001). They can form sentences that are eight or more words long. Children will also have learned to use various sentence structures, including complex sentences, negatives, questions, and sentences expressing causality. Finally, children will have learned important conversational rules, such as taking turns and taking the perspective of another. By the time a child is 5, he or she will have acquired most adult language forms (Bloom, 1991; McNeill, 1970); see Bloom (1991) for in-depth analysis of these forms.

Experts such as Aram and Hall (1989) state, "Speech and language development represents the major learning task of the preschool years and establishes the basis upon which most later academic achievement is accessed (through listening and reading) and demonstrated (through speaking and writing)" (p. 488). Regardless of the language they acquire, children pass through the sequence of its development at roughly the same ages (McNeill, 1970). Children in the 3- to 5-year range also make great strides in using language to organize their own ideas, and use language as a part of role playing and other symbolic activities during play. Language is critical to how these children display their emotions and to how they engage in interactions with others. Assessing language therefore needs to be a multistep process in which observation of the child's interacting systems is key. A rough outline of the typical language development of preschool children is presented in Table 10.1.

The Transactional Process of Early Language Development

Within every culture, people share a language through which they exchange experiences; thus language is an important source of one's cultural heritage and sense of identity. An innate ability (referred to as the *language acquisition device*; Chomsky, 1965; McNeill,

TABLE 10.1. A Rough Outline of Language Milestones

0–6 months

- Cries, coos in response to sounds; smiles.

6–12 months

- Recognizes voices; listens when spoken or sung to.
- Babbles; imitates some speech sounds ("ma-ma").
- Begins developing communicative functions, such as the ability to draw attention to self, direct the attention of others through the use of gestures.
- Understands/responds to some words (e.g., own name, "Mama," "Daddy"), although there is wide variation in the number.
- Produces first words (10–12 months), again with wide variation in the number (0–26 in Fenson et al., 1994).
- Responds to simple requests (e.g., "Touch your nose").

12–18 months

- Understanding of words increases greatly, although with wide variation (92–321 words in the Fenson et al. study).
- Production of words increases, again with wide variation (10–150+ in the Fenson et al. study).
- Begins to make requests.
- Use of gesture continues.
- Responds to facial expressions.

18–24 months

- Large burst in naming activity occurs.
- Combines words.
- Begins to name familiar objects.
- Can point appropriately.
- Follows simple one-step commands.
- Comprehends numbers.
- Begins to recognize syllables in words and rhymes.

2–3 years

- Begins to understand turn taking.
- Burst of expressive vocabulary occurs.
- Receptive vocabulary increases to 500–900 words.
- Learns suffixes (most by 30 months).
- Learns irregular nouns and past-tense verbs.
- Learns the basics of language for forming sentences and carrying out conversations.
- Uses *why* questions.
- Understands basic concepts such as *big*, *up*.
- Points to pictures in books and responds to questions about them.

3–4 years

- Basics of the sound system are acquired.
- Great growth occurs in both receptive vocabulary (1,200–2,000 words) and expressive vocabulary (800–1,500 words).
- Uses sentences 4–8 words long.

(continued)

TABLE 10.1. *(continued)*

3–4 years *(continued)*

- Engages in conversations.
- Asks *who*, *what*, *where*, and *why* questions; some confusion with *when* questions.
- Can tell a simple story.
- Follows two-step commands.
- Uses many relational concepts, such as *over* and *under.*
- Can sing simple songs and learn rhymes.

4–5 years

- Receptive language increases to 2,800–4,000 or more words.
- Expressive language increases to 900–2,000 words.
- Syntax is almost completely developed.
- Begins to understand the relationship between letters and sounds.
- Uses various sentence structures, such as negatives, questions, expressions of causality, and complex sentences.
- Uses language to express ideas, and also as part of role playing and symbolic play.
- Follows conversational rules, such as taking turns and taking perspective of another.
- Recounts stories.
- Understands most simple questions.
- Understands and uses facial and hand gestures.

5–6 years

- Has now acquired most adult language forms.
- Blends sounds.
- Frequently asks questions.
- Follows two- and three-part commands.
- Has expressive vocabulary of 5,000–8,000 words.
- Can have a receptive vocabulary of 14,000 words.
- Sentences can be 8 or more words long.
- Shares experiences and expresses ideas verbally.
- Uses conventional aspects of communication, including pitch and inflection, appropriately.
- Understands most relational terms, such as *before* and *after, first* and *last*, and *same* and *different.*
- Understands story narratives.

Note. Data from Bloom (1974, 1991); Bredekamp and Copple (1997); Fenson et al. (1994); Goswami (2002); Hart and Risley (1999); Lahey (1988); Linder (1996); McNeill (1970); Miller (1981); Olswang and Bain (1988); and Wetherby and Prizant (1992).

1966) allows children to acquire language early in life as they interact with people around them, who provide their language acquisition support system (Bruner, 1983a, 1983b; Dyson & Genishi, 1993). The developing brain is wired to process the visual and auditory information the child experiences in his or her culture. The development of language is thus a complex process that begins during infancy and evolves as the child interacts with parents, caregivers, siblings, and playmates—first through crying, other intonations, gestures, and facial expressions with others, and then through babbling and pointing to communicate desires and needs. Clearly, the contexts and the specific socialization interactions a child experiences play an important role in language development, and learning language is closely tied to learning how to feel and think. According to Locke (1994), “It is probably the social and emotional aspect of language rather than the need to convey information that motivates the infant to talk" (p. 473). The roots of early speech thus are social, with the functions of early interactions being to maintain and develop the interpersonal relationship between the child and his or her family, and to organize and comment on the situations in which they find themselves and the activities in which they engage (Wells, 1985, p. 56). Since language depends on the social interactions that take place between a child and others, the child needs to learn to adjust to the needs of the situation and the rules of carrying out conversations, such as turn taking.

A transactional model of infant development best describes the process of early communication (McLean, 1990; Sameroff, 1975; Sameroff & MacKenzie, 2003). Within this model an "infant's observable responses are seen to serve as both the antecedent events that evoke subsequent responses from the environment and as consequent events that either reinforce or punish (i.e., increase or decrease the rate of) those subsequent environmental events. Similarly, environmental events, consisting primarily of caregiver responses, also serve dual functions as both antecedent and consequent events, evoking and rewarding (or punishing) the infant's responses" (McLean, 1990, p. 14). This transactional process obviously continues as the child develops language in the preschool years, during interactions with teachers and other children as well as with caregivers. In each case, each party in a conversation influences the messages to and from the other. For example, a preschool teacher seeks to see whether the child understands a request; the child seeks to make his or her intentions known; and each party adjusts his or her messages to the nature of the situation. Each member of the dyad needs to be considered during assessment and intervention (McLean, 1990).

The transactional process is clearly illustrated in the work of Hart and Risley (1995, 1999), who observed children from 42 families (largely European American and African American) representing professional/managerial, working-class, and welfare backgrounds once a month in their homes for 2½ years. In their book *Meaningful Differences in the Everyday Experiences of Young American Children*, Hart and Risley (1995) demonstrated that while all families in their study provided sufficient support for competent language development, there were great differences in the amount of talk between family members, regardless of a child's gender or a family's race. There were enormous differences by SES in the utterances per hour. Parents in the professional families addressed an average of 487 utterances to their children per hour, families in working-class families 301 utterances, and families on welfare 178. Professional families also used more words and more different words, more multiclause sentences, and more grammatical forms than did the families from working-class and welfare families. The cumulative difference in language experiences was enormous—not only in regard to the number of words addressed to a child (3 million per year in welfare families to 11 million per year in professional families), but in regard to the provision of encouraging feedback versus discouragements.

Despite these data supporting the relationship between family SES and the amount parents talked, the data [also] showed "that no matter what the family SES, the more time parents spent talking to their child from day to day, the more rapidly the child's vocabulary was likely to be growing and the higher the child's score on an IQ test was likely to be at age 3" (Hart & Risley, 1999, p. 3). The differences in family talk did not occur during routines necessary to daily living, such as eating, dressing, and safety; they occurred during the "extra, optional talk" (p. 3) that took place when parents and children were partners in play or other shared activities (doing a puzzle, folding laundry). During these activities, parents were more likely to comment on nuances or elaborate on what was said, thus providing children with exposure and practice. But children also contributed importantly as conversational partners, with each child "listening and speaking, following and leading, locked into the ways language works between people," and learning the "social dance of his or her own family culture that governs what its members talk about, how much, and in what circumstances" (Hart & Risley, 1999, p. 4). The more talkative the parents, the more opportunity children had to participate in the "social dance," encouraging their talkativeness. Hearing many words also contributes to other skills, such as phonemic awareness. According to Goswami (2001), the more words children hear, the better able they are to make distinctions between similar sounds in words, which is a natural part of their language learning.

The Interaction of Language Development with Cognitive Development

The development and use of language, as illustrated above in Figure 10.1, are interdependent with all other psychological domains of development—cognitive/information-processing, sensory–motor, and socioemotional. Bloom (1991) points out that since language serves the dual purposes of *expressing* thoughts to others and *interpreting* past and present objects and events, "how language is acquired depends very much on how children think and what they know" (p. 4) based on their past experiences. Thus, according to Bloom, language development and cognitive development are inextricably intertwined. Some of the early cognitive precursors to language acquisition include recognizing that things exist, even if they are not present; cause–effect relationships; symbolic activities such as pointing, gesturing, and labeling; and recognizing pictures as symbols for objects. Bloom's work documents that by the time a child is 3 years of age, he or she already has developed a substantial set of cognitive abilities, including object permanence, the use of symbols (words/signs) to represent thoughts, and the ability to perform tasks with intentionality and represent situations through symbolic play (all areas for assessors to observe). Children are able to draw upon their experiences and to organize their ideas mentally. Other cognitive skills children are learning relate to understanding categories, sequencing events, and following directions of increasing length and complexity. The works of Piaget (1969), Bruner (1983a, 1983b), and Vygotsky (1962, 1978), among others, provide important understanding regarding the interaction between language and cognitive development. Aspects of cognitive growth and their interaction with language development are covered in Chapter 11.

Developing Communicative Competence

In developing communicative competence, the child is actually developing three closely interrelated sets of skills: production, comprehension, and dyadic/discourse skills (McLean, 1990, p. 14). Each of these areas needs to be accounted for in assessment. Through *production* skills, including both verbal and nonverbal forms, a child conveys meaning and intent to others. *Comprehension* skills allow the child to derive meaning from communicative and environmental events. Comprehension skills include understanding spoken language (i.e., the task, word meaning, phrases, questions), as well as deriving meaning from both symbolic (e.g., books) and nonsymbolic (e.g., tone of voice) forms of communication. *Dyadic/discourse* skills allow a child to communicate appropriately and effectively with others (i.e., the *pragmatic* skills discussed later). A child's communicative competence is closely related to many disorders of early childhood.

> For example, Alex is a 4-year-old child with autistic disorder. His language abilities, with the exception of pragmatic knowledge, are all intact and developing normally. However, due to Alex's severe lack of interpersonal connectedness, his true language abilities are rarely revealed. He does not initiate contact with his peers or the adults he comes into contact with unless verbally prompted. His verbalizations often consist of incoherent combinations of meaningful words, echolalic interactions with adults, and imperceptible utterances with no discernable meaning to others. He also exhibits stereotyped repetitive motor mannerisms, such as handclapping and spinning.

Prizant and Wetherby (1990) note the close link between the early development of communication (including both gestures and language) and the growth of socioemotional competence, as in the example above. Despite the reciprocal development of competence in these areas, researchers and clinicians often focus on either one or the other, leading to a fragmented picture of early development in these two related fields. A review of studies documenting the co-occurrence of communication disorders and emotional–behavioral disorders in children is presented by Prizant et al. (1990). This topic is detailed in Chapter 13. Assessment practices are often fragmented as well; this leads in turn to disjointed intervention strategies that do not connect language development and socioemotional development (Prizant & Wetherby, 1990). Achenbach and Rescorla (2000b) have attempted to address this issue by including a Language Development Survey (consisting of a parent-completed checklist of 310 words in 14 categories the child says spontaneously and 5 examples of phrases of two or more words the child uses) in the latest version of the Child Behavior Checklist for Ages 1½–5, a widely used parent rating scale for identifying emotional and behavioral disorders in young children (see Chapter 14 for a review of this well-researched instrument).

Assessment needs to take into account not only the nature of children's communicative difficulty, but with whom it occurs and the extent to which the children can persist and correct their language interactions. People in the child's environment need to provide the opportunity for the child to develop vital communicative functions—that is, to communicate in order to get others to do things (behavior regulation), to draw attention to him- or herself (social interaction), and to direct the attention of others to objects and events (joint attention, such as when a child brings a classroom assistant to look at a hamster playing) (Wetherby & Prizant, 1992). These communicative functions emerge by the end of a normally developing child's first year of life and before the child's first words. Researchers stress that it is important for parents, teachers, medical personnel, and other early interventionists to be aware of these early signs of communicative competence (Wetherby & Prizant, 1992).

Wetherby and Prizant (1993) have developed the Communication and Symbolic Behavior Scales (CSBS) to measure early stages of language acquisition in children between 8 months and 2 years of age (or up to 6 years if developmental delays are present). Components of the CSBS include a caregiver questionnaire, a videotaped behavior sample of caregiver interaction with the child, and a Behavior Sample Rating Form. The CSBS measures both communicative behavior and symbolic development. Use of the scales gives early interventionists the opportunity to develop intervention activities, document change over time, and assess older children with severe delays.

The prevailing opinion in the research literature, which we endorse in this chapter, is that language assessment needs to include multiple formal and informal procedures, including observation in natural contexts, norm-referenced and criterion-referenced tests, interviews, developmental scales, elicited responses, dynamic assessment activities, and adaptive teaching. Observation, when possible in a play situation, needs to have the central role. Furthermore, since context is very important to the content of the language samples obtained, assessment needs to occur across contexts.

> For example, José, age 4-6 years, is being raised in a Spanish–English bilingual home. In school, José has difficulty when it comes to following his teacher's directions in the classroom and learning new things such as the alphabet. However, in social situations, such as on the playground, José's language abilities appear to be better developed.

Language assessment also needs to be considered an ongoing process, with goals modified as interventions are employed and the child develops skill. During in-depth assessment, an interdisciplinary team approach is advocated; the persons involved should include the speech–language specialists, preschool school psychologist, early childhood teachers, and parents.

The Interacting Components of Language

Language consists of multiple interactive components, including (1) *phonology*, the sound system of language; (2) *semantics*, the content of language, including the meaning of words and the relations between words that are structured into phrases and sentences; (3) *morphology*, the smallest bits of meaning a word can be broken down into; (4) *syntax*, the grammatical rules for ordering words and sentence structure; and (5) *pragmatics*, the use of language in everyday social contexts, such as turn taking during conversations. Each of these components contributes to the whole of language, which is greater than the sum of the parts (Olswang & Bain, 1988) that "come together in understanding and saying messages" (Lahey, 1988, p. 15). Bloom and Lahey (1978), in their description of the interacting components of language, characterized the sounds and syntax of language as *form*, the semantics of language as *content*, and the pragmatics of language as *use*. This theoretical position is used as the framework for organizing this portion of the chapter.

Another important distinction should also be mentioned here: that between the language we comprehend (*receptive*) and the language we both comprehend and produce (*expressive*). Difficulties in either of these aspects will impede further acquisition and sharing of ideas in the preschool and in the classroom, and later will be evidenced in all school subject areas requiring reading and writing (Aram & Hall, 1989, p. 488). In addition, children's developing information-processing capacity allows them to perceive information in their environment, organize and remember it, and retrieve ideas from memory, along with the associated words to express these ideas (Aram, Ekelman, & Nation, 1984; Kaminski & Good, 1996; Scarborough & Dobrich, 1990).

Form

The form a specific language takes includes the sound system of that language (*phonology*), and the organization of these sounds by the grammar of the language (*syntax*). Form is thus the means for connecting sounds with meaning (Lahey, 1988).

PHONOLOGY (THE SOUND SYSTEM)

The sound system consists of three components: (1) *phonemes*, the smallest units of discrete speech sounds; (2) *combinations of phonemes*, which are governed by phonological rules to form syllables; and (3) *prosodic elements*, or intonation and stress patterns (Menyuk, 1972; Myers, 1988). The English language consists of 43+ phonemes. There is general agreement regarding the ages at which these phonemes are acquired. These data have been detailed by authors such as Davis (1938), McCarthy (1930), and Templin (1957). The results of five commonly cited studies were summarized by Newman, Creaghead, and Secord (1985) and are presented in Table 10.2. As can be seen from this table, the ages from 3 to 6 are critical for developing this mastery.

Across languages, front consonants, (e.g., *b*) and back vowels (e.g., *e*) provide a starting point for speech (McNeill, 1970). McNeill (1970) indicates that the development of a phonemic system is the result of filling in the gap between two sounds, which are increasingly differentiated through the process of development. Consonants and vowels are combined into syllables as a child begins to babble ("da da") at about 6 months of age, regardless of language. Children continue to acquire phonological rules for many years. Stages of sound development are detailed by Ingram (1981), Newman et al. (1985), and Lund and Duncan (1993). The works of Carroll, Snowling, Hulme, and Stevenson (2003), Cisero and Royer (1995), Goswami (2001), Liberman and

TABLE 10.2. Ages of Phoneme Development across Five Studies

	Wellman et al. (1931)	Poole (1934)	Templin (1957)	Sander (1972)	Prather et al. (1975)
m	3	3½	3	before 2	2
n	3	4½	3	before 2	2
h	3	3½	3	before 2	2
p	4	3½	3	before 2	2
f	3	5½	3	3	2–4
w	3	3½	3	before 2	2–8
b	3	3½	4	before 2	2–8
ŋ		4½	3	2	2
j	4	4½	3½	3	2–4
k	4	4½	4	2	2–4
g	4	4½	4	2	2–4
l	4	6½	6	3	3–4
d	5	4½	4	2	2–4
t	5	4½	6	2	2–8
s	5	7½	4½	3	3
r	5	7½	4	3	3–4
tʃ	5		4½	4	3–8
v	5	6½	6	4	4
z	5	7½	7	4	4
ʒ	6	6½	7	6	4
θ		7½	6	5	4
dʒ			7	4	4
ʃ		6½	4½	4	3–8
ð		6½	7	5	4

Note. From Newman, Creaghead, and Secord (1985). Published by Allyn & Bacon, Boston, MA. Copyright 1985 by Pearson Education. Reprinted by permission of the publisher.

Shankweiler (1985), Stanovich, Cunningham, and Crammer (1984), and Torgesen and Wagner (1998), among others, provide a basis for a theoretical understanding of phonemic development.

Allen (1989, p. 443) notes, "It is relatively easy to identify children who present with disturbances in sound production since such deficits are readily accessible to direct observation." It is more problematic, however, to determine whether phonological errors represent linguistic deficits, speech articulation problems, or mild hearing loss. Allen makes the following distinction: A child is considered to have a phonology problem when there are unusual, inconsistent, or unpredictable sound substitutions (e.g., saying "fool" for *school*), omissions, or distortions, or when they are breakdowns in longer sequences of consonants but isolated consonants are used spontaneously and are accurately imitated. Such difficulties can be assessed informally across assessment activities (such as where the child can or cannot be understood) or more formally by a speech–language specialist if a problem is suspected. These difficulties contrast with patterns of developmental misarticulations in younger or linguistically immature children (e.g., saying "aminal" for *animal*). Children from linguistically and culturally diverse backgrounds may display other patterns. Tests have been developed to assess phonological processes, such as the Fluharty Preschool Speech and Language Screening Test—Second Edition (Fluharty-2; Fluharty, 2001). Tests such as these are not discussed in detail in this chapter (but are summarized in Appendix 10.1), since they are typically administered by a speech pathologist (see Lund & Duncan, 1993; Owens, 1995; R. Paul, 2001; and Shipley & McAfee, 1998, for reviews).

With increasing age, the intelligibility of sound productions increases, as does children's ability to discriminate between sounds—a process referred to as *phonological awareness*. Children can encounter difficulties in discriminating the sounds that make up words they hear (such discrimination is an important aspect of receptive language). Phonological awareness of individual sounds in words is crucial for later success in reading, such as word identification, and allows children to decode words rapidly and focus their attention on comprehension (see Chapter 7). Since phonological awareness may have a significant impact on later learning and is an important predictor of reading skill in the early grades (Bradley & Bryant, 1985; Goswami, 2001; Kirby et al., 2003; Liberman & Shankweiler, 1985; Stanovich et al., 1984; Wagner & Torgesen, 1987), it is important for all assessors to observe behaviors related to language forms (see Table 10.3). A speech–language pathologist can determine whether physical reasons for deficits exist, along with the nature of the difficulties in the child's productions, and appropriate intervention strategies. However, it is important for the school psychologist and assessors representing other disciplines to observe and report these difficulties during the assessment process.

Phonological awareness involves three forms of awareness: awareness of (1) syllables; (2) onset (the beginning consonant or consonant cluster) and rime (the vowel and remaining sounds that provide meaning, such as "ap" in *cap* and *lap*); and (3) individual phonemes (e.g., the word *purses* has three phonemes, *pur/se/s*) (Cisero & Royer, 1995). For preschool children, rime detection is easier than detecting initial and final phonemes (Carroll, Snowling, Hulme, & Stevenson, 2003; Goswami, 2001). This may be due to children's greater exposure to rhyming activities and the fact that rime detection involves a holistic judgment, not knowledge that words have separate sounds. Phonological skills also transfer from one's native language to another (Cisero & Royer, 1995). If a child can rhyme in Spanish, he or she can quickly learn to rhyme in English.

The 5- or 6-year-old child also needs to understand how letters and sounds are related, and that spoken words are divisible into speech sounds. The ability to blend these

TABLE 10.3. Assessor's Observations of Language Behaviors

1. Does the child appear to have a language delay?
2. Does the child appear to have an articulation problem?
   - Is the child understandable?
   - Does the child make sound substitutions? Distortions?
3. Does the child understand what was said?
   - During warm-up activities or relatively open tasks?
   - Task directions?
   - Task items?
4. Does the child respond spontaneously? With words/phrases/sentences/gestures?
5. How does the child respond to you? Words/phrases/sentences/gestures?
6. Does the child appear to have difficulty expressing ideas?
   - Limited vocabulary?
   - Problems with retrieving words or expressing meanings precisely?
   - Difficulty maintaining word order?
   - Problems with using appropriate grammar?
7. Does the child ask questions?
8. Does the child engage in turn taking with you during conversation?
9. Does the child make irrelevant comments?
10. Does the child use nonverbal communicative behaviors (e.g., gestures) instead of words?

sounds into words is an indicator of phonemic awareness. Many of these skills are developed prior to kindergarten. A child's degree of phonological awareness development can be informally assessed by examining a number of skills, such as rhyming, segmenting, and blending. For example, can children "hear" a compound word, such as *birthday*, and divide it into two parts? Can they hear the syllables in the word *apple* or the distinct sounds in the word *cat*? Can they add *p* to *an* to make *pan*? These skills can be assessed informally through such activities as making up nonsense words, singing songs, and reading together rhyming books. A more formal measure is the Pre-Reading Inventory of Phonological Awareness (PIPA; Dodd et al., 2003), which includes six subtests: Rhyme Awareness, Syllable Segmentation, Alliteration Awareness, Sound Isolation, Sound Segmentation, and Letter–Sound Knowledge. This inventory (see Appendix 7.1 for full details on it) was developed for children 4-0 through 6-11 years old. It can be administered by teachers and paraprofessionals as well as speech pathologists, thus providing observational data across contexts. Adams, Foorman, Lundberg, and Beeler (1998), in their book *Phonemic Awareness in Young Children*, provide excellent phonological activities for preschool children and an extensive bibliography of rhyming stories. In sum, young children need to comprehend as well as produce the sounds of language and understand their function in words.

SYNTAX

"Between sound and meaning stand *syntax*. The relation between sound and meaning is, therefore, understood to the degree that the syntax of the language is understood" (McNeill, 1970, p. 1146). Syntax provides the rules for combining words into larger units, including phrases, clauses, and sentences—the grammar of the language. The combination and location of words reflects changing relationships between components (tense, inflections, and the use of auxiliaries such as *will* or *may*), as well as purpose (statement vs. question) and the context of the utterance. Deficits in syntax usually result in two forms of difficulty—omission of required grammatical forms and misapplication of learned grammatical "rules" (Allen, 1989, p. 444)—as well as difficulty in using complex sentences. Regardless of the child's home language, the sequence of syntax development is as follows: Normal children "babble at 6 months, utter their first 'word' at 10 to 12 months, combine words at 18 to 24 months, and acquire syntax almost completely at 48 to 60 months" (McNeill, 1970, p. 1062) or by the time they enter kindergarten. Thus it is important to observe the grammatical forms a child uses.

> For example, observation of Sally, a child 3-6 years of age, during free play at home indicated that she used various types of sentences. She used the declarative when she announced that she had completed a puzzle, and the imperative when she told her friend to stop singing. Sally used a negative sentence when she stated that she did not need to use the bathroom. She also asked many *wh*-questions (e.g., "Why are you writing that?").

An important aspect of syntax is *morphology. Morphemes* are the smallest segments of speech that carry meaning, including individual words (morphological units) and grammatical inflections (i.e., plurals, tense, prefixes, suffixes) that change words in specific ways. For example, inflections "modulate the meaning of a sentence" (Lahey, 1988; Brown, 1973) by indicating past or present time (tense), the number of objects or actors (singular or plural), and negation. These inflections are accounted for when determining a child's mean length of utterance (MLU, to be discussed later in the chapter) or through analyzing language samples. Brown (1973) identified 14 grammatical morphemes that children begin to acquire between 24 and 30 months of age. de Villiers and de Villiers (1973) detailed the order of acquisition of these morphemes.

There are two broad classes of words that Brown (1973) refers to as "the major building blocks" of meaning: (1) *content words* (nouns, verbs, adjectives, and adverbs) and (2) *function words* (articles, conjunctions, and prepositions), which connect content words. Both types need to be accounted for during assessment.

Content (Semantics)

The *content* (or *semantics*) of language includes vocabulary, the various aspects of meaning conveyed in a word (i.e., a cat is also an animal), classes and categories, and relational information (Lahey, 1988). Lahey (1988) details the primary categories of content:

1. Objects (including particular objects, such as cars, and classes of objects, such as vehicles).
2. Relations between objects, such as "one object on top of another."
3. Relations between events (temporal, causal, epistemic [what user knows or thinks], such as "Marty washed her hands before she ate her snack."

Children who have difficulties with content have difficulty both comprehending language and expressing themselves through language. They may, for example, overextend the meanings of words (e.g., using "kitty cat" to refer to both cats and dogs). Since comprehension is a cognitive task, when a child has difficulties in this area, it is important to distinguish whether (1) the child has a general cognitive deficit; (2) the lack of comprehension is related to the child's range of experience; (3) the language sample obtained is limited and possibly not representative of the child's knowledge; or (4) linguistic and dialect differences (such as a second-language background) are influencing performance. Each of these factors can be assessed in a number of ways, such as having the child point to pictures as they are named, respond to questions during storybook reading (e.g., identify what happened before or after another event in a story sequence), or follow directions.

Use (Pragmatics)

Pragmatics is the term used to refer to the *use* of language in social contexts. First of all, children learn how to take turns in conversation (one person speaks at a time), how to maintain the flow, and how to read the signals of others that indicate they wish to start or conclude a conversation. A child's use of language thus needs to take into account and integrate a number of interrelated features, including (1) the purpose or function of the utterance; (2) the context in which language takes place (as the context shifts, speakers need to adjust their language appropriately); (3) what has previously occurred or been said; and (4) the social conventions that govern interpersonal communication in the child's culture. Children's pragmatic difficulties can include making irrelevant comments; missing the point of questions directed to them; violating of conversational turn-taking rules; difficulty initiating, maintaining, or ending conversations or topics under discussion; not recognizing cues parents or teachers use; and not determining what information the listener needs to know. In contrast, appropriate practices include asking for food or desired objects, interacting verbally with peers during play, attending to others while they speak, initiating conversations with teachers or peers, and engaging in turn taking during conversations. Each of these behaviors can be observed by members of the assessment team.

Making sense out of events is another indicator of pragmatic skill. Lund and Duncan (1993) provide a framework for assessing a child's "sense making," including (1) the ability to maintain the flow of events from beginning to end with an adult or peer; (2) attention to and involvement in activities; and (3) intentionality (e.g., pretending to feed a doll, using an empty cup). Observation of young children in everyday activities is the best way to collect information relevant to these issues.

> For example, while playing with a toolbox (a favorite activity), Noah, age 4-8 years, demonstrated appropriate use of language in a number of ways. These included requesting action ("Can I have that hammer?"); commenting on an object ("This saw is so cool!"); acknowledging another's speech ("Uh-huh," "Okay"); requesting objects and information ("How does that work?"); providing information ("See, this is how you do it"); and personal reactions ("I like that saw"). Other discourse skills were also evidenced. Noah was able to attend to the speaker and demonstrated consistent eye contact. He initiated conversations, took turns speaking, maintained a topic over time by adding information or requesting information, and used questions to extend conversation ("What's this for?") or to ask for clarification ("What did you say?")

In a clinic setting, the assessor can gain information about the child's use of language from the parent and teacher through interviews and checklists. The assessor can also observe such behaviors as the child's response to greetings and warm-up activities, ability to make eye contact (if culturally appropriate), spontaneous comments, ability to follow commands, take turns, and stay on task.

Sources of Variability in the Language Behaviors of Young Children

Preschool children are by nature highly variable in their behavior, and this variability is particularly evidenced in their language behavior. Several sources of variability need to be accounted for during the assessment process, including context, adult input and interaction, and cultural/linguistic diversity.

The Influence of Context

The importance of context is an issue raised by most experts who focus on language development and its measurement. Critical context variables include (1) the person with whom the child is communicating; (2) the activities and settings in which, and time at which, a language sample is collected; and (3) the mood and motivation of the child when the language sample is obtained. Considering the contexts in which language is acquired and used is essential both for understanding a child's language development and for planning intervention. In particular, the individual communicating to the child (i.e., parent, sibling, relative, peer, teacher, assessor) can influence the child's language output (Gallagher, 1987; Olswang & Bain, 1988; Olswang & Carpenter, 1978). Prizant et al. (1993) point out that assessing the child's interaction with familiar others (communicative partners) also provides information on the strategies these individuals use to support or hinder a child's communicative growth. For example, conversation partners may or may not react to a child's signals, know how to capture the child's attention, or know how to provide experiences that contribute to word learning. Supportive partner strategies include those that facilitate interaction, "such as responding contingently to child behavior, providing developmentally appropriate communicative models, maintaining the topic of child initiations, and expanding or elaborating on communicative attempts" (Prizant et al., 1993, p. 271).

Other context variables, such as setting, are important as well. Language samples collected in the home are different from those collected in a structured setting, such as the typical clinic setting (Bloom & Lahey, 1978; Coggins, Olswang, & Guthrie, 1987). Olswang and Bain (1988), for example, reviewed studies indicating that many child behaviors, such as pointing, verbally indicating possession, and requesting information, occur infrequently in testing situations, which makes comprehensive sampling of language difficult. In the longitudinal study reported by Wells (1985), there was considerable variation in the amount of speech produced according to the conversational setting in which it occurred, as well as the time of day and the child's gender. In order to obtain a representative sample of a child's language as indicated at the beginning of this chapter, it is important to use multiple measures and approaches; these include observation in the natural contexts of home and/or school, and with different partners (Lahey, 1988; Myers, 1988; Olswang & Bain, 1988; Owens, 2004; R. Paul, 2001; Wells, 1985). Multiple observations carried out over time, activity type, and setting can address issues such as these:

- Different language forms children use across activities, such as play, snack, and teacher–child exchanges.
- How children use language in conversation (e.g., whether they can extend the conversation, maintain the topic across several successive utterances with an adult or another child, ask questions, or make comments).

- How caregivers and peers initiate and respond to the communicative efforts of children (e.g., whether they give the children enough time to respond or reinforce their efforts).
- The particular strategies a child employs to communicate with others (e.g., turn taking, pointing, grabbing, asking for objects).
- How children interact during play that involves role playing or shared storybook reading.

Such descriptive information of children's language in natural settings can be used to help (1) confirm or reject the existence of a problem in communication; (2) provide explicit examples of language content, form, and use, along with other cognitive and socio-emotional behaviors; (3) provide information about the nature of the interaction with others across settings and/or activities; and (4) formulate the goals and strategies of intervention.

The Importance of Adult Input

As the discussion above suggests, closely related to context are both the amount and form of adult input as children acquire language. Children learn from the examples of speech they hear (or, for deaf children growing up with deaf parents, the signs to which they are exposed) and gradually assimilate these examples into their own grammars. Each individual gains cues from the other. Bloom (1991) views context in an interpersonal sense, in which children learn very early about conversational turn taking and about connecting discourse to previous discourse. Although there is not complete agreement, the evidence supports a reciprocity between children and caregivers: Parents and other adults modify the complexity of their speech when speaking to children, and gain cues from children's comprehension and subsequent actions. This interaction was clearly illustrated in the studies by Hart and Risley (1995, 1999) cited earlier in this chapter. Situations also differ in terms of communication possibilities and constraints. Thus assessment and intervention need to include familiar others who interact with the child.

Although children need to have developed the cognitive basis to acquire linguistic structures (Slobin, 1973; Snow, 1977), development of cognitive structures is not in itself sufficient for production of linguistic categories (Wells, 1985). Children therefore need to experience repeated examples of the forms and uses of language, and to have opportunities to practice and extend their mastery. McNeill (1970), citing the classic work of Cazden (1965) and Brown, Cazden, and Bellugi (1968), details the ways this occurs: *expansion*, *prompting*, *commenting*, and *modeling*. Through expansion, an adult improves a toddler's telegraphic sentences by using the child's words and adding the parts he or she thinks the child has omitted, given the contextual situation. When prompting, the adult begins with a *wh-* question that, if not answered, can be repeated in another form. When commenting, the adult remarks on what the child says but does not use the child's own words. When modeling, the adult uses typical language forms. Wells (1985) demonstrated that the adult variable showing the most consistent pattern of significant association with child gain scores (independent of the amount of speech addressed to the child) was the percentage of *extending* utterances (ones that incorporated all or part of the child's utterances and added new but related semantic content—in other words, expansion as described above).

Adult input continues to play an important role for children in the 3- to 5-year range. For example, a child's language learning and shared experiences with caregivers during activities such as storybook reading are important for both language learning and the early development of literacy. Snow and Ninio (1986) underscore the point that repeated book reading "provides a child with exposure to more complex, more elaborate, and more decontextualized language than almost any other kind of interaction" (p. 118). Extensive evidence also supports the importance of mealtime conversations for the development of such forms of language as recounting events, expressing feelings and concerns, and discussing plans (Dickenson & Snow, 1987; Dickenson & Tabors, 1991, 2001).

In a study of early conversations with caregivers, Bloom, Margulis, Tinker, and Fujita (1996) present evidence in support of the *intentionality model* of language development proposed by Bloom (1993), in which the child plays a primary role. According to this model, the child "provides the driving force for language, in general, and in conversations, in particular, from the beginning of word learning" (Bloom et al., 1996, p. 3154), building on his or her inner resources. This model contrasts with the *scaffolding model* described by Bruner (1983a, 1983b) and Vygotsky (1978), which emphasizes the role of adults in providing the needed guidance for a child to be successful in language exchanges originally beyond the child's capacity. Bloom et al. (1996) point out a number of challenges in the literature to the scaffolding model, such as the extent to which mothers and children in different cultures participate in highly structured and conventional routines, games, and joint picture book reading.

The way adults talk to and interact with children may also affect language delay (Dumtschin, 1988). Whereas children's language development is positively related to parents' use of questions, acknowledgments, expansions, or restatements, it is negatively related to parents' use of controlling, directive speech (Cross, 1984)—a finding supported by Hart and Risley (1995). Mothers of children with language delays, for example, often use more disapproval (Bondurant, Romeo, & Kretschmer, 1983) or try to impose adult speech (i.e., they correct their children, rather than encourage their attempts or approve appropriate speech; Schodorf & Edwards, 1983). It is unclear whether these mothers are responding to children's delays or whether their behavior is contributing to them.

Teachers and other caregivers, as well as parents, play a vital role in language development. Roberts, Bailey, and Nychka (1991), for example, studied 31 teachers working in developmental daycare centers and tallied their use of facilitation strategies found in the literature to promote the communication of preschool children with disabilities. The investigators used the Teacher–Child Communication Scale (TCCS; Bailey & Roberts, 1987), a 5-point rating scale that measures the quantity and quality of nine teacher facilitation strategies: (1) engages the child in a communication interaction; (2) comments on events; (3) prompts for higher level of response; (4) responds to communicative attempts; (5) waits for a response: (6) expands child's utterances; (7) promotes peer interactions; (8) prompts communication to replace undesirable behaviors; and (9) modifies the environment to promote communication. Results indicated that these teachers were highly involved with their students in encouraging communication. They frequently engaged, responded, and waited for children to respond, with high-quality use of these strategies. However, they infrequently expanded on children's utterances, prompted for a higher level of response, prompted peer interactions, or modified the environment to promote communication. These results suggest that teachers may benefit from training in these areas facilitative of communication strategies. The TCCS appears to be a very useful scale for evaluating the environment of young children with communication delays, and could provide important information as a component of an assessment battery.

The Influence of Cultural and Linguistic Diversity

As we have discussed at length in Chapter 9, an increasing number of children in the United States come from families who speak languages and dialects other than standard American English. These children often demonstrate differences that are not necessarily reflective of language difficulty (Jitendra & Rohena-Diaz, 1996). Brown (1973) and Slobin (1973), along with many other researchers, summarize cross-cultural research on language acquisition (which is beyond the scope of this chapter). Across cultures, the interactions available to the maturing infants within their social and physical worlds are basically similar. Thus "there will be very great similarity in the meanings that the child understands and seeks to encode in his [or her] early utterances, whatever the culture in which he lives" (Wells, 1985, p. 57). However, the lexical items and grammatical structures in which meanings are encoded will vary across different language communities, and differences as well as similarities are to be expected in children's acquisition of different languages. Considerable variation also exists within language communities in the importance that adults attach to children's language development and in the function of language in family interactions (Wells, 1985).

Growing up bilingual is of particular relevance as an assessor seeks to understand a child's communication strengths and needs. Stokes and Duncan (1989) point out that the assessment needs of monolingual and bilingual children are the same, and that the same thorough assessment protocol can be implemented with a bilingual child as with a monolingual child but "must be carried out in both (all) the child's languages" (p. 114). As discussed in Chapter 9, carrying out procedures in both or all the child's languages often requires the use of a translator if the assessor is not bilingual in the child's language; the use of an informant familiar with the child's language and culture to respond to interview questions in consultation with the parent; and the use of translated language measures for which norms often are not available (except increasingly in Spanish) and in which the examples used may vary in difficulty level or be inappropriate. The use of standardized norms for English speakers is not appropriate. A standardized test in English for children for whom English is their second language will only reflect the children's language abilities in their second language, not their overall language skills (Stokes & Duncan, 1989). Therefore, it is important whenever possible to use measures translated and normed in English and the child's home language, as well as dynamic assessment techniques. The challenge is to differentiate actual language disturbances from children's difficulties in understanding or expressing themselves in a second language. For example, they may engage in code switching from their native language to English, where errors may occur. Such errors are a natural aspect of language acquisition and should not be viewed as reflecting a language deficiency (Jitendra & Rohena-Diaz, 1996). The challenge is exacerbated by the wide diversity of languages and dialects young children in the North American school system speak, as well as by the lack of available measures. Stokes and Duncan (1989) clearly state the issue: "The practitioner will continue to be faced with the difficulty of assessing a child whose first language is unfamiliar to [him or] her, for whom there is no interpreter/co-worker and about which language [he or] she has no information" (p. 118). R. Paul (2001), in her text *Language Disorders from Infancy through Adolescence*, presents an excellent table (p. 182) of dimensions to be considered in assessing the communicative competence of such a child, using methods sensitive to cultural practices; she also provides an overview of measures available in languages other than English. Important phonemic contrasts between standard English and African American, Hispanic American, and Asian American English are presented by Owens (2004) and R. Paul (2001), along with forms the speech–language specialist might use for reporting the language skills of these children.

An extensive literature exists for assessing and treating communicative disorders in culturally and linguistically diverse populations (e.g., Cole, 1985; Gallagher, 1991; Mattes & Omark, 1984; Oller & Damico, 1991; Owens, 2004; R. Paul, 2001; Taylor, 1986). Assessors need to determine the language dominance of a referred child and the language(s) in which assessment should take place through observation, questionnaires, interview, and review of case history information. If a child is identified as having language skills significantly below those of other children from similar backgrounds, collecting and analyzing a spontaneous speech sample may be more representative of the child's language skills (R. Paul, 2001). It is also important to collect data regarding the child's pragmatics both in his or her home language (e.g., with friends on the playground) and in American English in the classroom and at home. Dynamic test–teach–test procedures such as those reported by Lidz (2003) and Lidz and Pena (1996), which focus on the extent to which adult mediation (support) influences the child's learning of new material, can be helpful as well. Finally, criterion-referenced materials translated into the child's first language (see Chapter 7) can be used by the assessment team prior to referral for intervention services (Pena, Quinn, & Iglesias, 1992), as well as by the speech–language specialist (Owens, 2004; R. Paul, 2001).

Forms of Disability That Affect Language Development

The major childhood disorders in which there are communication difficulties or language delays include mental retardation, learning disabilities (LD), autism spectrum disorders (ASD), visual impairment/blindness, hearing impairments/deafness, and some disorders not covered in this chapter (e.g., motor problems). Specific disorders confined to communication difficulties may also exist, though these are more controversial (see below). As indicated below, many labels are used to describe children's communication problems, and many experts express concern about applying these labels at all, unless they are needed for children to qualify for services. Whatever the problem, learning and using language are closely related to cognition and require important information-processing skills, including the abilities to (1) attend to and encode relevant incoming stimuli, (2) remember the stimuli and store them in long-term memory, (3) understand the requirements of a task, (4) retrieve appropriate experiences from memory, (5) use available environmental supports, (6) interact with others appropriately, and (7) respond using appropriate communicative forms (Owens, 2004; R. Paul, 2001). Difficulty with any of these activities needs to be identified and addressed during intervention. This section covers issues regarding terminology and labeling, the prevalence of language disorders among preschool children, and the particular language-learning difficulties seen in children with different disability conditions. Table 10.4 presents a summary of these difficulties by disability area.

TABLE 10.4. Overview of Language Behaviors by Disability Condition

Disability condition	Language behaviors: Content	Form	Use
Specific language impairment (SLI)	• Slower and more restricted vocabulary development, including basic relational concepts • Word-finding problems	• Late and slow development of form • Similar order of emergence as in normally developing children • Phonological difficulties • Some grammatical errors along with more mature forms • Less difficult and less complex sentence constructions—fewer morphemes	• Less frequent talk when playing around another child, but respect for turn taking • Speech more like that of younger child • Difficulty understanding others/making themselves understood
Mental retardation	• Possible impairment in comprehension • Slow vocabulary growth • Use of more concrete words • Less extensive variety of verbs • Poorer receptive language skills • Difficulty with relational terms • Use of more immature forms • Poorer short-term memory skills	• Later emergence of language structures, although in same order as in normally developing children • More concrete word mechanics • Shorter, less complex sentences	• Less developed communicative exchanges • Difficulty with perspective taking, seeking clarification • Display turn taking and maintain the topic
Language-related learning disability (LD)	• Normal receptive vocabulary • Word-finding difficulties, such as recalling specific words, making word substitutions • Slower rate of naming and circumlocutions • Difficulty with relational terms (*before–after*, etc.) • Possible inattention	• Difficulty with phonological awareness (skills important for early reading) • Difficulty with more complex syntactic structures • Difficulty with morphological markers (negatives, passive forms, tenses)	• Inappropriate turn taking • Possible difficulty responding to questions or requesting clarification • Possible attention problems
Autism spectrum disorders (ASD)	• Delay in onset of expressive language • Difficulty with receptive language • Frequent difficulty with nonverbal communication and the spontaneous use of gestures • Word-finding problems • Inappropriate responses	• Inappropriate use of many word forms • Use of less complex sentences	• Poor communication skills • Difficulty with conversation • Failure to get the point of questions directed to them • Stereotypic use/repetitive use of words; perseverance • Failure to take listener into account • Conversations often not contingent • Lack of emotional tone; voice quality often unusual • Inappropriate relating to others • Inappropriate comments; echolalia • Frequent absence of speech

(continued)

TABLE 10.4. *(continued)*

Disability condition	Language behaviors		
	Content	Form	Use
Visual impairment/ blindness	• Limited receptive and expressive language • Slower concept development, especially temporal relational concepts and spatial prepositions	• Some delays in syntactic forms • Substantial improvement with intervention and once children learn Braille	• Inability to perceive visual cues • Less child-initiated dialogue with caregivers • Fewer spontaneous verbalizations • Possible difficulty maintaining topic
Hearing impairment/ deafness	• Great variability, depending on timing and level of loss • Need for careful monitoring to determine whether skills are keeping up to date	• Use of fewer compound and complex sentences • Articulation differences, depending on timing of loss, level of loss, age when interventions began, and whether or not parents have learned ASL • Syntactic development normal but slower • Great difficulty with modifiers, inflectional morphemes, adverbs, and prepositions • Frequent development of own syntactic rules	• Less communicative behavior • Difficulty in understanding severely hearing-impaired children

Note. Data from Allen (1988); Aram (1991); Dumtschin (1988); German (1989); Lahey (1988); Owens (2004); P. V. Paul (2001); Koenig and Holbrook (2000); and Riccio (1992).

Issues Regarding Terminology and Labeling

There is no consensus regarding the terminology used to describe children who are not learning language effectively in comparison with other children of the same age and background. Terms used include *language disorder*, *deviant language*, *language delay*, *language disability*, and "language impairment." Lahey (1988) uses the following operational definition: "Disordered, or deviant, language development can be described as any disruption in the learning or use of language content, form, or use or in the interaction among these components" (p. 22). Many different kinds and patterns of disruption are possible. The term *specific language impairment* (SLI) is often used to describe language problems in children with normal nonverbal intelligence, without emotional or sensory problems, who are developing normally in other areas (Dumtschin, 1988). Based on a review of the literature, Dumtschin (1988) found that methodological inconsistencies across research studies have precluded an agreed-upon specific description of the nature of SLI. Characteristics of children with SLI are summarized in Table 10.4.

Despite normal nonverbal intelligence, they also may have difficulty processing incoming information, difficulty with comprehension of more extended discourse, problems with short-term auditory sequential memory, and difficulty with solving complex problems (R. Paul, 2001; Owens, 2004; Rescorla & Lee, 2001). Language specialists caution, however, that there is great variation among children with SLI (several subtypes seem to exist); that the most outstanding characteristic of this difficulty is late and slow development of form, with better development of content and use interactions; and that the SLI label does not inform intervention (see, e.g., Aram, 1991; Lahey, 1988; Owens, 2004; and R. Paul, 2001).

The *Diagnostic and Statistical Manual of Mental Disorders*, fourth edition, text revision (DSM-IV-TR; American Psychiatric Association, 2000) defines five types of communication disorders that are based on low scores on individually administered standardized tests, and that interfere with academic achievement:

1. *Expressive language disorder*, characterized by "scores on standardized individually administered measures of expressive language development substantially below those obtained from standardized measures of both nonverbal intellectual capacity and receptive language development" (p. 58). Phonological difficulties are the most common associated feature of this disorder in younger children.
2. *Mixed receptive–expressive language disorder*, characterized by both receptive and expressive language development substantially below nonverbal intellectual capacity. In addition to the difficulties associated with expressive language disorder, children also have "difficulty understanding words, sentences, or specific types of words" (p. 62). This disorder may be developmental or acquired after a period of normal development as a result of a neurological or medical condition.
3. *Phonological disorder*, characterized by the "failure to use developmentally expected speech sounds that are appropriate for the individual's age and dialect" (p. 65).
4. *Stuttering*, characterized by "a disturbance in the normal fluency and time patterning of speech that is inappropriate for the individual's age," including "frequent repetitions or prolongations of sounds of sounds or syllables" (p. 67). A large proportion of individuals with this problem recover, many spontaneously.
5. *Communication disorder not otherwise specified* (e.g., a voice disorder).

A concern for many speech–language specialists is possible bias when standardized tests are used to evaluate children from diverse backgrounds (Bloom, 1991; Warner & Nelson, 2000). The diagnostic categories yielded do not indicate the etiology of the condition, explain the nature of the language disorder, or specify behaviors that should be developed in intervention. Furthermore, labels may be the source of great concern for parents and have a negative effect on children (Warner & Nelson, 2000). Except to obtain services where categorization may be required, most experts focus on the need to describe children's specific language behaviors, including their strategies and strengths, as well as their limitations across the areas of form, content, and use. Such information can contribute to intervention planning as well as early identification. We endorse this perspective.

Prevalence of Language Disorders among Preschool Children, and the Importance of Early Identification

Many children served under IDEA 2004 in the age range of 3–5 years are classified with speech and/or language disorders. During 1999–2000, more than 1 million students in the public schools' special education programs were categorized as having speech or language impairment as a primary problem (National Institute of Child Health and Human Development [NICHD], 2003). Wetherby and Prizant (1993) indicate that 70% of all children ages 3–5 identified with disabilities have speech and language problems. These researchers further indicated that, given the wide variability in the age at which children say their first word, preschool children with communication problems usually are not identified until after 3 years of age, except for those with severe developmental disabilities (family members may disagree on whether a problem exists, and primary healthcare providers may delay referral). There is also substantial evidence that these early language difficulties persist despite intervention (Aram & Nation, 1980; Aram & Hall, 1989; Lahey, 1988; Wetherby & Prizant, 1996). It is quite understandable for preschool children with language disorders to be at risk for later learning difficulties, since using language to encode/decode messages is central to problem solving, reading, and writing. Furthermore, a large proportion of preschoolers with speech and language problems will continue to present some degree of language problems during the school years, to experience some form of academic learning problems, and to be at risk for emotional or behavioral difficulties (Aram & Hall, 1989; Owens, 2004; R. Paul, 2001; Wetherby & Prizant, 1993).

Wetherby and Prizant (1993) point out that the challenge for professionals is "to distinguish a child who is late in beginning to talk but who will catch up spontaneously from one who will have persisting language problems" (p. 291), and many children slow to start talking do catch up. Thus professionals are cautious about referring children before they are 3 or 4 years old (R. Paul, 2001). R. Paul (2001) points out that children with mild to moderate SLI may resolve many of their language problems before beginning their formal education. However, as the demands of learning require more complex language skills, these problems may "resurface" and "grow" into LD (p. 157). Since a large number of children do not "outgrow" their language problems, Aram and Hall (1989) have pointed to the need for a long-term perspective on language disorders and intervention. Although preschool intervention may not prevent later difficulties, many speech and language impairments may be correctable during the preschool years (Glascoe, 1991).

Mental Retardation

Most children with low cognitive skills exhibit disruption in all areas of language, as well as delays in most areas of development. (A detailed discussion of children with mental retardation is presented in Chapter 12; the focus here is on issues related to language development.) Quantitative analyses have pointed to slower vocabulary growth and the use of more concrete words; use of a less extensive variety of verbs; later emergence of language structures, although these appear in the same developmental sequence (after babbling) of content and form as in children without mental retardation until the mean length of utterance has reached 3 (R. Paul, 2001); and less developed communicative interactions with others, such as the use of gestures. There are no specific, unique patterns of language dysfunction among children with low-level cognitive skills. Furthermore, the diagnosis of mental retardation does not lead to the identification of specific language-learning needs or to specific procedures for teaching language (Lahey, 1988). These children should always be assessed for language comprehension in order to plan and implement intervention.

Based on their work with students with mental retardation, Abbeduto and Nuccio (1989, p. 502) present a model of communication, which requires assessment in four domains that may help guide some areas of intervention:

1. Linguistic ability (i.e., mastery of vocabulary, syntax, and phonology).
2. Cognitive ability (e.g., memory).
3. Social skills (e.g., perspective taking).
4. Pragmatic competence (i.e., knowledge and skill specific to the process of communication with others, such as knowing when one should answer questions).

Learning Disabilities

The LD category includes a broad range of learning difficulties in children with normal intelligence and without other disabling conditions, such as sensory difficulties or emotional problems. This category is not widely applied at the preschool level, where the even broader term *developmental delay* is more frequently used. Lahey (1988) points out that the syndrome of LD closely resembles that of SLI. Riccio (1992) reviewed research indicating that many preschoolers (up to 45%) with speech and/or language disorders, despite intervention, are later identified as having LD, particularly children who demonstrate both receptive and expressive language problems. Furthermore, there is a high prevalence of communication disorders among the population with LD (up to 90%), and such difficulty is frequently associated with a reading disability (Riccio, 1992; Snyder & Downey, 1991). These children often have word-finding difficulties, such as inaccurate production of names of pictures, difficulty recalling specific words to communicate ideas, slower rate of naming, circumlocutions, and difficulty with complex syntactic structures (Bowers & Swanson, 1991; German, 1989; Lahey, 1988). Poor word naming (word retrieval) in kindergarten is predictive of reading difficulty in later years (Jansky & de Hirsch, 1972; Wiig & Semel, 1984). Word-finding difficulties may reflect deficient vocabularies and may result in a need for longer time to respond, as well as in communication breakdowns such as word substitutions or insertions (Owens, 1995). Teachers and other assessors need to be alert to such problems and request observation by a speech–language specialist. Most children with LD have difficulty with phonology, which contributes to their decoding or word retrieval difficulties (Riccio, 1992). These children also have difficulty with synthesizing the rules of language (Owens, 2004).

Autism Spectrum Disorders

Difficulties with both verbal and nonverbal communication are among the critical features of ASD. Among the specific difficulties are (1) oddities in the use of gesture or other forms of nonverbal communication; (2) difficulties in receptive language; (3) stereotypical or repetitive use of language (e.g., echoing back what they have heard); (4) difficulty in reading the verbal and nonverbal signals of others (e.g., eye contact); and (4) lack of use of language for social communication. As described in detail in Chapter 13, the language of autistic children is clearly *deviant*, as opposed to just *delayed*. What distinguishes these children from children with developmental language disorders children are behaviors other than language, such as deficits in relatedness (they may miss the point of questions directed to them, and their speech may lack emotional tone) and stereotypic or perseverative behaviors and preoccupations (Allen, 1989). The onset of language is late for most of these children, and markedly so for those with IQs below 70. Allen (1988) cautions that because of their pervasive social and cognitive problems, the specific language problems in children with ASD are often overlooked or are not addressed in intervention. (Again, see Chapter 13 for greater detail.)

Visual Impairments/Blindness

Children with visual deficits often demonstrate delays in the onset of language and have limited receptive and expressive language. The reasons for such delays are multifaceted. For example, toddlers without visual impairments learn 60% of their information through their incidental visual experiences with the environment (Bishop, 1986; Koenig & Holbrook, 2000). Lacking visual input, children with visual difficulties need to explore their environment through sound and touch. Systematic exposure to their environment, with objects and events labeled by adults (techniques that parents learn through early intervention), is essential to stimulate language learning (Ferrell et al., 1990). The need for these children to develop high awareness of their surroundings through tactile and auditory channels adds to their attention and memory load. Lacking visual input, they miss the gestures and nonverbal cues of others, such as pointing and smiles or other signs of affective behavior.

Given their more circuitous avenue of learning, children with visual impairments may be delayed in acquiring vocabulary (Lahey, 1988). Concepts develop more slowly, particularly those that involve sensory–motor interactions and abstract ideas. Even young children who appear typically verbal often do not have a cognitive understanding of many terms, because they will never be able to get the "whole" cognitive picture of objects as they appear in the everyday environment. With preschool and early-school-age children, for example, this difficulty is pronounced with temporal relational concepts, such as *before–after* and *more–less*, which are important for following teacher directions and complying with instruction (Boehm, 1986, 2001; Stolarski & Boehm, 2006). Children with visual impairments also have difficulty with spatial prepositions (e.g., *over*), since they do not see the spatial images that these prepositions code and do not have access to the many nonverbal cues that are conveyed in pictures. (However, some concepts such as *right* and *left* become more salient at an earlier age, as children learn to explore from left to right.) They do not necessarily develop a language disorder, but may use linguistic forms without full knowledge of their meaning (i.e., extend them beyond the context in which they were learned). Although the meanings coded in the single-word utterance phase are similar to those of children without visual impairments, delays in syntactic constructions can occur (Lahey, 1988). At the kindergarten level and above, good Braille teaching will introduce correct grammatical constructions in printed form. Some children with visual impairments may have limited motivation to explore (Koenig & Holbrook, 2000) and may have more difficulty maintaining conversational topics (R. Paul, 2001).

Assessing preschool children with visual impairments is a challenge. For example, we (Stolarski & Boehm, 2006; Stolarski, Boehm, & Boisvert, 2006) are developing versions of the *Boehm Test of Basic Concepts—Third Edition* (BTBC-3) and of its preschool counterpart (Boehm-3: Preschool) for blind and visually impaired children. Enlargements of test items have been developed from the original computer representations in combination with digital images for the Boehm-3 (Stolarski & Boehm, 2005) and with raised figures for the Boehm-3: Preschool (Stolarski et al., 2005). This process is more difficult than it sounds. For example, the outlines of enlarged figures become fuzzy, and the contrast between colors may not be adequate. The raised figure version is being developed with a few carefully chosen target objects and geometric figures that a child needs to explore tactually. For a young child, such modifications may change the complexity of the verbal directions given and/or the difficulty level of the item.

It is particularly important to use elicitation procedures during assessment. The assessor who has had specialized training in visual impairment and blindness, for example, needs to go back and query the child's understanding of missed items ("Tell me what that feels like," "Describe it"). Finally, the assessor needs to have additional objects at hand (e.g., cubes, ball, doll, shoebox) to probe the child's understanding ("Pick up the ball. Put it under the box") and explore the forms of adult assistance needed. As Koenig and Holbrook (2000) state, "The goal is to modify what is necessary to make the assessment tool fair, but not to change the difficulty level and validity of the task" (p. 42). All such changes must be recorded and described.

Hearing Impairments/Deafness

As might be expected, children with moderate to severe hearing impairments have great difficulty in learning the auditory/vocal aspects of language, as compared to the use of gestures and other symbolic forms. These children may or may not display a language disorder, depending on the environment in which they are raised (signing or nonsigning) (Lahey, 1988). Deaf children of nonsigning parents have particular difficulty. Such parents' acceptance of their child's hearing loss plays an essential role. As Marschark, Lang, and Albertini (2002) state, "Perhaps the two most important variables in the development of deaf children are parental attitudes toward hearing loss and the quality of parent–child communication" (p. 91).

Meier (1991) presents a number of lines of argument to illustrate that children isolated from speech acquire linguistic skills in much the same way as children who hear if they have appropriate stimulation. He presents evidence to support the position set forth by Chomsky (1988) that children have a biologically based capacity to learn language. In the typical language-learning environment, children receive linguistic input that is auditory and accessible from birth. Deaf children of hearing parents may hear little or none of their parents' speech. If parents do not use ASL or other sign language, the children are not consistently exposed to language and, as a result, are linguistically deprived. According to Meier (1991), "More than 90% of prelingually deaf children are born to hearing parents" (p. 62) and are thus often deprived of exposure to sign language. Interestingly, children who are thus deprived usually invent their own system of communication through gestures, which they combine to form sentences. These invented gestures and orders of gesture are used consistently (Meier, 1991). Meier proposes, as a possible explanation for this resiliency, that children are biologically prepared to acquire these linguistic properties.

Meier and Newport (1990) documented that deaf children born to deaf parents who use ASL pass through the language-learning milestones in very much the same way (same sequence and same age) as normally hearing children—producing their first words at about 12 months, combining words between 18 and 24 months, and using inflectional word endings by 30 months. Meier and Newport also provided evidence to support the importance of early exposure to ASL. Intervention during the early years of life (before age 3) is particularly important for deaf children of hearing parents, who sometimes wait or do not know they need to seek services. This problem may now be partially resolved through federal legislation that authorizes hearing screening, evaluation, and intervention for all newborn and infants (the Newborn and Infant Hearing Screening and Intervention Act of 1999). Children of immigrant parents, however, may not receive these services.

There is conflicting evidence that early recurrent mild hearing or intermittent hearing loss, such as otitis media, can affect language learning for some children (Downs & Blager, 1982; Lahey, 1988; Wallace, 1986). Otitis media often causes a temporary hearing loss, which in turn may affect a young child's attention and early language development. Lahey (1988) suggests that children with this difficulty should be considered "at risk" for language-learning problems, and cautions that these children may miss incidental learning experiences. She recommends careful monitoring of progress to determine whether a child's skills are developing normally; if not, extra language stimulation may be needed.

Lonigan, Fischel, Whitehurst, Arnold, and Valdez-Menchaca (1992) studied the effects of medically documented otitis media on two groups of children: those classified as having developmental expressive language disorder without other impairments, and those progressing normally. There was no difference in frequency of occurrence or duration of otitis media between the disordered group and the normal control group. However, otitis media appeared to be related to the development of expressive language disorder, particularly when children were starting to talk (12–18 months). The researchers also found that children experiencing more, or more severe, episodes of otitis media between 18 and 24 months had significantly poorer articulation than those who experienced fewer episodes of otitis media; however, these problems with articulation resolved spontaneously when the infection subsided. These authors concluded that a history of otitis media is one of the important variables in expressive language disorder, particularly during the age span of 12–18 months (a critical period for the development of expressive language). However, spontaneous improvement of language development is likely as the infection passes. Language difficulties may be more long-lasting with prolonged, recurrent otitis media, including problems with auditory processing and expressive language, attention and behavioral problems, and difficulty in communicating intentions (Prutting, 1982). Therefore, along with monitoring language development when children are experiencing recurrent otitis media, parents and teachers need to speak slowly and directly to these children and to provide stimulating language experiences as required (Lahey, 1988).

Although deaf children can follow much the same developmental route in acquiring language as children without hearing loss, it is often greatly delayed in deaf children of hearing parents, as noted above. Some differences include engaging in less communicative behavior; using different types of early verb forms; being less sophisticated in auditory/vocal forms expressed or understood; and having difficulty with concept words and words with multiple meanings (Lahey, 1988; P. V. Paul, 2001). Depending on the age at which intervention is started, "inflectional morphemes, adverbs, prepositions, quantifiers, and indefinite pronouns seem to be especially difficult" for these children (P. V. Paul, 2001, p. 124). Distinct differences from typical speech are observed in the oral linguistic productions of all severely hearing impaired children, except those who become deaf after having acquired language. They are difficult to understand and have a distinctive voice quality. Children with hearing impairments often do not have difficulty with pragmatics and communicate effectively with others; the greater the hearing loss, however, the more difficulty these children have with pragmatics. Some parents communicate in a directive manner with their hearing-impaired children, which can interfere with the children's language development. Assessors need specialized training in hearing impairment and deafness to evaluate these conditions thoroughly. However, all assessors need to be sensitive to possible hearing loss in young children, and possibly slow down their presentation of tasks to allow more time for working memory.

Research in this area (Kretschmer & Kretschmer, 2001; Lahey, 1988; Marschark et al., 2002; P. V. Paul, 2001; Quigley & Kretschmer, 1982) indicates the following:

1. The timing of loss of hearing affects language development. Children who lose hearing *after they learn language* are superior in both speech and language skills to those with prelinguistic hearing loss.
2. The degree of hearing loss is related to the level of language skills acquired.
3. The age at which intervention begins is particularly relevant, with intervention begun before age 3 having greater positive effects for deaf children of hearing parents.
4. The form of intervention (oral, total, or manual) has no differential effects, depending on the quality and timing of intervention.
5. Deaf children of hearing parents have better speech production skills than deaf children of deaf parents, whereas this latter group has better language skills.
6. Providing an environment with frequent storybook reading and exposure to print and writing contributes importantly to literacy development.
7. Literacy development is a slow process, with the majority of deaf students leaving high school still reading at a fourth- to sixth-grade level (Marschark et al., 2002).
8. The difficulty in acquiring language for most students with severe to profound hearing impairment has pervasive effects on their cognitive and psychosocial development (P. V. Paul, 2001).

ASSESSMENT APPROACHES AND PROCEDURES

Assessment of language development, like assessment of other areas, needs to be an ongoing process. Language assessment may occur for a number of reasons and under different circumstances: as part of (1) developmental screening covering all domains (see Chapter 6), when a problem is suspected to exist or when a child is making a transition from one program to another (typically at age 3 from early intervention to preschool, or at age 5 from preschool or daycare to kindergarten); (2) diagnostic evaluation, to determine whether a problem exists, and if so, whether a child qualifies for special education services; (3) in-depth diagnostic evaluation, to determine the child's current baseline level of functioning across language functions of comprehension and production (R. Paul, 2001) and to identify the child's strengths and limitations; (4) establishing the nature of the intervention and intervention goals in areas of concern; and (5) charting progress, testing hypotheses, and adjusting goals. If a parent, teacher, or healthcare provider is concerned about a child's language development and makes a referral, the first step is to interview the parent and gain a developmental and medical history of the child. It is essential to determine whether a recent hearing evaluation has taken place and, if so, how extensive that evaluation was. The assessor then needs to observe the child engaged in a play activity with a familiar toy (or with other children). Depending on the outcome of these activities, the assessor may then wish to have the parent complete the Vineland Adaptive Behavior Scale, Second Edition (Vineland-II; Sparrow et al., 2005) to rule out possible mental retardation or other interpersonal problems. The Vineland-II has a strong communication domain and this information could be used with a language test to determine whether the child has a language delay and qualifies for services. If the child qualifies for services, the next step is in-depth evaluation by a speech–language specialist to determine the nature and extent of the problem along with intervention goals and procedures. See Figure 10.2 for an overview of assessment activities that need to occur, depending on the assessment purpose.

Step 1: Schoolwide developmental screening.	Step 1 (alternative): Referral by parent, teacher, or healthcare provider.
• Use brief test such as ESI-R or DIAL-3 (see Chapter 6). • Obtain identifying information about child and family. • Perform vision/hearing/health check. • Use questionnaire to gain information on socioemotional behaviors not covered on screening tests. • Three possible screening outcomes: 1. No difficulty—feedback to parents and teachers. 2. Retest—child moves to step 2. 3. Refer—child moves to step 3.	Child moves automatically to step 3.

Step 2: If language problem suspected, observation.

1. Observe in classroom child's use of language in play and other activities that encourage communication over time.
2. Engage in ongoing observation of child to understand language strengths and areas needing development, including:
   - Discourse skills: Gains the attention of others, communicates appropriately and effectively with others.
   - Intelligibility of what child says.
   - Requests for information.
   - Expression of ideas and feelings.
   - Ability to follow directions of increasing length and complexity.
3. Look for:
   - Violation of turn taking.
   - Difficulty initiating, maintaining, or ending conversations.
   - Not recognizing cues teachers/parents use.
   - Not attending to others when they speak.
4. Document observations:
   - Provide enrichment activities (i.e., prereferral interventions).
   - Involve parents in providing language enrichment activities at home.
   - Offer all parents organized programs/workshops, as well as activities to support language development.
5. Check out observations with parents and gain their input.

If difficulty is observed and continues, child moves to step 3.

Step 3: Evaluation to determine eligibility for services.

1. Obtain medical and developmental history through interview or questionnaire and ensure that a thorough hearing evaluation has taken place.
2. Interview parent or guardian.
3. Administer Vineland-II to rule out possible presence of mental retardation or other mental disorders as well as get parent perception of communicative competence.
4. Determine whether recent hearing evaluation has taken place.
5. Engage child in play activities with familiar toys.
6. Administer Boehm-3: Preschool to make sure child understands basic concepts, and a test such as PLS-4 or CELF Preschool-2 to get a broad picture of language functioning.
7. Observe in classroom, if possible.

Factors to be taken into account:

1. Language spoken at home by child.
2. Whether assessment is carried out in child's first language.
3. Child's personality and style.

If difficulty is observed and continues, child moves to step 4.

(continued)

FIGURE 10.2. Assessment activities from screening to in-depth language evaluation.

Step 4: In-depth evaluation to determine nature and extent of problem, along with intervention goals and procedures (carried out by a speech–language specialist).

1. Review records.
2. Interview parents to gain a history of child's language development and day-to-day communicative activities.
   - Determine how family members perceive the child and what their concerns are.
   - Possibly have parent(s) complete appropriate questionnaire (e.g., Ages and Stages).
3. Double-check that a recent hearing evaluation has taken place.
   - Possibly administer audiological measures.
4. Rule out mental retardation (if not already done) and determine interplay of other emotional or medical problems.
5. Observe child in critical environments of home and school to identify not only child needs, but possible environmental adaptations.
   - If class observations not possible, ask teacher to complete questionnaires and rating scales.
6. Gain a representative language sample to determine mean length of utterance (MLU), and/or analyze language structures through elicitation tasks.
   - Engage child in play with toys of high appeal.
   - Use elicitation tasks as needed (e.g., play with puppets).
   - Observe parent interacting with child.
7. Administer normative assessment tasks to focus on a particular language area of concern.
8. Depending on the child's presenting problem and age, review areas such as the following to determine the nature of the child's communicative strengths and difficulties, as well as the influence of context:
   - Receptive and expressive language.
   - Use of symbols (words, gestures, signals) to express thoughts.
   - Size of vocabulary, including content words, objects, relations between objects, events, verbs, adjectives, basic relational concepts, adverbs, function words (articles, conjunctions, prepositions), and unusual words.
   - Ability to follow directions of increasing length and complexity.
   - Story comprehension (picture content, what happens before/after/next, story characters).
   - Syntax: Use of morphemes (suffixes, plurals, possessives, past tense); use of auxiliaries, other grammatical forms; complex sentences.
   - Phonology: Speech sounds, use of phonemes (sounds that make up words); awareness of individual sounds in words; rhymes; relationships between letters and sounds; production of speech sounds; omissions, substitutions, distortions, blending, intonational patterns.
   - Use of language in social situations: turn taking in conversations, verbalizations in play activities; expression of ideas; ability to gain attention of others; ability to get others to do things.
   - Memory and information processing: Attention and concentration; ability to retrieve words and ideas from memory; ability to persist and correct errors.
   - Environmental issues: Responses of adults to child's efforts (whether they model, expand on, prompt, comment on what child says); other supportive or nonsupportive strategies used by parents and teachers.
   - Other factors: Dialect differences versus developmental language difficulties; home language and culture; disability conditions; child personality/style.
9. Develop short- and long-term goals, along with intervention plan.

Step 5:

1. Engage in ongoing assessment and modify activities as child progresses.
2. Evaluate intervention effectiveness.

Step 6: Evaluate intervention effectiveness.

FIGURE 10.2. *(continued)*

In addition to the fact that no one instrument or battery can provide a comprehensive picture of form, content, and use functions across contexts, at no one point in time is the child going to produce all the forms of language in his or her repertoire. The approaches used need to be based on the needs of the child to be assessed. Individual measures and procedures sample different behaviors and may or may not tap what a child knows and can do. Moreover, since language use varies over contexts, it is widely agreed that in-depth assessment using descriptive approaches needs to take place across situations. A multidimensional plan needs to be developed that takes into account the child's functioning across all developmental areas; all of the child's language experience contexts; and all aspects of language comprehension and production. These factors are summarized in Figure 10.3 and presented in the sections that follow.

Involving Parents

Because the input of parents as expert informants is particularly important, assessors need to have highly refined interviewing skills (Prizant et al., 1993). Such skills are also necessary to build the rapport needed to engage parents in intervention activities. For a referred child, it is important for the assessor to (1) obtain a history of the child's language development; (2) obtain information about the child's day-to-day communicative activities; (3) determine whether there has been a recent hearing evaluation, as noted above; and (4) determine the interplay of mental retardation, emotional problems, and other medical problems. Since there is substantial evidence that there is a familial basis for developmental speech and language disorders (American Psychiatric Association, 2000; Riccio, 1992), family history needs to be investigated during the interview as well. It is also important for the interviewer to gain a picture of how the family perceives the child (e.g., friendly, bright, annoying) and the family's own fears and concerns (Lund & Duncan, 1993).

After identifying information and each parent's immediate concerns have been elicited, this interview might include questions such as those presented in Table 10.5. Depending on the presenting problem (such as visual impairment), other questions could be added to this list. For some families, many of these questions could be built into a preassessment questionnaire, allowing the assessor to follow up on important areas. Gallagher (1983) has suggested such a questionnaire, in which caregivers and teachers are asked (by mail, phone, or interview) about the influence of various contexts on the child's communicative behaviors, the words and phrases the child uses or other language behaviors of interest, and the activities and toys the child enjoys. This information will allow the assessor to make best use of the relatively short periods of direct observation. Filling out such a questionnaire, however, may be difficult for some families. A number of parent-completed checklists of the child's receptive and expressive language use are also available, such as the second edition of the Ages and Stages Questionnaires (ASQ; Bricker & Squires, 1999) and the MacArthur Communicative Developmental Inventories (Fenson et al., 1994) (see below).

Exploring Language Use across Contexts

Procedures for assessing language use across contexts include (1) determining in what activities the child is most likely to use language, through a questionnaire or interview with a parent or other adult (such as a teacher or caregiver); and (2) observing the child's use of language while engaged in these activities. Developmental norms can then be used

Child factors		
Cognitive ability	Physical/Sensory Condition	Socioemotional factors
• Verbal and nonverbal intelligence • Symbolic play • Ability to organize and remember information • Ability to retrieve words and ideas from memory • Ability to follow directions of increasing length and complexity	• Physical well-being • Hearing • Other possible disabling conditions	• Personality • Affective state • Motivation and interests • Attention • Interactions with others • Play behaviors

Contexts of language experience				
Home	School/daycare	Community	Medical	Particular Activity
• Culture • Language spoken • Opportunities for language exchanges • Adults present	• Staff • Materials • Activities	• Services available • Cultural network	• Medical problems • Persistent history of otitis media	• Play • Book sharing/ story retelling • Elicited samples of behavior • Formal tests

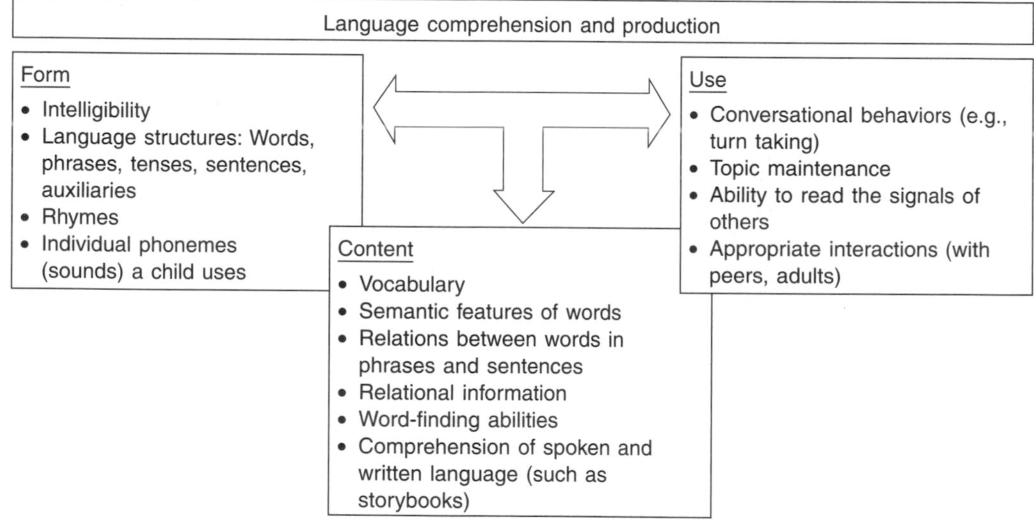

(continued)

FIGURE 10.3. Factors to be accounted for in the assessment process.

1. Does a language problem exist in one or more areas? If so, what is the extent/nature of the problem?
2. Is there an interaction with other problems?
3. Has there been a sampling of infrequent language behaviors?
4. Has the influence of context been taken into account (i.e., has a representative sample been taken across contexts)?
5. Is there familiarity with the child's culture and past experiences?
6. Has information been gained on the nature of language transactions occurring between child and adults?
7. Have both comprehension and production been evaluated?
8. Have multiple interactive components of language been examined: content, form (phonology and syntax), and use (ability to communicate effectively with others, express thoughts, engage in interactive play)?
9. Have behaviors used by adults to help children develop language been examined?
10. Have specific intervention activities been suggested? If so, have they been attempted and with what results?

FIGURE 10.3. *(continued)*

to assess the possible need for intervention. Possible adaptations/supports that might allow the child to be successful can also be identified through observation (Downing, 1989). Moreover, it is important to identify which persons (parents, teachers, or other caregivers) interact with the child on a regular basis, and to identify the strategies that support or interfere with the child's communicative interactions (Prizant et al., 1993). Thus, when possible, it is important to observe a parent (and/or teacher/childcare provider) interacting with the child (e.g., engaging in a play activity). The communicative behaviors used by each dyad can inform diagnosis and intervention. Whenever possible, such an activity should be built into the assessment process.

Given the interaction of all developmental domains, it is not surprising that there is considerable overlap in assessment tasks across these domains, particularly at the preschool level (e.g., a child's vocabulary will be assessed in both cognitive and language domains). This overlap allows various members of an assessment team to contribute importantly to the process. Furthermore, it is difficult to engage in most forms of assessment (except direct observation) without the use of language; whether or not a child needs to respond verbally to certain tasks, the child needs to be familiar with the vocabulary and concepts used by the assessor. Thus, as indicated above, most language specialists recommend using a variety of techniques to obtain a representative language sample and to understand the child's interactions with other individuals across contexts (Cole, 1982; Downing, 1989; Davis-McFarland & Dowell, 2000; Lahey, 1988; Lund & Duncan, 1993; Olswang & Bain, 1988; Owens, 1995, 2004; R. Paul, 2001; Roberts & Crais, 1989; Wells, 1985).

After collecting identifying information about the child and his or her family, taking a medical and developmental history, determining whether or not a recent hearing evaluation has been completed, and reviewing the child's level of nonverbal intelligence (and in some cases adaptive behavior), the assessor should pursue as many of the following basic strategies described in the literature for collecting language data as possible:

TABLE 10.5. Possible Areas to Be Covered in Parent Interview

General

- What concerns do you have about your child's language development?
- During which activities is your child most likely to talk or interact with you?
- What toys does your child enjoy?

Receptive understanding of language

- What language do you generally speak at home?
- Does your child understand what you say? How does he or she let you know?
- Is your child able to follow the directions that you give? If your child has difficulty, give an example.
- Does your child enjoy storybook reading? How does he or she respond to your questions or prompts?

Expressive use of language

- When did your child first begin using words?
- What are some of the words your child uses?
- Does your child use phrases/sentences? If so, what are some examples?
- If your child watches television or videos, does he/she make comments?
- Does your child participate in conversations, such as at mealtime? How?
- Does your child comment during play with you or other children? When you read storybooks? If so, how?

Medical or physical problems that might interfere with learning language

- Does your child have frequent colds or ear infections?
- Has this happened for a long time?
- About what age was your child when these problems began?
- Does your child have trouble hearing you?
- Are there other medical problems?
- Has your child had a recent hearing evaluation? If so, when? What were the the outcomes?

Attention or behavior problems

- Does your child have difficulty paying attention? In what ways?
- How does your child get along with other children?
- How does your child communicate with other children when playing?
- How does your child communicate with you when you play?

Prior assistance

- Has your child had a language evaluation in the past?
- What were the outcomes?
- Has your child received assistance before?
- What were the outcomes?

The present evaluation

- What activities can be used to best understand how your child uses language?

1. Direct observation of language use, either spontaneously in familiar activities or through the use of elicitation tasks. The first line of assessment is to observe children at play. Depending on the information provided the assessor earlier, may ask the parent to bring in some of the child's favorite toys. Or collections of toys may be used to elicit desired language behaviors. Newman et al. (1985), for example, suggest four sets of toys (a total of about 35) associated with a doll, dishes, house, and garage, which represent nearly all phonemes in two positions. These authors also suggest creating stories for children to retell that include desired language behaviors. It is recommended that such assessment activities be audiotaped for later review whenever possible.

2. Indirect observation through parent or teacher interview, or by using developmental scales or checklists. For example, the Vineland-II (Sparrow et al., 2005), a parent semistructured interview scale with excellent technical characteristics (see Chapters 12 and 13), helps assessors determine the presence or absence of cognitive, language, motor, and social/emotional problems. The second edition of the ASQ (Bricker & Squires, 1999; see Chapter 4) is a screening system that consists of 19 parent-completed questionnaires covering the age span of 4–60 months that covers five developmental areas (Communication, Gross Motor, Fine Motor, Problem Solving, and Personal–Social). Extensive data are provided regarding the technical characteristics of the scale.

Several other scales are widely used to assess a child's level of language development. For instance, the MacArthur Communicative Developmental Inventories (Fenson et al., 1994) are parent-completed, research-based developmental inventories of children's language and communication skills, including both "Words and Gestures" and "Words and Sentences." The Language Development Survey from the Child Behavior Checklist for Ages 1½–5 (Achenbach & Rescorla, 2000b) is a parent-completed checklist of words the child uses or understands. The parent also provides examples of phrases used by the child. (See Chapter 14 for a review of the Child Behavior Checklist.)

3. Interview with at least one teacher/childcare provider regarding this person's concerns and the child's day-to-day language behaviors.

4. Formal norm-referenced measures and criterion-referenced tests, to assess particular language behaviors not directly observed or to track progress. Some assessment devices focus on just one component of language. For instance, the Peabody Picture Vocabulary Test—Third Edition (PPVT-III; Dunn & Dunn, 1997), focuses on receptive vocabulary, and the Boehm-3 and Boehm-3: Preschool (Boehm, 2000a, 2001) and Bracken Basic Concepts Scale—Revised (Bracken, 1998) on understanding of the receptive understanding of important relational concepts used across language tasks. Others, such as the Preschool Language Scale—Fourth Edition (PLS-4; Zimmerman et al., 2002) and the Clinical Evaluation of Language Fundamentals Preschool—Second Edition (CELF Preschool-2; Wiig, Secord, & Semel, 2005) cover multidimensional aspects. An overview of several selected measures is presented in Appendix 10.1. Another group—the Battelle Developmental Inventory, Second Edition (BDI-2; Newborg, 2004), the Hawaii Early Learning Profile (Furuno et al., 1994), and the Developmental Profile II (DP-II; Alpern, Boll, & Shearer, 1986), among others (see Appendices 6.1 and 7.1 for some of these), are broad-based tests that cover the major developmental domains, including language.

5. Play-based assessment. The assessment of children at play is essential, and many measures have been developed to look at different aspects of language development. The Transdisciplinary Play-Based Assessment approach detailed by Linder (1996) embeds many of the procedures described above (direct observation of free play alone

and with another child; elicited activities provided by a facilitator; parent interview and feedback from parents as integral members of the team). Linder also provides excellent guidelines and forms for recording observed behaviors. See Chapter 4 for greater detail.

6. Elicitation activities, such as story retelling or responding to puppets.
7. Dynamic assessment procedures, to determine the ways in which adult mediation and test–teach–test procedures influence a child's language use, and to inform intervention.

The first, second, and fourth categories above are described more fully in the sections that follow. Each approach has its strengths and limitations and serves different purposes. The goal is to understand the child's competencies, difficulties, strategies, and adult supports needed for success, in order to determine the need for special services and develop intervention strategies.

Direct Observation and Description

It is not possible, except through watching and listening, to assess young children's verbal expressive language, use of gesture, or other forms of expression. Ongoing observation of a child's spontaneous use of language in the natural environment of the home or preschool setting provides the best opportunity to gain a representative understanding of a child's functional use of language in everyday situations, such as during play (as described earlier). Through observing play activities the assessor can describe the child's productive language performance, along with cognitive skills, make-believe activities, and social interaction with others.

Observation in everyday settings provides the assessor with important ongoing information regarding not only the content and form of language, but the child's *use* of language—both to achieve interpersonal objectives and to meet his or her basic daily needs. The influence of various speakers and activities can also be accounted for in language use, and the bridge from assessment to intervention is more direct. For example, it is possible to describe how the child's language behaviors in different contexts and in different types of tasks are modified to meet the child's needs or in relationship to the difficulty of activities, and to adjust intervention strategies accordingly as the child makes gains or encounters difficulty. In addition, the observer will want to note the child's use of gestures (such as pointing), spontaneous labeling, off-topic statements, turn-taking activities, memory, speed of processing, and so forth. Although different contextual settings and the assessor's familiarity with cultural differences influence the amounts of language data obtained and the types of language behaviors observed, they do not affect the types of language structures observed in young children (Lahey, 1988; Olswang & Carpenter, 1988; Stokes & Duncan, 1989). Observation not only provides the assessor with the opportunity to sample the regularities and inconsistencies of a child's language behavior in a natural setting; it provides information needed to confirm or reject the existence of a problem, understand the strategies a child uses, clarify the nature of interactions with others, determine the role of the adult in providing the prompts necessary for the child to succeed, verify comments made by parent/teacher, and obtain descriptive information relevant to goals of intervention.

Collecting and analyzing a representative language sample, however, are labor-intensive tasks. Given the assessment question and the characteristics of the child, the assessor or assessment team needs to decide ahead of time how and when to collect a rich language sample—that is, *when the child is most likely to engage in communicative events*. In the home setting, this might be during general play, interactions with a parent or sibling, or mealtimes. It is important to interview the teacher prior to observing in a classroom to determine the typical schedule and find out which activities planned for the day of observation, since different language interactions are likely to occur during show and tell, in the housekeeping area, during block building or other forms of free play, and during snacktime.

If a problem is suspected and prereferral activities have not been successful, the next step is to administer a formal test such as the CELF Preschool-2. If the outcomes of this test confirm a problem, the child is generally referred for in-depth evaluation. One of the first steps during in-depth evaluation is to collect a language sample while the child is engaged in a familiar activity (see later section for greater detail).

Videotaping or high-quality audiotaping is the preferred method for recording observations, to provide an accurate record of vocal interactions; handwritten notes can be used to provide details about context. These recordings can be reviewed and, if needed, followed by print transcripts. While one is collecting this sample, it is important to be as unobtrusive as possible, to keep one's own talking to a minimum, and to use open-ended questions (Owens, 1995).

Mean Length of Utterance

Most authors cite *mean length of utterance* (MLU), which was given significance by Roger Brown (1973), as one rough measure for understanding a child's development of spoken language. Brown's findings have been extended through 5 years of age by Miller and Chapman (1981), who describe the following stages:

Stage	Age	MLU
I	1 to 2-2 years	1.0–2.0
II	2-3 to 2-6 years	2.0–2.5
III	2-7 to 2-10 years	2.5–3.0
IV	2-11 to 3-4 years	3.0–3.75
V	3-5 to 3-10 years	3.75–4.5
	3-11+ years	4.75+

MLU is determined by following these steps after collecting a language sample:

1. Counting consecutive words (utterances) spoken by the child during an observation period (typically about 50).
2. Counting the total number of morphemes used in this language sample. A morpheme is the smallest unit of sound that has meaning, such as a base word, affix, or inflection (e.g., *-s* or *=ed*). A base word counts as one morpheme; a word plus an inflection counts as two.
3. Dividing the total number of morphemes by the total number of utterances (e.g., 180 morphemes divided by 50 utterances = 3.6 MLU).

Lund and Duncan (1993) provide detailed examples of what to exclude and include in the MLU count. Rules for computing MLU for Spanish-speaking children are detailed by Linares (1981).

Up to an average of 4.0, MLU is cited as a good measure of language maturity and is reached by a typically developing child at about age 4 (Owens, 2004). However, many researchers (e.g., Chapman, 1981; Bloom, 1991; Lahey, 1988; Muma, 1985; and Wells, 1985) are careful to point out that MLU has limited value once a level of 3.0 has been achieved, is not a substitute for more detailed analysis, and does not discriminate between various types of linguistic development. Miller (1981) presented a table of the predicted ages ±1 *SD* for each MLU at each stage of development described by Brown (1973), and indicated that children 1 *SD* or more below the mean require further study.

As children get older, they have an increasingly large range of options available to them in their linguistic systems; thus correlations with MLU drop and become less useful. A slowing down occurs in the rate of MLU increase from about 42 months onward (Wells, 1985) as children use various strategies to make their utterances more concise. Variation also relates to a child's temperament and style (responsive, passive), conversational opportunities, and adult interaction styles. Muma (1986) states that "when MLU exceeds 4.0, knowledge of formal grammatical mechanisms can no longer be indexed by increments in MLU" (p. 214) and contends that the sequence of acquisition and use of grammatical structures is a more useful measure. Language specialists in general caution that MLU should never be used as the single basis for determining a child's developmental status, and that it should be used in combination with an analysis of structural errors and appropriate use of grammatical forms.

R. Paul (2001) cites evidence that MLU can be a useful developmental measure into the school years when used as a baseline to target other areas of language development during assessment. For example, MLU can be used to track growth over time in syntax and intervention effectiveness. However, she also points out that computing MLU is a time-consuming process that is not needed for every language sample, and she recommends that speech–language specialists who are pressed for time use other analysis procedures (e.g., elicitation tasks) that yield more information relevant to intervention planning. Finally, Hirsh-Pasek et al. (2005) caution that MLU is not comparable across dialects, such as African American English, where use of the past tense is optional. These researchers indicate that sentence diversity is more sensitive to emerging language abilities.

Elicitation Tasks

In order to assess particular language interactions, and to get at aspects of language that occur infrequently or may not occur in spontaneous speech, elicitation tasks may be used. The speech–language specialist can suggest tasks (e.g., games, role playing, story retelling) that are familiar and interesting to the child, and can then use probes based on the child's responses, such as asking the child to describe what he or she is doing (e.g., "What are you going to give the baby for supper?") or to give directions to puppets. Or the examiner may request the child to repeat phrases or sentences that vary in structure and complexity (i.e., desired language behaviors are modeled for the child). Lund and Duncan (1993) present a list of helpful ideas for getting a reluctant talker to talk; such tasks have the advantage of ensuring that the child will attempt specific constructions (Bryan, 1986). The examiner then needs to transcribe the resulting language interactions, to account for their context, and to analyze them in terms of the question at hand about the child's language use. Since this also is a time-consuming task, R. Paul (2001) recommends that speech sample analysis be carried out only if it has been established (from her perspective, based on the results of standardized testing) that the child has a productive language deficit. For the trained speech–language specialist, she recommends the more practical approach of listening to tape-recorded speech samples and using worksheets to analyze phonological and syntactic production.

Structured elicitation tasks can yield information about how a child's language development compares to that of other children. They do not give information about a child's rule system for content–form–use interactions, and they may elicit language in ways that are not representative of the child's normal mode of processing and using language in everyday settings (Lahey, 1988). They do, however, serve as a useful tool and allow analysis of children's production strategies. The technique used needs to be determined by the assessor's knowledge of the child. Miller (1981) provides multiple procedures and examples of elicited production and elicited imitation. Detailed procedures for structural analysis of a child's productions are provided by Lund and Duncan (1993), Lahey (1988), Miller (1981), Owens (2004), and R. Paul (2001). Computer programs for transcript analysis are described by R. Paul (2001).

In sum, most experts recommend collecting spontaneous language samples as a young child engages in familiar activities, or eliciting samples in the context of a semistructured play interview with the child, as an appropriate alternative to formal testing. Appealing representational toys are used so that children can reenact real-life situations. Puzzles and constructional toys are also available for children who cannot or do not choose to play symbolically. The speech–language specialist also must be prepared to use probe-like questions to elicit language behaviors that may not occur spontaneously. "The amount of language used, fluency, intelligibility, rate, and topic maintenance are all readily observable in this kind of setting, as is the child's ability to initiate and respond within a conversational mode" (Allen, 1989, p. 443).

Developmental Scales and Checklists

As noted earlier in this chapter, substantial research documents the order in which language milestones are achieved, along with the expected variability in the ages of mastery of these milestones (Bloom, 1991; Bloom & Lahey, 1978; Cole, 1982; Hart & Risley, 1999; Lahey, 1988; Linder, 1997; Olswang & Bain, 1988; for comprehensive summaries, see Coggins & Carpenter, 1981; Miller, 1981; Owens, 2004; R. Paul, 2001). Many measures of language are developmental scales and checklists based on these milestones, which are used to help identify language behaviors that the child has developed. Such scales may be more or less finely tuned. As Myers (1988) points out, "The scales are only as good as the milestones in development they sample and a prospective user should examine these milestones very carefully" (p. 39). Scales that report developmental ages also differ in the span of intervals in which milestones are reported; for example, some report developmental age in 3-month intervals, others in 6- or 12-month intervals. The number of language behaviors included in each interval also varies considerably, which can result in omission of important behaviors.

The accuracy with which developmental scales are completed, based either on direct observation or on knowledge of the child (in the case of parents or teachers), also depends on the adequacy of the observational sample obtained before completing the scale. Typically, those completing the scale indicate whether the behavior is present or absent, or give a numerical rating regarding the extent of that behavior. Sometimes the scale also requests a description of the observed language behavior (e.g., the Vineland-II). Only infrequently is specific information requested about the contexts in which these behaviors were observed. Some developmental scales were designed to be used over time, such as the Assessment, Evaluation, and Programming System for Infants and Children, Volume 4 (Bricker & Pretti-Fontczak, 1996). This scale is particularly useful to establish goals and monitor progress; suggestions are also provided for intervention activities.

In general, however, developmental scales and checklists focus on a child's achievements and fail to focus on the strategies the child uses; the nature of the child's interaction with the other member of the communication dyad; the influence of environmental characteristics and the value placed on language use in the child's culture; and the nature of the activity. Developmental scales may or may not be standardized, and also vary along a continuum of objectivity. Finally, those completing such scales often have only limited knowledge about the child's language functioning across language contexts. Assessors can address this last issue by having the same scale completed by different individuals (i.e., parents, teachers, childcare providers, and the assessors themselves) across contexts; by completing the scale after spending some time with the child; and by making use of repeated observations (e.g., completing the scale after a period of time working with the child). Teacher rating scales and checklists have the advantage of allowing teachers to assess communication behavior over time in the classroom, and take into account the needs of children who are culturally and linguistically diverse. Developmental scales and checklists are generally used in the context of other assessment information and can be useful in identifying children's relative strengths and areas needing development. If used over time, they can help chart progress.

Formal Tests

In language development as in other areas, the use of standardized tests allows comparison of a child's performance with that of other children of the same age. Standard, detailed procedures are followed for administering and scoring items. Detailed data regarding normative data, reliability, and validity are presented. Some tests also yield criterion-referenced information. Use of such tests may be important for children to qualify for services and for placement purposes. Often there is considerable item similarity between norm-referenced or criterion-referenced tests on the one hand and developmental scales or checklists on the other. Although many commonly used standardized language tests can provide a useful overview of functioning, some are not sufficiently precise to identify the richness and complexity of language production or comprehension problems; more recently revised tests seek to address this issue. In what follows, we review specific areas of language development and describe formal procedures that have been developed for their measurement.

Measures of Receptive and Expressive Language Comprehension

Children reveal their comprehension through the words and grammatical forms they know and use, or through such activities as pointing to and describing pictures ("Show me the picture of . . ., " "Tell me what the dog is doing") or pointing to or manipulating objects ("Touch your nose," "Throw me the ball"). These types of tasks are included on many language measures, as are responses to *wh-* questions. *Receptive comprehension* requires a child to encode and remember stimulus questions; understand what is required; retrieve from memory appropriate experiences; and manipulate toys, produce actions, or select from pictorial representations. Receptive comprehension can be tapped in a number of ways:

- Assessing receptive understanding of single words through asking the child to point to the picture that best represents the word spoken by the assessor. Examples include such tests as the PPVT-III (Dunn & Dunn, 1997), The Boehm-3 and Boehm-3: Preschool (Boehm, 2000a, 2001) and the Receptive One-Word Picture Vocabulary Test—2000 Edition (ROWPVT; Brownell, 2000b). Here the child demonstrates the ability to retrieve the meaning of words with which he or she has had experience from memory. Hirsh-Pasek et al. (2005) point out, however, that tests such as these do not provide insight regarding how the child uses the words assessed or how the words assessed are related to other words—that is, "the kinds of processes that earmark sophistication in vocabulary acquisition" (p. 6).
- Having the child manipulate toys in response to the assessor's oral commands.
- Having the child respond to directions of increasing length and complexity.
- Asking the child to point to pictures that represent the antonyms of spoken words.
- Asking the child to answer questions about a story.

In contrast, *expressive comprehension* requires a child not only to encode and remember stimulus questions, understand what is required, and retrieve from memory appropriate experiences, but to formulate appropriate answers through spoken or sign language. Expressive comprehension is assessed by having the child do such things as the following:

- Respond (verbally or in signs) to comprehension questions.
- Produce antonyms or synonyms to spoken words.
- Repeat (or imitate, without verbatim repetition) sentences of increasing length or complexity.
- Retell a story.
- Respond to tasks that require categorization.
- Demonstrate the expressive use of words through such tests as the Expressive One-Word Picture Vocabulary Test—2000 Edition (EOWPVT; Brownell, 2000a).

Of particular interest is the child's word diversity, or the number of different words used. Hirsh-Pasek et al. (2005) note that according to Tabors, Roach, and Snow (2002), the "density of rare words used and understood was the most predictive factor in further word learning" (p. 7). These researchers also indicate that learning how to add suffixes and prefixes greatly helps children expand their vocabulary.

A number of recently revised tests that measure receptive and expressive comprehension with acceptable technical data are now described briefly (technical data are presented in Appendix 10.1). These measures, in general, assess such areas as vocabulary, grammatical morphemes, and syntactic structures. The core subtests are brief (generally 30–45 minutes) and are intended to be used as part of the initial assessment process (which would include collecting case history, parent and teacher questionnaires, parent interview, accounting for the status of a child's hearing, and other test and observational data detailed earlier) as well as in-depth evaluation. Many of these tests do not indicate the nature of specific problems, however (McCauley & Swisher, 1984) or do they provide guidance for intervention planning (Salvia & Ysseldyke, 2004). More recent tests include supplemental parent/and or teacher questionnaires to cover the pragmatic component of language functioning (see also "Measures of Pragmatic Skills," below) and have sections addressed to issues of diversity.

Oades-Ses and Alfonso (2005) present a critical review of the psychometric integrity of 21 preschool language tests published between 1994 and 2004. Outcomes of this review indicate that significant improvements have been made in the technical adequacy of these tests in most areas other than test–retest reliabilities and test floors. In addition to the technical adequacy of measures, assessors need to consider the underlying processes children use as they acquire language (Hirsh-Pasek et al., 2005).

CLINICAL EVALUATION OF LANGUAGE FUNDAMENTALS—FOURTH EDITION

The CELF-4 (Semel, Wiig, & Secord, 2003) is a diagnostic battery that moves beyond making a diagnosis for eligibility purposes to identify strengths and weaknesses in receptive and expressive language for individuals 5–21 years of age. The CELF-4 Assessment Process Model includes four levels of subtests, to do the following:

Level 1: Identify whether or not there is a language disorder.
Level 2: Describe the nature of the disorder.
Level 3: Evaluate underlying clinical behaviors.
Level 4: Evaluate language and communication in context.

The core subtests used to determine the Core Language Score were chosen for their ability to distinguish language disorders. At level 1 for ages 5–8, these include Concepts and Following Directions, Word Structure, Recalling Sentences, and Formulating Sentences. By administering two additional subtests at level 2 (Word Classes 1 and Sentence Structure), assessors may be able to determine the nature of the disorder and obtain two additional index scores (Receptive Language and Expressive Language). Extension testing activities are provided for each subtest. At level 3, additional supplemental subtests are selected and administered (depending on the child's need) to determine the skill deficits or behavior underlying the disorder; these lead to four additional index scores, Language Structure, Language Content, Language Memory, and Working Memory. At level 4, an Observational Rating Scale (completed by the assessor, teacher, or parent) and a Pragmatics Profile provide information about the child's language use in the everyday contexts of home and school.

The CELF-4 is a comprehensive system that encompasses observational procedures. The administration and scoring of some subtests will require considerable practice. A computer scoring assistant is available to help assessors calculate the Core Language Score, to provide norm-referenced indices, and criterion-referenced cutoff scores and to provide interpretive reports (if desired). An interactive training CD is also available, including case studies and training handouts.

The four-level format of the CELF-4 should address many concerns of critics of standardized testing. The test content, however, will be very difficult for many 5-year-old children and inappropriate for those with developmental problems. Some of these issues are addressed in the preschool version of the test.

CLINICAL EVALUATION OF LANGUAGE FUNDAMENTALS PRESCHOOL—SECOND EDITION

The CELF Preschool-2 (Wiig et al., 2005) is a downward extension of the CELF-4 to help assessors identify, diagnose, and perform follow-up evaluations of language deficits in children 3-0 to 6-11 years of age. The subtests parallel those of the CELF-4, and some share items. Seven subtests are norm-referenced measures that yield scale scores, and two are supplemental norm-referenced measures that yield criterion-referenced or percentile ranges. In addition, two norm-referenced checklists can be used to gain information about the child's skills outside the testing situation. Three subtests are used to obtain the Core Language Score to determine whether a language disorder is present (Sentence Structure, Word Structure, and Expressive Vocabulary). Once a problem has been identified, a number of paths can be followed to (1) diagnose the nature of the disorder, (2) evaluate early classroom literacy skills, and (3) evaluate language and communication in context. A supplemental section addresses dialect variations and sensitivity to culture. The instructions and scoring procedures are clear. Training is needed to use this test effectively. The four levels of the test can be used independently to serve the needs of many preschool assessors.

FLUHARTY PRESCHOOL SPEECH AND LANGUAGE SCREENING TEST—SECOND EDITION

The Fluharty-2 (Fluharty, 2001) yields Receptive Language, Expressive Language, and a General Language Quotient. Subtests include Articulation, Repeating Sentences, Following Directives and Answering Questions, Describing Actions, and Sequencing Events. The test was developed for children ages 3-0 to 6-11 years and requires 10 minutes to administer. Items are scored as correct or incorrect except for Sequencing Events, which is scored based on the number of steps included and topic maintenance. A teacher questionnaire is available. The test is easy to administer and score by trained assessors and is useful for screening purposes.

PRESCHOOL LANGUAGE SCALE—FOURTH EDITION

The PLS-4 (Zimmerman et al., 2002), developed to identify children who have a language disorder or delay, yields Auditory Comprehension, Expressive Communication, and Total Language Scores. The test, developed for children from 2 weeks to 6-11 years of age, requires 20–45 minutes (depending on the age of the child). Starting points are provided by age, and basal and ceiling rules apply. The Auditory Comprehension subtest items cover different aspects of attention, play, and gesture (appropriate for children up to 2-11 years of age); semantics (vocabulary and qualitative, quantitative, spatial, and time/sequence concepts); language structure (morphology and syntax); integrative language skills; and phonological awareness. Expressive Communication items cover vocabulary, gesture, semantics, language structure, integrative language skills, and phonological awareness. A profile on the response form indicates items that are included in each area. An Articulation Screener can also be used and is included on the response form. A Language Sample Checklist and a Caregiver Questionnaire are other supplemental measures provided. Instructions for administration, scoring, and interpretation are clear and concise. A separate Spanish version with Spanish norms is available.

TEST OF AUDITORY COMPREHENSION OF LANGUAGE—THIRD EDITION

The TACL-3 (Carrow-Woolfolk, 1999) measures receptive spoken vocabulary, grammar, and syntax. The test was developed for children ages 3-0 to 9-11 years, to identify auditory comprehension deficits and clarify the strengths and weaknesses in a way that can lead to intervention planning. It requires 15–25 minutes to administer. Subtests assess three categories of language abilities: Vocabulary (nouns, verbs, adjectives, and adverbs); Grammatical Morphemes; and Elaborated Phrases and Sentences (three- and four-word phrases, and phrases combined by *and* into compound sentences and complex sentences including prepositions, pronouns, noun number and tense, verb number and tense, derivational suffixes). The child selects one of three pictures that best matches the stimulus provided by the examiner. Subtest results are strongly related to age and differentiate children with and without disabilities affecting auditory comprehension of language. Factor-analytic studies support a single factor, General Auditory Comprehension of Language. This measure should be used in combination with other methods of assessing children's language functioning. It requires formal training in test administration, but is easy to administer and score.

TEST OF EARLY LANGUAGE DEVELOPMENT—THIRD EDITION

The TELD-3 (Hresko, Reid, & Hammill, 1999) measures Receptive, Expressive, and Overall Spoken Language. The test was developed for children ages 2-0 to 7-11 years to identify children who may benefit from early intervention, as well as to identify individual strengths and weaknesses in language. It requires 15–40 minutes to administer. Reviewers suggest that the test is better used as a screener for potential problems than as a diagnostic tool. Entry level is determined by age, with basal and ceiling levels provided. Two forms of the test are available.

TEST OF LANGUAGE DEVELOPMENT—PRIMARY, THIRD EDITION

The TOLD-P: 3 was developed by Newcomer and Hammill (1997) for children ages 4-0 to 8-11 years to identify delays in language proficiency, and to assess strengths and weaknesses in language skills. The test requires 30 to 60 minutes to administer with basal and ceiling rules provided for every subtest. The six subtests include Picture Vocabulary, Relational Vocabulary, Oral Vocabulary, Grammatic Understanding, Sentence Imitation, and Grammatic Completion, as well as three supplemental subtests, Word Discrimination, Phonemic Analysis, and Word Articulation. Combinations of these subtests yield composite scores for Listening, Organizing, Speaking, Semantics, Syntax, and Spoken Language. Procedures for administering and scoring the test are clearly presented. Formal training in test administration is required. Items at the 4-year-old level may be very difficult for children with developmental delays.

Tests such as these need to be followed up through interview to understand the strategies a child uses to select responses, and through observation to determine whether the child uses these words and desired grammatical forms in their expressive exchanges and across contexts.

Measures of Word-Finding Difficulties

Some children with good receptive language have difficulty in expressing themselves. One such difficulty is with word finding. Word-finding problems (i.e., problems recalling desired words to express ideas or respond to questions) are frequently observed among individuals with language-learning difficulties (Denckla & Rudel, 1976; German, 1983; Wiig & Semel, 1984). Word-finding difficulties are also evidenced through such behaviors as longer response times to come up with desired words, talking around desired words, repetitions, substitutions, and insertions (German & Simon, 1991). Hall and Jordan (1987) cited the need for a word-finding task during language screening and reviewed several techniques for assessing word-finding difficulties: observation of a child's conversational speech; observation of the child's ability to name a sequential series of words; having the child complete open-ended sentences; confrontational naming of common pictures (called *confrontational* because an individual must produce the precise name when confronted with a specific pictorial stimulus); rapid automatized naming (RAN) of a small number of stimuli; and spontaneous generation of words within a specific time period in a given category (e.g., animals). Denckla and Rudel (1976) designed an RAN test that requires naming 50 familiar symbols (e.g., letters, digits) as rapidly as possible. Since this test might be difficult for many preschoolers, an RAN task of animals was developed by Catts (1991) for the kindergarten level; this is particularly useful at the beginning of the academic year. Rathvon (2004) cautions that RAN tasks should be distinguished from confrontational naming tasks, which do not have stringent time limitations. Measures of confrontational naming of words a child knows include the Boston Naming Test—Second Edition (Kaplan, Goodglass, & Weintraub, 2000), and the Test of Word Finding—Second Edition (German, 2000). RAN tasks are also components of other tests, such as the Comprehensive Test of Phonological Processing (CTOPP; Wagner, Torgesen, & Rashotte, 1999). Again, these tests in general are appropriate beginning at age 5, but may be difficult for many children at the beginning of kindergarten (Rathvon, 2004, provides useful reviews of these measures). A teacher checklist for word-finding problems is presented by German (1983).

Assessment of Phonology

As might be expected, both the articulation abilities of preschool children and their discrimination of sounds improve as they grow older. These skills are essential for children to produce and receive messages, and are necessary for gaining the skills associated with early reading. Factors that affect the number and type of misarticulations observed include "familiarity of the listener with the child, and whether the listener has an idea of what the child is talking about" (Lund & Duncan, 1993, p. 130). Children who have articulation deficits also tend to have poor speech sound discrimination (Myers, 1988). A sample of a child's phonological productions can be gathered during conversations, play activities, or elicited tasks. Supplementary articulation subtests are now available in many standardized tests. Steps that a speech–language specialist might use for taking a phonological inventory and for understanding phonological processes used by young children (such as substitutions and deletions) have been detailed by Ingram (1981), Lund and Duncan (1993), and Newman et al. (1985), among others. Articulation tests that measure a variety of dimensions of speech production, such as place and manner of articulation and presence of voicing, are reviewed by McCauley and Swisher (1984) and R. Paul (2001). A recent screening measure, the Diagnostic Evaluation of Language Variation—Screening Test (Seymour, Roeper, & de Villiers, 2003b), was developed to assist clinicians in distinguishing normal and developmental language changes among children 4–12 years old who speak a variation of mainstream American English. The test assesses syntax, morphology, and phonology. The Diagnostic Evaluation of Language Variation—Criterion Referenced (Seymour, Roeper, & De Villiers, 2003a), a criterion-referenced version of the test, provides a more comprehensive evaluation.

As noted both in Chapter 7 and in this chapter, phonological awareness is an important precursor to success with early reading activities in normally developing children (Bradley & Bryant, 1985; Goswami, 2001; Perfetti et al., 1988; Rack, Hulme, Snowling,

& Wightman, 1994; Torgesen, 2002; Wagner & Torgesen, 1987). It involves "an awareness of the phonological sequences in a spoken word and the ability to manipulate those segments" (Chafouleas et al., 1997, p. 334). Chafouleas et al. (1997), in their comprehensive study of the performance of 171 children in grades K–2 on several tasks of phonological awareness, found an ordering of tasks by difficulty and age. In order of difficulty (from least to most) were tasks involving *rhyme* (providing a rhyming word for a target word, determining words that did not share a common rhyme); *alliteration* (identifying the initial, middle, and final sounds of words); *blending* (combining individual phonemes into a word); *segmentation* (counting phonemes by using manipulatives, naming individual phonemes in a word); and *manipulation* (deletion of initial phoneme, deletion of final phoneme, substitution of initial/middle/final sounds, reversal of sounds). Success on tasks increased with age: Rapid growth was seen in 6-year-old children, and most children reached mastery by grade 2. A recent study by Carroll et al. (2003) has focused on the development of phonological awareness in preschool children. These researchers provide evidence that there is a progression in development, with the awareness of large units (syllables and rimes) occurring before that of small units (phonemes), and that these are separable skills. Furthermore, phoneme awareness was predicted by measures of large-unit awareness and articulation skill, confirming the continuum provided by Adams (1990) and underscored by Goswami (2001) (see Chapter 7). These results can help preschool assessors evaluate those skills that are the precursors to success with phonological tasks and develop activities (e.g., word games that involve rhyming) for both home and school.

A child's ability to discriminate sounds and associate them with letters is essential for early learning. A number of tests designed to identify the child's strengths and needs in this area are available, such as the Lindamood Auditory Conceptualization Test—Revised (Lindamood & Lindamood, 1991), the Phonological Abilities Test (Mutter, Hulme, & Snowling, 1997), the PIPA (Dodd et al., 2003), and the Test of Phonological Awareness (Torgesen & Bryant, 1994) (see Appendix 7.1 for several of these).

Measures of Syntax

Using syntactic structures of increasing diversity and complexity to combine words into phrases and sentences is an important aspect of language development. The speech–language specialist will use multiple procedures to evaluate syntax, including several tasks described earlier in this chapter (e.g., spontaneous speech samples and elicitation tasks). Scarborough (1990) developed an Index of Productive Syntax to identify the complexity of sentences used. Observing the types of *wh-* questions children understand and use also reveals their developing syntactic abilities (Hirsh-Pasek et al., 2005). Sentence completion tasks and cloze procedures are used as well. Lund and Duncan (1993), Owens (2004), and R. Paul (2001), among others, provide excellent summaries and worksheets for analyzing and summarizing these structures.

Measures of Pragmatic Skills

Measures of pragmatic competence in everyday social situations are still relatively few (Abbeduto & Nuccio, 1989). The Let's Talk Inventory for Children (Bray & Wiig, 1987), which presents topics for children to discuss, is one example. According to Abbeduto and Nuccio (1989), such measures need to include tasks representative of everyday communicative interactions, including these:

- Taking turns at speaking.
- Managing the referential function of language (making messages clear to others and as a listener, searching for the intended referent).
- Expression and comprehension of speech acts.
- Knowing what linguistic forms are needed to convey thoughts and ideas.
- Recognizing situations when politeness is appropriate and what forms are needed.
- Knowing how speakers behave (e.g., not asking a question if they already know the answer, being contingent).
- Staying on topic, contributing so that the discussion of the topic progresses, and introducing new topics as appropriate.
- Repairing conversational failures, such as requesting clarification of messages not understood.
- Using language to accomplish social goals, such as talking to persuade, tease, and apologize.
- Adjusting communicative behavior to the nature of the situation.

Pragmatic assessment also needs to focus on aspects of the adult–child interaction, such as the following:

- Who is communicating with the child (parent, sibling, caregiver, teacher, peer, assessor)?
- What prompts do adults provide (questioning, expanding, commenting, rewording) to help children interact and respond?
- What actions do adults use to support (or interfere) with a child's communicative attempts, and to provide objects and experiences that contribute to vocabulary growth?
- How do adults help children explore their environment with activities that contribute to emergent literacy?
- In what ways do adults break down tasks into doable units and give children time to respond?
- In what ways to do adults use questions to engage, but not correct or judge, the child?
- In what ways do adults reinforce the child's attempts?
- In what ways do adults promote communication to solve problems?

Interacting appropriately during everyday tasks is an important issue for individuals with a variety of developmental disorders, including mental retardation, LD, ASD, and SLI. Gallagher (1991) details multiple procedures for tapping a child's pragmatic use of language.

In order to find out *how* the child uses language, with whom, and under what circumstances, teacher and parent report measures (often rating scales) are generally used; these should be followed up by interview. Observations of children engaged in everyday activities, and repeated use of developmental checklists, are also key to documenting these behaviors. The goal is to identify what pragmatic behaviors need to be practiced and then transferred to everyday contexts. Critical dyadic discourse skills are detailed by McLean (1990), Prizant and Wetherby (1990, 1992), and Prizant et al. (1993). As noted in an earlier section, the CSBS (Wetherby & Prizant, 1993), while focused on infants and toddlers 8 months to 2 years of age, can be used with children up to 6 years of age if delays are present.

Linking Assessment to Intervention

As stressed throughout this chapter (and this book), assessment needs to be linked to intervention and to be viewed as an ongoing process. This begins with specifying and sequencing both immediate and long-term goals. Lahey (1988) presents a content/form/use goal plan for language learning, based on knowledge of normal language development. A useful format for summarizing information obtained through multiple measures and procedures used in language assessment is presented by Olswang and Bain (1988). Samples of performance across the components of form, content, and use are summarized and profiled.

When assessors are interpreting discrepancies in the results for these components, Olswang and Bain (1988) are careful to caution that not all children have the potential to achieve expected age norms, and that the amount of individual variation that is acceptable across language components has not yet been determined. Several different measures need to be used; these will allow an assessor to construct a profile showing where a child's development is relatively strong or delayed. Since communication skills are critical basic skills used continuously throughout the day, intervention needs to take place in a familiar context as often as possible, using toys and activities of interest to a child. This is particularly true for a children with a severe disability. Training activities practiced in isolation, or in an individual session with a therapist outside the preschool or child care setting, may not transfer into the child's use of language across situations in everyday life. Therefore, it is important to develop activities as close as possible to the real-life experiences in which the child needs to use the desired language behaviors. Intervention needs to target practical behaviors that have many opportunities for practice and reinforcement in everyday situations (Cole & Crais, 1989), and to include a systematic plan for ongoing communication with the parent and teacher. It is also important to plan graduated interventions in various skill areas, beginning at a level where the child is functioning and providing a bridge to the next higher skill level (Cole & Crais, 1989).

The speech–language specialist, preschool special educator, or school psychologist can help teachers and parents recognize potential communicative opportunities that naturally exist in the activities of the classroom or the home. Examples include extending the time they wait for a response; asking open-ended questions; and using multiple modes of communication, such as signing, pointing to pictures, eye gaze, gestures, tone of voice, and use of objects. Assessment needs to target all these modes of receiving and communicating a message, in order to understand a severely disabled child's ability to interact with others. Several other considerations are also involved in developing interventions with parents:

1. Review (and, where possible, alter) factors that interfere with a child's language learning, such as hearing loss or illness.

2. Discuss results with parents and work together to establish goals. If needed, engage parents in a support group to help them deal with their reactions to the child's speech delay.

3. Develop workshops and activities that deal with the amount and types of language modeling parents can provide. We know from the research reviewed in this chapter that the more time parents spend talking with children on a daily basis, the more their vocabulary and their sensitivity to the sounds in words increase; this increase in turn contributes importantly to their comprehension and emerging literacy skills. Parents can learn to prompt children to tell what they know (labeling, greeting, recounting events);

ask for what they want or don't have; and use language for learning (labeling, pretending, comparing).

4. Another area regards how parents initiate and respond to a child's communicative efforts. Develop workshops and activities that help parents understand the important role they play by *expanding* on what the child says; *prompting* the child to say more; *commenting* on what the child says or on objects, pictures, and story events; *modeling* typical language forms; *responding* to the child's signals; and *reinforcing* the child's efforts. These interactive behaviors can take place any time during the day at home or during outings (to the store, post office, park, etc.). Such activities provide children with opportunities to learn the characteristics of objects, the relations between events, and the relations between objects. Through these interactions children also learn how to take turns in conversation, maintain the flow of conversation, respond to the signals of others, and adjust speech to the context of the situation. Many examples can be provided to help parents capture the child's attention, build on the child's interests, encourage him or her to persist, and make activities fun. Parents need to be guided not to use controlling speech and impose adult forms, but rather to encourage their child's attempts. Bricker and Pretti-Fontczak (1996) provide useful examples of how to use home and school routines to develop activity plans.

5. Joint storybook reading and toy play interactions provide wonderful opportunities to use language to interact with the child. Books representing different genres (prediction, rhyming, feelings, etc.) allow children to learn many forms and uses of language. Kaderavek and Sulzby (2000) present a useful table of scaffolding behaviors used by parents during storybook reading and underscore the importance of repeated book reading.

Many of these same considerations apply to the preschool or daycare environment. In the study reported by Roberts et al. (1991), for example, teachers frequently engaged preschool children with disabilities in communicative interactions, responded to the children, and waited for the children to respond. However, they infrequently expanded on the children's responses, prompted for higher-level responses, promoted peer interactions, prompted communication to replace undesirable behavior, or modified the environment to promote communication. These infrequently used behaviors can be developed through in-service training activities or through routine observation and feedback by another teacher, a speech–language specialist, or the school psychologist.

Multiple activities and materials have been developed for speech–language specialists to use with parents, teachers, and children; these target each of the areas covered in this chapter, but are beyond the scope of the chapter to review. Increasingly, intervention activities are suggested in test manuals and associated materials (e.g., Linder, 1993). Major texts covering language disorders (e.g., Owens, 2004; Olswang & Bain, 1988; R. Paul, 2001) and journals such as the *Journal of Speech and Hearing Research* describe research supported intervention approaches. Lahey (1988) urges that the focus of intervention be on language itself. The procedures used can be treated as hypotheses, which can be tested through diagnostic teaching and interactive activities.

SUMMARY

The ages of 3–5 years are a time of great language development, which takes place in the social and cultural contexts of home, childcare, and preschool. The nature of a child's communicative exchanges with adults is a critical component of the developmental process that needs to be considered during assessment. Children following the normal path of development will acquire the forms needed for carrying out conversation. When difficulties are present, it is important to determine with whom and under what circumstances these disruptions occur. The multiple interactive components of language, described in this chapter within the broad categories of form, content, and use, are demonstrated through the child's receptive and expressive uses of language. Difficulties in any of these areas can impede a child's day-to-day communication at home, during play, and in the preschool, as well as his or her early learning activities in reading, writing, and mathematics.

Language development and use are interconnected with all areas of development and are disrupted in different ways across childhood disorders such as mental retardation, behavioral and emotional problems, and sensory deficits. Essential considerations are how well children's information-processing capabilities allow them to perceive, organize, and retrieve from memory their past experiences, and how disturbances in these capabilities contribute to disruptions in language learning.

An interdisciplinary team (often composed of a parent, a teacher, a speech–language specialist, and the school psychologist) is important to identify language delays. Each team member will contribute observations of language interactions. While the school psychologist can identify the presence of mental retardation or an emotional problem, the speech–language specialist will delve into the phonemic, grammatical, and pragmatic aspects of language. Parent and teacher observations are critical to understanding language use in everyday contexts. Language assessment is thus a collaborative process across disciplines, using multiple approaches to answer questions such as these:

- How does a child use language and other communicative forms across contexts?
- In what ways do the important adults in the child's life interact with the child to foster or hinder language growth?
- Does a child in fact have a language problem? If so, what is its nature?
- In what contexts and in what ways does language break down?
- How does the language problem interact with other problems (e.g., ASD, hearing impairment)?
- What adult supports are needed to help the child develop needed language forms or their appropriate use in social contexts?
- What are the goals of intervention? What activities are needed to achieve these goals, and who will carry them out?
- How will the success of intervention be periodically evaluated?

An overview of procedures used for assessing language behaviors has been presented. Many of these are carried out by a speech–language specialist, including tasks to elicit spontaneous language samples. Norm-referenced tests, used to compare a child's performance with that of other children of the same age, are often needed for children to qualify for services and have also been reviewed. These tests in general provide global information about relative strength and weakness in receptive and expressive language, although more recent tests offer additional ways to analyze more specific language forms, along with teacher or parent observational checklists and/or articulation surveys. Such information is needed (or required) as part of in-depth analysis of language samples by the speech–language specialist, or to justify continuation of these services. Finally, suggestions linking assessment to intervention have been provided.

APPENDIX 10.1. Review of Measures

Measure	Bankson Language Test—Second Edition (BLT-2). Bankson (1990).
Purpose	Serving as a norm-referenced survey of language skills; providing an informal diagnostic inventory of strengths and weaknesses; and serving as a research tool when language assessment is desired.
Areas	Semantic Knowledge, Morphological/Syntactical Rules, Pragmatics (optional).
Format	Subjects are presented with black-and-white line drawings and verbal cues in question form or cloze sentences. Test items are scored 1 if correct or 0 if incorrect. Screening procedure is available that utilizes 20 items from the full BLT-2.
Scores	Percentiles and standard scores available for Semantic Knowledge and Morphological/Syntactical Rules subtests. A sum of these standard scores may be converted to a composite Language Quotient. A comparison of standard scores to this quotient allows overall performance to be categorized as very poor, poor, below average, average, above average, superior, or very superior.
Age group	3-0 to 6-11 years.
Time	20–30 minutes.
Users	Trained examiners.
Norms	Data collected on over 1,200 children in 19 states. Demographics are representative of the national population on such important characteristics as sex, residence, race, geographic region, and family income.
Reliability	Internal reliability, .91–.97 across age groups; test–retest, not reported.
Validity	Concurrent validity assessed by correlations with the Screening Children for Related Early Educational Needs yielded coefficients ranging from .43 to .74 (*n* = 22). Construct validity is suggested by correlations between raw scores and chronological age that appear to demonstrate this measure's ability to capture the developmental aspect of language. This measure may also distinguish between language-delayed and normally developing children; however, not enough information is provided to allow one to judge the predictive validity of it.
Comments	Predictive validity of the test has not been established. Reliability and validity, although improved, are still not strongly evidenced. The screening procedure, a 20-item test composed of selected items, is potentially useful to identify areas in need of further evaluation.
References consulted	Gilliam (1992); Towne (1992). See book's References list.

Measure	Boehm Test of Basic Concepts—Third Edition (Boehm-3) and Boehm Test of Basic Concepts—Third Edition: Preschool (Boehm-3: Preschool). See Chapter 7, Appendix 7.1.

Measure	Boston Naming Test—Second Edition (BNT-2). Kaplan, Goodglass, and Weintraub (2000).
Purpose	Measuring confrontational naming abilities.
Areas	Expressive Vocabulary.
Format	60 items, full form; 15-item, short form. Subject is presented with black-and-white line drawings, ordered from easy to difficult, which he or she is asked to

	name. Responses must be given within 20 seconds; after this time, the examiner follows a prompting procedure that starts with a stimulus cue and follows with a phonemic cue if needed. A multiple-choice portion is administered after completion of the test; only items that were incorrect after a phonemic cue are given at this point. Error codes are recorded for the different types of paraphasic errors. Start and end points are provided.
Scores	Total score consists of total number of correct responses given spontaneously or after a stimulus cue. Summary of scores also yields totals for the number of stimulus cues given, the number of phonemic cues given, the number of correct responses following phonemic cues, and the number of multiple choices given. There is also space to tally the paraphasia types observed.
Age group	Designed for use with adults but has been used with children.
Time	10–20 minutes.
Users	Trained professionals.
Norms	Limited information available for children. Norms published in record booklet are based on a sample of 356 children ranging in age from 5-0 to 12-5 years. These norms were established as part of a master's thesis (1987).
Reliability	No information available.
Validity	No information available.
Comments	This measure has very limited information regarding its psychometric properties. It is better utilized as a qualitative measure that provides information about children's expressive abilities, such as expressive vocabulary, retrieval difficulties, and signs of brain damage.
References consulted	Test manual.

Measure	**Bracken Basic Concept Scale—Revised (BBCS-R). Bracken (1998). See Chapter 7, Appendix 7.1.**

Measure	**Clinical Evaluation of Language Fundamentals—Fourth Edition (CELF-4). Semel, Wiig, and Secord (2003).**
Purpose	Identifying and diagnosing language disorders quickly and accurately.
Areas	Syntax, metalinguistics, morphology, semantics, semantic classes, working memory, phonology, preliteracy, pragmatics, classroom performance/social interaction.
Format	Individually administered. Consists of 20 total subtests with four core subtests making up the Core Language Score. Subtests differ in format with some being visually presented and others being orally presented.
Scores	Scaled scores, standard scores, percentiles, age equivalents; Core Language Score, Receptive Language Index, Expressive Language Index, Language Structure Index, Language Context Index, Language Memory Index, Working Memory Index (supplemental).
Age group	5-0–21 years.
Time	30–45 minutes for core subtests.
Users	Must have training in assessment.

Norms	Data collected on over 4,500 individuals. English was the primary language spoken by all, and 9.5% of the standardization population received services for being gifted/talented or disabled. The sample was stratified by parent education level and representative of 2000 U.S. Census data for the following variables: race/ethnicity, parent educational level, age, sex, and geographic region.
Reliability	Test–retest (7–35 days; n = 320) subtest average corrected stability coefficients range from .70s to .90, with most in the .80s; composite average corrected stability coefficients are .88 (4 composites), .89 (1 composite), and .92 (2 composites); percent of decision agreement for criterion measures ranges from .87–.98 (mean). Mean internal consistency alphas range from .69 to .91 for subtests and .87 to .95 for composites; mean alphas for criterion measures range from .73 to .98. Mean split-half reliabilities range from .71 to .92 for subtests and .87 to .95 for composites; mean split-half reliabilities for criterion measures range from .74 to .98. Mean alphas across clinical groups range from .83 to .97; mean split-half reliabilities across clinical groups range from .85 to .98. Interrater reliabilities range from .90 to .99 on subtests requiring scorer judgment.
Validity	Evidence provided based on content, response process, internal structure, intercorrelational studies, and factor analytic studies. Concurrent validity with the CELF-3 is high between composite scores, and high to moderate between subtests across normal and clinical groups. Significant differences were found on subtests and composites between LLD and non-LLD samples. The sensitivity and specificity of the measure ranges from good to excellent; for LLD sample scoring –1, –1.5, and –2 standard deviations below the mean, sensitivity ranges from .87 to 1.00 and specificity ranges from .82 to .96.
Comments	This new version of the CELF distinguishes itself from the third edition by laying out a four-step assessment model. It also offers a core battery of four subtests that were chosen for their ability to distinguish language disorders as well as new index scores. Although reviewers of the previous edition commented on marginal subtest reliabilities, this version offers reliabilities that are only slightly improved. Supplemental subtests include: Phonological Awareness (ages 5–12), Word Associations (ages 5–21), Rapid Automatic Naming (ages 5–21), and Working Memory subtests (Number Repetition and Familiar Sequences). The manual provides a good description of what these skills relate to and when administration of these subtests is warranted. Other supplemental material includes: Observational Rating Scale (examiner, parent, and student self-report forms); Pragmatics Profile; extension testing procedures are provided in manual for all subtests. Scoring Assistant computer program available.
References consulted	Test manual; Boehm review.

Measure	**Clinical Evaluation of Language Fundamentals Preschool—Second Edition (CELF Preschool-2). Wiig, Secord, and Semel (2005).**
Purpose	Identifying, diagnosing, and performing follow-up evaluations of language deficits in preschool children. A downward extension of the CELF-4.
Areas	Sentence Structure, Word Structure, Expressive Vocabulary, Concepts and Following Directions, Recalling Sentences, Basic Concepts, Word Classes, Recalling Sentences in Context, and Phonological Awareness. A Pre-Literacy Rating Scale and Descriptive Pragmatics Profile can be used to gain information about the child's skills outside the testing situation.

Format	Individually administered. Children are presented with items either orally in sentences or visually in multiple-choice format, and respond by pointing. Items are scored 1 or 0; ceiling rules apply. Rating system consists of 0, 1, 2, or 3 points, depending on subtest.
Scores	Core Language Score and four index scores: Receptive Language, Expressive Language, Language Content, and Language Structure. Scaled scores for seven subtests, with a mean of 10 and *SD* of 3; age equivalents for subtests with scaled scores. Percentile ranks and percentile rank confidence intervals for the Pre-Literacy Rating Scale and the Descriptive Pragmatics Profile.
Age group	3-0 to 6-11 years. Two age levels: 3-0 to 4-11, 5-0 to 6-11.
Time	15–20 minutes for the three core subtests.
Users	Speech–language pathologists, school psychologists, special educators, and trained diagnosticians.
Norms	800 children, 100 at each of eight 6-month age groups, stratified by U.S. geographic location (Northeast, North Central, West, and South), age, gender, race/ethnicity, and education of primary caregiver. Children had to have the ability to use spoken language to communicate; 13% of the sample were reported to be receiving special services.
Reliability	Internal consistency, .73–.96; test–retest (based on 13–17 children from each age group after 2–24 days, corrected for the variability of the standardization group), .77–.92 for subtests and .91–.94 for composite scores.
Validity	The manual indicates that items were selected to reflect the development of language skills sampled in the research literature and were reviewed by experts. Correlations between the CELF-Preschool and CELF Preschool-2, CELF-4, and PLS-4 were moderate to high for composite scores and for subtests. Sensitivity of the Core Language Score was reported as .85; the specificity as .82.
Comments	Materials are colorful and attractive to children. The record form is organized well, facilitating accurate administration and scoring. Guidelines for administration, scoring, and interpretation are discussed in the manual in detail. Little information is provided with regard to item selection (how and why items were selected). The CELF Preschool-2 has adequate reliability and validity data, which suggests that a clinician can use this test confidently for the identification of language problems in preschool children.
References consulted	Norris (1998); Thompson (1998); Boehm review. See book's References list.

Measure	**Diagnostic Evaluation of Language Variation—Criterion Referenced (DELV). Seymour, Roeper, and de Villiers (2003a).**
Purpose	Distinguishing children who are developing speech and language normally from those who are not.
Areas	Pragmatics, Syntax, Semantics, Phonology.
Format	Individually administered.
Scores	Criterion referenced.
Age group	4-0 to 9-0 years.
Time	45–50 minutes.
Users	Experienced speech language specialists.

Norms	Criterion referenced.
Reliability	Criterion referenced. Content validity documented.
Validity	Criterion referenced.
Comments	Contains items specifically designed to limit the effect of variations in Mainstream American English (MAE) on children's performance in order to tap true language abilities. Screening version of the DELV is designed to "distinguish language differences from language disorders." This measure identifies children at-risk for developing a language disorder.
References consulted	Test manual.

Measure	**Early Language Milestone Scale—Second Edition (ELM Scale-2). Coplan (1993).**
Purpose	Assessing the development of speech and language in infancy and early childhood.
Areas	Auditory Expressive, Auditory Receptive, and Visual.
Format	43-item scale, completed on basis of parental history, direct testing or incidental observation. A pass–fail method or a point-scoring system is used to score items. The point-scoring system assigns 1 point for each item passed. The pass–fail method is the most efficient for screening. A child must pass all three subtests, and those items that 90% of children in the population are expected to pass. The ELM Scale-2 identifies the lowest 10% of children in terms of speech and language.
Scores	Percentiles, standard scores, and age equivalents. A Global Language score can also be computed.
Age group	0–36 months.
Time	1–10 minutes.
Users	Examiners with knowledge in child language development.
Norms	Normative data were originally obtained for the first edition of the scale on 191 pediatric patients 0–3 years of age, and subsequently validated on several groups of developmentally delayed children.
Reliability	Test–retest, .74–.94; interrater, .93–.99.
Validity	Between 83% and 100% of the sample population was identified correctly as having or not having speech/language delays when the ELM Scale-2 was compared with other measures of language.
Comments	Instructions for administration provided in the manual are very clear and include many examples of scoring items at different age levels. Validity studies appear to be adequate. This instrument relies heavily on the reporting of parents. Parental rating may be affected by inaccurate memory of behaviors or desire to portray a particular image of a child. It appears that this instrument is useful in screening children with delays in speech and language development, particularly for children from birth to 12 months.
References consulted	Backlund (1998); Waterman (1998). See book's References list.

Measure	**Expressive One-Word Picture Vocabulary Test—2000 Edition (EOWPVT). Brownell, R. (Ed.). (2000a).**
Purpose	Measuring an individual's English-speaking ability.
Areas	Ability to use language in speaking and writing (expressive).
Format	The test administrator presents the examinee with a series of illustrations representing objects, concepts, or actions.
Scores	Standard scores, percentiles, and age equivalents. Charts in the test manual demonstrate converting standard scores to NCEs, *T*-scores, scaled scores, and stanines.
Age group	Ages 2–18 years.
Time	10–15 minutes.
Users	May be administered by trained examiners. Must be interpreted by individuals with training in psychometrics.
Norms	Original normative sample of 3,661 was pared to 2,327 randomly selected examinees to create a demographic "balance." In contrast to standardization procedures for earlier editions of the EOWPVT, testing was conducted in a wide range of locations (32 states and 220 sites).
Reliability	Internal consistency, .93–.98; split-half, .98; test–retest (20 days), .77–.90.
Validity	High correlations (.93–.98) validate the strength of the relationship between item order and item difficulty. Correlations with 12 other vocabulary measures are not overly high (median .79). The construct validity evidence is extensive. Correlations between the EOWPVT and various measures of other constructs, such as cognitive ability and academic achievement, are also not overly high and suggest the narrow scope of the assessment. There is a stronger relationship between the former and current editions of the EOWPVT.
Comments	The current edition of the EOWPVT has national norms and was conormed with the Receptive One-Word Picture Vocabulary Test (ROWPVT).
References consulted	Longo (2003). See book's References list.

Measure	**Expressive Vocabulary Test (EVT). Williams (1997).**
Purpose	Measuring expressive vocabulary skills.
Areas	Expressive Language.
Format	Individually administered. Two item types: labeling and synonym. Only items that approximate ability level are administered. Subject is presented with stimulus picture and stimulus word(s) within a carrier phrase; examinee is asked for a one-word response; teaching and prompting instructions are provided.
Scores	Age-based standard scores, percentiles, stanines, normal curve equivalents, test-age equivalents, and Expressive Vocabulary domain score.
Age group	2-6 to 90 years and up.
Time	15 minutes.
Users	Trained professionals.

Norms	Data collected on 2,725 subjects (out of 3,726 who participated in standardization) ranging in age from 2-6 to 90 years and up across 268 sites in the United States. Sample representative of 1994 U.S. Census data and controlled for age, gender, race, geographic region, SES/parent education, and community size. The sample included subjects who were learning disabled, speech impaired, mentally retarded, hearing impaired, gifted and talented, and mentally retarded adults ages 25 and up. The EVT was conormed with the PPVT-III.
Reliability	Internal consistency, .90–.98 (median .95); split-half, .83–.97 (median .91); test–retest, .77–.90.
Validity	Intercorrelations with PPVT-III Form A range from .62 to .88 (median .79) and PPVT-III Form B range from .61 to .88 (median .77). Criterion-related validity established with OWLS for two age groups (mean age 4-8 years and mean age 10-3 years); listening comprehension, .47 and .69; oral expression, .60 and .86; oral composite, .57 and .85. Also established with measures of cognitive ability (WISC-III, K-BIT, KAIT) with correlations ranging from .54 to .84. Significant differences were found between the following clinical groups and control groups: language delay, language impairment, mental retardation, learning disability (reading), hearing impairment.
Comments	This measure is easy to administer and score. Items are presented in full color. Because it is conormed with the PPVT-III, comparisons may be made between receptive and expressive language abilities. Special care was taken to increase cultural sensitivity and eliminate bias within the measure.
References consulted	Bessai (2001a); Wasyliw (2001a). See book's References list.

Measure	**Fluharty Preschool Speech and Language Screening Test—Second Edition (Fluharty-2). Fluharty (2001).**
Purpose	Identifying young children who need a comprehensive speech and language assessment.
Areas	Includes 5 subtests: Articulation, Repeating Sentences, Following Directives and Answering Questions, Describing Actions, and Sequencing Events.
Format	Items scored as either correct (1) or incorrect (0).
Scores	Receptive Language, Expressive Language, and General Language Quotients. Scores from each subtest are compared with age-appropriate cutoff scores. A child fails the screening test if one or more of the subtest scores fall below the cutoff scores.
Age group	3-0 to 6-11 years.
Time	10 minutes.
Users	Trained examiners.
Norms	Data collected on 2,147 children, stratified by age, race/ethnicity, SES, and geographic regions.
Reliability	Interrater, .87–1.00 for the subtests.
Validity	A .90 correlation between a child's screening test performance (pass–fail) and the implications of his or her speech evaluations (needs therapy vs. does not need therapy) supports the validity of cutoff scores (n = 211).

Comments	All test materials are supplied except for a hat, paper bag, and 10 cards. The manual provides clear and simple directions, which makes the test easy to administer and score. However, the manual's statement of validity is somewhat confusing and makes it difficult to determine whether the measure is valid or not. This measure is recommended if a rapid screening measure of communication skills is desired. A real strength of the measure is its efforts to make the normative sample and scoring more sensitive to children with a range of regional and cultural dialects.
References consulted	Hurford (2003b); McCauley (2003). See book's References list.

Measure	**Illinois Test of Psycholinguistic Abilities—Third Edition (ITPA-3). Hammill, Mather, and Roberts (2001).**
Purpose	Identifying children at risk for school failure, determining specific strengths and weaknesses among linguistic abilities, documenting development of language as a result of intervention, and using data for research.
Areas	General Language, Spoken Language, and Written Language.
Format	Individually administered. Consists of 12 subtests (6 within spoken language and 6 within written language). Verbal or written stimuli/response depending on subtest.
Scores	Standard scores, quotients, percentiles, age equivalents, grade equivalents, and composite scores (general language, spoken language, written language).
Age group	5-0 to 12-11 years. Written subtests administered only to ages 6-6 and older.
Time	45–60 minutes.
Users	Trained professionals.
Norms	Data collected on nationally representative sample (n = 1,522) of individuals from 27 states ranging in age from 5 to 12 and reflective of projected 2000 U.S. Census data in terms of geographic region, gender, race, rural/urban, ethnicity, family income, parental educational background, and disability status. Testing occurred during 1999 and 2000.
Reliability	Internal consistency, .79–.99 across 8 age levels; test–retest (n = 30), .86–.99; interrater (n = 30), .95–.99.
Validity	Strong evidence of content validity demonstrated by five methods including differential item functioning analysis showing little to no bias in test items; criterion-related validity (concurrent only) is evidenced by comparisons with tests of same abilities (e.g., WJ-R) where correlations with all but one subtest of the General Language Composite exceeded .75; strong evidence provided for construct validity as well.
Comments	The revised ITPA-3 shows several improvements over the previous version including updated norms and improved reliability and validity data. It is easy to administer and score, but requires additional knowledge for meaningful interpretation of results. Additionally, although this is a comprehensive measure, certain constructs are measured with only 2 subtests, and therefore should be explored further with other measures if a child demonstrates potential deficits. Only selected subtests appropriate at the 5-year-old level. Tasks would be very difficult for children presenting language problems.
References consulted	Towne (2001). See book's References list.

Measure	Kindergarten Language Screening Test—Second Edition (KLST-2). Gauthier and Madison (1998).
Purpose	Screening test of language abilities for children.
Areas	Receptive and Expressive Language.
Format	18 individually administered items. Last item requires examiner to give subjective rating (good or poor) of intelligibility, attention to ask, willingness to communicate, gestural communication, response rate, fluency, and voice.
Scores	Total score, percentiles, stanines.
Age group	4-0 to 6-11 years.
Time	5 minutes.
Users	Professionals.
Norms	Data collected on 519 children from 16 states. Sample was representative of 1990 U.S. Census data but lacked adequate geographical representation.
Reliability	Internal consistency, .81–.90 across ages; test–retest (1–3 weeks), .83–.98; interrater, .99 (based on results obtained by two PRO-ED staff members on 30 randomly selected protocols).
Validity	Content validity is provided in authors' discussion of rationale for inclusion of items; biserial correlations of greater than or equal to .30 suggest that this measure might be able to discriminate between high- and low-scoring children. Criterion-related validity established with PLS-3, TOLD:P-3, CELF-P (moderate to high correlations). Construct validity studies support ability to differentiate groups and specificity of measure.
Comments	This measure is quick and easy; however, it provides an extremely cursory assessment.
References consulted	Eastman Lukin (2001); Konold (2001). See book's References list.

Measure	Peabody Picture Vocabulary Test—Third Edition (PPVT-III). Dunn and Dunn (1997).
Purpose	Measuring receptive vocabulary for standard English.
Areas	Receptive vocabulary.
Format	Two forms are available, IIIA and IIIB. Each form has 204 items, grouped in 17 sets of 12 items. Starting point depends on examinee's age. Basal and ceiling rules.
Scores	Age-referenced normative scores, standard scores, percentiles, stanines, normal curve equivalents, and age equivalents.
Age group	2.6 to 90+ years.
Time	No time limits; administration takes about 11–12 minutes.
Users	Technicians; does not require specialized training.
Norms	Data collected on 2,725 examinees (Form IIIA, 1,476; form IIIB, 1,249), representative of 1994 census data. Variables taken into account: gender, geographic location, ethnicity and educational level. Individuals with limited language ability or hearing/vision impairments not included. Norms are in 2-month intervals for children ages 2-6–6-11 years.

Reliability	Extensive data are provided. Internal consistency ranged from .92 to .98. Alternate-form reliability was derived from administration of two different test forms to the same groups of subjects. The coefficients computed from standard scores ranged from .88 to .96, with a median of .94. Test–retest reliability (carried out over a broad span of time) coefficients ranged from .91 to. 93. Split-half reliability from forms IIIA and IIIB ranged from .86 to .97, with a median of .94.
Validity	Stimulus words were selected from a pool of words that primarily consisted of entries in various editions of *Webster's New Collegiate Dictionary* (1953, 1967, 1981). Correlations with the WISC-III ranged from .82 to .92 for Verbal IQ, with the highest correlation for the Vocabulary subtest. Correlations with the Kaufman Adult Intelligence Test (KAIT) ranged from .76 to .91. Correlations with the Kaufman Brief Intelligence Test (K-BIT) ranged from .62 to .82.
Comments	This well-known measure is easy to administer and score. Pronunciation guidelines are provided. Although it is widely used as a test of verbal ability, this test should not be used as a measure of intelligence. Test floors are good across both forms. A Spanish version is available (Test de Vocabulario en Imagenes Peabody; TVIP) for assessment of Spanish vocabulary, but the scores are not comparable to the PPVT-III scores. The reliability data for the Spanish version is internal consistency, .92; test–retest (6–9 days), .53.
References consulted	Bessai (2001b); Rathvon (2004); Wasyliw (2001b). See book's References list.

Measure	**Preschool Language Scale—Fourth Edition (PLS-4). Zimmerman, Steiner, and Pond (2002).**
Purpose	Assessing language development in young children; identifying children with language disorders or delay.
Areas	Auditory Comprehension and Expressive Communication.
Format	68 items, but almost every item contains two to eight related subitems.
Scores	Standard scores, percentiles, and age equivalents for Auditory Comprehension (AC), Expressive Communication (EC), and Total Language (TL) Score.
Age group	Birth to 6-11 years.
Time	20–45 minutes.
Users	Professionals with experience and training in assessment.
Norms	Data collected on 1,900 children in four U.S. geographic locations (Northeast, North Central, South, and West). The sample was stratified on the basis of age, gender, race/ethnicity, and education of the primary caregiver.
Reliability	Internal consistency, .68–.94 (n = 1,900); test–tetest (2–14 days), .82–.94 (n = 85); interrater, .98 (n = 80).
Validity	The correlation between the Expressive Communication and Auditory Comprehension subscale standard scores was .64. The correlation between the PLS-3 and the PLS-Revised ranged from .66 to .88 (n = 29). The correlation with the CELF-R ranged from .69 to .82 (n = 58). PLS-4 gathered evidence for validity from content, response processes, internal structure, relationships with other variables, and consequences. It is probably used best as a quick language assessment measure for 3- to 5-year-old children.
Comments	The record form provides ample space for recording and scoring responses. Instructions for administration, scoring, and interpretation are discussed in a clear and concise manner. Materials needed but not included in the test kit are

	a cellophane sheet, a teddy bear, a shoebox, a ball, keys on a key ring, three plastic spoons and cups, a white sock, a watch with a second hand, and age-appropriate toys and books.
References consulted	Flowerday (2005). See book's References list.

Measure	**Receptive One-Word Picture Vocabulary Test—2000 Edition (ROWPVT). Brownell, R. (Ed.). (2000b).**
Purpose	Assessing English hearing vocabulary.
Areas	Receptive Language.
Format	Individually administered. Subjects are presented with a word spoken by the examiner and four pictures; subject responds by pointing or stating the number of the picture that represents the meaning of the stimulus word. Start points determined by age.
Scores	Percentiles, standard scores, age equivalents, normal curve equivalents, scaled scores, *T*-scores, and stanines.
Age group	2–18 years.
Time	10–15 minutes.
Users	Trained professionals for administration. Interpretation by psychometrically trained individual.
Norms	Data collected on random sample of 2,327 individuals (of 3,661 that were involved in standardization) in 32 states. Sample included only primary English speakers in norming sample that were stratified by age and representative of school-age population with regards to region of country, race–ethnicity, gender, parent education level, urban/rural, and disability status. Conormed with EOWPVT.
Reliability	Internal consistency coefficient alphas range from .95 to .98 across age groups. Split-half coefficients range from .96 to .99. Test–retest (average of 20 days) reliabilities for the entire sample range from .78 to .93 (mean of .84). Interrater reliability was assessed by evaluating the consistency with which examiners were able to follow the scoring procedure after test administration (n = 30); this method yielded 100% agreement among novice scorers, trained scorers, and computer scoring.
Validity	Criterion-related validity established with 12 other measures of receptive language (coefficients range from .44 to .97), and other, broader tests of language (coefficients range from .45 to .92). Correlation with PPVT-III was .71. Speaking to the sensitivity of the measure, children in the standardization sample with disabilities commonly associated with vocabulary delays scored significantly lower than the population mean, whereas children with disabilities not usually associated with vocabulary delays did not.
Comments	Offers quick and easy administration and scoring. The manual is well designed and clearly presents information about administration, scoring, and test characteristics. This measure is strictly limited to assessment of single-word receptive vocabulary knowledge. Conormed with EOWPVT (see review in this Appendix) to allow for comparisons between receptive and expressive vocabulary. If administered together, EOWPVT should be given first to avoid a learning effect. New features of current version include updated norms, improved psychometric properties, full-color items to increase interest, lower and upper levels combined to cover larger age range, instructions for examiner prompts and cues included, and many items replaced or added.

References consulted	Fairbank (2001b); Pratt (2001). See book's References list.

Measure	**Reynell Developmental Language Scales—Third Edition. Reynell (1997).**
Purpose	Assessing verbal comprehension and expressive language skills in children.
Areas	Verbal Comprehension and Expressive Language.
Format	67-item Verbal Comprehension scale and 67-item Expressive Language scale. The Verbal Comprehension scale has two versions, one in which only pointing responses are required and a second in which simple oral responses are required.
Scores	Standard scores (mean = 100 and *SD* = 15).
Age group	1-0 to 6-11 years.
Time	30 minutes.
Users	It is recommended that only experienced speech pathologists use this instrument, because their diagnostic/therapeutic knowledge is likely to mitigate the possibility of misinterpretation as a result of insufficient psychometric data.
Norms	Data collected on 619 children, selected on a nonrandom basis with regard to the following demographic variables: geographic region, ethnicity, parental education level, and gender.
Reliability	Internal reliability coefficients for the two scales cluster around .90, with some in the .80s for children ages 1-0 to 3-5 and ages 1-0 to 1-11. Internal reliability coefficients for children ages 3-6 to 4-11 are generally in the .80s and typically fall below .80 for children ages 5-0 to 6-11.
Validity	Limited evidence is available for construct validity. Internal consistency reliability coefficients were used to support the unitary nature of language development underlying this instrument. The criterion-related validity evidence (concurrent and predictive) reported in the manual is weak, as the studies are outdated and were conducted using the British revised edition.
Comments	Children will find the stimulus cards interesting and engaging. Detailed guidelines for scoring and interpretation, as well as case examples, are available for each of the two scales. Guidelines are also available for children with hearing impairments/deafness. Most of the validity studies are based on the British version. This instrument is most useful and reliable for the assessment of young children.
References consulted	Flanagan (1995); McCauley (1995). See book's References list.

Measure	**Sequenced Inventory of Communication Development—Revised Edition (SICD-R). Hedrick, Prather, and Tobin (1984).**
Purpose	Quantitatively measuring communication development in children.
Areas	Receptive Scale and Expressive Scale.
Format	Rating scale (yes–no) and parent interview. A Spanish version is available.
Scores	Receptive Communication Age (RCA) and Expressive Communication Age (ECA). RCA and ECA are calculated at the point at which the child has 75% or more successful responses.
Age group	4 months to 4 years.
Time	20–40 minutes.

Users	Examiners need to know normal language development as well as individualized testing practices to make appropriate interpretations.
Norms	Original sample consisted of 252 white children in the Seattle area, equally divided among low, middle, and high SES. Revised edition includes a sample of 609 children; 276 black children with an age range of 31–48 months were added to the sample. The norms for the revised edition for children between 4 and 30 months are based exclusively on white children.
Reliability	Interrater, mean of .96 (n = 16); test–retest, mean of .93 (n = 10).
Validity	Correlations of RCA and ECA with the original PPVT, . 81 and .76, respectively.
Comments	The manual provides clearly written instructions for scoring and administration. Materials are easily carried in the tackle-type box provided and are appealing to children. Norms for the Spanish version are not available. The normative sample has great limitations with regard to size and composition. Meticulous selection of test items provides evidence of content validity. However, the manual provides no evidence of predictive or concurrent validity. Reliability data were strong, but were based on a limited sample size. These psychometric limitations are compelling enough to suggest that this instrument not be the only source of data for deciding on the presence of a language delay. A Spanish version is available.
References consulted	Mardell-Czudnowski (1989); Pearson (1989). See book's References list.

Measure	**Test for Auditory Comprehension of Language—Third Edition (TACL-3). Carrow-Woolfolk (1999).**
Purpose	Measuring receptive spoken vocabulary, grammar, and syntax as well as identifying auditory comprehension deficits.
Areas	Vocabulary (word classes), Syntax (understanding of grammatical morphemes), Elaborated Phrases and Sentences (understanding of syntactically based word relations and elaborated phrase and sentence constructions).
Format	Individually administered. Subject is presented with a picture plate while examiner reads verbal cue; subjects respond by pointing to correct picture; ceiling rules for each section are provided; correct responses are scored 1 and incorrect are scored 0.
Scores	Percentiles, standard scores, and age equivalents available for the three subtests and total score; quotients with descriptive ratings.
Age group	3-0 to 9-11 years.
Time	15–25 minutes.
Users	Trained professionals.
Norms	Data collected on representative sample of 1,102 children from 24 sites relative to projected 2000 U.S. Census data. The sample was stratified by age relative to ethnicity, gender, race, and disability. Norms extend to age 9-11. Sample included children with learning disabilities and speech–language disorders.
Reliability	Internal consistency reliabilities fall in the .90s across subtests and ages, with the exception of Vocabulary at ages 5 (.89) and 9 (.84). Interrater reliability fell below .90 for two subtests; evidence of consistency across various subgroups; however, this is based on a small and limited sample. Test–retest based on 29 second- and third-grade students was .86 to .97.

Validity	Group differentiation studies lend support to the validity of the measure: individuals with speech and language delays, hearing impairments, and mental retardation scored lower than other groups. Factor analysis yielded one factor and subtest correlations that show a positive relationship, yet remains small enough to support the idea that each subtest measures a distinct aspect of auditory comprehension. Convergent validity was established with the CREVT showing that the TACL-3 correlates more highly with the Receptive than Expressive Vocabulary subtest. No predictive validity studies with TACL-3 are provided.
Comments	The TACL-3 is easy to administer and score. It appears to be a valid and reliable measure of the specific constructs it purports to measure. The new version includes full-color pictures, updated norms, and strong psychometric properties.
References consulted	Manikam (2001); Novak (2002). See book's References list.

Measure	**Test of Children's Language (TOCL). Barenbaum and Newcomer (1996).**
Purpose	Measuring important aspects of spoken language, reading, and writing.
Areas	Spoken Language, Reading, Writing.
Format	Most of the assessment is conducted throughout the reading of a storybook; questions are asked by the examiner before/after reading the pages; includes having child read the last three pages of the storybook if capable and having the child rewrite the story from memory.
Scores	Seven component scores (one is for language), four combined scores (Spoken Language Quotient, Reading Quotient, Writing Quotient, Total Language Quotient); standard scores, quotients, age equivalents, percentiles, stanines.
Age group	5-0 to 8-11 years.
Time	30–40 minutes.
Users	Trained professionals.
Norms	Data collected on 908 children. The sample was representative of 1990 U.S. Census data.
Reliability	Internal consistency, greater than .80 and .90 in most instances; test–retest (14–21 days) (n = 45 in one age group), .82–.98; Reading Comprehension, .77. No interrater reliability information provided.
Validity	Criterion-related established with other measures of reading and language ability (correlations range, .56–.83); total score on TOCL correlates .84 and .88 with other measures. Construct validity evidence: increasing means with age; total score correlates .86 with WISC-R Full Scale IQ, subtests correlate significantly with WISC-R subtests (the only exception being the writing subtests). Validity evidence indicates that the spoken language and reading aspects of this test may be too easy for older children (i.e., 7–8-year-olds), and that the writing tasks are too hard for young children.
Comments	Due to the questionable validity of the measure with older and younger children, it may be most useful with children ages 6 and 7. This measure is labor intensive for the examiner.
References consulted	Graham (2001); Wolf (2001). See book's References list.

Measure	**Test of Early Language Development—Third Edition (TELD-3). Hresko, Reid, and Hammill (1999).**
Purpose	Identifying early strengths and weaknesses in language, documenting the progress of students in intervention programs, and aiding in the direction of instruction.
Areas	Receptive Language, Expressive Language. Each version includes semantic and syntactic items in each area.
Format	Two versions, A and B. Each version has 76 items; scores are based on report, direct observation, and responses to prompts.
Scores	Overall Language Quotient; percentiles; NCEs.
Age group	2-0 to 7-11 years.
Time	15–40 minutes.
Users	Trained administrators.
Norms	Data collected on 2,217 children (1990–1991, 1996–1997) from four regions of the country representing 35 states. Variables: geographic area, gender, race, urban–rural location, ethnicity, income, educational background of the parents, disability status, and age.
Reliability	Several types of reliability are demonstrated to be strong. Average subtest coefficients > .90 for both forms; split-half reliabilities between forms A and B > .80, with two exceptions; adequate 2-week test–retest reliability.
Validity	Content, construct, and criterion-related validity are all strongly supported.
Comments	TELD-3 now has two subtests, Receptive Language and Expressive Language, and yields an overall Spoken Language score. The test is quick and easy to administer and includes all necessary manipulatives. Below the age of 3-0 years, only a small number of items are administered largely based on confirmatory report or observation. Assessors need to determine where problems occur.
References consulted	Backlund (2001); Morreale-Sherwin (2001); Suen (2001); Boehm review. See book's References list.

Measure	**Test of Language Development—Primary, Third Edition (TOLD-P: 3). Newcomer and Hammill (1997).**
Purpose	Identifying children with language deficiencies, and assessing strengths and weaknesses in language skills.
Areas	Picture Vocabulary, Relational Vocabulary, Oral Vocabulary, Grammatic Understanding, Sentence Imitation, Grammatic Completion, Word Discrimination (optional), Phonemic Analysis (optional), and Word Articulation (optional).
Format	Individually and orally administered; basal and ceiling rules provided for every subtest. Total of nine subtests (six core subtests measure semantics and syntax; three supplemental subtests measure phonological processes). Following is a description of the 6 core subtests for the TOLD-P:3. Picture Vocabulary: 30 items; assesses a child's understanding of the meaning of words; Relational Vocabulary: 30 items; requires a child to state the relationship between two words; Oral Vocabulary: 28 items; requires a child to define words given by the examiner; Grammatic Understanding: 25 items; a child selects the one picture out of three that corresponds to a sentence given by the examiner; Sentence Imitation: 30 items; a child is asked to repeat a sentence stated by the examiner;

	Grammatic Completion: 28 items; a cloze technique is used in asking a child to complete a sentence begun by the examiner for which the final word is missing. The three supplemental subtests are Word Discrimination, Phonemic Analysis, and Word Articulation. Word Discrimination: 20 items, a child is presented with word pairs and asked whether the words are the same or different; Phonemic Analysis: 14 items; a child is asked to break words into smaller phonemic units; Word Articulation: 20 items; pictures of common objects are accompanied by a sentence or two to prompt the child to say a particular word.
Scores	Standard scores, percentiles, age equivalents, six composite scores, and one global score.
Age group	4-0 to 8-11 years.
Time	30–60 minutes for the core battery; 30 minutes for supplemental subtests.
Users	Professionals with graduate training.
Norms	Data collected on 1,000 children between the ages of 4 and 8, with characteristics approximating 1997 U.S. population. Variables: geographic region, gender, race, rural versus urban status, ethnicity, educational attainment of parents, and disability status. Slight overrepresentation of lower-income families. Presented in 6-month intervals; 153 children at age 5.
Reliability	Internal consistency ranges from .80 to low .90 for all subtests and is > .90 for composites; Spoken Language Composite has internal consistency of .95 or greater for all age groups; 4-month test–retest reliability based on a sample of 33 children ranges from .81 to .92; interrater reliability is .99 across all scales.
Validity	Overall, content validity is supported qualitatively and quantitatively; however, there are some limited floors on some subtests for ages 4 and 5, and ceiling effects for older ages. There is little support for divergent validity, and evidence of construct validity is limited.
Comments	Administration and scoring procedures are presented clearly in the manual. Pronunciation guides are provided for the Word Articulation items. Evidence for the reliability and validity of this measure makes it useful for its intended purpose. However, it is important to be aware of the floors and ceilings when testing children at either extreme of the age range. There is limited sampling of phonological processing skills. Subtest floors below age 6-6 are inadequate for some subtests and age 5-6 for others. Thus, care needs to be used in interpreting results for young children. The small sample limits its use for intervention planning.
References consulted	Madle (2001b); Stutman (2001); Rathvon (2004); Salvia and Ysseldyke (2004). See book's References list.

Measure	**Test of Word Finding—Second Edition (TWF-2). German (2000).**
Purpose	Assessing children's word-finding skills.
Areas	Four naming sections (Nouns, Sentence, Completion, Verbs, Categories)
Format	Consists of standardized and informal portions. Standardized portion requires subjects to provide names for things presented visually with verbal cue; comprehension check allows examiner to distinguish between naming errors and word-finding errors. Informal portion consists of supplemental analyses to assess: (1) percent of responses delayed greater than or equal to 4 seconds; (2) tally of behaviors that often accompany word-finding difficulty; (3) phonemic cueing procedure; (4) imitation procedure with previously failed items; and (5) response analysis of errors on noun and verb sections.

Scores	Standardized portion: Word-Finding Quotient, percentile; Informal portion: percent of responses delayed, tally of secondary characteristics, pass/fail for phonemic cueing and imitation procedures, response analysis.
Age group	4-0 to 12-11 years.
Time	20–30 minutes.
Users	Formal training is not necessary; however, examiner should have experience and knowledge in test administration, scoring, and interpretation.
Norms	Data collected on 1,836 children from 27 states (four geographic regions); representative of 1997 U.S. Census data and stratified by geographic area, gender, race, urban/rural, ethnicity, family income, educational attainment of parents, disability classification.
Reliability	Internal consistency ranges from .71 to .91 across ages (means: Preprimary, .76; Primary, .87; Intermediate, .87); mean Cronbach's alphas for subjects who demonstrated word-finding difficulties are .84 (Preprimary), .88 (Primary), and .91 (Intermediate). Test–retest (n = 61; 10–14 days) is .80; one-year delay (n = 24) yielded correlation of .71. Interrater reliability is .99 (two PRO-ED staff members scored 10 completed protocols for each level of the test.)
Validity	Concurrent validity with the EOWPVT (see review in this table) is .53; with TWF-2 is .69 (synonyms subtest) and .66 (antonyms subtest). Predictive validity with CELF-3 is .57. Construct validity demonstrated by factor analysis, evidence of developmental trend, and discrimination studies showing the test's ability to differentiate between students with and without word-finding difficulties.
Comments	This test is easy to administer and score. The stimulus book is well laid out and provides clear examiner instructions. Record form is clear regarding scoring of supplemental procedures. Three forms of test: Preprimary (Pre-K and K), Primary (grades 1 and 2), Intermediate (grades 3–6).
References consulted	Olmi (2001). See book's References list.

Measure	**Token Test for Children. DiSimoni (1978).**
Purpose	Evaluating receptive language dysfunction in children.
Areas	Receptive language.
Format	61 items grouped into five parts of increasing difficulty. The first four parts each contain 10 items requiring the subject to touch the tokens designated. The 21 items in the fifth part also require the subject to touch, to pick up, to put down, or to take designate objects.
Scores	Standard scores for the total score and for each subtest.
Age group	3-0 to 12-6 years.
Time	15 minutes.
Users	The test may provide useful for experienced speech–language pathologists, though they are cautioned against using it as a norm-referenced measure.
Norms	Data collected on 1,304 children ranging in age from 3-0 to 12-6 years. Children were excluded from the sample if they had a known language problem, had failed a grade, were suspected of having a learning problem, "was not reading satisfactorily on grade level," or were "suspected of exhibiting any peculiarity of receptive language." Understanding of the concepts

	circle, *square*, *large*, and *small*, as well as the five colors of the tokens, was also required for participation, The author states, "This procedure greatly reduced the number of three and four-year-old children who could participate."
Reliability	Not reported in manual.
Validity	Not reported in manual.
Comments	Detailed instructions for administration and scoring are provided in the manual. The standard scores do not follow a typical score distribution (i.e., a mean of 500 and an *SD* of 5). Technical limitations suggest that a clinician should use this measure with caution.
References consulted	Reynolds (1985); Salvia (1985). See book's References list.

Measure	**Utah Test of Language Development—Fourth Edition (UTLD-4). Mecham (2003).**
Purpose	Identifying children with language problems, determining the severity of problems, and determining whether special education services are needed.
Areas	Picture Identification, Word Functions, Morphological Structures, Sentence Repetition, and Word Segmentation.
Format	Rating system.
Scores	Five subtests, three composite scores, and total score; percentiles, age equivalents, standard scores, descriptive ratings.
Age group	3-0 to 9-11 years.
Time	30–45 minutes.
Users	Professionals trained in the assessment of language development children.
Norms	Data collected on 841 children from 14 states in which 93% of the sample had no disability, 5% had speech and language disabilities, and 2% had "other" disabilities. The normative sample was weighted, which resulted in a sample very similar to the demographic characteristics of the U.S. population.
Reliability	Internal consistency, .75–.98; test–retest (2 weeks), .78–.93
Validity	Content validity, criterion-related validity, and construct validity are all supported.
Comments	The UTLD-4 measures two different aspects of language—Language Comprehension and Language Expression—in a brief, easy-to-administer test. The psychometric properties of this measures are reasonably strong; however the poor design of some items and the overlap of certain competencies on the form and content tasks can make interpretation difficult. The test does not assess areas such as Morphology and Syntax, and, therefore, needs to be supplemented with a language measure that assesses functional communication.
References consulted	Hurford (2005); Johnston (2005). See book's References list.

Chapter 11

Cognitive Assessment

SUSAN VIG
MICHELLE SANDERS

Cognitive assessment helps to identify young children's strengths and difficulties in intellectual development, and leads to intervention that optimizes this development. So that this process can occur with maximum effectiveness, preschool assessors need to be familiar not only with cognitive assessment procedures, but with young children and their developmental characteristics. This chapter is intended to be a practical guide for assessors working with children 3–6 years of age. Through careful observation (in preschool, childcare, and home settings), standardized testing, and alternative assessment approaches, much can be learned about young children's cognitive status and intervention needs.

REASONS FOR COGNITIVE ASSESSMENT DURING EARLY CHILDHOOD

Jenny is a 5-year-old girl who has been attending kindergarten for 4 months. The teacher has concerns about Jenny's learning difficulties and says that she is not able to keep up with the classroom work. Jenny can name only two letters of the alphabet, counts by rote only to 5, does not count objects with one-to-one correspondence, and cannot write her first name. Even with a lot of repetition and demonstra-

Susan Vig, EdM, PhD, is Director of the Early Intervention Training Institute at the Rose F. Kennedy Center, and Director of Allied Health Training for the Children's Evaluation and Rehabilitation Center, as well as Professor of Clinical Pediatrics at the Albert Einstein College of Medicine, New York.

Michelle Sanders, MSEd, PsyD, is a Clinical Instructor in the Department of Pediatrics at the Albert Einstein College of Medicine. She works with young children and their families at the Center for Babies, Toddlers, and Families.

tion, Jenny does not seem able to master early kindergarten skills. The teacher further reports that Jenny seems immature; she gets up and wanders around the room while her classmates are working.

The teacher invites Jenny's parents to come in for a conference, and shares her concerns. The parents say that they too have been concerned, because Jenny appears to learn more slowly than her older brother did at her age. Even with a lot of extra help, she seems confused about her homework and cannot manage the assignments. After the parent–teacher conference, Jenny's parents decide to have her tested by the school district to find out why she is having such a hard time learning.

The case of Jenny illustrates a common concern that leads to cognitive assessment, as a component of multidisciplinary assessment, for children under age 6. In what follows, we address specific reasons for cognitive assessment. All of these reasons (identifying and differentiating developmental problems, determining eligibility for services, planning intervention, developing expectations, and monitoring progress) are applicable to the case of Jenny.

Identifying and Differentiating Developmental Problems

Cognitive assessment can help to differentiate the developmental problems experienced by young children, so that appropriate intervention can be planned. Many young children are referred for evaluation because someone becomes concerned about their language development. It is important to know whether a child's language problems are due to specific language impairment or to global cognitive delay (Vig & Jedrysek, 1996b). In a study by Field, Fox, and Radcliffe (1990), 42% of children evaluated for developmental problems were referred because of delayed speech, but only 14% of the children received a final diagnosis of developmental language disorder; most were found to have cognitive limitations. Similarly, assessment teams must sometimes decide whether a child's short attention span, impulsivity, or high activity level represents an attentional disorder or is instead characteristic of functioning at an earlier developmental level. Cognitive assessment and its information about developmental levels can help to clarify these issues. A 4-year-old with a mental age of 30 months is apt to be active and unable to sit and do table-top activities for more than a few minutes, because he or she is functioning at an earlier developmental level.

Assessment teams evaluating kindergartners must sometimes determine whether a child's failure to acquire early academic skills is due to cognitive limitations or to specific learning deficits. In the latter case, finding that a child has normal cognitive ability, despite learning difficulties, can be a great relief to parents.

Determining Eligibility for Services

Federal legislation (Public Law 99-457, the original IDEA, IDEA 1997, and now IDEA 2004) has mandated multidisciplinary assessment of young children to document eligibility for intervention services. With its emphasis on early identification of abilities related to early reading, the NCLB Act of 2001 has created an increased need for cognitive assessment (Ford & Dahinten, 2005).

Cognitive assessment during early childhood is often undertaken to document children's eligibility for services. Publicly funded school-based services require documentation through multidisciplinary assessment, including cognitive assessment. Entitlements, such as Supplemental Security Income for children with significant cognitive limitations, are based in part on the documentation provided by standardized testing. Children's eligibility to participate in accelerated or gifted programs, or to be admitted to selective independent schools, also depends on the results of cognitive assessment. Sattler (2001) has noted that standardized tests of cognitive ability provide objective standards for such determinations and can prevent misplacement of children.

Planning Intervention

Cognitive assessment contributes to effective intervention planning. In order to plan intervention that will best meet a child's developmental needs, information about the child's potential for learning and anticipated responsiveness to intervention is essential. Understanding the child's cognitive functioning can help assessment teams decide what kind of instructional pace will be appropriate, how much adult assistance may be needed for skill acquisition, which types of instructional goals are realistic, and what rate of progress can be expected (see below). A lack of information about cognitive status and its implications for daily functioning can lead to frustration, failure, or too much assistance with tasks that are developmentally too advanced. Too much adult scaffolding, in which an adult provides hand-over-hand assistance or other help with novel tasks, deprives the child of valuable exploration and discovery experiences.

Cognitive assessment can also help early childhood professionals predict how young children will respond to particular interventions. For example, a child must have a mental age of approximately 15–18 months to use an augmentative communication device, such as a communication board, for spontaneous, self-structured communication. (This is the point at which prerequisite symbolic understanding and finger pointing should have developed.)

Developing Expectations for Progress and Behavior

Cognitive assessment can help families, teachers, and others develop realistic expectations for progress and behavior. A 4-year-old whose cognitive functioning resembles that of a 3-year-old cannot be expected to draw a recognizable picture, build representational block structures, or tell a sequenced story in a preschool classroom. If a child's cognitive impairment is not identified, families and school personnel may believe that an intervention program will "cure" the child's developmental problems, and may become frustrated and angry when this does not occur. Families may blame the school or intervention program when the child continues to have developmental problems despite intervention. For example, without cognitive information, a preschool teacher might become discouraged when the 4-year-old just mentioned disrupts play in the block corner and cannot be persuaded to build houses with classmates. A parent might be annoyed with a 3-year-old who spills a good deal when using a spoon, attributing this to willful misbehavior rather than recognizing that the child is functioning at an earlier developmental level.

Families can be helped to understand the implications of cognitive impairment for behavior as well as progress. A 5-year-old who functions more like a 3-year-old may lack judgment about sources of potential danger (oncoming traffic, sharp scissors), or may act out distress behaviorally with a temper tantrum rather than discussing it verbally. The child may require more supervision than same-age peers or may benefit from behavior management approaches suitable for younger children.

Monitoring Progress

Once children have been placed in preschool or intervention programs, cognitive assessment helps to monitor their progress. Although IQ changes over time are not expected for the majority of children with cognitive impairments (Field et al., 1990; Keogh, Coots, & Bernheimer, 1995; Vig, Kaminer, & Jedrysek, 1987), gains have been reported for some young children at biological or environmental risk (Infant Health and Development Program, 1990). Periodic cognitive assessment (triennial reevaluation, or reevaluation at the time of transition from early intervention to preschool or from preschool to elementary school) can help document the need for new services, or for the continuation or modification of current services. What is discussed less frequently and less comfortably is the issue of discontinuing services that are no longer helpful to a child. Cognitive assessment can help early childhood professionals decide whether an intervention is helping the child to progress or has reached a point of diminishing returns.

CHALLENGES OF COGNITIVE ASSESSMENT

Cognitive assessment presents a number of challenges for assessment teams. Assessment approaches and instruments must be selected with particular sensitivity to the needs of young examinees who are members of culturally and linguistically diverse groups, including those who speak English as a second language (ESL) and those with limited English proficiency (LEP). There is a lack of instruments normed in languages other than English. In addition, most nonverbal tests are inappropriate for preschoolers, and many tests for preschool children lack adequate floor (easy items) for examinees with cognitive limitations. Moreover, assessors are sometimes limited in selection of approaches by local guidelines that specify which measures may, or may not, be used. Additionally, assessors must be able to manage the challenging behaviors often presented by preschoolers.

The use of labels based on the results of cognitive assessment is particularly controversial in regard to preschool children. Opponents of labeling assert that labels may alter adults' interactions with such young children and may negatively affect expectations for their progress. Proponents of labeling argue that labels positively influence adult expectations by reducing unrealistic behavioral demands or instructional goals. Personal beliefs about these issues can jeopardize the collaborative dimension of team functioning.

Another challenge is the need to prioritize strengths as well as difficulties in describing young children's developmental status. Although intervention should ameliorate weaknesses and deficits, it should also capitalize on the strengths identified though cognitive assessment. For example, a child with strength in visual processing may benefit from pictorial support when learning to tell a story that has a beginning, middle, and end.

Meeting all of these challenges requires flexibility in the selection of assessment approaches, sensitivity to children's backgrounds and behavioral characteristics, and respect for the ideas and expertise of other team members.

PREDICTIVE VALUE OF COGNITIVE ASSESSMENT

Standardized tests for young children are sometimes criticized for having poor predictive value. The stability of test scores prior to the elementary school years is questioned (Kranzler, 1997). In evaluating the issues of stability and prediction, it is important to distinguish between infant and preschool tests, and between children with typical development and children with developmental disabilities.

Results of infant testing do not correlate well with subsequent cognitive functioning. Comparing developmental assessment with information-processing measures for infants under 1 year of age, Bornstein and Sigman (1986) found that the developmental assessment had little predictive value; habituation of attention and novelty preference were more strongly associated with subsequent cognitive competence between 2 and 8 years. Although such infant information-processing capacities as focused attention (Ruff & Dubiner, 1987) and cross-modal matching (Rose & Wallace, 1985) are associated with subsequent cognitive competence, those capacities are not generally measured by the kinds of items found in developmental tests for infants. Sattler (1988, 2001) has explained that infant tests have limited predictive power for most young children because they actually present perceptual–motor, rather than cognitive, content. When children reach a mental age of 18–24 months, their cognitive abilities begin to be addressed by test items (pointing to named body parts, objects, and pictures; labeling; combining words; finding hidden objects). Prediction based on test scores then begins to improve. Finally, prediction based on test scores is stronger for children with developmental disabilities than with typical development (Sattler, 1988, 2001; see also Chapter 12).

THEORETICAL FOUNDATIONS FOR COGNITIVE ASSESSMENT

Theoretical models of intelligence and information processing have been developed to explain children's cognitive functioning. Many of the tests used for cognitive assessment of older children are based on these models. Evidence from factor-analytic studies, and from practical knowledge of child development, suggests that models of intelligence and cognitive processing may be more relevant to older individuals than to preschool children. Factor analysis of tests commonly used for cognitive assessment consistently show that there are fewer factors for preschoolers than for older children (Buckhalt, 1991; Delugach, 1991; Elliott, 1990; Keith, 1990; Laurent, Swerdlik, & Ryburn, 1992; Stone, Gridley, & Gyurke, 1991; Thorndike, 1990). Factor analysis has thus failed to support multidimensional models of intelligence for children under age 6.

As an example, the Stanford–Binet Intelligence Scale: Fourth Edition (SB-IV; Thorndike, Hagen, & Sattler, 1986a, 1986b) is based on Horn and Cattell's (1966) model of *fluid* and *crystallized* intelligence. Comprehensive descriptions of the model are found in Horn (1985), Horn and Noll (1997), and McGrew (1997). This three-level model proposes general reasoning ability at the apex; crystallized abilities, fluid analytic abilities, and short-term memory at the second level; and the areas of verbal reasoning, abstract/visual reasoning, quantitative reasoning, and short-term memory at the base. According to the model, crystallized abilities are thought to include verbal and quantitative reasoning; fluid analytic abilities include abstract/visual reasoning; and short-term memory includes both verbal and nonverbal memory. This model has not been supported for children under age 6. Based on a review of validity research, Laurent et al. (1992) concluded that confirmatory factor analysis supports only two factors (verbal reasoning and abstract/ visual reasoning) for children 2–6 years of age.

Due to limited differentiation of cognitive abilities during the preschool years, the cross-battery approach described by Flanagan and McGrew (1997) and McGrew (1997), which is useful for older children, may not be relevant to preschool children. Profile analysis may involve inferences based on characteristics of instruments, rather than abilities of children.

The *planning, attention, simultaneous, and successive* (PASS) cognitive processing model is described by Naglieri, Braden, and Gottling (1993), Naglieri (2005), and Naglieri and Das (2005). According to the model, intelligence comprises three components: attentional processes, planning processes, and information processes. Attentional processes focus cognitive activity through arousal and selective attention to relevant stimuli. Planning involves the generation of problem-solving plans. Information is coded both simultaneously (relating each component of a stimulus to an entire array) and successively (ordering stimuli in a chain-like progression.)

The PASS model has been operationalized as the Cognitive Assessment System (Naglieri & Das, 1997), designed for children ages 5–17 years. Its tasks may be too difficult for many 5-year-olds, suggesting that the model may not be useful for young children. For example, one task requires children to identify big and small animals based on actual sizes in nature, rather than the sizes represented on a stimulus page.

Although theories of intelligence may be useful for thinking about assessment in a general way, practical information about child development may be more useful for answering referral questions about a particular child and reporting assessment results to parents and others.

DEVELOPMENTAL FOUNDATIONS FOR COGNITIVE ASSESSMENT

Influences of Caregiver–Child Attachment on Cognitive Development

In addition to being knowledgeable about early childhood development, assessors should be familiar with the influences of caregiver–child attachment on cognitive development. Comprehensive assessment of young children should always include the exploration of attachment influences. All team members can help to identify family/caregiver strengths or challenges that can be addressed in planning intervention.

Secure attachment with important or special people (attachment figures) encourages children to explore and master their environments (see Walters & Cummings, 2000). Children who lack this encouragement, and have low mastery motivation in preschool, enter kindergarten not only with lower mastery motivation but also with lower achievement (Turner & Johnson, 2003). Sensitive parenting provides children with a secure base from which to explore, and helps them "think aloud" about their own behavior (Symons & Clark, 2000). In a study by Fivush and Vasuveda (2002), mothers who reported a secure attachment bond with their preschoolers engaged in more elaborate reminiscing (structuring conversations about past events) than mothers who did not report secure attachments. This kind of interaction encourages thinking and learning, and optimizes children's cognitive development. Positive parent–child attachment also provides emotional support for cognitive development. In a study of mother–infant interaction, Feldman and Greenbaum (1997) found that affect regulation and synchrony observed in a play context were precursors of children's subsequent symbolic competence. On the other hand, negative relationships with caregivers can inhibit or disrupt children's mental state reasoning (Repacholi & Trapolini, 2004).

The take-home message for assessment teams is that young children must be viewed not only in terms of their own cognitive competencies or difficulties, but also within the context of their attachment relationships, which can have either a positive or negative impact on cognitive development. Assessors can gain relevant insights by observing children interacting with their caregivers, and by asking parents or other caregivers about home activities, learning experiences provided for children, and disciplinary practices.

Early Childhood Development as a Context for Assessment

During the course of early cognitive development, the child initially focuses on his or her own body, then turns attention toward the outside world, and finally becomes able to represent that world mentally. In contrast to motor or language skills, cognitive processes such as discrimination, categorization, or symbolic representation cannot be observed directly. They must instead be inferred from what the child says or does with objects. Features of early childhood development that are relevant to cognitive assessment, briefly described below and summarized in Table 11.1, are based on the work of experts who have studied the development of young children and/or have published instruments used to assess their abilities (Bayley, 1993, 2006a, 2006b; Frankenburg et al., 1990; Griffiths, 1970; Huntley, 1996; Ireton, 1992; Molnar & Kaminer, 1985; Sparrow, Balla, & Cicchetti, 1984). Features seen in children under age 3 are included, because many older children seen for cognitive assessment are found to function at earlier developmental levels.

- *1–6 months.* Infants achieve state regulation and begin the process of attachment with their parents or other primary caregivers. By 6 months, they show interest in environmental sights and sounds.
- *6–12 months.* Fine motor skills and hand–eye coordination permit active exploration of objects. Focused attention during object manipulation allows the infant to derive maximum information by touching or mouthing an object or by viewing it from different spatial perspectives. This correlates with subsequent cognitive ability (Ruff & Dubiner, 1987). By 8 months, infants demonstrate a capacity for mental representation, which forms a basis for many cognitive and linguistic processes (understanding or using symbols in the form of words, pictures, and referential gestures).
- *12–18 months.* This is a time of transition from sensory–motor skills to more cognitively based skills. Children begin to use words; they also begin to understand that pictures and dolls represent real entities, and are not just things to hold, pat, drop, or slide across a surface.
- *18–24 months.* Assessment results begin to be predictive of subsequent cognitive functioning. By 24 months, children should understand multiword utterances, combine at least two words when speaking, understand and use representational gestures, understand pictures, and combine toys on the basis of representational properties (e.g., use a toy spoon to pretend to feed a doll).
- *24–36 months.* Children's language becomes more complex, and they can talk about remote events as well as the current situation. Children also begin to copy very simple forms from a pictorial model, rather than relying on movement cues provided by an adult's demonstration.
- *36–48 months.* Children acquire temporal concepts and use past and future tenses when speaking. They begin to understand the concepts of *same* and *different.* Their play shows evidence of planning ("They're gonna have dinner") and decontextualization (substituting one object for another, or requesting absent objects to use in mentally formulated scenarios).
- *48–60 months.* Children use full sentences, create narratives based on temporal order, and use internalized language to mediate behavior ("First I'll get some juice, then I'll play with my trucks"). In play, they set up complex scenarios without realistic props and create extensive dialogue for dolls. They draw recognizable pictures of people.

TABLE 11.1. Developmental Skills Relevant to Cognitive Assessment

Age	Skill	Assessment item
1–6 months	• Looks at objects. • Shows interest in sounds. • Begins to grasp objects.	• Follows moving object. • Turns head when bell is rung. • Holds rod in hand.
6–12 months	• Uses hand–eye coordination to explore objects. • Grasps objects. • Forms mental representation of object.	• Manipulates bell. • Picks up spoon by handle. • Looks for hidden object.
12–18 months	• Relates pencil to paper. • Represents two or more ideas through language.	• Scribbles. • Combines two or more words.
18–24 months	• Represents simple form, using pencil and paper. • Understands words for body parts. • Uses words to represent objects. • Uses phrases to express ideas. • Combines toys according to function rather than physical properties.	• Imitates vertical line drawn by adult. • Points to several named body parts. • Names objects and pictures. • Uses phrases of four or more syllables. • Relates doll-size furniture and table utensils to doll.
24–36 months	• Defines words by function. • Imitates simple block construction. • Copies simple geometric forms without need for movement cues.	• Responds to "What do you do with a chair?" • Builds eight-block tower. • Copies vertical and horizontal lines from pictorial model.
36–48 months	• Imitates two-dimensional block construction modeled by adult. • Understands simple questions. • Asks questions to obtain information. • Matches colors. • Represents person through drawing.	• Builds three-component bridge with blocks. • Gives name or age when asked. • Asks questions that begin with *what*, *where*, *who*. • Sorts red, yellow, and blue blocks. • Draws recognizable human figure with head and limbs.
48–60 months	• Represents experiences verbally. • Sequences ideas.	• Relates personal experiences in detail when asked. • Tells simple story with beginning, middle, and end.

Note. Data from Bayley (1993); Griffiths (1970); Frankenburg et al. (1990); Ireton (1992); Molnar and Kaminer (1985); and Sparrow, Balla, and Cicchetti (1984).

ASSESSMENT APPROACHES

Cognitive assessment during early childhood should be based on multiple sources of information: abilities demonstrated spontaneously, response to structured tasks, and information provided by the caregiver. Best practice requires flexible use of more than one assessment approach. The following sections explore several approaches: standardized testing, observation of play with objects, assessment of adaptive behavior, copying and drawing as estimates of cognitive ability, and dynamic assessment.

Standardized Testing

General Considerations

PROS AND CONS OF STANDARDIZED TESTING

The use of standardized tests with young children has been the subject of considerable discussion and controversy. In a survey of psychologists experienced in early childhood assessment, 43% of respondents reported that intelligence tests were "useless" for young children and that alternative methods should be used instead (Bagnato & Neisworth, 1994). Preschool tests have been criticized for inadequate norms, test floors, and item gradients, as well as for inappropriate materials, tasks, and procedures (Alfonso & Flanagan, 1999; Bagnato & Neisworth, 1994; Neisworth & Bagnato, 1992). The behavioral characteristics of preschool children (short attention spans, tendency to become oppositional) have also been described as barriers to testing.

Despite these criticisms, many experts support the use of standardized tests with young children. Bracken (1994) and Gyurke (1994) have stated that standardized intellectual assessments and alternative assessments are not mutually exclusive, and that alternative methods have not been empirically validated. Standardized testing provides a context for obtaining maximum information within a short time. Gyurke (1994) suggests that observing a child in a semistructured situation, doing the well-defined tasks of standardized tests, should be one of the multiple sources of information constituting comprehensive assessment.

Standardized testing is a useful and important component of preschool assessment if the following conditions can be met:

1. Developmentally appropriate instruments are selected.
2. Clinical usefulness is not sacrificed for psychometric priorities when ideal instruments do not exist for a particular child.
3. Several different standardized instruments are available to assessors.
4. Standardized testing is supplemented by other assessment approaches (play observation, caregiver interviews).
5. Standardized instruments are administered by assessors with a background in early childhood (internalized norms for development and behavior, based on experience with young children of different ages and different kinds of developmental competencies); knowledge of developmental disabilities and their characteristics during early childhood; and developmentally appropriate techniques for managing young children's behavior during assessment sessions.

Some other issues that need to be considered when selecting and administering tests, and interpreting the results of standardized testing, are summarized next.

NOVELTY VERSUS PRACTICE

The issue of novelty versus learning or practice is especially important during the preschool years. The best measures of cognitive ability present activities that are new to a child. The child must both conceptualize a task and organize him- or herself to complete it. A background in early childhood development will enable assessors to recognize the stages at which specific kinds of tasks are apt to be novel to young children, and subsequent stages during which the tasks cease to be novel because they have been practiced repeatedly at home or at preschool. Novel tasks make strong cognitive demands for grasping what is expected and envisioning how behavior can be organized toward achieving a goal. Tasks mastered through repeated practice do not require as much cognitive activity and are less useful for determining a child's cognitive potential. When a parent who may be observing an assessment of a young child comments, "She hasn't learned that yet," or "He hasn't done that yet at school," the assessor can explain that the child's responses to unfamiliar activities are of greatest interest and value in understanding the child's cognitive functioning.

By way of illustration, consider the block-stacking task included in many preschool tests. For a 2-year-old, building a tower of two to four blocks is apt to be a new kind of activity, requiring an understanding of what is expected and organization of the necessary motor schemas (grasp and release patterns) to achieve the cognitively envisioned goal of building a tower. If the same task is presented to a 5-year-old with mental retardation, who functions at a much earlier developmental level, the task will have ceased to be novel. The 5-year-old will have practiced block stacking at school. The learned task will no longer be a good measure of cognitive capacity, and may result in score inflation.

COGNITIVE LOADING OF TEST ITEMS

In standardized cognitive assessment of preschoolers, it is useful to think about the cognitive demands or so-called "loading" of individual test items. Considering items' demands for conceptualization and self-organization is helpful, whether the assessment team is reviewing new materials for possible purchase, selecting an appropriate instrument for an assessment session, or interpreting test results.

The way test materials are presented to the child can increase or decrease the cognitive loading of apparently similar tasks. Inset formboards, for example, are presented differently on different tests. For a simple formboard of the Bayley Scales of Infant Development—Third Edition (Bayley-III; Bayley, 2006a, 2006b), the examiner hands insets to the child one by one. In early items of the Stanford-Binet Intelligence Scale, Fifth Edition (SB5; Roid 2005), insets are placed in correct receptacles by the examiner, then removed and placed on the table in front of the child. On the Griffiths Mental Development Scales (Griffiths, 1970), insets are stacked in front of the board so that visual matches are not immediately apparent. The child must take the cognitively more advanced step of unstacking the piles of insets before visual matches can be made. In thinking about assessment tasks, it is useful to consider the degree of visual guidance provided, as well as the amount of self-organization and problem solving required of the child.

Test Characteristics to Consider in Making a Selection

In selecting tests for young children, it is important to think about the interests and behaviors typical of this age group. Selecting tests with developmentally appropriate materials, formats, and procedures will help to avoid "untestability" and produce valid assessments.

MATERIALS

Young preschoolers, and older preschoolers functioning at earlier developmental levels, like to manipulate toys, blocks, and other materials. They are apt to maintain their best involvement with tests providing objects to hold, touch, and manipulate. Schematic drawings and easel formats may be less appealing to them.

FORMAT AND PROCEDURES

Preschoolers have short attention spans and become frustrated by formats requiring several consecutive failures of the same kind of item. They do best with procedures that allow mixing different kinds of items (verbal and nonverbal, easy and difficult).

LANGUAGE DEMANDS

The language demands of assessment procedures affect developmental suitability. This issue is relevant not only for monolingual speakers of English, but also for examinees who speak ESL or have LEP that is not necessarily apparent in informal conversation. Slight changes of wording can introduce higher levels of abstraction and thereby impose stronger cognitive demands. For example, a 4-year-old with typical development should have no trouble providing a functional definition of an object ("What do you do with a cup?"). The same 4-year-old, and even a 5-year-old, may have trouble with a more abstract attributive definition ("What is a cup?").

Because the wording of instructions can affect test suitability, the length and complexity of test instructions should be evaluated for both nonverbal and verbal assessment tasks. Flanagan, Alfonso, Kaminer, and Rader (1995) systematically studied the basic concepts used in preschool test instructions. They used the original Boehm Test of Basic Concepts (Boehm, 1986) and the original Bracken Basic Concepts Scale (Bracken, 1984) to identify which of the specific concepts used in test instructions were understood by preschoolers. They found, for example, that the concept *another*, used in all five tests reviewed, was understood by only 11% of 3-year-olds, 30% of 4-year-olds, and 48% of 5-year-olds. Thus, if unfamiliar concepts are embedded in the task instructions, outcomes are dubious.

As emphasized throughout this book and particularly in Chapter 9, cultural/linguistic fairness is essential. Ortiz and Dynda (2005) have pointed out that standardized tests of cognitive ability sometimes become tests of English proficiency for members of culturally and linguistically diverse groups. These experts further note that nonverbal tests do not eliminate this problem, and state that nonverbal tests or subtests often present inherent language demands. Nonverbal tests generally involve a verbal interaction between examiner and examinee, and instructions are sometimes presented verbally rather than pantomimed.

RECENCY OF TEST NORMS

Because some clinically useful tests were normed many years ago, the issue of norming recency should be considered in test selection. Based on an analysis of 73 studies involving more than 7,500 participants, Flynn (1984) concluded that IQ scores increase 3 points per decade. Kranzler (1997) noted that the use of older tests can result in inflated scores and may underidentify mental retardation. When older instruments are used, potential score inflation should be considered in test selection.

Technical versus Clinical Features

Used judiciously, standardized assessment can provide important information about young children's cognitive abilities. Ideally, assessment instruments should be both technically adequate and clinically appropriate. In the real world, however, most preschool tests are not equally strong in both areas (see Chapter 3). Bracken (1987) proposed the following guidelines for the technical adequacy of preschool instruments: median subtest reliabilities of .80 or greater; total test internal consistency and stability coefficients of .90 or greater; subtest and total test floors extending at least 2 *SD* below test means; subtest item gradients of no fewer than 3 raw score items per standard score deviation; and evidence of validity. In an expanded version of these guidelines, Bracken and Walker (1997) stated that test floors of 3–4 *SD* below test means are preferable. This would make tests more suitable for children with mental retardation.

Unfortunately, most preschool assessment instruments are not equally strong in both psychometric and clinical properties. In assessment situations, this poses a dilemma. Should the assessor use an instrument with excellent technical features, but with materials and activities that have little appeal or tasks that are too difficult for young children? Will the resultant lack of interest, withdrawal of effort, or oppositional behavior yield a clinically valid assessment? Will the child be described as "untestable"? On the other hand, will the assessor be criticized for selecting clinically and developmentally appropriate instruments with weaker technical features? Is it permissible to use a test that has older norms or a less than adequate norming sample, but that has adequate floor, presents appealing activities, and results in full testability? These issues are particularly critical for young children with cognitive disabilities or autism spectrum disorders (ASD), who are often referred for comprehensive diagnostic assessment.

The following review of commonly used tests includes technical information, but emphasizes clinical features that are (and are not) appropriate for preschoolers. These commonly used tests, and additional tests of cognitive ability, are summarized in Appendix 11.1. As this book was in its final stages of preparation, publication of a new edition of the Differential Ability Scales (Elliott, 2006), for individuals ages 2-5–17-11 years, was expected. More detailed information about the technical adequacy of preschool tests is provided by Alfonso and Flanagan (1999), Bracken and Walker (1997), Flanagan and Alfonso (1995), Flanagan and Harrison (2005), Sattler (2001), and Sattler and Dumont (2004).

Bayley Scales of Infant and Toddler Development—Third Edition

The Bayley Scales of Infant and Toddler Development—Third Edition (Bayley-III; Bayley, 2006a, 2006b) assesses the developmental functioning of infants and young children aged 1–42 months. In contrast to the many preschool instruments that extend test formats designed for older children downward into a younger age range, the Bayley-II is specifically designed for infants and very young children. The test includes Cognitive, Language, Motor, Social–Emotional, and Adaptive Behavior scales. Composites are available for each scale and for all subtests (receptive and expressive language, fine and gross motor, 10 specific areas of adaptive behavior). Discrepancy comparisons are available for each scale. This represents a substantial change from the Bayley Scales of Infant Development—Second Edition (BSID-II; Bayley, 1993), which included Mental and Motor Scales, but did not present subtests within those areas. The Bayley-III provides developmental age equivalents for subtests. Growth scores, based on an equal interval scale, may be used to track the progress of individual children over time. The test manual discusses adaptations and modifications for testing children with special needs.

The Bayley-III was normed on 1,700 children ages 1–42 months. Stratification variables included sex, parent education, race/ethnicity, and geographic region. A stability coefficient of .81 for all ages is reported for the Cognitive Scale; coefficients of .87 and .83 are reported for the Language and Motor Scales, respectively. Coefficients for internal consistency range from .86 to .93. Test–retest reliability improves with increasing age. Coefficients of .67 to .80 are reported for ages 2–4 months, .77 to .86 for 9–13 months, .71 to .88 for 19–26 months, and .83 to .94 for 33–42 months. The relation between the Bayley-III and other tests has been explored to establish validity. The test manual reports coefficients representing the relation between the Bayley-III Cognitive Composite and the BSID-II Mental Development Index (.60); WPPSI-III Full Scale IQ (.79); Preschool Language Scale—Fourth Edition, Total Language score (.57); Peabody Developmental Motor Scales—Second Edition, Total Motor score (.45); and Adaptive Behavior Assessment System—Second Edition, Parent Form General Adaptive score (.36). As further evidence of validity, the test manual presents data for use of the Bayley-III in diagnostic assessment of special groups: children with Down syndrome, pervasive developmental disorder, cerebral palsy, specific language impairment, risk of developmental delay, asphyxiation at birth, prenatal alcohol exposure, status as small for gestational age, and premature or low birth weight. The manual notes that these data should be interpreted cautiously, due to small sample sizes and nonrandom selection.

The lowest composite scores available are 55 for the Cognitive Scale and 45 for the Language and Motor Scales. Although this degree of test floor is adequate for most children, being able to obtain even lower composites would be preferable for children with more significant delays.

For purposes of cognitive assessment, the Cognitive Scale is of primary interest. Although cognitive and motor skills should be considered as separate areas, some items of the Bayley-III Motor Scale's Fine Motor subtest (e.g., replicating a block bridge, copying a plus sign with paper and pencil) are cognitively loaded so that a child's motor performance may be affected by cognitive factors. By identifying possible cognitive influences, the psychologist can help a multidisciplinary team decide the extent to which motor deficits should be addressed in intervention.

ISSUES TO CONSIDER IN USING THE BAYLEY-III TO ASSESS PRESCHOOL CHILDREN

The materials and format of the Bayley-III are developmentally appropriate and highly appealing to young children. There are plenty of toys and materials to handle. Toys, puzzles, pegs, and blocks are easily washed. Tasks using pictures are interspersed with other activities. The test format presents continually varying item types. For example, at one level on the Cognitive Scale, the child listens to a story, completes an inset formboard, assembles a two-component puzzle, completes a pegboard, assembles another puzzle, matches pictures, and engages in representational play. The examiner has flexibility in determining the order of subtest presentations, as long as basal and ceiling rules are followed. Many demonstrations and trials are permitted. Verbal instructions have been simplified in this edition. All scales, color coded for easy identification, are included in one record form.

By presenting separate scales for cognitive, language, and other areas, the Bayley-III provides a more appropriate assessment of children with language problems than did previous editions of the test. (The BSID-II included language as part of its global Mental Development Index, which penalized children with significant language impairments.) Because separate scores are available for each of the scales and subtests, assessors can readily identify specific areas of strength or weakness, and plan well-targeted intervention.

Basal and ceiling rules have been simplified in the Bayley-III. The examiner begins testing at a designated start point corresponding to a child's chronological age. If the child attains success on the first 3 consecutive items administered, basal is established. If the child fails to obtain 3 consecutive successes, the examiner drops back to the previous starting point. If the child achieves successes on the first consecutive items at the lower start point, basal is established. If not, the examiner keeps dropping back to previous start points until basal is established. Ceiling is defined as 5 consecutive failures. Because each test item presents a different kind of task, the child is not apt to become frustrated by this discontinuation procedure.

The Bayley-III is often used to assess the development of children born prematurely. An adjustment for prematurity, based on a 40-week gestation period, may be used when converting raw scores to standard scores. The test manual and record form provide guidance in adjusting for prematurity through 24 months. Within the field of early childhood assessment, however, there is not full agreement about the age at which the adjustment should be discontinued. In an informal poll of psychologists experienced in BSID-II administration, Ross and Lawson (1997) found that while most practitioners discontinued correction at 24 months, some advocated discontinuation at 12, 18, or 30 months, or at school age. If adjustment for prematurity is used with the Bayley-III, best practice suggests reporting both corrected and uncorrected scores.

Due to its strong psychometric and clinical properties, the Bayley-III is the best choice for assessing children up to 42 months of age.

Stanford–Binet Intelligence Scales, Fifth Edition

The Fifth Edition of the Stanford–Binet (SB5; Roid, 2003a, 2003b) is an intelligence test normed for individuals between 2 and 85+ years of age. The SB5 comprises 10 subtests, which yield an overall Verbal IQ, Nonverbal IQ, and Full Scale IQ. There are five factors embedded in the Verbal and Nonverbal Domains: Fluid Reasoning, Knowledge, Quantitative Reasoning, Visual–Spatial Processing, and Working Memory. These five factors are based on the Cattell–Horn–Carroll theory of intellectual abilities (see Sattler, 2002, for description). This hierarchical model proposes three levels or strata. A narrow stratum comprises the specific abilities used in processing mental information (e.g., visualization, speech discrimination). A second, broader stratum includes eight factors: fluid intelligence, crystallized intelligence, general memory and learning, broad visual perception, broad auditory perception, broad retrieval capacity, broad cognitive speediness, and processing speed (Sattler, 2001). The third stratum, at the apex of the hierarchy, is a general factor.

The Stanford–Binet Intelligence Scales for Early Childhood (Early SB5; Roid, 2005) is a specialized version of the SB5 developed for use with children ages 2-0–7-3 years. Advanced items have been eliminated from subscales. The SB5 was normed on a sample of 4,800 individuals, stratified by age, gender, ethnicity, geographic region, and SES. Although the sample included some individuals with special needs, no special accommodation was made for them, and the sample excluded those with significant medical conditions, LEP, severe communication or sensory deficits, and severe emotional or behavior disorders (Johnson, 2003).

The SB5 has test–retest reliability coefficients ranging from .92 to .95 for the Verbal, Nonverbal, and Full Scale IQs. The SB5 Full Scale IQ correlates with other intelligence measures. Correlation coefficients are .90 for the SB-IV Test Composite, .83 for the WPPSI-R Full Scale IQ, and .78 for General Intellectual Ability on the Woodcock–Johnson III.

In establishing the SB5's validity, studies were completed with individuals representing special populations, including individuals with attention-deficit/hyperactivity disorder (ADHD), autism, LEP, giftedness, learning disabilities, orthopedic/motor problems, speech–language impairment, deafness/hearing impairment, and serious emotional disturbances. Although preschool children were included in several of these groups, results are not reported separately for preschoolers.

ISSUES TO CONSIDER IN USING THE SB5 TO ASSESS PRESCHOOL CHILDREN

The SB5 presents materials and activities appealing to preschoolers. There are manipulatives, toys, and brightly colored pictures that portray objects, people, and activities interesting to young children. Discontinuation based on failure of any two items within a series of three to six items at a particular level is less frustrating to young children than the multiple consecutive failures required for discontinuation required by other tests of cognitive ability. Test instructions are usually worded with simple vocabulary and syntax. The test provides demonstration and practice items.

One of the principal disadvantages of the SB5 for preschoolers is the sequence of subtest administrations. Administrative guidelines state that all Nonverbal subtests should be given first. This is followed by administration of all Verbal subtests. Although it is a good idea to start testing with a nonverbal activity requiring no expressive language and little social interaction with the examiner, completing all Nonverbal subtests before beginning the Verbal subtests may be frustrating for children. Children with disabilities (the group most likely to be tested during the preschool years) usually have language problems and often become less cooperative for language-based tasks than they are for performance-based (nonverbal) tasks.

Another important issue to consider in using the SB5 with preschoolers is the language skills it requires. Although the test clearly differentiates between the Nonverbal and Verbal Domains, some nonverbal activities have a significant verbal component. According to Bain (2005, p. 94), "most of the nonverbal subtests do require some degree of receptive and expressive language, rather than relying on completely nonverbal directions." A receptive understanding of verbal commands and comparative relational concepts is required for some nonverbal subtests. For example, initial items of the nonverbal Quantitative Reasoning subtest require an understanding of the concepts *bigger* and *more* (the latter is embedded in a sentence of eight words). Preschoolers with language impairment, ASD, or mental retardation may not be successful with such "nonverbal" tasks.

The SB5 also lacks sufficient floor for 2-, 3-, and some 4-year-olds with cognitive limitations. For example, the first item of the Nonverbal Routing subtest (which is also the first item of the entire test) requires an understanding of the concept *same* and expects the child not to touch appealing objects presented in the stimulus array. Both of these expectations may exceed the conceptual and behavioral capacities of examinees functioning at very early developmental levels. (In contrast, Bayley-III instructions remind assessors that very young children should be given the opportunity to touch and hold stimulus materials.)

In short, the SB5 may be most useful for testing 4- and 5-year-olds with mild cognitive or language difficulties, and preschoolers of all ages who are being tested for accelerated or gifted programs.

Wechsler Preschool and Primary Scale of Intelligence—Third Edition

The WPPSI-III (Wechsler, 2002) is normed for children ages 2-6 to 7-3 years. This age range is divided into two age groups: 2-6 to 3-11 years, and 4-0 to 7-3 years. There are different test batteries for each age group. For ages 2-6 to 3-11 years, core subtests include Receptive Vocabulary, Information, Block Design, and Object Assembly. A supplemental Picture Naming subtest is also available. For ages 4-0 to 7-3 years, core subtests are Information, Vocabulary, Word Reasoning, Block Design, Matrix Reasoning, Picture Concepts, and Coding. Supplemental subtests include Symbol Search, Comprehension, Similarities, and Object Assembly. The manual provides specific guidelines about substitution of supplemental subtests for core subtests. Optional Receptive Vocabulary and Picture Naming subtests provide additional information about language abilities for ages 4-0 to 7-3 years, but may not be substituted for core subtests. The WPPSI-III provides Verbal, Performance, and Full Scale IQs. A General Language Composite is available for both age groups, and a Processing Speed Score is available for the older group.

The WPPSI-III was normed on a sample of 1,700 children, representative of the U.S. population as based on the 2000 census. Stratification variables included age, sex, parental education, race/ethnicity, and geographic region. Internal consistency coefficients across all ages range from .89 to .96 for composites, and .83 to .95 for subtests. Stability coefficients for the Full Scale IQ are .92 for ages 2-6 to 3-11 years, but are less stable (less than .80) for ages 4-0 to 5-5 years (Sattler & Dumont, 2004).

Factor analysis has identified two factors (Verbal and Performance) for the younger age group and three factors (Verbal, Performance, and Processing Speed) for the older group. In factor-analytic studies reported in the technical manual, the nonverbal Picture Completion and Picture Concepts subtests loaded on the Verbal factor. Investigators inferred that verbal mediation might be involved in these tasks.

In validity studies, WPPSI-III correlations with other tests resulted in coefficients of .85 for the WPPSI-R, .80 for the BSID-II Mental Scale, and .87 for the DAS. Validity studies described in the technical manual included administration of the WPPSI-III to special groups: children previously identified as intellectually gifted, and children with mild or moderate mental retardation, developmental delays, developmental risk factors, autism, expressive language disorder, mixed expressive–receptive language disorder, LEP, ADHD, and motor impairment.

ISSUES TO CONSIDER IN USING THE WPPSI-III TO ASSESS PRESCHOOL CHILDREN

The WPPSI-III presents a number of features contributing to ease of administration. Most younger preschoolers can complete the test within 45 minutes, and older preschoolers within an hour. There are separate sections in the administration and scoring manual for the two age groups. Full administrative instructions for all subtests are presented in each section, which eliminates the need to switch back and forth between sections for those subtests administered to both age groups. The record form is easy to use. Verbal instructions have been simplified and are easier for young children to understand than WPPSI-R instructions.

Materials include blocks and colorful pictures, but no toys. So that difficulties with fine motor coordination will not affect measurement of cognitive ability, time bonuses have been eliminated from Block Design and Object Assembly subtests in this edition. Scoring guidelines permit slight gaps and misalignments.

The format and conceptual demands of some WPPSI-III subtests are too complex for many preschoolers with disabilities. Hamilton (2003) has suggested that the conceptual demands of both the Matrix Reasoning and Picture Concepts subtests may be problematic for preschool children. Picture Concepts requires the child to select two (and in more advanced items, three) pictures, presented in linear arrays, that "go together." Although the pictures are clear and highly appealing to young children, inherent demands for changing the bases of categorization (e.g., perceptual features, functional characteristics) from item to item exceed the cognitive capacities of many preschoolers. They are apt to select responses on the basis of personal preference ("I like this one and this one!").

Another drawback is that most WPPSI-III subtests require four or five consecutive failures of the same type of item before the subtest can be discontinued. Although this procedure is generally tolerated by older children and more able preschoolers, young children with developmental problems tend to become frustrated. They sometimes show their frustration by becoming inattentive, active, or oppositional.

In short, the WPPSI-III has many attractive features: an expanded age range, simple verbal instructions, and appealing pictures and activities. Some tasks and formats may be too complicated for children with disabilities. The test has strong psychometric properties and may be most useful for 3-, 4-, and 5-year-olds who are being assessed for accelerated or gifted programs or have close to normal cognitive ability, and 5-year-olds with mild cognitive difficulties.

Griffiths Mental Development Scales

The Griffiths Mental Development Scales (Griffiths, 1970; Huntley, 1996), a British test, is discussed here because it exemplifies the kinds of clinical features needed for cognitive assessment of preschool children with developmental disabilities. The Griffiths is used for children ranging in age from birth to 8 years. There are five scales for children up to age 2, and six scales for children over age 2. Scales for the younger group include Locomotor, Personal–Social, Hearing and Speech, Eye and Hand Coordination, and Performance; scales for children over age 2 include these five plus a Practical Reasoning Scale. Developmental quotients, based on ratios of mental ages to chronological ages, can be calculated for individual scales as well as for the test as a whole. The 1996 revision of the birth to age 2 test provides percentiles as well as developmental quotients and age equivalents.

The 1970 edition of the Griffiths, which is still used for children ages 3–8 years, was normed on a sample of 2,260 British children. There were over 200 children in each of eight age groups for years I through VII, and 77 children in the year VIII group. The sample was not random, nor was it stratified for gender, ethnicity, or SES. The 1996 restandardization sample for the birth to age 2 group is stratified by gender, ethnicity, SES, urban/rural area, and geographic region.

According to information provided in the Griffiths administrative and technical manual, correlation coefficients representing the relationship between the overall General Quotient and each of the six subscales range from .64 to .77. Test–retest reliability is .77. Validity studies described in the manual have documented correlation coefficients of .77 to .81, for years III through VI age groups, between the Griffiths General Quotient and Terman–Merrill (Form L) IQs. Aldridge Smith, Bidder, Gardner, and Gray (1980) examined interrater reliability and found high rates of reliability for the Eye and Hand Coordination, Performance, and Practical Reasoning scales, and lower rates for the Locomotor, Personal–Social, and Hearing and Speech scales. In examining item reliability of individual scales for all age groups, Hanson (1982) concluded that "very little of the test is seriously unreliable" (p. 160), with relatively poorest reliability reported for the Personal–Social scale.

RESEARCH WITH THE GRIFFITHS

Due in part to a format yielding separate standard scores for all scales, and an extensive age range permitting retesting with the same instrument in longitudinal studies, the Griffiths has been used for research (Slone, Durrheim, Lachman, & Kaminer, 1998).

Hanson and Aldridge Smith (1987) examined young children's attainment on the Griffiths by comparing overall scores of children tested in 1960 with scores of children tested in 1980. Results indicated that young children mastered test items at a considerably younger age in 1980 than they did in 1960. The researchers noted that social class (i.e., SES) bias did not account for the results. The research also indicated that the usefulness of the Griffiths was greatest up to age 4 for children with normal or near-normal intelligence.

Conn (1993) examined the relationship between the Griffiths scores children achieved at ages 4-0 to 4-11 years and selected educational outcomes (placements based on their Griffiths scores). Results of the study indicated that Griffiths scores achieved at these ages had predictive validity for educational outcomes at 7+ years.

Luiz, Foxcroft, and Stewart (2001) examined the construct validity of the Griffiths for a sample of 430 South African children from four ethnic groups (described as white, mixed-race, Asian, and black), who ranged in age from 54 months to 83 months. The sample was stratified for age, gender, language, and SES. Results indicated that the pattern of correlations between the South African groups was consistent with, and similar to, the pattern of correlations found by Griffiths in 1970 with the British standardization sample. Factor analysis indicated that the Hearing and Speech, Eye and Hand Coordination, Performance, and Practical Reasoning scales demonstrated a strong level of concurrence between each of the groups in terms of the construct measured for each group.

ISSUES TO CONSIDER IN USING THE GRIFFITHS TO ASSESS PRESCHOOL CHILDREN

Griffiths materials and activities are highly appealing to young children, including those with significant cognitive difficulties. There are many toys (miniature car, dog, cat, horse, chair, etc.) and manipulatives (puzzles, blocks, beads, screw-top jar, color plaques, cylinders of different weights). Most of the materials can be washed. For a picture-naming task, there are small, brightly colored pictures for the child to hold and, if desired, place in a small box. A particularly appealing nonverbal task is having the child first replicate a three-component "bridge" constructed with wooden boxes by the examiner, and then replicate a "train" constructed of several blocks and pass it under the bridge. The item is scored at different developmental levels, depending on the degree of success with the task components. Young children enjoy watching the demonstration and hearing the examiner say, "Choo choo. Here comes the train!" while passing the train back and forth under the bridge.

Tasks presented on the nonverbal Performance scale are truly nonverbal. Instructions can be pantomimed. Children with ASD or other developmental disabilities who do not speak, or who refuse tasks involving interaction with the assessor, can often be persuaded to become involved in the performance-based tasks (filling boxes of cubes, stacking cubes, completing formboards of varying complexities, replicating block patterns and structures). This involvement results in an actual score indicating cognitive ability within a nonverbal context, rather than the description of "untestability" that is apt to result from use of a clinically or developmentally inappropriate instrument.

Due to an age range extending downward to the age of 1 month, and its appealing materials and activities, the Griffiths is an excellent instrument for 3- and 4-year-olds with mild cognitive delays and 5-year-olds with significant cognitive delays (for whom other tests provide inadequate floor). Renorming the Griffiths on an American sample would greatly benefit the field of early childhood cognitive assessment.

Nonverbal Tests of Cognitive Ability

Nonverbal tests are useful for older children with communication disorders, hearing impairment, LEP, traumatic brain injury, and other conditions. If response demands are limited to direction of eye gaze, nonverbal tests can sometimes be used for children with cerebral palsy. Unfortunately, few of these tests are appropriate at the preschool level.

Nonverbal tests of cognitive ability do not eliminate the problem of inadequate floor. Some make explicit or inherent demands for understanding language. Although normed for children as young as 2-0 years, the Leiter International Performance Scale—Revised (Roid & Miller, 1997) presents many tasks that are too difficult for preschoolers.

The Naglieri Nonverbal Ability Test (NNAT; Naglieri, 1997) is a well-known test of nonverbal abilities that has been used with a variety of populations (Lohman, 2005; Naglieri, 1997, 2003; Naglieri, Booth, & Winsler, 2004; Naglieri & Ronning, 2000), including white, black, Hispanic, and gifted students. However, because the NNAT was normed on children from 5 to 18 years of age, it is not an appropriate instrument to assess cognitive functioning in preschool children.

Challenges for Assessors Using Standardized Tests

Standardized testing yields important cognitive information for assessment teams, provided that assessors can meet the many challenges inherent in a standardized testing approach for preschool children. Assessors must select tests that are culturally and linguistically fair, are consistent with examinees' developmental and behavioral capacities, and do not make conceptual or linguistic demands (both explicit and implicit) far exceeding children's competency levels.

Because standardized testing can be challenging for early childhood assessors, alternative approaches and additional sources of information are essential. Standardized testing should constitute just one component of comprehensive cognitive assessment, and should be supplemented by other approaches. All members of assessment teams play crucial roles in obtaining cognitive information from multiple sources. The following sections review several additional approaches.

Play Assessment

Uses of Play Assessment

ESTIMATING COGNITIVE COMPETENCE

Play is a natural, enjoyable activity for young children. Watching them play with representational toys is a wonderful way to learn about their cognitive abilities. By observing how a child combines toys, introduces themes, creates dialogue, and makes comments, the assessor can determine the child's mental representational capacities and corresponding developmental levels. This serves as a check on the validity of standardized test results, as well as providing good information about cognitively influenced behaviors: focusing attention, organizing actions to meet self-conceptualized goals, and flexibly in changing schemas to incorporate new material. Although "untestability" is not usually an issue if developmentally appropriate instruments are used for standardized assessment, the assessor may occasionally encounter a child who refuses so many imposed tasks that scores cannot be calculated. Play observation permits estimation of developmental levels for such a child.

OBSERVING BEHAVIOR TO IDENTIFY AND DIFFERENTIATE DEVELOPMENTAL PROBLEMS

Play provides a useful context for observing children's behavior in a self-structured situation, and for comparing it to the adult-structured context of formal standardized testing. Marked differences in activity level, concentration, and compliance are sometimes seen in the two situations. Thinking about reasons for the differences (e.g., capacity for self-organization, comfort with imposed demands) can yield useful diagnostic information. A child with an ASD may become overactive and disorganized under the stress of imposed tasks, but may show good attention and focus during self-structured play. In this situation, observing free play helps the assessor differentiate attentional problems associated with ADHD from attentional problems resulting from distress about imposed demands. Play observation thus contributes to the process of differential diagnosis.

Investigators have studied the characteristics of object play in young children with specific developmental conditions: autism (Baron-Cohen, 1987; Rutherford & Rogers, 2003; Sigman & Ungerer, 1984); blindness/visual impairment (Troster & Brambrig, 1994; Hughes, Dote-Kwan, & Dolendo, 1998); deafness/hearing impairment (Spencer, 1996); Down syndrome (Lender, Goodman, & Linn, 1998; Linn, Goodman, & Lender, 2000; Ruskin, Mundy, Kasari, & Sigman, 1994); language impairment (Casby, 1997; Rescorla & Goossens, 1992); and mental retardation/cognitive delay (Gowen, Johnson-Martin, Goldman, & Hussey, 1992; Malone & Stoneman, 1990; see also Vig, in press). Assessors of cognitive development should become familiar with features of play in children with a variety of developmental conditions, in order to identify those that do and those that do not signal possible cognitive problems. (See Chapter 12, which discusses what to look for in young children with mental retardation.)

OBTAINING A LANGUAGE SAMPLE

Play provides a good opportunity to obtain a sample of spontaneous language. Most children talk while they are playing. Many speak more freely during play than during formal testing, and may show their best syntactic competence in a play situation. Comparing the spontaneous language used in play with the reactive or "demand" language required in conversation and formal testing gives insight about children's cognitive and linguistic competence.

Sequential Development of Play Skills

A number of investigators (Belsky & Most, 1981; Bond, Creasy, & Abrams, 1990; Jarrold, Boucher, & Smith, 1993; McCune-Nicholich, 1981; Westby, 1980, 1991, 2000) have described the sequential acquisition of play skills. Children initially explore the physical properties of toys (12–17 months). They then begin to recognize the representational characteristics of toys (i.e., they being to understand that toys represent real people and things). They initially relate toys to themselves (e.g., pretend to drink from a miniature bottle), and subsequently relate toys to dolls (e.g., pretend to give a doll a drink from a miniature bottle), from 17 to 24 months. They begin to chain actions together (e.g., prepare "food," seat a doll on a chair by a table, and feed the doll) from 24 to 36 months. Children create more elaborate themes, substitute objects for one another (e.g., pretend that a piece of bread represents an airplane), and ask for absent objects needed for imagined scenarios from 36 to 42 months. They then engage in planning and implementing fantasy play (36–48 months), and finally become able to coordinate play events, develop complex scenarios without realistic props, and create extensive dialogue for dolls (48–60 months). By becoming familiar with these play milestones and anchoring observations with a play scale, assessors can estimate children's developmental levels.

Play Assessment Approaches

Play assessment can be done in preschools, childcare centers, center-based early intervention programs, clinical settings, and homes. Transdisciplinary Play-Based Assessment (TPBA; Linder, 1996), appropriate for children from birth to 6 years, was developed for group settings and includes parents in the planning process. (See Chapter 14 for a description of TPBA.) Lowe and Costello's (1988) Symbolic Play Test—Second Edition, a British test for children ages 12–36 months, utilizes specific toy sets and scoring procedures. Its use is described in Paolito (1995) and in Power and Radcliff (2000). The Westby Scales (Westby, 1980, 1991, 2000) provide developmental anchors for play and language skills, and show the parallel development of play and language as different manifestations of underlying representational capacities. Assessors using the Westby Scales have a great deal of flexibility in their choice of materials and the time spent observing a child play. The Westby Scales are thus appropriate for assessors with diverse professional backgrounds, assessment purposes, and assessment settings, and for examinees representing diverse cultural/linguistic groups. They are an excellent resource for cognitive assessment of preschoolers of all ages and ability levels.

Assessment of Adaptive Behavior

Cognitive assessment of preschool children should include a measure of adaptive behavior, particularly if mental retardation or an ASD is suspected. *Adaptive behavior* refers to skills of daily living (e.g., at the preschool level, dressing, using table utensils, or helping with little household jobs). Information is obtained from someone who knows a child well. The American Association on Mental Retardation has specified that adaptive behavior, as well as standardized assessment of intelligence, should be used in identifying mental retardation (Grossman, 1983; Luckasson et al., 1992, 2002). Adaptive behavior and intelligence correlate more highly in children than in adults, with the strongest associations shown for young children with disabilities (Atkinson, Bevc, Dickens, & Blackwell, 1992; Dykens, Hodapp, Ort, & Leckman, 1993; Loveland & Kelly, 1991; Perry & Factor, 1989; Sparrow, Balla, & Cicchetti, 1984). In a study of adaptive behavior in young children with disabilities, Vig and Jedrysek (1995) obtained a correlation coefficient of .75 representing the relation between adaptive behavior (Vineland Adaptive Behavior Composite) and cognitive ability (composite score on one of several standardized tests of cognitive ability) for a sample of 497 children under age 6. A correlation coefficient of .89 was obtained for age equivalents. Due to the strong relationship between adaptive behavior and intelligence for preschool children, adaptive behavior can serve as a validity check on standardized testing, and can be used to estimate the developmental level of an untestable or partially testable child. The recent revision of the Vineland Adaptive Behavior Scales (Vineland-II; Sparrow et al., 2005) and other measures are discussed in Chapter 12.

Copying and Drawing as Estimates of Cognitive Ability

Comprehensive cognitive assessments often include a measure of copying and/or drawing for older preschoolers and kindergartners. Copying and drawing correlate positively with intelligence (Beery, 1989; Beery, Buktenica, & Beery, 2004; Koppitz, 1975). For example, Beery (1989) reported a correlation of .56 between the original Beery Test of Visual–Motor Integration and the Wechsler Intelligence Scale for Children—Revised (WISC-R) Full Scale IQ for children ages 6–11 years. Due to this positive association, copying and drawing can be used to help estimate children's developmental levels. This nonverbal assessment approach is especially useful for children who have language problems or are not fully testable with standardized tests of cognitive ability.

It is important to find out whether copying and drawing have been trained and practiced extensively at home or in preschool, thus reducing novelty and cognitive demands for grasping what is expected. If a 5-year-old, for example, draws a surprisingly mature picture of a person—one that is not developmentally consistent with the results of standardized testing, play observation, and assessment of adaptive behavior—it may be a good idea to see whether he or she can also draw a house (which is generally practiced less).

Beery–Buktenica Developmental Test of Visual–Motor Integration, Fifth Edition

The Beery–Buktenica Test of Visual–Motor Integration, Fifth Edition (Beery et al., 2004) can be used for children ages 2–18 years. The test consists of geometric designs arranged in order of increasing difficulty. There is a short test booklet (21 figures) for children ages 2–7 years. The Fifth Edition was normed on a sample of 2,512 children. Split-half reliability for children ages 2–5 ranges from .90 to .93. A correlation of .89 between the test and chronological age for the total norming sample suggests adequate construct validity.

The Fifth Edition extends age norms downward to age 2. Very young children imitate simple forms demonstrated by the assessor (vertical and horizontal lines and a circle). The test manual provides clear scoring criteria, accompanied by many examples of credited and noncredited responses. The manual also presents the sequence of developmental prerequisites for each design, making it a useful tool for new practitioners.

Human Figure Drawing

During the course of normal development, children begin to draw pictures of human figures between 3 and 4 years of age. Before they can do so, they must acquire the symbolic understanding that a drawing is a representation of a real entity. Early drawings consist of tadpole-like figures containing a large circular head and an additional stroke or two representing a limb or limbs. Psychodynamic interpretations of developmentally appropriate features (large head, no hands) should be avoided for preschool children or older children functioning at early developmental levels.

Although there are scoring systems used to determine standard scores or age equivalents based on the number of features included in drawings, most of these systems are not appropriate for preschoolers. The Draw A Person: A Quantitative Scoring System (Naglieri, 1988), designed for children ages 5–17 years, may be appropriate for kindergartners with close to normal development. The older Goodenough–Harris Drawing Test (Goodenough & Harris, 1964) is designed for children 3–15 years of age. Koppitz (1968) introduced a similar scoring system, known as the Koppitz Developmental Inventory. In a sample of 125 children ages 5–12 years, Abell, Von Briesen, and Watz (1996) compared children's performance on these two measures with their functioning on standardized tests of intelligence. Although they found that interrater reliability was good for both measures, the researchers described the relationship between figure drawing and intelligence as inconclusive. Due to such findings, as well as to their older norms, these scoring systems should be used with great caution (if at all) for preschoolers.

An Alternative Approach: Dynamic Assessment

Dynamic assessment refers to a variety of procedures that use a test–intervene–retest format and embed interaction with a child as part of the assessment process. The approach is based on Vygotsky's theory of proximal development, which explores what children can do with the assistance of others; it was developed by Feuerstein, Feuerstein, and Cross (1997) and Lidz (1997). In dynamic assessment, the assessor first analyzes the cognitive processes required by an assessment task (e.g., memory, attention, perception), and the learner's current skill levels. The assessor decides which skills the learner needs to develop in order to master the task, and which instructional procedures would best facilitate development of the needed skills. The assessor then provides instructional strategies and observes the child's response to instruction. Finally, retesting is used to determine whether the child has achieved competency.

In a review of the current status of dynamic assessment, Lidz (2005) has noted that the approach addresses the concepts of responsiveness to intervention and evidence-based practice. Lidz suggests that the child's response to the intervention embedded within the assessment procedure provides evidence upon which to build an instructional design.

Although used more frequently with older children, dynamic assessment procedures have been adapted for preschool children. The Preschool Learning Assessment Device (Lidz, 1990; Lidz & Thomas, 1987) applies mediated learning experiences to the Triangles subtest of the original Kaufman Assessment Battery for Children (K-ABC; Kaufman & Kaufman, 1983). The assessor tries to determine the problem-solving strategies or response styles that account for a child's failures, then provides mediated (adult-scaffolded) learning experiences illustrating the child's modifiability. The procedure requires approximately 60–90 minutes. The Application of Cognitive Functions

Scales (described in Lidz, 2005), appropriate for children functioning in the 3- to 5-year age range, presents six tasks incorporating the processes of classification, auditory memory, visual memory, pattern sequencing, planning, and perspective taking. The content, presented in a pretest–intervention–posttest format, corresponds to that of typical preschool curricula. With standardized instructions, and with both prescribed and semiscripted interventions, the approach is suitable for research and diagnostic screening.

Dynamic assessment can be used to supplement traditional standardized testing ("static" assessment), or as an alternative approach for both English-speaking children and members of linguistically and culturally diverse groups. The approach can be useful for identifying specific instructional strategies and developing well-targeted supports for children with cognitive difficulties.

ISSUES TO CONSIDER IN LINKING ASSESSMENT TO INTERVENTION

The Assessment Process as an Important Intervention

Identification of a child's developmental status through multidisciplinary assessment, including cognitive assessment, is itself an important intervention (Werner, 2000). Meisels and Atkins-Burnett (2000) have noted that acquiring appropriate expectations for a child's development may be the only intervention needed by some families. Vig and Kaminer (2003) have suggested several reasons why interdisciplinary evaluation constitutes intervention: providing a context for parent–professional observation of a child, confirming suspicions of developmental problems, providing diagnostic clarification, identifying child and family strengths, and helping parents develop new ways of interacting with a child. All team members, each with special expertise, make significant contributions to the process.

Sharing Assessment Results with Families

A key step in linking assessment to intervention is informing the family of a child's developmental status, including cognitive capacities. Intervention will not occur unless the family members understand the reasons for it and believe that the plan will be helpful to their child. Conveying sensitive information about significant cognitive difficulties can be challenging for assessors and upsetting to families. Suggestions for reporting to families and optimizing support for them are discussed in Chapter 12.

Relating Intervention Goals to Assessment Results

When cognitive assessment identifies superior cognitive ability in young children, intervention can make strong conceptual demands, and instruction can proceed at a fast pace with little need for extensive practice and review. Children will generalize new ideas without much need for explicit teaching. Expectations are for rapid progress.

When, on the other hand, assessment identifies cognitive difficulties, plans for intervention and expectations for progress are very different. Many developmental disabilities are chronic and lifelong, and will persist despite intervention. Kaminer and Robinson (1993) have suggested that the goal of intervention in such a case should be to help a child become a participating member of the family and community, rather than to "cure" a disability.

MULTIDISCIPLINARY ASSESSMENT: IT'S A TEAM EFFORT

Sources of Information

Cognitive assessment of preschool children is frequently implemented by multidisciplinary teams in school or clinical settings. In both settings, good assessment requires information from many sources. Johnston and Murray (2003) suggest that assessment has two components: a *multimodal* component, in which information is gathered by various methods (e.g., standardized tests, parent interviews, teachers' reports, rating scales); and a *multi-informant* component, in which information is gathered from a variety of sources (child, parents, teachers). All team members address both components.

Competencies of Assessors

Multicultural Competency

While members of assessment teams each have areas of specialization and expertise, an essential commonality is multicultural competency. *Multiculturalism* has been defined as "recognizing the broad scope of dimensions of race, ethnicity, language, sexual orientation, gender, age, disability, class status, education, religious/spiritual orientation, and other cultural dimensions" (American Psychological Association, 2003, p. 380). It is important for professionals working with children and families to be sensitive to multicultural issues, but often the tools needed to equip professionals with such information are not readily available (Nilsson et al., 2003). Stuart (2004) has made a number of suggestions that may help professionals to enhance their multicultural competence. Some have particular relevance to preschool assessors: developing skills in uncovering each person's cultural outlook; acknowledging and controlling personal biases by articulating one's own world view and evaluating its sources and validity; developing sensitivity to cultural issues without overemphasizing them; and developing a sufficiently complex set of cultural categories.

Checklist of Competencies Related to Cognitive Assessment

Early childhood professionals involved in cognitive assessment should demonstrate mastery of the following competencies:

1. Multicultural competency.
2. Appreciation of the family perspective.
3. Knowledge of early cognitive development.
4. Knowledge of developmental disabilities and other developmental conditions in young children.
5. Observational skills.
6. Familiarity with cognitive assessment instruments and approaches appropriate for young children.
7. Understanding of what different levels of cognitive ability mean for learning and behavior.
8. Respect for the contributions of all team members.

Team Implementation of Cognitive Assessment: Steps to Follow

Cognitive assessment is usually a component of more comprehensive multidisciplinary assessment during the preschool years. Although team composition and procedures may vary across settings, most cognitive assessments include the following steps:

Referral and screening

1. Identify the nature of the referral concern.
2. Determine who has the concern (family member, teacher, pediatrician, child welfare professional).
3. Respond to the concern by taking action. This may include formal screening with a screening instrument, informal observation of the child, gathering preliminary information from the parent, or referral for comprehensive assessment.

Assessment

4. Observe the child in classroom and/or assessment settings.
5. Obtain information from the family: current concerns about the child, the child's developmental skills and behavior, the family's cultural practices.
6. Explore parent–child attachment as a context for cognitive development: Observe parent–child interaction, and discuss the parents' ideas about parenting this particular child.
7. Implement multiple assessment approaches (standardized testing, play observation, language sample, copying/drawing, and/or dynamic assessment).
8. Identify the child's strengths as well as difficulties.
9. In medical settings, explore etiology.

Linking assessment to intervention

10. Recognize that the assessment process is itself an important intervention.
11. Create a formal description of the child's developmental status, and/or make a formal diagnosis.
12. Develop an intervention plan addressing cognitive and other issues.
13. Share assessment results with the family.
14. Take steps to implement the intervention plan.
15. Monitor the child's progress and response to intervention (IEP review in a school setting, developmental follow-up in a clinical setting).

Case Example of Team Process

As discussed at the beginning of this chapter, 5-year-old Jenny has been referred for assessment because of concerns about her learning difficulties in kindergarten.

Preliminary Exploration

After consulting with Jenny's teacher, members of the assessment team (educational specialist, school psychologist, social worker, speech–language specialist) meet to plan Jenny's evaluation. At Jenny's school, all assessors regularly enter classrooms for observation and consultation. Team members individually spend some time in Jenny's classroom, observing her interactions with her teacher and classmates, and her responses to instructional tasks. The assessors are impressed with Jenny's friendliness and her eagerness to communicate with children and adults. The educational specialist offers Jenny some help with a new task, and finds that Jenny tries hard but remains confused.

Assessment

Team members implement multidisciplinary assessment for Jenny. The school psychologist attempts to administer the WPPSI-III, but finds that Jenny achieves no correct responses for the first subtest, only one correct response for the second subtest, and no correct responses for the third subtest. The psychologist decides that the WPPSI-III is to difficult for this particular child, and switches to the SB5, which provides more floor (developmentally easy items). The psychologist also asks Jenny to copy Beery designs and draw a picture of a girl. Next, the psychologist administers the Vineland-II to Jenny's parents. By asking routine Vineland questions about communication, self-care, socialization, and motor skills, the psychologist learns a good deal about the home environment and the parents' expectations for Jenny. The social worker obtains additional information about the family: structure of the family unit, siblings, extended family involvement, employment status, and sources of support. The speech–language specialist administers standardized tests of speech and language development, and observes Jenny's toy play both with and without adult scaffolding. The educational specialist administers tests of academic achievement, switching to a preschool test when Jenny is unsuccessful with kindergarten tasks. The educational specialist also spends time doing trial teaching, as well as reviewing Jenny's school notebook.

After completing these activities, team members meet to discuss their findings. Jenny has attained a Nonverbal IQ of 59, Verbal IQ of 62, and Full Scale IQ of 58, indicating that she functions cognitively within the range of mild mental retardation. SB5 index scores range from 62 for Fluid Reasoning to 68 for Working Memory. Vineland-II composites range from 56 for Motor Skills to 65 for Daily Living Skills. The educational specialist finds that Jenny lacks developmental readiness for early kindergarten tasks. The educational specialist reports that Jenny could not manage kindergarten-level assessment tasks, but achieved successes with preschool tasks (color matching, shape identification). The speech–language specialist obtains standard scores comparable to those of the SB5, and finds that Jenny's play skills are emerging at a level of 3 to 3-6 years. All team members comment on Jenny's cheerful disposition and eagerness to communicate.

Team members formulate a diagnosis of mild mental retardation and recommend intervention based on that diagnosis. In their contacts with Jenny's parents, they have learned that the parents provide a loving home, language stimulation, and plenty of cognitively enriching activities (picture books, cause-and-effect toys, materials lending themselves to pretend play). They do not pressure Jenny to achieve more than she can manage. Team members decide that Jenny will do best in a small special education class for children who do not have behavior problems or more significant mental retardation, but cannot manage the instructional pace of an integrated or inclusion class. Because the speech–language specialist's findings show that Jenny's language skills are consistent with her general developmental level, her speech is easy to understand, her communicative intent is excellent, and she receives optimal language stimulation at home, the team members also decide that Jenny does not presently need speech–language services at school.

Linking Assessment to Intervention

The school psychologist and educational specialist meet with Jenny's parents to share the team's findings and recommendations. As expected, the parents are upset to learn that the reason for Jenny's learning difficulties is that she has mild mental retardation. In sharing findings, the assessors describe Jenny's interest in communicating and interacting with other people as very positive aspects of her development. The assessors emphasize that assessment results are helpful for planning during the next 2 or 3 years, and say that Jenny will be retested in 3 years to determine her developmental status at that time. The parents agree that a more appropriately paced class will reduce frustration for Jenny and enable her to achieve successes with preacademic activities. The assessors explain the IEP process, with 3-month reviews, as a way of monitoring Jenny's progress. The parents ask the assessors for suggestions about ways they can learn more about mental retardation, and the assessors recommend a book and the websites of several national organizations.

COGNITIVE ASSESSMENT FOR SPECIAL POPULATIONS

Cognitive assessment is usually required, as a component of multidisciplinary assessment, to document developmental disabilities qualifying young children for publicly funded intervention services or other entitlements. In some other cases, cognitive assessment is undertaken to establish eligibility for accelerated or gifted programs. The following section describes some of the issues involved in identifying common disabilities and giftedness.

Autism Spectrum Disorders

Cognitive assessment of young children with ASD can be particularly challenging for assessors. Because children with ASD do not readily imitate the actions of others, they may not be willing to replicate demonstrated activities. Due to self-absorption, a preference for following their own agenda, and discomfort with imposed demands, it can be difficult to engage these children initially in assessment tasks. Once engaged, they may drift into activities of their own choosing and may use test materials in their own way. Although some children with ASD may be only partially testable, it is important to obtain as much information as possible about their cognitive status, so that intervention can be targeted to their developmental level.

Children with ASD tend to cooperate best for tests that impose minimal demands for language processing and social interaction with the examiner. For example, instructions for the Performance scale of the Griffiths Mental Developmental Scales can be pantomimed, and some scoring is done on the basis of what the child does spontaneously with test materials. Observations of behavior and object play are crucial to the identification of autism. Samples of language, which may have a pedantic quality or reflect preoccupations, contribute to the identification of Asperger syndrome or higher-functioning autism. Cognitive assessment should be supplemented with checklists or other instruments designed specifically for the identification of ASD. The California Department of Developmental Services (2002) and New York State Department of Health (1999) have published useful guidelines for the assessment of children with autism. (See also Chapter 13.)

> André is 3-6 years of age. His parents have been concerned about his failure to speak as well as other children of his age. He uses only two words (*no* and *juice*). Members of the assessment team learn from André's parents that he takes little interest in the activities of other children. He looks away when people look at him or speak to him. He screams in protest if his toys are moved to a different location. The school psychologist decides that André will not understand the verbal instructions and task demands of most standardized tests, and selects the Griffiths Mental Development Scales as an instrument providing adequate floor (easy items) and making minimal demands for understanding complex verbal instructions. Although he tries to use test materials in his own way, André is eventually able to involve himself in tasks within his competence range. He completes a three-hole inset formboard in a standard but not a rotated presentation, and scribbles on paper but does not imitate a circle. He touches materials in a repetitive manner and puts some of them into his mouth. When given toys for free play, he places them in a row, then loses interest. His par-

ents say that he also does this at home. A Griffiths General Quotient of 50 (mental age of 21 months) indicates global cognitive potential within the range of moderate mental retardation. André's language skills are below the 15-month level, and his nonverbal skills are also well below age expectancy (24–28 months). The assessment team determines that André meets diagnostic criteria for autistic disorder. A program serving children with ASD and cognitive limitations, speech–language therapy to improve communicative intent, and potential use of augmentative communication are recommended.

Giftedness

Although indications of special abilities can be seen in very young children, giftedness is not usually identified formally until children make the transition from preschool to kindergarten. Sattler (2002) summarizes characteristics of giftedness in preschoolers. These children meet developmental milestones early. They show curiosity, ask many questions, make up stories and songs, create complex block constructions, and assemble difficult puzzles. They are apt to become interested in a particular topic and to take initiative and sustain interest in learning about it. The children use language to exchange ideas, handle conflict, or influence other children's behavior. They learn quickly and can understand abstract concepts. They often have a sense of humor. Torrance (2000) discusses creativity as an aspect of giftedness, stating that preschool children with creative giftedness have large vocabularies and know a lot about many different topics. Like Sattler (2002), Torrance emphasizes curiosity, humor, and deep involvement in areas of personal interest. In identifying preschoolers who may eventually be eligible for gifted programs, these characteristics may serve as useful markers.

Formal eligibility for gifted programs is usually established through standardized intelligence testing. The criterion for admission to some gifted programs is cognitive potential at least 2 *SD* above the mean of an intelligence test (IQ of 130 or above for tests with an *SD* of 15). Other programs and many selective independent schools require an IQ of at least 120, indicating cognitive ability within the superior range.

Short forms of standardized tests of intelligence are sometimes used to identify children who may qualify for participation in programs for the gifted. There are several drawbacks to this approach. Sattler (2001) and Sattler and Dumont (2004) have pointed out that short forms are less reliable, provide less information about examinees' strengths and weaknesses, and reduce opportunities to observe examinees' problem-solving approaches. According to Sattler and Dumont (2004), the only legitimate uses of short forms of the WPPSI-III are for screening, research, or obtaining an estimate of a child's cognitive status when a precise IQ is not needed. Short forms should not be used for classification or documenting eligibility for programs or services.

Veronica, age 4-6 years, is attending a community childcare center. She will soon enter public school kindergarten. The teacher has been impressed with Veronica's verbal skills, rapid skill mastery, and creative play. Veronica finds common themes among the stories the teacher reads aloud, asks why the story characters behave in particular ways, and suggests that the characters might have solved their problems differently. When playing in the doll corner, Veronica creates complicated, well-sequenced fantasy stories and assigns roles for her classmates to play with the dolls. Veronica's mother and the teacher wonder whether Veronica might qualify for a publicly funded program for gifted students, and decide to have her tested. A school psychologist tests her and obtains a Full Scale IQ of 128 on the WPPSI-III. Veronica has strong motivation, a mature vocabulary, and the ability to provide additional or alternative explanations for test items requiring an understanding of cause and effect. Members of the assessment team learn from Veronica's mother and teacher that she is liked by other children and has many friends. A decision is made, on the basis of her cognitive potential and emotional maturity, to accept Veronica for a program serving gifted kindergarten children during the forthcoming school year.

Language Impairment

Language impairment is best identified by an assessment team that includes a speech–language pathologist or specialist. Cognitive assessment is also needed to determine whether a child's language deficiencies are due to global delay or constitute an isolated area of weakness. Tests that represent cognitive potential with a single quotient (e.g., the BSID-II) are less useful for children with language impairment than tests that provide separate quotients for verbal and nonverbal abilities (the Bayley-III, Griffiths, the SB5, the WPPSI-III). In selecting instruments for children suspected to have language impairment, it is particularly important to think about linguistic demands of test instructions and tasks. In addition to obtaining scores, it is essential to describe a child's speech and language qualitatively. All members of the assessment team can address the following questions: Is the child's speech intelligible? Does the child use age-appropriate phrases and sentences? Does the child use general rather than specific terms? Can an older preschooler sequence ideas in relating an anecdote? All assessors should record many examples of the child's language. Standardized testing and informal conversation provide examples of reactive or "demand" language (language used in response to the language of another person). Free play with toys gives an opportunity to record the child's spontaneous language. The examples are helpful in documenting language impairment. (See also Chapter 10.)

Walter is a 4-year-old boy whose preschool teacher is concerned about his unclear speech and immature language. He mispronounces simple words and has trouble relating his experiences. The teacher has to ask many questions in an effort to understand what he is trying to communicate. The teacher encourages Walter's parents to have him evaluated by a multidisciplinary assessment team. The school psychologist administers the SB-5 and finds that Walter has normal intelligence (Full Scale IQ of 105). However, his attainment on most language-based subtests is well below what he achieves on nonverbal subtests. He manages simple naming activities, but has trouble with tasks requiring more complex verbal explanations. The speech–language specialist finds that Walter obtains verbal standard scores well below his nonverbal scores obtained in standardized assessment of cognitive ability. All members of the team note and document Walter's use of short phrases and of general rather than specific words (e.g., "the thing" instead of "the puzzle"). They find that his speech is only 50%–75% intelligible when context is not known. Based on his speech and language impairments as documented by cognitive and other assessments, Walter qualifies for publicly funded speech–language services. Walter's parents state that they are very pleased to learn of his normal intelligence, noting that they had thought he might be delayed in all areas. They express their expectation that the speech–language services will be very helpful to him.

Mental Retardation

Many preschool tests of cognitive ability do not present adequate floor for young children with mental retardation. The best choices for this population are tests with norms that extend downward to infancy (e.g., Bayley-III, the BSID-II, the Griffiths, Merrill-

Palmer—Revised, described in Appendix 11.1) or below 2 years (the Mullen Scales of Early Learning, described in Appendix 11.1). A test of adaptive behavior must also be administered for a formal diagnosis of mental retardation. Issues relevant to young children with mental retardation are discussed more fully, and case examples are provided, in Chapter 12.

CONCLUSION

Cognitive assessment is an essential component of multidisciplinary assessment. The challenge for assessors is to conduct assessments that are multiculturally and linguistically appropriate, are sensitive to the priorities and concerns of families, and incorporate developmentally appropriate assessment approaches. In linking assessment to effective and well-targeted intervention, assessors should combine assessment results with their general understanding of children's cognitive status and what it means for responsiveness to intervention.

To provide cognitive assessment that represents best practice for young children, assessors should do the following:

1. Acquire background in early childhood development and behavior as a foundation for internalized norms.
2. Acquire knowledge of developmental disabilities and their characteristics during early childhood.
3. Think about the child within the context of the family, and include the family in the assessment process.
4. Use a combination of standardized testing and other assessment approaches.
5. Consider clinical features as well as technical adequacy in test selection.
6. Use results of cognitive assessment to plan intervention that accurately and realistically addresses the needs of the child and concerns of the family.

Incorporating these principles will result in cognitive assessment that is truly beneficial to young children.

APPENDIX 11.1. Review of Measures

Measure	**Bayley Scales of Infant and Toddler Development, Third Edition (Bayley-III). Bayley (2006).**
Purpose	Identifying infants and children with developmental delay, and providing information for intervention planning.
Areas	Five scales: Cognitive, Language, Motor, Social–Emotional, and Adaptive Behavior Scales.
Format	The Bayley-III is an individually administered assessment. The child and examiner are seated at a table for most of the assessment; however, the Motor Scale allows for the child to move about the room to demonstrate different gross motor movements.
Scores	Scaled scores, composite scores, percentile ranks, developmental age equivalents, and growth scores.
Age group	1–42 months.
Time	50–90 minutes.
Users	Users should have training and experience in the administration and interpretation of comprehensive developmental assessments. In addition, they should have experience testing young children whose ages and cultural background match those of the population under assessment. Most users have completed some formal graduate or professional training; however, a trained technician can administer and score the Bayley-III with supervision.
Norms	Data collected on 1,700 children ages 16 days to 43 months 15 days, in addition to a special group of children (including ones with Down syndrome, cerebral palsy, pervasive Developmental Disorder, premature birth, language impairment, and risk for developmental delay).
Reliability	Internal consistency, .86–.93; test–retest, .67–.80 (2–4 months, .77–.86 (9–13 months), .71–.88 (19–26 months), and .83–.94 (33–42 months); interrater, determined for the Adaptive Behavior Scale only, with adaptive domains averaging .79 and skill areas averaging .73.
Validity	Convergent and discriminant validity, established; content validity, established. Concurrent validity was established using the BSID-II, WPPSI-III, PLS-4, Peabody Developmental Motor Scales, Second Edition, and Adaptive Behavior Assessment System, Second Edition Parent/Primary Caregiver Form.
Comments	The third edition demonstrates excellent concurrent validity, utilizing several commonly used assessments for comparison, with moderate to strong correlations. Much work went into establishing test content validity by demonstrating an adequate range of items/tasks for the intended age ranges and maintaining application to the constructs being measured. The Bayley-III still exemplifies outstanding standardization practices and a remarkable establishment of reliability. The examiner's materials have been updated to reflect a more contemporary style. The record form, which used to be two separate forms, is now one document; it is well designed, with plenty of space for comments and observations. The stimulus book has a fresh new look, with enlarged and updated illustrations, and appears even more engaging and colorful.
References consulted	Bayley (2006a, 2006b). See book's References list.

Measure	**Griffiths Mental Development Scales. Griffiths (1970). Griffiths Mental Development Scales from Birth to 2 Years: 1996 Revision. Huntley (1996).**
Purpose	Testing young children's cognitive abilities.
Areas	Scales: Locomotor, Personal–Social, Hearing and Speech, Eye and Hand Coordination, Performance, and (for children over age 2) Practical Reasoning.
Format	Infants tested on blanket or caregiver's lap. Children sit at a table for most tasks, move about for gross motor activities.
Scores	Subquotients and general quotient for all ages. Percentiles available for birth to 2 years.
Age group	Birth to 8 years.
Time	45–60 minutes.
Users	Health professionals who have undergone training in use and application of this instrument.
Norms	Data collected on 2,260 British children ages 1 month to 8 years. Sample not random or stratified. The 1996 restandardization for birth to age 2 based on 665 British children aged 1 to 24 months. Sample stratified for gender, ethnicity, SES, urban/rural area, geographic region.
Reliability	Correlation of subscales with General Quotient .64–.77; stability for General Quotient, .77; interrater, high.
Validity	Correlations of .79–.81 with Terman–Merrill (Form L); predictive validity as a tool to identify young children with learning difficulties; adequate construct validity.
Comments	Highly appealing materials (including toys) and activities. Flexible order of item presentation. Excellent clinical properties for assessing preschoolers with disabilities. Adequate floor. Psychometric drawbacks include British norming sample.
References consulted	Conn (1993); Griffiths (1970); Huntley (1996); Luiz, Foxcroft, and Stewart (2001); Aldridge Smith, Bidder, Gardner, and Gray (1980). See book's References list.

Measure	**Kaufman Assessment Battery for Children, Second Edition (KABC-II). Kaufman and Kaufman (2004).**
Purpose	Testing children's cognitive abilities.
Areas	Visual Processing, Short-Term Memory, Fluid Reasoning, Long-Term Storage and Retrieval, Crystallized Ability.
Format	Child seated at table. Test items presented primarily in easel format.
Scores	Age-based standard scores, age equivalents, percentile ranks.
Age group	3-0 to 18-11 years.
Time	25–70 minutes.
Users	Trained professionals who have completed graduate (usually doctoral) program that includes coursework and supervised practical experience in administration and interpretation of clinical tests.
Norms	Data collected on 3,025 children, stratified by sex, race/ethnicity, SES, parental education, geographic region, special education status.
Reliability	Split-half, in the mid-.90s for the Global Score (Mental Processing Composite and Fluid–Crystallized Index combined).

Validity	Construct validity supported by factor-analytic studies; positive correlations with the WISC-IV, Woodcock–Johnson III, Wechsler Individual Achievement Test—Second Edition, Peabody Individual Achievement Test—Revised/ Normative Update.
Comments	Assessor has flexibility in types of subtests administered to comprise Global Score. Correct Spanish-language responses provided.
References consulted	Kaufman, Kaufman, Kaufman-Singer, and Kaufman (2005). See book's References list.

Measure	**Leiter International Performance Scale—Revised (Leiter-R). Roid and Miller (1997).**
Purpose	Nonverbal test of cognitive ability.
Areas	Visualization and Reasoning, Attention and Memory.
Format	Child seated at table. Easel presentation of stimulus items. Few manipulatives.
Scores	Standard scores, percentile ranks, age equivalents, growth scores.
Age group	2-0 to 20-11 years.
Time	25–40 minutes.
Users	4-year degree in psychology, counseling, or related field; specialized training and coursework in test administration and interpretation.
Norms	Data collected in 1,719 individuals stratified for gender, race, ethnicity, parents' education, and geographic region.
Reliability	Internal consistency, .75–.90 for Visualization and Reasoning, .67–.87 for Attention and Memory.
Validity	Correlations of .86 and .83 with WISC-III in two studies of children ages 6–16 years. Data provided about using test for classification of disability groups for children age 6 and older.
Comments	Test lacks adequate floor for children ages 2–6 years with disabilities. Many test items present complex formats and require a high degree of abstract conceptualization.
References consulted	Athanasiou-Schicke (2000); Bradley-Johnson (2001); Roid and Miller (1997). See book's References list.

Measure	**Merrill–Palmer—Revised Scales of Development. Roid and Sampers (2004).**
Purpose	Assessing general cognitive development and other developmental areas.
Areas	Cognitive, Language, Motor (fine and gross), Social–emotional, Self-help, Adaptive.
Format	Infant tested on mat and in adult's lap. Child seated at table. Toys available up to 30-month level; manipulatives and easel format for older children.
Scores	Standard scores, percentile ranks, age equivalents, criterion-referenced change-sensitive growth scores.
Age group	1 month to 6-6 years.
Time	45 minutes.
Users	4-year degree in psychology, counseling, or related field; specialized training in test interpretation or appropriate licensure/certification.

Norms	Data collected on 1,068 children, including 250 described as "atypical." Sample stratified by gender, ethnicity, parental education, geographic region.
Reliability	Internal consistency, .97–.98 for Developmental Index across age groups.
Validity	Correlations of .92 with BSID-II, .97 with Leiter-R, .76–.90 with SB5 for two age groups.
Comments	Instructions printed in English and Spanish. Test comes in rolling case. Colorful toys and manipulatives. Expressive Language not included in core Cognitive Battery. Flexibility in establishing entry point. Discontinuation based on cumulative, rather than consecutive, errors. Administrative guidelines presented in complicated format.
References consulted	Roid and Sampers (2004). See book's References list.

Measure	**Mullen Scales of Early Learning: AGS Edition. Mullen (1995).**
Purpose	Testing young children's cognitive abilities.
Areas	Gross Motor, Visual Reception, Fine Motor, Expressive Language, Receptive Language.
Format	Child seated for tabletop activities, can move about for assessment of gross-motor skills.
Scores	*T*-scores, percentile ranks, age equivalents for scales. Standard scores and percentile ranks for Composite.
Age group	0–68 months.
Time	15 minutes (1 year); 25–35 minutes (3 years); 40–60 minutes (5 years).
Users	Doctorate or master's degree in psychology or related field, including training in clinical assessment of infants.
Norms	Standardized on 1,849 children. Sample approximates 1990 Census, only for gender. More limited correspondence for ethnicity, community size, SES.
Reliability	Internal consistency, .83–.95; test–retest reliability coefficients below .80 for children aged 25–56 months.
Validity	Correlation of .70 with Bayley Scales of Infant Development. High correlations of Mullen Language scales with the Preschool Language Assessment (1979), and Mullen Fine Motor scale with Peabody Fine Motor Scale (1983).
Comments	Test provides toys and developmentally appropriate activities. Most pictures are black and white, and not particularly appealing to children. Examiners must provide some of their own materials. Lengthy discontinuation procedures avoided. Adequate clinical floor.
References consulted	Bradley-Johnson (2001); Dumont, Cruse, Alfonso, and Levine (2000). See book's References list.

Measure	**Stanford–Binet Intelligence Scales, Fifth Edition (SB5). Roid (2003a, 2003b). Stanford–Binet Intelligence Scales for Early Childhood (Early SB5). Roid (2005).**
Purpose	Testing cognitive abilities in persons of all ages.
Areas	Fluid Reasoning, Knowledge, Quantitative Reasoning, Visual–Spatial Processing, Working Memory.
Format	Child seated at table for all activities.
Scores	Standard scores, percentile ranks, age equivalents, change-sensitive scores.

Age group	2-0 to 85+ years.
Time	SB5, 45–75 minutes for full battery; Early SB5, 30–50 minutes for full battery.
Users	Graduate degree in psychology or related field. Training and supervised experience in administration and interpretation of intelligence tests.
Norms	Data collected on 4,800 individuals, stratified by age, sex, ethnicity, geographic region, SES.
Reliability	Average internal consistency .95–.98 across all age groups.
Validity	Correlations of .78–.90 for Full Scale IQ with similar composites on Woodcock–Johnson III Tests of Cognitive Abilities, SB-IV, WPPSI-R.
Comments	Colorful toys, manipulatives, and pictures. Lengthy discontinuation procedures avoided. Lacks adequate clinical floor for younger and less able preschoolers. Understanding and use of language required for some nonverbal activities. The Early SB5 is a specialized version of the SB5 designed for use with children ages 2-0–7-3 years. Difficult items have been dropped from subscales, so the instrument is not appropriate for children with above-average intelligence.
References consulted	Roid (2003a, 2003b). See book's References list.

Measure	**Wechsler Preschool and Primary Scale of Intelligence—Third Edition (WPPSI-III). Wechsler (2002).**
Purpose	Testing cognitive abilities in preschoolers and primary school students.
Areas	Verbal, Performance, and Full Scale IQs. Subtests for ages 2-6 to 3-11 years: Receptive Vocabulary, Information, Block Design, and Object Assembly (core) and Picture Naming (supplemental). Subtests for ages 4-0 to 7-3 years: Information, Vocabulary, Word Reasoning, Block Design, Matrix Reasoning, Picture Concepts, and Coding (core); Symbol Search, Comprehension, Similarities, and Object Assembly (supplemental); and Receptive Vocabulary and Picture Naming (optional).
Format	Child seated at table. Primarily easel format with a few manipulatives.
Scores	Standard scores, percentile ranks, age equivalents.
Age group	2-6 to 7-3 years.
Time	25–35 minutes for younger age group. 45–50 minutes for older age group.
Users	Doctorate in psychology or related field, or licensure. Relevant training in assessment.
Norms	Data collected on 1,700 children, stratified by age, sex, parental education, ethnicity, geographic region.
Reliability	Internal consistency, .89–.96 for composite scores. Stability, .92 for ages 2-6 to 3-11 years, .80 for ages 4-0 to 5-5 years.
Validity	Correlations of .80–.87 with DAS, WPPSI-R, BSID-II Mental Scale.
Comments	Colorful pictures and manipulatives. Simple wording for most instructions. No toys. Discontinuation procedures are lengthy. Some initial items too complex for younger and lower-functioning preschoolers. The test presents one set of subtests for children ages 2-6 to 3-11 years, and another set for children ages 4-0 to 7-3 years. Because the scoring tables for the earlier section cannot be used for the older group, the test has limited usefulness for children with mental retardation.
References consulted	Sattler and Dumont (2004); Wechsler (2002). See book's References list.

Measure	**Woodcock–Johnson III Tests of Cognitive Abilities. Woodcock, McGrew, and Mather (2001b).**
Purpose	Testing cognitive abilities in persons of all ages.
Areas	Verbal ability, thinking ability, cognitive efficiency.
Format	Child seated at table. Easel format.
Scores	Standard scores, percentile ranks, age and grade equivalents.
Age group	2–90 years.
Time	35–45 minutes.
Users	Graduate degree in psychology, education, or related field. Coursework and supervised experience in test administration and interpretation.
Norms	Conormed with Woodcock–Johnson III Tests of Achievement. Data collected on 8,818 individuals, including 1,143 preschool children. Sample stratified by geographic region, community size, sex, SES, ethnicity.
Reliability	Internal consistency, .81–.94 for Standard Battery. Stability, .70–.96 for timed subtests for individuals age 7 years or older.
Validity	Correlations of .72–.76 with DAS, WPPSI-R, SB-IV.
Comments	No toys or manipulatives. Tasks and verbal instructions much too complicated for many preschoolers. Inadequate clinical floor for preschoolers with disabilities. May be used to supplement other tests if information is needed about specific cognitive processes for older and more able preschoolers. Examiner must provide cassette player and headphones for subtests presented on prerecorded tape. The test cannot be hand-scored.
References consulted	Sandoval (2003). See book's References list.

Chapter 12

Assessment of Mental Retardation

SUSAN VIG
MICHELLE SANDERS

William is a handsome 3-year-old boy attending a childcare center. His teacher notices that he does not speak as well as his classmates. He runs and climbs well, but expresses himself mostly by pointing and using single words and a few two-word phrases. William's mother has also become concerned about his limited use of language.

Olivia is a pretty 4-year-old girl attending a community preschool. Her teacher reports a number of behavior problems: Olivia does not listen to the teacher's requests, gets up to wander around the classroom during circle time, throws puzzle pieces on the floor when asked to complete a puzzle, and tries to grab other children's toys. However, Olivia loves to sing and enjoys singing and dancing activities.

William's language difficulties and Olivia's behavior problems represent two common reasons why preschool children are referred for the multidisciplinary assessment that may eventually result in a diagnosis of mental retardation. Because the children are physically attractive and have adequate motor skills, their teachers and families do not suspect mental retardation as a possible reason for their language and behavior problems.

Young children are frequently referred for multidisciplinary assessment because someone becomes concerned about their failure to achieve expected developmental milestones. Often the expected milestones involve speech or language. Sometimes there is a concern about behavior problems, such as poor listening, noncompliance, or temper tantrums. Cognitive assessment helps to clarify whether a child's failure to speak as expected for his or her age is due to a specific speech or language impairment, or is instead part of a more global delay. Similarly, cognitive assessment can help to clarify whether a child's frequent tantrums represent an emotional or behavioral disorder, or are instead due to frustration caused by unrealistically high adult expectations. Some of the children referred for assessment will be found to have cognitive limitations or mental retardation.

The diagnosis of mental retardation is based on standardized cognitive testing by a qualified psychologist, and administration of an adaptive behavior scale. All assessment team members obtain valuable information about a child's family circumstances, behavior, play skills, speech and language abilities, and response to learning tasks. The perspectives of all team members contribute to comprehensive understanding of a young child's developmental status, and lead to intervention plans that can optimize the child's development.

For preschoolers with cognitive limitations, as well as those with other developmental conditions, family involvement in the assessment process is essential. The family provides a child's first language and learning experiences. Parent–child attachment (the emotional bond between a child and parent or primary caregiver) can either enhance or negatively affect a young child's development (Osofsky & Thompson, 2000; Thompson, 1999; Zeanah & Boris, 2000). Assessment for children with cognitive difficulties should therefore include exploration of the family environment and attachment influences, so that the intervention plan can capitalize on family strengths, or offer support and assistance if attachment is less than optimal (Kelly & Barnard, 2000). Assessors' responsiveness to cultural and linguistic diversity is also crucial. Assessment results must be interpreted within the context of the child's and family's culture. (See Chapters 8, 9, and 11 for further discussion of family and cultural/linguistic diversity issues.)

When children attend childcare or preschool programs, information from teachers and other service providers is useful as well. Providing simple forms for teachers to complete facilitates the process.

This chapter provides background for assessors serving young children with mental retardation and their families. The chapter addresses the following topics: (1) terminology and definitional issues; (2) etiology; (3) co-occurring conditions; (4) characteristics of young children with mental retardation; (5) myths about such children; (6) reasons for identifying mental retardation; (7) issues and practices related to cognitive, play, and adaptive behavior assessment; and (8) linking assessment to intervention.

TERMINOLOGY AND DEFINITION

Within the field of developmental disabilities, there has been a good deal of controversy about use of the term *mental retardation*. A number of alternatives have been proposed: *general learning disorder*, *intellectual disability*, and *cognitive–adaptive disability* (Baroff, 1999; Gelb, 2002; Walsh, 2002).

Discomfort with the term *mental retardation* in some settings is suggested by increasing use of the term *learning disability* (LD) for individuals with cognitive limitations. In a study of school-age children by MacMillan, Gresham, Siperstein, and Bocian (1996), only 6 of 43 children with IQs at or below 75 were classified as having mental retardation; 18 were classified as having LD. According to data from the U.S. Department of Education, cited by Baroff (1999), the number of children classified as having LD increased 202% from 1994 to 1997, while the number classified as having mental retardation decreased by 38%.

Despite controversy over terminology, the term *mental retardation* continues to be widely used. The American Association on Mental Retardation periodically provides official definitions of mental retardation. According to the 1992 definition (Luckasson et al.,

1992), a diagnosis of mental retardation was to be based on subaverage intelligence (IQ of 70–75 or below by standardized testing) and limitations in two or more specified adaptive skill areas: communication, self-care, home living, social skills, community use, self-direction, health and safety, functional academics, leisure, and work. The definition eliminated IQ severity levels (mild, moderate, severe, profound) and replaced them with intensities of support. However, the definition was criticized for difficulty in operationalizing levels of support (King, State, Shah, Davanzo, & Dykens, 1997); and poor relevance of adaptive skill areas to children (Gresham, MacMillan, & Siperstein, 1995; Vig & Jedrysek, 1996a).

The American Association on Mental Retardation published a new definition of mental retardation in 2002 (Luckasson et al., 2002). The 2002 definition specifies that a diagnosis of mental retardation must be based on limitations in intelligence (functioning approximately 2 *SD* below the mean of an intelligence test), and adaptive behavior (functioning at least 2 *SD* below the mean in conceptual, social, or practical types of adaptive behavior). The 2002 definition prioritizes classification based on intensities of supports as a preferred direction for the field, but acknowledges that IQ-based classification levels (mild, moderate, severe, profound) are sometimes more useful.

ETIOLOGY AND ITS IMPLICATIONS FOR INTERVENTION

There are many causes of mental retardation. Earlier theorists proposed a "two-group" theory of etiology (Burack, 1990; Zigler, Balla, & Hodapp, 1986). According to the theory, individuals with an "organic" etiology have IQs below 50, an unusual physical appearance, and siblings with normal intelligence. Individuals in the larger "cultural/familial" etiology group have IQs between 50 and 70, a normal physical appearance, low SES, and at least one relative with lower intelligence.

In recent years, it has been thought that the "two-group" theory may oversimplify the causes of mental retardation. Human genome research has identified many genetic causes of mental retardation previously believed to be "familial." In describing genetic research findings from the Human Genome Project, Plomin and Spinath (2004) have concluded that cognitive problems seldom show single-gene effects, and are instead caused by multiple genes and environmental factors. These investigators further note that the same genes may affect diverse cognitive processes.

Maternal alcohol use has been associated with children's cognitive limitations, whether or not the physical features characteristic of fetal alcohol syndrome are present (Mattson, Riley, Gramling, Delis, & Lyons Jones, 1998). Maternal use of crack cocaine or other drugs may cause premature birth and associated cognitive problems (Mayes, 1999; Yolton & Bolig, 1994). Prenatal substance exposure is apt to be accompanied by environmental and psychosocial risk factors.

Due to complex interactions of genetic, other biological, environmental, and psychosocial risk factors, experts currently propose a "multifactorial" (multiple-risk-factor) model of etiology (Luckasson et al., 2002). The following list, based in part on the work of Durkin and Stein (1996), Luckasson et al. (2002), and Sattler (2002), suggests some of the common causes of mental retardation:

1. Single-gene abnormality (e.g., fragile X syndrome, tuberous sclerosis).
2. Chromosomal abnormality (e.g., Down syndrome).

3. Fetal malnutrition.
4. Prenatal maternal infections (e.g., rubella, HIV, syphilis).
5. Prenatal substance use (drugs, alcohol).
6. Premature birth.
7. Postnatal exposure to lead.
8. Postnatal encephalitis or meningitis.
9. Postnatal head injury.
10. Severe child neglect or deprivation.

Although causes can be identified for the majority of individuals with IQs below 50, specific causes cannot be identified for many individuals with IQs above 50 (Durkin & Stein, 1996).

Etiology has implications for intervention, which may target biological, environmental, and/or psychosocial issues. For example, genetic syndromes have been associated with specific medical or behavioral problems. Down syndrome is associated with obesity, as well as with cardiac, endocrine, vision, and learning problems (Hayes & Batshaw, 1993). Intervention involves pediatric monitoring, medical procedures, and genetic counseling, in addition to developmental services and family support. Prader–Willi syndrome is characterized by compulsive overeating and requires weight management and special behavioral support (Fiedler & Hodapp, 1998).

Fragile X syndrome is the most common hereditary cause of mental retardation (Hagerman, 1996). Boys with fragile X typically have mild mental retardation in childhood, but will have moderate mental retardation in adulthood, suggesting a decline in cognitive performance over time. Girls tend to be less affected, and fewer will experience IQ decline with age (Hagerman, 1996). Loesch et al. (2003) have documented cognitive executive function impairments associated with a specific protein deficit in individuals with fragile X syndrome. Goldson and Hagerman (1992) have described characteristics of the disorder over time, as well as the interventions that will be needed. As infants and toddlers, children with fragile X syndrome tend to be hypotonic and temperamentally difficult. They benefit from early intervention programs, developmental therapies, and support for their parents that emphasizes understanding the disorder and dealing with the children's behavior problems. At school age, medication may be helpful to address attentional problems seen at that time. Researchers have found that the genes causing fragile X syndrome grow larger over time, and that symptoms worsen from generation to generation (Kolata, 1992). Genetic counseling for parents is therefore an essential component of intervention.

Clearly, knowing the cause of a child's mental retardation helps early childhood professionals plan well-targeted intervention to address characteristics associated with specific etiological conditions. Knowing about etiology also helps professionals and families know what to expect over time and which interventions may be needed in the future.

CO-OCCURRING CONDITIONS

Many children with mental retardation have other developmental problems. Concurrent problems for young children include cerebral palsy, autism spectrum disorders (ASD), and behavioral difficulties. These other conditions may constitute children's primary diagnoses. Sometimes clinicians, educators, and families focus on the other problems and do not recognize the significance of mental retardation for the child's current and future functioning.

Cerebral Palsy

It has been estimated that 50% of children with cerebral palsy have cognitive delays (Huang, Hunter, Reinert, & Wishon, 1992), and that 25% have mental retardation (Rice, 1993). Due to the children's physical limitations, standardized cognitive assessment may require modifications (e.g., administration of verbal portions of tests, or use of nonverbal tests in which responses are made through eye gaze). Occupational therapists may be asked to help position children for testing, using adaptive seating or other approaches to ensure the children's comfort and optimal performance.

Autism Spectrum Disorders

An overlap between ASD and mental retardation has been extensively documented. Many people with ASD have mental retardation, and many people with moderate to profound mental retardation have autistic features. Using slightly different diagnostic criteria, investigators have identified IQs below 70 for 75% of individuals with autism (Lord & Rutter, 1994) and 70%–90% of children with autistic behavior (Myers, 1989), as well as developmental delays in 68% of 18-month-olds at risk for autism (Baron-Cohen et al., 1996). Autistic features have been identified in 30%–50% of children with IQs below 50 (Capute, Derivan, Chauvel, & Rodriguez, 1975; Deb & Prasad, 1994; Nordin & Gillberg, 1996; Wing, 1981b). Focusing specifically on young children, Kaminer, Jedrysek, and Soles (1984) documented autistic features in 42% of 2- to 6-year-olds with moderate to severe mental retardation.

Mental retardation can affect expression of autistic symptomatology in young children. Some of the behaviors used as diagnostic criteria for ASD (echolalia, lack of symbolic play, resistance to changes of routine) may not occur in young children functioning at early developmental levels (Vig & Jedrysek, 1999). For example, a 3-year-old with mental retardation may not have enough language to echo what others say. The child may not have sufficient conceptual ability to perceive patterns of activity, and therefore may not become distressed by changes of routine.

Behavior Problems

Mental retardation in young children is frequently accompanied by behavior problems. These children are at higher risk for maladaptive behavior than are those with typical development (Semrud-Clikeman & Hynd, 1993). Some behavior problems represent identifiable psychiatric conditions (e.g., mood disorders, attachment disorders, traumatic stress reactions). Other problems may not represent mental disorders, but create challenges for family life or preschool adjustment.

Research studies have documented the co-occurrence of behavior problems and cognitive limitations in large samples of children (Baker, Blacher, Crnic, & Edelbrock, 2002; Dietz, Lavigne, Arend, & Rosenbaum, 1997; Merrell & Holland, 1997). Crnic, Hoffman, Gaze, and Edelbrock (2004) have found that different kinds of behavior problems are seen in children with different degrees of cognitive impairment. Children with borderline intelligence and mild mental retardation tend to have attention-deficit/hyperactivity disorder (ADHD) and oppositional defiant disorder; those functioning in lower ranges of mental retardation tend to have stereotypic behavior (hand mannerisms, repetitive motor actions). These investigators suggest that oppositional behavior requires higher cognitive functioning, while stereotypies do not require cognitive planning.

CHARACTERISTICS OF YOUNG CHILDREN WITH MENTAL RETARDATION

Subaverage Intellectual Ability

Children with mental retardation have subaverage intellectual ability. Degrees of mental retardation are determined by scores obtained on standardized tests of intelligence. When based on tests with an *SD* of 15, mental retardation is classified as mild (IQ 55–69), moderate (IQ 40–54), severe (IQ 25–39), and profound (IQ below 20). Approximately 85% of individuals with mental retardation have mild, 10% have moderate, 3.5% have severe, and 1.5% have profound mental retardation (Sattler, 2002).

It is often useful to discuss preschool children's cognitive difficulties in terms of developmental levels corresponding to mental ages. Many tests provide specific age equivalents. When this information is not available, an informal rule of thumb is that a child with mild mental retardation functions at approximately two-thirds of his or her chronological age. Children with moderate, severe, and profound mental retardation function at approximately one-half, one-third, and less than one-quarter of their chronological ages, respectively. For example, the skills of a 4-year-old with moderate mental retardation will resemble those of an 18- to 24-month-old. (For specific skills expected in children of different ages who have different levels of mental retardation, see Berk, 1993; Grossman, 1983; Jacobson & Mulick, 1996; and Sattler, 2002)

Behavioral Characteristics

Young children with mental retardation not only function below their chronological ages, but also exhibit behavioral characteristics that all members of assessment teams should look for. Sometimes the behaviors are subtle and not easy to identify. The following list, based in part on the work of Gioia (1993) and Kozma and Stock (1993), outlines what to look for in observing preschoolers with cognitive difficulties. Compared to typically developing peers, a young child with mental retardation:

1. Shows less curiosity about his or her surroundings.
2. Engages in less exploration to discover the function of objects.
3. Engages in more general manipulation of objects (sliding across a surface, banging, touching, holding, throwing, mouthing).
4. Exhibits less cognitive flexibility (e.g., perseverates on initial orientation when an inset formboard is rotated).
5. Gets stuck in an earlier pattern even when new skills have been acquired (e.g., communicates by pointing or gesturing even after words are acquired).
6. Shows restricted repertoire of play behaviors (does the same thing over and over).
7. Benefits less from incidental learning opportunities (needs explicit teaching).
8. Demonstrates less competence in problem solving (gives up, repeats unsuccessful strategies).

9. Does not generalize a learned skill to new situations.
10. Forgets new skills if they are not practiced regularly.

MYTHS ABOUT CHILDREN WITH MENTAL RETARDATION

Myth: Children with Mental Retardation Have a Stigmatized Physical Appearance

Children with mental retardation who have syndromes or genetic anomalies may look different from other children. However, the majority of children with mental retardation, including those with significant degrees of impairment, do not have an unusual physical appearance. Burack (1990) distinguishes between individuals with "organic" mental retardation (IQs below 50 and an organic etiology, such as a chromosomal disorder or fetal alcohol syndrome), and those with IQs above 50, no organic etiology, and a normal physical appearance. Since, as Sattler (2002) has pointed out, approximately 85% of people with mental retardation have mild mental retardation (IQs above 50), the great majority of the young children with mental retardation seen by preschool assessors will look just like children with typical development. *Physical attractiveness does not preclude a diagnosis of mental retardation.*

Myth: Children with Mental Retardation Are Clumsy

Although some children with mental retardation have difficulties with gross and fine motor coordination, many do not. Grossman (1983) has stated that many people with profound mental retardation (IQs below 20) have moderate to good motor skills. Sattler (2002) reports minimal impairment in sensory–motor areas for children below 6 years of age who have mild mental retardation. Cognitive and motor abilities are separate areas of development. *Good motor skills do not preclude a diagnosis of mental retardation.*

Myth: Children with Mental Retardation Are Impaired in All Areas

Although many children with mental retardation have global impairment, some have isolated areas of good functioning. Experts have described areas of special ability, often referred to as "savant" or "splinter" skills, in individuals with mental retardation (many of whom have concurrent ASD): musical abilities; mental calculation skills; unusual memory for places and routes; puzzle skills; hyperlexia (word decoding); drawing skills; special competence in finding embedded figures; calendar memory; and the ability to recite lists, poems, television commercials, and segments of dialogue from videos and television programs (Frith & Baron-Cohen, 1985; Heaton & Wallace, 2004; Miller, 1999; Sacks, 1995; Wing, 1985, 1998). Suggested explanations for these special skills include differences in attentional processes (Baron-Cohen, 1987; Miller, 1999) and inherent talent plus genetic factors (Heaton & Wallace, 2004).

In preschoolers with mental retardation (and often concurrent ASD), strong rote memory skills frequently involve rote counting; alphabet recitation; repetition of television commercials or dialogue; memory for places and routes; and number, letter, color, or shape naming. These competencies often mislead adults into thinking that the children have strong cognitive ability when in actuality they have mental retardation. This can result in no intervention or inappropriate intervention. *The presence of splinter skills should not preclude a diagnosis of mental retardation.*

Addressing the Myths

Erroneously believing that a normal physical appearance, good motor skills, or strong rote memory skills mean that a child should not be given a diagnosis of mental retardation does a disservice to both the child and the family. Failure to identify a child's mental retardation can lead to frustration when the child cannot meet adult expectations, or to instructional goals that exceed the child's capacities. Educating parents and professionals about mental retardation, including the strengths seen in many children with mental retardation, can result in developmentally appropriate expectations and intervention plans.

REASONS FOR IDENTIFYING MENTAL RETARDATION IN YOUNG CHILDREN

Many early childhood professionals are uncomfortable about the concept of mental retardation and are reluctant to make that diagnosis for young children. Realization that mental retardation is a lifelong condition may contribute to the discomfort. Other professionals believe that diagnostic precision can be beneficial to young children and their families. When members of assessment teams have different points of view, open discussion and clarification of this sensitive issue can help smooth the way for effective team functioning. Some of the potential benefits of identifying mental retardation are listed below:

1. Documenting children's eligibility for programs, services, and entitlements.
2. Explaining a child's failure to meet expected developmental milestones.
3. Explaining a slow rate of progress despite intervention.
4. In some instances, providing an explanation for language or behavior problems.
5. Setting parameters for intervention approaches.
6. Reducing risk of maltreatment.
7. Helping families, teachers, and service providers formulate appropriate expectations for progress and behavior.
8. Helping families gain access to relevant literature, support groups, and other resources.

COGNITIVE ASSESSMENT

Predictive Value of Cognitive Assessment

Once children have reached the developmental stage in which cognitive abilities (rather than earlier sensory–motor skills) can be assessed, results of preschool assessment become predictive of subsequent functioning. Prediction based on cognitive assessment has been found to be even better for young children with developmental disabilities, including mental retardation, than for those with typical development (Sattler, 1988).

Results of longitudinal studies show that young children's IQs (or IQ equivalents) remain stable over time. Vanderveer and Schweid (1974) found that all children with mental retardation or borderline intelligence at age 24 months continued to have those cognitive impairments at 45 months. Vig et al. (1987) studied a group of young children with borderline intelligence or mild mental retardation, who were initially tested at 2–4 years and retested at 6–7 years. The mean IQs were 73 in initial testing and 74 at follow-up. In a longitudinal study by Bernheimer and Keogh (1988), the IQs of children initially tested at the age of 34 months, and retested at 52, 74, and 109 months, changed little over time (IQs of 67, 76, 71, and 70, respectively). Other investigators have provided similar documentation of IQ stability (Carr, 1988; Field et al., 1990; Keogh et al., 1995).

Results of longitudinal studies documenting IQ stability for young children with cognitive impairments can help assessors feel confident about test results and their implications for intervention and progress. Results of longitudinal studies also suggest that, despite special education services, most children identified with mental retardation when they are young will continue to have mental retardation as they grow older.

Challenges for Assessors

In addition to the general challenges presented in the cognitive assessment of preschoolers (see Chapter 11), there are issues especially relevant to the assessment of young children with mental retardation.

Lack of Appropriate Tests

Most tests with age norms extending into the preschool years do not present adequate floor (developmentally easier items) for young children with mental retardation. There is also a lack of appropriate instruments for examinees representing culturally and linguistically diverse groups, including those who speak English as a second language or have limited English proficiency. Local assessment guidelines, often based on test suitability for older or more proficient children, specify tests that may or may not be used. This may mean that no clinically appropriate instrument is available for assessors. Since the diagnosis of mental retardation depends on administration of a standardized test of cognitive ability, a good deal of advocacy by assessors may be needed to obtain appropriate instruments, so that children can receive the services to which they are entitled.

Score Inflation

The issue of score inflation is especially relevant to children with mental retardation. One potential source of score inflation is the use of older tests (which may be the only clinically appropriate tests available for children functioning at early developmental levels). Consistent with Flynn's (1984) finding of 3-point IQ increases per decade, older tests may yield inflated scores. The use of older tests may underidentify mental retardation (Kranzler, 1997) and reduce eligibility for services.

Score inflation may also occur when tests designed for infants and very young children are administered to older preschoolers. Older children with cognitive impairments, who function at earlier developmental levels, may have had a good deal of practice with activities appropriate to those earlier levels. For example, copying a circle may be novel for a 3-year-old, but will not present much mental challenge for a 5-year-old functioning at an earlier developmental level, who has practiced the activity frequently at school.

Examinees Who Experience Environmental/Psychosocial Risk

Interpretation of test results can be particularly challenging when examinees and their families experience environmental/psychosocial risk factors that can compromise their development: poverty; educational deprivation; social isolation; unemployment; and/or parental substance abuse, mental illness, or intellectual limitations (Christian, 1999; Emery & Laumann-Billings, 1998; Jaudes & Shapiro, 1999; Knutson, 1995). Does the mental retardation identified in these children represent a chronic, lifelong disability, or rather a temporary condition caused by a lack of cognitive and linguistic stimulation? Is it fair to these children to avoid identifying their cognitive limitations because of concern about stigmatizing them with labels, and thereby to deprive them of services that could ameliorate the effects of environmental risk? Some assessment teams successfully resolve this dilemma by identifying cognitive limitations so that the children can receive intervention services, monitoring the children's development, and retesting in the future.

Standardized Tests of Cognitive Ability

When assessing young children with mental retardation, it is important to keep them both interested and safe. Tests permitting flexibility in item administration, and presenting many different kinds of tasks, best ensure children's involvement and cooperation. Materials should include toys and manipulatives, and should be washable and large enough to prevent choking. They should also be sturdy enough to withstand being mouthed, dropped, or thrown.

The problem of inadequate test floor (psychometric and clinical) is especially pertinent to the cognitive assessment of young children with mental retardation. Many preschool tests do not have norms permitting identification of moderate to profound mental retardation. Even when an IQ equivalent can be obtained, it is sometimes done on the basis of only a few credited items if a test has inadequate clinical floor. This represents a poor sampling of cognitive ability. Instruments providing a sufficient number of developmentally early items, which a child can handle comfortably, will give a better picture of cognitive functioning.

Some tests for preschoolers present items, formats, and instructions that are much too difficult for children under age 5 who have significant mental retardation. For example, the first item of the Early Reasoning subtest of the Stanford–Binet Intelligence Scales, Fifth Edition (SB5; Roid, 2003a, 2003b) asks a child to describe a complex picture. The format for the Matrix Reasoning subtest of the Wechsler Preschool and Primary Scale of Intelligence—Third Edition (WPPSI-III; Wechsler, 2002) requires pointing to a response choice, selected from an array, to complete a matrix. The WPPSI-III coding subtest requires a child to make linear and circular marks corresponding to five different geometric shapes. These examples suggest that assessors who use standardized tests must be familiar with the specific cognitive and linguistic competencies of children functioning at very early developmental levels. Table 12.1 summarizes desirable features of tests. Tables 12.2 and 12.3 provide case examples.

The following section describes the Bayley Scales of Infant and Toddler Development—Third Edition (Bayley-III; Bayley, 2006a, 2006b) in detail as an example of a test often used to assess children who function at early developmental levels. Appendix 12.1 describes the suitability of other standardized cognitive tests used for assessment of preschool children with mental retardation (many of which have been covered at greater length in Chapter 11 and Appendix 11.1). As this book was in its final stages of preparation, publication of a new edition of the Differential Ability Scales (Elliott, 2006) for individuals ages 2-5–17-11 years, was expected.

TABLE 12.1. Desirable Clinical Characteristics of Tests Used to Assess Young Children with Mental Retardation

Materials include toys

- Bayley Scales of Infant Development—Third Edition
- Griffiths Mental Development Scales
- Merrill–Palmer—Revised Scales of Development
- Mullen Scales of Early Learning
- Stanford–Binet Intelligence Scales, Fifth Edition

Age range starts at infancy

- Bayley Scales of Infant Development—Third Edition
- Griffiths Mental Development Scales
- Merrill–Palmer—Revised Scales of Development
- Mullen Scales of Early Learning

Instructions for nonverbal tests may be pantomimed

- Griffiths Mental Development Scales
- Merrill–Palmer—Revised Scales of Development

Flexibility of item administration (verbal, nonverbal, difficult, easy)

- Bayley Scales of Infant Development—Third Edition
- Griffiths Mental Development Scales
- Merrill–Palmer—Revised Scales of Development
- Mullen Scales of Early Learning

Tasks understandable to preschool children with a mental age of less than 2 years

- Bayley Scales of Infant Development—Second Edition
- Griffiths Mental Development Scales
- Merrill–Palmer—Revised Scales of Development
- Mullen Scales of Early Learning

Lengthy discontinuation procedures avoided

- Bayley Scales of Infant Development—Third Edition
- Griffiths Mental Development Scales
- Merrill–Palmer—Revised Scales of Development
- Stanford–Binet Intelligence Scales, Fifth Edition

TABLE 12.2. Assessment of a Child with Mild Mental Retardation

Angel is a 5-year-old boy referred to the child study team at his school because of his behavior problems. His kindergarten teacher describes him as inattentive, active, impulsive, disobedient, defiant, and moody. The teacher reports that he provokes other children, and often crawls under his desk or runs around the classroom. She says that he has made virtually no academic progress, and notes that his speech is unclear.

The school psychologist administers the Stanford–Binet Intelligence Scale: Fifth Edition (SB5) and obtains the following scores:

	Standard score	Age equivalent
Nonverbal IQ	62	3-0 years
Verbal IQ	61	3-2 years
Full Scale IQ	60	3-1 years
Fluid Reasoning	65	3-1 years
Knowledge	72	3-1 years
Quantitative Reasoning	64	3-1 years
Visual–Spatial Processing	62	3-0 years
Working Memory	65	3-3 years

The psychologist also administers the Vineland-II, with Angel's mother as informant, to assess adaptive behavior. The following scores are obtained:

	Standard score
Communication	61
Daily Living Skills	64
Socialization	61
Motor Skills	67
Adaptive Behavior Composite	61

Adaptive levels for subdomains range from moderately low to low.

Test results indicate that Angel's cognitive potential is within the range of mild mental retardation. For a 5-year-old functioning cognitively more like a 3-year-old, the SB5 has provided adequate floor and the child is fully testable.

The speech–language pathologist obtains standard scores and age equivalents that are comparable to the cognitive scores, but finds that Angel's articulatory difficulties are worse than what would be predicted on the basis of his mental age. The assessment team's educational specialist observes Angel in his classroom and does some trial teaching with him. The specialist reports that he lacks developmental readiness for kindergarten work, and notes that his behavior problems seem to occur when demands are made that he does not understand and cannot meet. The team social worker meets with Angel's parents and, in discussing disciplinary practices, finds that they are punishing him for "acting like a baby" and refusing to do his kindergarten homework.

The assessment team recommends a readiness program that has an appropriate instructional pace and a small student–teacher ratio, as well as speech therapy to remediate articulatory difficulties. The team also suggests several parent education resources and supports. Once these interventions are put into place, Angel begins to experience success in the classroom, and his behavior gradually improves. His parents and the school staff regularly monitor his progress through IEP reviews.

TABLE 12.3. Assessment of a Child with Severe Mental Retardation

Carla is a 4-year-old girl brought by her parents to a developmental clinic for diagnostic clarification. Carla had previously been evaluated through her state's early intervention system, and at 18 months of age was found to be eligible for early intervention services. She attended a high-quality center-based early intervention program until age 3, and was then moved to an excellent special preschool program. She received speech–language therapy and occupational therapy in both programs.

Carla's parents express disappointment about her lack of expected progress. They report that despite over 2 years of speech–language therapy, Carla is not yet saying words. She has not yet acquired toilet training. The parents say that when initially told by previous assessors that Carla had developmental delays, they had hoped that intervention would help Carla "catch up" to children of her age.

The psychologist administers the Griffiths Mental Development Scales, which provide very early developmental activities if needed, as well as separate standard scores for language and nonverbal abilities. The following scores are obtained:

	Quotient	Mental age
Locomotor	AQ = 59	29.5 months
Personal–Social	BQ = 34	17 months
Hearing and Speech	CQ = 15	7.5 months
Eye and Hand Coordination	DQ = 36	18 months
Performance	EQ = 35	17.5 months
General Quotient	GQ = 36	17.9 months

During psychological assessment, Carla is able to dump cubes out of a box, place a circular inset in a form board, and scribble on paper. She rings a bell and turns several pages of a sturdy cardboard book designed for children under 2 years of age. Carla vocalizes with phonemic differentiation, but does not say words.

The psychologist also administers the Vineland Adaptive Behavior Scales, Second Edition, with the parents as informants, and obtains the following scores:

	Standard score
Communication	42
Daily Living Skills	43
Socialization	42
Motor Skills	28
Adaptive Behavior Composite	38

The adaptive levels for all subdomains are rated as low. The psychologist notes in the psychological report that these findings should be interpreted with great caution. Due to Carla's functioning at a very early developmental level, some subdomains (e.g., Written Communication) yield raw scores of zero. Although the test manual states that this is to be expected, the psychologist decides to report scores, but to emphasize qualitative descriptions of Carla's adaptive behavior skills and areas in which intervention could be helpful.

When given a doll family, utensils, and doll furniture for free play, Carla picks up several toys and looks briefly at each. She throws two dolls into the air, bangs them on the table, then loses interest and wanders away.

Test results indicate that Carla functions globally within the range of severe mental retardation by *SD* norms. Her nonverbal skills are commensurate with severe mental retardation. Her language skills are well below other areas.

(continued)

TABLE 12.3. *(continued)*

Other members of the assessment team also evaluate Carla and obtain information from her parents. The audiologist identifies normal hearing. The social worker learns that Carla's parents are worried about her lack of progress, but enjoy caring for her. They play with her and provide activities and stimulation appropriate to her developmental level. The developmental pediatrician completes a neurodevelopmental assessment and finds that Carla has microcephaly (a small head size). The speech–language pathologist does an oromotor assessment, discusses feeding practices with her parents, and learns that Carla does not swallow easily and rejects many foods.

Following comprehensive multidisciplinary assessment, the psychologist and pediatrician meet with Carla's parents to present her diagnosis of severe mental retardation, and to share team recommendations for intervention. The intervention plan includes a special education class with emphasis on acquisition of life skills, participation in a feeding group to address oromotor issues, and further exploration of reasons for Carla's small head size. The parents ask whether Carla will eventually "catch up" and function at her age level. The clinicians explain that a child diagnosed with severe mental retardation at age 4 is likely to continue to function well below age expectancy even with high-quality intervention. The parents ask how they can learn more about mental retardation, and they are given information about organizations, literature, and Internet resources. The clinicians offer developmental follow-up in the future to help monitor Carla's development and service needs.

During one of the follow-up sessions, the parents say that although Carla's diagnosis was initially difficult to accept, they appreciated having a name for her problem and a reason for her slow progress.

Bayley Scales of Infant and Toddler Development—Third Edition

The Bayley-III is used for infants and younger preschoolers. The norms cover a range of 1–42 months. Although the norming sample did not include children with mental retardation, the test manual states that supplementary studies, involving small samples and nonrandom selection of participants, provide evidence of validity for children with Down syndrome, pervasive developmental disorder, cerebral palsy, and other conditions placing them at risk for mental retardation.

Because early portions of the test assess sensory–motor skills rather than cognitive abilities, scores obtained for infants do not correlate well with subsequent measures of cognitive potential. Although the majority of infants with Down syndrome eventually test within the range of moderate mental retardation (Hayes & Batshaw, 1993), testing with the Bayley-III may indicate little delay. Parents need to know that infant testing based on assessment of sensory–motor skills tends not to be predictive of subsequent ability. Prediction improves between 24 and 42 months of age.

The Bayley-III provides composite scores for Cognitive, Language, Motor, Social–Emotional, and Adaptive Behavior areas. (See Chapter 11 for more detailed information.) There is no global index of developmental functioning. The test is characterized as a developmental test, rather than a test of intelligence. Mental retardation and its classification levels are not discussed. The technical manual describes composite scores of 69 and below as "extremely low." The lowest Cognitive composite available is 55. Because the Bayley-III lacks a global index, and composite scores extend only 3 SDs below the mean, it is difficult to make a formal diagnosis of significant mental retardation on the basis of assessment with this instrument. Assessors may wish to tell families of older examinees that a Cognitive composite of 69 or below would represent mental retardation for an older child assessed with an intelligence test. Use of the developmental ages provided in the test manual can be helpful in explaining degrees of delay. A 36-month-old who attains a developmental age of 12 months would probably function within the range of severe mental retardation when subsequently assessed with an intelligence test.

The Bayley-III has excellent clinical floor (developmentally early items). Each test item presents a new activity. Although discontinuation is based on five consecutive failures, the fact that each item involves a different activity greatly reduces potential frustration for the child as ceiling is established. Bayley-III materials are colorful and highly appealing to young children. Most are washable. Test procedures are developmentally appropriate. A 3-year-old with significant delay might be expected ring a bell, look at pictures with interest, pick up blocks, search for missing objects, and remove blocks from a cup.

Because of the developmentally early items available in the Bayley-III, the test may be used to assess children above 42 months of age who have significant delays. The test manual states that an older child's performance can be described only in terms of developmental age equivalents. The manual cautions that because age equivalents do not represent equally spaced units throughout the scale, small raw score changes may result in large changes in age equivalents.

Although cognitive assessment, represented by the Bayley-III Cognitive Composite, has greatest relevance to mental retardation, motor assessment should be mentioned. Assessors should know that the Motor Scale is not a pure measure of motor skills. Some of the tasks presented by the Bayley-III Motor Scale, especially its Fine Motor subtest, contain a substantial cognitive component. A child with intellectual limitations may fail to conceptualize what is expected, and may therefore fail cognitively loaded motor items (e.g., replicating a block structure resembling steps). Failure to recognize cognitive dimensions of Motor Scale tasks may erroneously lead to a recommendation for remediation of motor deficits for a child with mental retardation who does not have motor problems.

PLAY ASSESSMENT

Watching young children play with toys gives valuable information about their developmental status. Play assessment can be implemented by any members of assessment teams. As explained more extensively in Chapter 11, play assessment provides a way to estimate children's developmental ages, and thereby serves as an informal validity check for standardized testing. Toy play is also a useful context for behavioral observations that help assessors differentiate children's developmental problems. Young children often talk while playing with toys, so toy play is a good source of language samples as well.

In order to implement play assessment effectively for young children with mental retardation, assessors need to be familiar with the sequential development of play skills (described in Chapter 11) in order to anchor observations developmentally. They should also be knowledgeable about the special characteristics of object play seen in children with mental retardation.

Characteristics of Object Play in Children with Mental Retardation

Studies of young children with mental retardation have documented qualitative differences in play behavior, and less sophisticated play patterns, as compared to children with typical development (Beeghley, Weiss-Perry, & Cicchetti, 1989; Cunningham, Glen, Wilkinson, & Sloper, 1985; Fewell, Ogura, Notari-Sylverson, & Wheeden, 1997; Gowen et al., 1992; Hill & McCune-Nicholich, 1981; Lender et al., 1998; Linn et al., 2000;

Malone & Landers, 2001; Malone & Stoneman, 1990; Ruskin et al., 1994). The following list of play characteristics associated with mental retardation is based on the work of these experts.

1. Interest in physical, rather than representational, properties of toys.
2. More time spent in nonspecific manipulation (holding, fingering, sliding, throwing).
3. Less sustained involvement with toys.
4. Less varied play schemas.
5. More repetition.
6. Fewer toys combined.
7. Fewer sequential combinations of toys.
8. Less elaboration of play themes.

Conducting a Play Observation Session

Procedures for observing the toy play of a child with mental retardation are the same as for other examinees. Materials should include one or more doll figures (a family of dolls is ideal), furniture, dishes, and utensils. Although cars and trucks are appealing to young children, and may be used to establish rapport, activities undertaken with vehicles do not lend themselves well to developmental analysis. Miniature toys are easily portable and well suited to small observation spaces. Toys are presented in random order, and the child is invited to play with them. Most preschoolers with mental retardation can be expected to sustain concentration for at least a few minutes; this is ample time for anchoring observations developmentally by watching what a child does with the toys. The assessor should simply present the toys, but should not become involved in the child's play. The assessor should refrain from suggesting toy combinations or themes (e.g., he or she should not place a chair near a table or suggest that a doll wants to eat). While the child plays, the assessor should record everything the child says, and everything the child does with the toys. This record provides a basis for developmental analysis (see Table 12.4 for examples of recorded observations).

Assessment Instruments

The Symbolic Play Test—Second Edition (Lowe & Costello, 1988), designed for children ages 12–36 months, presents four different sets of toys. Scores are given for specific toy combinations, and an age equivalent is determined by the total score for all four sets. In a review of the test, Paolito (1995) notes that the dolls presented in the toy sets are fragile. The Westby Play Scales (Westby, 1980, 1991, 2000) provide general age levels for various kinds of toy combinations and activities. Although the Symbolic Play Test has been used for research (e.g., Power & Radcliff, 2000), the Westby Scales do not require special materials and provide an easy way to anchor observations developmentally in preschool classrooms, assessment settings, and homes.

ASSESSMENT OF ADAPTIVE BEHAVIOR

Adaptive behavior includes two basic concepts: (1) self-sufficiency in carrying out activities of daily living, and (2) social competence (Demchak & Drinkwater, 1998; Sparrow, Balla, & Cicchetti, 1984). A diagnosis of mental retardation, and determination of eligi-

TABLE 12.4. Examples of Object Play in Young Children with Mental Retardation

Crystal

Age: 4-9 years
IQ: 66 (mild mental retardation)

Play observations

Pretends to give baby a bottle.
- "Let her sleep. He doesn't fit there. Put this stuff right here. Top the bed."

Piles toys.
Places table upside down, bed on top of shelves, foods in bed.
- "Put this here till they finish. (*Pause*) What's this?"

Extends jar of "instant coffee" to examiner. Looks at baby.
- "That's on the top. (*Pause*) Nobody hit. Don't hit this baby. Don't break her."

Points to design on spoon.
- "Somebody put this sticker on here."

Places spoon and coffee in bed (which has been piled on top of shelves).
- "Put this stuff in here, too."

Puts girl doll in chair near general pile of objects.
- "Him sit here. (*Pause*) Oop, baby" (*speaks softly*). Baby go here."

Puts baby in bed with foods.
Removes foods and puts basket in bed and baby in basket.
- "Let her sleep. So she won't fall down. (*Pause*) The baby want some milk."

Gives baby doll a bottle.
- "She drink a lot of milk. She need a napkin."

Gets up and finds paper towel. Wipes own face.
- "My face is clean."

Comment

Crystal's play skills are representational, but below age expectancy. She does not elaborate the themes she introduces (e.g., putting the baby to bed), sequence play actions, or organize actions around a theme. Her play has a disorganized quality, and there is one instance of immature autosymbolic play (wiping her own face rather than the doll's face). Crystal's highest skills (at the level of 3-0 to 3-6 years) are verbalizing her intention to give the baby some milk (which provides evidence of planning) and requesting an absent object ("She need a napkin").

Tyrone

Age: 4-1 years
IQ: 20 (profound mental retardation)

Play observations

Reaches for doll.
Extends doll bed toward his mother.
Looks briefly at toys.
Grabs bottle. Releases it so that it falls to floor.
Loses interest in toys.

Comment

Tyrone's play skills resemble those of a young infant. He shows brief interest in the toys as objects to reach for, hand to someone, and drop. Tyrone demonstrates no understanding of the function of a miniature doll bed or bottle, and does not recognize that the doll represents a person.

bility for services based on that diagnosis, are based on adaptive behavior as well as intelligence. Adaptive behavior is age-related and increases in complexity as the child matures. For infants and young children, sensory–motor, communication, self-help, and socialization skills are primary (Demchak & Drinkwater, 1998; Grossman, 1983; Harrison & Boan, 2000). During later childhood and adolescence, basic academic skills and those requiring judgment and reasoning become important.

Assessment of adaptive behavior addresses the actual behavior and typical performance, rather than the underlying abilities, of the individual being assessed. For preschoolers, assessment usually involves asking a third party (parent or teacher) which skills a child has fully mastered, which skills are emerging, and which are not yet observed.

Relationship of Adaptive Behavior to Intelligence

A significant relationship between adaptive behavior and intelligence has been documented for young children with disabilities. Loveland and Kelly (1991) investigated the adaptive behavior of 32 children (ages 19–80 months) with Down syndrome or autism. They obtained coefficients of .63–.87 for correlations based on measures of adaptive behavior and intelligence. In a study of 497 preschool children with developmental disabilities, ranging in age from 15 to 72 months, Vig and Jedrysek (1995) obtained correlation coefficients of .75 (based on standard scores) and .89 (based on age equivalents) for measures of adaptive behavior and intelligence. It may be that for young children with disabilities, whose adaptive skills are just emerging, cognitive demands (for "catching on" to new adaptive tasks) are stronger than they are for older individuals who have been exposed to training and practice. Due to the strong association between adaptive behavior and intelligence for children functioning at earlier chronological and mental ages, measures of adaptive behavior can be used as a rough estimate of cognitive ability for untestable or partially testable preschoolers.

Results of intelligence testing establish parameters for the adaptive functioning of children with mental retardation. This is important for establishing teaching goals and helping families develop realistic expectations for skill acquisition. For example, a 4-year-old with moderate mental retardation will function developmentally more like a 2-year-old. The child cannot be expected to use all table utensils without spilling, or to speak in full sentences. Berk (1993), Grossman (1983), Jacobson and Mulick (1996), and Sattler (2002) have provided useful reviews of the specific adaptive skills that can be expected of children of different ages and levels of mental retardation. Grossman (1983) focuses on the 3-year, 6-year, 9-year, and 12-year age groups. According to Grossman, a 3-year-old with mild mental retardation can use a spoon for eating cereal or soft foods, but considerable spilling can be expected. A 3-year-old with severe mental retardation can be expected to finger-feed, but is not apt to manage a spoon.

Multicultural Issues

Adaptive behavior should be interpreted within the context of culture, ethnicity, and family expectations (Harrison & Boan, 2000). Child-rearing practices vary considerable among families representing diverse cultural groups. For example, some Hispanic families provide baby bottles for preschool children, while other groups encourage cup drinking in 15-month-olds (Zuniga, 2004). Some Korean families introduce toilet training when infants are 3–4 months old, while other groups may wait until children are between 3 and

4 years old (Chan & Lee, 2004). Many mothers in Japan encourage closeness and dependency in young children, while mothers in the United States prioritize independence and autonomy (Rothbaum, Weiss, Pott, Miyake, & Morelli, 2000).

Although assessors must recognize the importance of multicultural competence, they cannot be expected to be familiar with the practices and beliefs of all ethnic and cultural groups. It is always permissible, and indeed highly desirable, to question families respectfully about the child-rearing practices of their particular group.

Using Information about Adaptive Behavior for Intervention Planning

Assessment of adaptive behavior is useful for intervention planning. Identification of specific skill deficits can lead to IEP goals directed toward skill acquisition. Results of adaptive behavior assessment can be used to monitor the progress of individual children and the efficacy of intervention plans.

Results of intelligence testing are used to make inferences about underlying ability and potential for learning. Teaching a child the specific tasks not mastered on an intelligence test ("teaching to the test") is not ethical, may represent a violation of test security, and may lead to an artificial and erroneous overestimation of ability in future testing. In contrast, it is perfectly ethical and highly desirable to teach a child the tasks not mastered on a test of adaptive behavior. If a child is developmentally ready to put on a jacket but does not do it, the skill may be taught. Young children with mental retardation tend to be passive, and may lack the motivation, goal conceptualization, and initiative to acquire new adaptive skills or to practice skills already acquired. Specific instruction from an adult is helpful to them. Task analysis (breaking a new skill into small components and teaching mastery of each small step before introducing a new step) can be helpful. Pecukonis (1993) and Sattler (2002) present examples of task analysis applied to specific skills. Since children with mental retardation often forget what they have been taught, or fail to generalize a learned skill to new situations, plenty of practice and review in a variety of settings may be required for skill maintenance.

As is true for tests of cognitive ability, instruments used to assess adaptive behavior often lack sufficient psychometric and clinical floor for young children with mental retardation. The next section describes the Vineland Adaptive Behavior Scales, Second Edition (Vineland-II; Sparrow et al., 2005), which is the instrument most commonly used to assess children's adaptive behavior. The optional Bayley-III Adaptive Behavior subtest and Merrill–Palmer-R Self-Help/Adaptive rating scales are sometimes used for briefer assessment of this domain. Other instruments are discussed in Harrison and Boan's (2000) comprehensive review.

Vineland Adaptive Behavior Scales, Second Edition

The Vineland-II represents a substantial revision of the original Vineland Adaptive Behavior Scales (Sparrow et al., 1984). In addition to expanding the age range of the Vineland-II scales by adding new items, the developers have added new items in the birth to 3-year range to allow for greater differentiation during these early years of rapid development. The organization of items in developmental order by subdomain rather than domain, as well as the use of symbols to identify specific content areas, aids interviewers in formulating appropriate questions relevant to the specific content area. The new scales cover an age range from birth to 90 years. There are separate editions for home and classroom, including a Spanish edition. Information is obtained from parents, other caregivers, or teachers. Report forms provide explanations of domains, scores, and descriptive levels that facilitate the interpretation of results. For preschoolers, domains assessed include Communication, Daily Living Skills, Socialization, and Motor Skills. The Motor Skills domain is not assessed after a child reaches 6 years of age. Depending on the form used and the age of the child, administration time ranges from 20 to 60 minutes.

An optional Maladaptive Behavior Scale is available for individuals 3 years of age or older. Items address internalizing and externalizing behaviors (tantrums, sleep disturbance, crying, dependency, attention, activity level). The Maladaptive Behavior Scale yields a Maladaptive Behavior Index, which can be classified into three descriptive categories: average, elevated, and clinically significant. The clinically significant level indicates that the individual exhibits more maladaptive behaviors than 98% of those in the same age in the standardization sample. This score is best used as a screening device to determine the need for further comprehensive evaluation of maladaptive behavior. Because 3- and 4-year-olds with mental retardation function at earlier developmental levels, the Maladaptive Behavior Scale is not appropriate for them. Behaviors that might indicate maladaptive behavior in children with a mental age of at least 3 years may be more acceptable in children functioning at younger developmental ages. For example, crying too easily or sucking thumb and fingers in a child with a mental age of 2 or 3 years is not necessarily a cause for concern.

The Vineland-II was normed on a national sample 3,695 individuals ages birth through 90 years, including 1,325 children under age. The norming sample was stratified for age, sex, race/ethnicity, SES, geographic region, mother's educational level, community size, and educational placement. Children classified as exceptional and in need of educational placement included those with ADHD, emotional/behavioral disturbance, learning disability, mental retardation, speech/language impairment, and other conditions (sensory, physical, or health impairments; multiple impairments; autism; or traumatic brain injury).

Standard scores, *v*-scale scores, percentile ranks, age equivalents, stanines, as well as descriptive levels, are available. Composite standard scores extend downward to 20, suggesting adequate floor. Subdomain scores are reported in terms of *v*-scale scores (mean of 15, SD of 3) that range from 1 (4.66 SD below the mean) to 24 (3 SD above the mean), permitting finer differentiation at lower levels of functioning. The test manual notes, however, that for younger ages, zero is a fairly common raw score for some subdomains, requiring caution in interpretation of test scores. The reason for this is that very young children, or those functioning at early developmental levels, may not have acquired the skills assessed by some of the subdomains (e.g., Written Expression, Domestic, or Community Use). A very young child is not apt to distinguish letters from numbers, talk on the telephone, or assume responsibility for such household chores as feeding a pet. Despite the addition of more items for children under age 3, the instrument may lack adequate floor for young examinees with significant mental retardation.

Internal consistency reliabilities for Vineland-II composites are primarily in the .90s for ages birth through 5; subdomain scores are primarily in the .70s and .80s. Test–retest reliability coefficients are high, with most values exceeding .85, except for ages 14 through 21. Interviewer reliability is a concern for clinicians administering a semi-structured interview since examiner variability may contribute to variations in scores. For the birth through age 6 group, the interviewer reliability is .87 for the Adaptive Behavior Composite, and ranges from .66 to .87 for Socialization and Daily Living Skills domains, respectively, and from .48 to .92 for Play/Leisure Time and Written Expression subdomains, respectively.

Administration of Vineland-II items, particularly those of the Daily Living Skills domain, can be a nonthreatening way to obtain information about a child's home situation as well as his or her developmental skills. A few items of the Communication domain (e.g., questions about the child's use of various prepositional constructions) tend to be too technical for some parents. However, the inclusion of some scoring tips, as well as symbols organizing items into content areas, enables interviewers to formulate appropriate questions to probe further for accurate responses.

LINKING ASSESSMENT TO INTERVENTION

The process of linking assessment to intervention should result in appropriate developmental services for children with mental retardation, and in support for their families. Steps in the process include sharing developmental information with families, and identifying potentially beneficial services and resources.

Labeling

Following assessment of a young child, results are shared with families. When assessment reveals mental retardation, the question arises about what terminology to use for describing the disability. In settings where assessment is undertaken for purposes of educational planning and identification of service needs, general phrases and noncategorical labeling are often used ("preschool child with a disability," "child with special needs"). In clinical settings, where the purpose of assessment is diagnostic clarification, specific labels ("borderline intelligence," "moderate mental retardation") are more apt to be given.

At what age should the label "mental retardation" be used? The term "developmental delay" is often used for children under 3 years of age. Once cognitive abilities have emerged sufficiently to be assessed by standardized tests (between 24 and 36 months), the label "mental retardation" becomes meaningful. In settings in which diagnostic clarification is the primary goal of assessment, the label is used at 36 months or even earlier.

The issue of diagnostic labeling is controversial at all ages (see Vig, 2005), but particularly so during early childhood. Critics of labeling sometimes hope that a young child will "outgrow" developmental problems, and suggest that labeling may lead to tracking into a special education system from which the child is not likely to emerge. Occasionally children who have experienced severe neglect, deprivation, or trauma do show improvement when these circumstances are ameliorated. For the majority of children, however, longitudinal studies of IQ stability indicate that mental retardation is a lifelong disability. Although functioning can be optimized by intervention, the disability cannot be "cured." A child with mental retardation will need special education services throughout his or her schooling because of the chronic nature of the disability, not because of the label used to describe it.

Critics of labeling also say that the use of labels will be upsetting to the family and may cause the family to view the child negatively. Several studies of parental reactions to being informed of a child's disability suggest that this is not necessarily true. Parents have expressed a preference for prompt diagnosis and full information (including diagnostic labels), rather than delayed diagnosis and evasiveness (Abrams & Goodman, 1998; Quine & Pahl, 1986; Quine & Rutter, 1994).

Proponents of labeling emphasize that precise identification and labeling of a child's problems will lead to appropriate intervention planning and realistic expectations for progress and behavior. Realistic expectations mean that a child with mental retardation can experience plenty of success in an intervention program, thus strengthening self-esteem. The label "mental retardation" carries prognostic information and helps to predict rates of progress and responsiveness to intervention. If family members and intervention professionals know that a child has mental retardation, they will encourage small steps of progress and accept plateaus in development. There will be less tendency to blame the child, the family, or the intervention program when the child does not, despite everyone's best efforts, "catch up" to same-age peers.

Labels can even protect children from maltreatment. Children with mental retardation and other developmental disabilities are at greater risk of maltreatment (abuse and neglect) than those with typical development (Diamond & Jaudes, 1983; Jaudes & Shapiro, 1999; Verdugo, Bermejo, & Fuertes, 1995; Vig & Kaminer, 2002). Children with milder disabilities may be at greater risk than those with more severe disabilities, whose limitations are more obvious (Benedict, White, Wulff, & Hall, 1990; Jaudes & Shapiro, 1999; Sullivan, Brookhouser, Scanlan, Knutson, & Schulte, 1991; Verdugo et al., 1995). Crnic et al. (2004) have noted that children with milder delays have more behavior problems, including oppositional behavior, than those with more significant delays. The implication for preschoolers is that if mental retardation (especially mild mental retardation) is not identified and labeled, a child's disability-related functional and behavioral deficits may be interpreted as willful misbehavior. This in turn may increase the child's vulnerability to maltreatment.

Finally, labels can lead families to targeted information, resources, and support and advocacy groups. Parents who have learned that their child has mental retardation can gain access to articles, books, and Internet resources about this disability. They can also become involved in support and advocacy groups, and meet other families whose children have mental retardation. A list of national organizations with useful information for families is presented in Table 12.5. Family members who are told that their child has "special needs" will be deprived of these opportunities.

Sharing Developmental Information with Families

How can families best be informed about a child's mental retardation? The following suggestions for assessors are based in part on the work of Kaminer and Cohen (1988). The steps are designed for settings in which the label "mental retardation" is used, and may be modified for settings that use other labels.

1. Prepare for the reporting session by checking your own feelings about the information to be conveyed.
2. Anticipate possible reactions of families, and think about how you will address these reactions.
3. Speak frankly, and use the label "mental retardation" in a normal (rather than whispered) tone of voice and while making eye contact with family members.
4. Use the label "mental retardation" as often as possible during the reporting session, conveying the idea that this condition can be discussed openly and without shame or embarrassment.
5. Resist the temptation to minimize or take back the information if family members are upset.
6. Suggest intervention services that will optimize the child's development. (Do not promise a "cure" for the disability.)

TABLE 12.5. Resources for Families of Children with Mental Retardation

American Association on Mental Retardation (AAMR)
444 North Capitol Street NW, Suite 846
Washington, DC 20001-1512
800-424-3688
www.aamr.org

The Arc of the United States
1010 Wayne Avenue, Suite 650
Silver Spring, MD 20910
301-565-3842
www.thearc.org

The Council for Exceptional Children (CEC)
1110 North Glebe Road, Suite 300
Arlington, VA 22201
888-232-7733
www.cec.sped.org

National Dissemination Center for Children with Disabilities (NICHCY)
P.O. Box 1492
Washington, DC 20013
800-695-0285
www.nichcy.org

7. Describe procedures for obtaining services.
8. Suggest resources providing information and/or support, if desired by the family.
9. Offer developmental follow-up.
10. Recognize that discussing plans for intervention and ongoing support can reduce family distress, but do not expected such discussion to eliminate it.

Multicultural Issues

When assessors are reporting developmental information to families representing diverse cultural or ethnic groups, it is important for them to know something about the cultural groups' beliefs about disability and its causes. For example, some Native American families attribute disabilities to supernatural forces and may consult with traditional healers or participate in special ceremonies designed to prevent the condition from worsening (Joe & Malach, 2004). Some Hispanic families may believe that a child's illness or disability is due to the presence of evil in the environment, and may place an amulet around the child's neck or use other folk remedies to ward off evil (Zuniga, 2004). If assessors know about families' cultural beliefs about disability, they will understand that alternative remedies may be used in addition to, or instead of, recommended intervention. Open and respectful discussion of families' ideas about disability and its treatment will strengthen the parent–professional partnership necessary for implementation of intervention plans.

When assessors are reporting assessment results to families who do not speak English or who speak English with limited proficiency, the reporting must sometimes be done through an interpreter. Meeting privately with the interpreter, and reviewing the steps described previously, will help to ensure a successful reporting session. If the label "mental retardation" is to be used, this should be discussed in advance with the interpreter. The interpreter's role should be to serve as a neutral conduit, conveying information back and forth between the assessor and the family, and not interjecting personal beliefs and interpretations. Although the interpreter may be uncomfortable about a family's distress, he or she should not minimize the information or tell the family that the child "will be fine" (implying a potential "cure" for the disability).

Types of Interventions

Young children with mental retardation can benefit from many of the same kinds of interventions provided for other children with developmental challenges. Identification of mental retardation, through multidisciplinary assessment, is a primary intervention (see Chapter 11 for a more extensive discussion). In formulating plans for additional interventions, assessors must consider the child's developmental level. For example, a communication board may be helpful to a child who has cerebral palsy or autism as well as mental retardation, if that child has the developmental readiness to understand picture symbols or icons. Play therapy, utilizing verbal reflection, may not be helpful to a child who has not yet acquired the developmental readiness to understand cause and effect.

The following list suggests the many kinds of interventions that can be helpful to young children with mental retardation and their families. Family-oriented supports and services are especially important for this disability group (see Table 12.5 for a list of national organizations that families can contact). Although family members understandably want everything possible done to help their child, this does not necessarily mean that more services, or more frequent services, are best for a child's development. Kaminer and Robinson (1993) urge early childhood professionals to move past a "more is better" perspective.

1. Identification of child's developmental problems and contributory factors.
2. Developmental therapies: occupational, physical, and speech–language therapy.
3. Center-based early intervention program.
4. Specialized preschool program (developmental or therapeutic approach).
5. Integrated or inclusionary program.
6. Itinerant special education services provided within community-based preschools and childcare centers.
7. Home visiting/consultation.
8. Applied behavioral analysis.
9. Parent–child dyadic intervention (infant mental health approach).
10. Parent education/support/social services.
11. Genetic counseling.
12. Case management services.
13. Medication management.
14. Pediatric primary care and dental services.
15. Ongoing monitoring and developmental follow-up.

CONCLUSION

To provide assessment that represents best practice for young children with mental retardation, assessors should do the following:

1. Acquire a background in early childhood development for children with and without disabilities.
2. Learn about mental retardation, its etiology, and its manifestations over the life span.
3. Learn about developmental conditions that co-occur with mental retardation.
4. Acquire background in the child-rearing practices, and beliefs about disability, that characterize families from diverse cultural and ethnic groups.
5. Become familiar with the behavioral characteristics and learning styles of young children with mental retardation.
6. Select developmentally appropriate assessment instruments and procedures for evaluating young children with mental retardation.
7. Be knowledgeable about the kinds of developmentally appropriate services that can optimize the functioning of these young children.
8. Gain information about resources and supports for families of young children with mental retardation.
9. Build ongoing monitoring and support into the intervention plan.

Following these guidelines will help to ensure that assessment is relevant to the interests and abilities of young children with mental retardation, and will lead to intervention that fully supports their development.

APPENDIX 12.1. Tests of Cognitive Ability: Suitability for Preschool Children with Mental Retardation

Measure	**Bayley Scales of Infant and Toddler Development, Third Edition (Bayley-III). Bayley (2005).**
Age group	1–42 months.
Lowest scores available	55 for the Cognitive Scale and 45 for the Language and Motor Scales.
Comments	Highly appealing materials and activities for children functioning at early developmental levels. Scores for infants do not correlate well with subsequent cognitive potential, because early items assess sensory–motor skills. Can be used for assessment of preschoolers with mental retardation.

Measure	**Griffiths Mental Development Scales. Griffiths (1970); Huntley (1996).**
Age group	Birth to 2 years; 3 to 8 years.
Lowest scores available	Developmental quotient of 50 for the birth to 2 years group; quotients below 20, based on ratio of MA to CA, for 3 to 8 years group.
Comments	Separate quotients available for each subscale (Locomotor, Personal–Social, Hearing and Speech, Eye and Hand Coordination, Performance, for all ages; Practical Reasoning additionally available, for ages 3–8 years). Excellent clinical floor. Materials brightly colored and highly appealing. Psychometric drawbacks are that test has older norms and British norming sample. Test is useful for young children with all levels of mental retardation.

Measure	**Merrill–Palmer—Revised Scales of Development. Roid and Sampers (2004).**
Age group	1 month to 6-6 years.
Lowest scores available	Developmental Index scores of 10 or 11 for ages 23–78 months.
Comments	Adequate floor. Age equivalents go down to 1 month. Spanish instructions available. Appropriate tasks and materials for children functioning at early levels. Test is suitable for preschoolers with all levels of mental retardation.

Measure	**Mullen Scales of Early Learning. Mullen (1995).**
Age group	0–68 months.
Lowest scores available	Lowest Composite Score is 49.
Comments	Toys and manipulatives are appealing. Test is not an IQ test and is not appropriate for assessing children with moderate to profound mental retardation.

Measure	**Stanford–Binet Intelligence Scales, Fifth Edition (SB5). Roid (2003a, 2003b). Stanford–Binet Intelligence Scales for Early Childhood (Early SB5). Roid (2005).**
Age group	SB5: 2-0 to 85+ years; Early SB5: 2-0 to 7-3 years.
Lowest scores available	Full Scale IQ of 40 for all age groups.

Comments	Teaching and practice items provided. Toys, manipulatives, and pictures are appealing to young children. Initial tasks may be conceptually too demanding and formats too complicated, for 2-, 3-, and some 4- and 5-year-olds with mental retardation. Advanced items have been eliminated in subscales comprising the Early SB5.

Measure	**Wechsler Preschool and Primary Scale of Intelligence—Third Edition (WPPSI-III). Wechsler (2002).**
Age group	2-6 to 7-3 years.
Lowest scores available	Lowest Full Scale IQ of 45 at ages 2-6 to 3-11 years would be based on raw scores of 0 on four core subtests (Sattler & Dumont, 2004). Lowest Full Scale IQ ranges from 56 at ages 4-0 to 4-2 to 45 at ages 6-0 to 7-3.
Comments	Test is divided into two age groups (2-6 to 3-11, and 4-0 to 7-3 years). When children ages 4-0 and older who function at developmentally early levels are being tested, the section designed for younger children cannot be used to obtain an IQ. Blocks, cardboard puzzles, and brightly colored pictures, but no toys available. Some tasks for older age group have complicated formats and instructions. If used to diagnose mental retardation, the test is most appropriate for children over age 5.

Chapter 13

Assessment of Autism Spectrum Disorders

The purpose of this chapter is to provide assessors with the information they need to screen preschoolers for autism spectrum disorders (ASD), make a differential diagnosis in a referred child, and gather information relevant to designing an IEP for such a child. Early and accurate identification of young children with ASD is very important. Participation in a comprehensive, high-quality treatment program has been shown to be effective in increasing positive developmental outcomes in many children, some dramatically so; however, 2 years or more in such a program are needed during the preschool years (Filipek et al., 1999). Better outcomes are associated with earlier age of entry into a program (Dawson & Osterling, 1997; Rogers, 1998), probably because of the elasticity of the brain in early childhood (Huttenlocher, 1994).

CRITICAL FEATURES OF AUTISM SPECTRUM DISORDERS

Autism is a developmental disorder that is due to specific brain abnormalities attributed primarily to genetic factors that influence brain development very early in life (Szatmari, Jones, Zwaigenbaum, & MacLean, 1998). The precise causes are unknown, and no biological markers have been identified (Hill & Frith, 2004). Because autism is a developmental disorder, its behavioral manifestations vary a great deal according to age, ability level, and expressive language skills (Lord, Rutter, DiLavore, & Risi, 2002). The critical features of the disorder consist of deviance and delay in *socialization*, *communication*, and *imagination* (the last of these is referred to currently as "restricted repetitive and stereotyped patterns of behavior, interests, and activities"—American Psychiatric Association, 2000, p. 75). These three characteristics are known as "Wing's triad of social impairments" (Wing & Gould, 1979), and they have been embodied in the current diagnostic criteria for the autistic disorder in the *International Classification of Diseases*, 10th revision (ICD-10; World Health Organization, 1992) and the *Diagnostic and Statistical Manual of Mental Disorders*, fourth edition, text revision (DSM-IV-TR; American Psychiatric Association, 2000; see Table 13.1).

ASD is a label used to describe individuals with severe social impairments. As currently conceptualized, it includes five subgroups:

TABLE 13.1. DSM-IV-TR Diagnostic Criteria for Autistic Disorder

A. A total of six (or more) items from (1), (2), and (3), with at least two from (1), and one each from (2) and (3):

(1) qualitative impairment in social interaction, as manifested by at least two of the following:

(a) marked impairment in the use of multiple nonverbal behaviors such as eye-to-eye gaze, facial expression, body postures, and gestures to regulate social interaction
(b) failure to develop peer relationships appropriate to developmental level
(c) a lack of spontaneous seeking to share enjoyment, interests, or achievements with other people (e.g., by a lack of showing, bringing, or pointing out objects of interest)
(d) lack of social or emotional reciprocity

(2) qualitative impairments in communication as manifested by at least one of the following:

(a) delay in, or total lack of, the development of spoken language (not accompanied by an attempt to compensate through alternative modes of communication such as gesture or mime)
(b) in individuals with adequate speech, marked impairment in the ability to initiate or sustain a conversation with others
(c) stereotyped and repetitive use of language or idiosyncratic language
(d) lack of varied, spontaneous make-believe play or social imitative play appropriate to developmental level

(3) restricted repetitive and stereotyped patterns of behavior, interests, and activities, as manifested by at least one of the following:

(a) encompassing preoccupation with one or more stereotyped and restricted patterns of interest that is abnormal either in intensity or focus
(b) apparently inflexible adherence to specific, nonfunctional routines or rituals
(c) stereotyped and repetitive motor mannerisms (e.g., hand or finger flapping or twisting, or complex whole-body movements)
(d) persistent preoccupation with parts of objects

B. Delays or abnormal functioning in at least one of the following areas, with onset prior to age 3 years: (1) social interaction, (2) language as used in social communication, or (3) symbolic or imaginative play.

C. The disturbance is not better accounted for by Rett's Disorder or Childhood Disintegrative Disorder.

Note. Reprinted with permission from the *Diagnostic and Statistical Manual of Mental Disorders*, Fourth Edition, Text Revision.

1. *Autistic disorder* is the label used when children clearly meet the criteria specified in Table 13.1, but exhibit none of the other characteristics described below.

2. Children with *childhood disintegrative disorder* (CDD), formerly known as Heller's disorder, demonstrate normal development for a minimum of 2 years after birth (up to 10 years of age) before regressing significantly in multiple domains (e.g., motor, social relationships, toilet training, communication) and meeting criteria very similar to those for autistic disorder. Some cases have been attributed to encephalitis (Evans-Jones & Rosenbloom, 1978), but in most cases the cause is unknown even though nonspecific neurological signs may be present (e.g., seizures). Whereas "autistic regression" is relatively common at 15–24 months of age in children identified as having an ASD (Robbins, Fein, Barton, & Green, 2001), a CDD diagnosis is rarely given and may be dropped in the next revision of diagnostic criteria.

3. Children with *Rett's disorder* also have a period of normal development, but this period is shorter than in CDD (9–12 months), before meeting criteria very similar to those for autistic disorder. Identified only in girls, the disorder also includes a deceleration in head growth, loss of previously acquired hand skills, and poorly coordinated gait or trunk movements (see Hagberg, 2002, for a detailed description of the clinical manifestations of this disorder).

4. *Asperger's disorder* or *Asperger syndrome* is hard to distinguish from high-functioning autism (autism with a normal-range IQ). Indeed, many researchers do not consider it a separate disorder (e.g., Wing, 2000), given the presence of both disorders and PDDNOS (see below) in affected families (Bailey et al., 1995; Bolton et al., 1994), similar clinical presentations (Mayes & Calhoun, 2001), and similar long-term functioning (Gilchrist et al., 2001; Howlin, 2000). These children show the social impairment and restricted/stereotypic behaviors of autism, but not a language delay. (However, their language is not normal; they often show problems with the pragmatics of language, such as being unable to adjust their conversation to their listeners' interests and knowledge, using pedantic or scholarly language, and speaking in a monologue.) They must also demonstrate normal-range cognitive ability, exhibit age-appropriate self-help skills and adaptive behavior in all nonsocial areas, and be curious about the environment. Motor awkwardness or clumsiness is typically observed, as are onset or recognition after age 3 and higher Verbal than Performance IQ, but these are not part of the diagnostic criteria (Volkmar & Klin, 2000).

5. Finally, the category of *pervasive developmental disorder not otherwise specified* (PDDNOS), also known as *atypical autism*, is used for children who have severe and pervasive impairments in social interaction with either verbal or nonverbal communication impairments or stereotyped and repetitive behaviors or interests (American Psychiatric Association, 2000). It is also used for children who have impairments in all three areas, but who do not meet full criteria for autistic disorder or the other disorders described above.

In DSM-IV-TR, diagnosis of these disorders proceeds hierarchically. First a child is evaluated relative to the criteria for Rett's disorder and CDD. If the criteria are not met, then autistic disorder is considered. If a child does not meet criteria for autistic disorder, then Asperger syndrome is considered, and then PDDNOS. As Lord and Risi (1998) note, the boundaries between these categories are not always clear once language skills are taken into consideration. Whereas *autism* (the term we use in this chapter for autistic disorder, Rett's disorder, and CDD) can be clearly discriminated from the absence of ASD, it is difficult to discriminate clearly between autism on the one hand and Asperger syndrome or PDDNOS on the other side. Language skills (much lower in autism, at least early on) or loss of language after it has developed, and the severity of autistic symptoms, are what determine the difference in diagnosis.

Educational criteria for autism in the federal regulations implementing IDEA (Assistance to States for the Education of Children with Disabilities, 2000), which continue to be used in IDEA 2004, are written broadly enough to encompass all five disorders:

> *Autism* means a developmental disability significantly affecting verbal and nonverbal communication and social interaction, generally evident before age 3, that adversely affects a child's educational performance. Other characteristics often associated with autism are engagement in repetitive activities and stereotyped movements, resistance to environmental change or change in daily routines, and unusual responses to sensory experiences. The term does not apply if a child's educational performance is adversely affected primarily because the child has an emotional disturbance . . . (section 300.7(c)(1)(i))

The word *pervasive* in *pervasive developmental disorders* (PDD)—the label DSM-IV-TR uses for this group of disorders—was chosen to draw attention to the breadth of distortion in the developmental process, which makes it different from specific developmental disorders (e.g., speech–language problems or specific learning disabilities). However, the PDD label presents difficulties because, although the disorders do affect a range of developmental processes, often some domains are spared. Characteristic strengths of children with ASD are a focus on detail independent of context and include auditory memory, visual–spatial thinking, procedural memory (how to do things), and visual–motor coordination (Siegel, 2003). Some children with high-functioning autism may have Performance IQs within the normal range and show relatively intact intellectual ability (Rutter & Schopler, 1987). Although many children with autism fall in the mentally retarded range (about 25%–40% have IQs < 70), the 60%–75% who do not demonstrate the independence of social impairments from intellectual and language ability (Hill & Frith, 2004).

Throughout this chapter, as noted above, we use the term *autism* to refer to autistic disorder, Rett's disorder, and CDD, as the clinical presentations for these three are quite similar. Asperger syndrome and PDDNOS are referred to either by name or collectively as *nonautism ASD*. *ASD* is used to describe all five of the categories described above.

At this point, let us consider a case example and use it to illustrate the diagnostic criteria for autism, associated features, and alternative diagnoses.

Seth, age 4-10 years, was referred to the special education preschool program in his school district when he was age 2-11 years by his pediatrician because of suspected rheumatoid arthritis. He had been developing normally until the age of 2-4, when he developed a fever while on an antibiotic prescribed by his physician. His fever persisted, and he was hospitalized for a week. A full medical evaluation was unable to identify any cause for the fever or for the subsequent marked change in Seth's behavior. His mother reported that he became a totally different child after his illness. Originally a loving and typical 2-year-old, he was now a moody, difficult, and unusual child who had shown a dramatic regression in development. He had been using two- to three-word sentences and gestures to communicate effectively with his parents and two older sisters, expressed affection and interest in family members, and displayed age-appropriate play with same-age cousins and other children in his nursery group at temple. He was being reevaluated at age 4-10 because of staff dissatisfaction with his diagnosis and the need for a new IEP as he prepared to make the transition into a new school for kindergarten.

With an IQ of 44 (mental age of 2-8 or 32 months), Seth met criteria for moderate mental retardation and CDD. However, he was given the diagnosis of autistic disorder rather than CDD because in practice the CDD diagnosis is rarely, if ever, used. In terms of a *qualitative impairment in social interaction* (two criteria must be met in this area for a diagnosis of autistic disorder), he demonstrated impairments in four out of four areas:

1. Marked impairment in the use of multiple nonverbal behaviors, such as eye to eye gaze, facial expression, body postures, and gestures to regulate social interaction. While Seth would make eye contact, he did not use gaze, facial expression, or gestures to convey social information such as his feelings or desires.

2. Failure to develop peer relationships appropriate to developmental level. With a mental age of 32 months, Seth should have played well with two to three children in a group and engaged in associative play (sharing toys with other children and communicating about play activities, even though their play agendas might be different). Instead, his peer relationships were both delayed relative to his mental age and deviant. For example, across three playground observations, he did not play with other children or show any interest in them, except as targets of his physical aggression. His interactions with other children consisted of pushing children ahead of him in line, or punching or pinching them if they got near him when he attempted to climb across bars or go down the slide or up the stairs. During the three classroom observations (12 students, one teacher, and one aide), he initiated an average of four unprovoked assaults per session.

3. Lack of spontaneous seeking to share enjoyment, interests, or achievement with other people. These behaviors typically develop midway through the first year of life, and their absence is one of the first signs of autism. While these behaviors were typical of Seth prior to his fever, neither Seth's parents nor his teacher nor the speech pathologist could think of a single example of showing, bringing, or pointing out objects he found interesting, an achievement, or an experience he enjoyed. It was also not observed during three 30-minute observations and several hours of individual testing.

4. Lack of social or emotional reciprocity. Seth did not participate in simple social play or games unless they were part of a class activity and his response depended on physical prompting from his aide. He played alone, using people as objects to push out of the way or attack. His parents report that he was much more likely to hit them in the face or pinch than to seek affection, generally treating them "like a piece of furniture." He seemed to be aware of the feelings of others only when they were angry. He sometimes smiled appropriately when someone said something nice to him, but he also smiled at other times for no discernible reason.

In terms of verbal and nonverbal communication (one criterion must be met in this domain), Seth demonstrated impairments in four out of four areas:

1. Delay in, or total lack of, the development of spoken language (not compensated for by the use of gesture or other forms of communication). In making this determination in children with some language, mental age is critical. With a mental age of 2-8 (32 months), Seth had a language age of about 1-7 (19 months), based on the Communication subscale of the Vineland Adaptive Behavior Scales, Second Edition (Vineland-II) given to his mother and on the speech pathologist's assessment. This was a significant delay. He did not use gestures, such as nodding for "yes" or shaking his head for "no," to compensate for his language delay. He understood the word "yes," had some understanding of the word "no," had a vocabulary of at least 10 words, and was partially able to

follow simple instructions. Expressively, he used sentences of four or more words, but most were echolalic (i.e., he repeated back what was said to him or what he heard someone else say). He knew his own first, but not last, name; indicated preference by taking what he wanted; and used the names of some of the other children in the class (after an intensive instructional program to teach him the names).

2. Marked impairment in the ability to initiate or sustain conversation with others. Seth could answer some simple questions (e.g., he would say "yes" if he was asked whether he wanted a cookie), but would not initiate or respond to a second language turn to maintain a conversation (e.g., "Which cookie would you like?" when given a choice of two kinds).

3. Stereotyped and repetitive use of language or idiosyncratic language. Seth's language was very limited, and, as noted above, he displayed immediate echolalia. For example, when the aide asked him, "What's the matter?", he said "The matter"; when asked to give a sentence describing himself in group speech class, he repeated the last part of what the boy next to him had just said, "Jump in the pool."

4. Lack of varied, spontaneous make-believe play or social imaginative play appropriate to developmental level. At a mental age of 32 months, Seth should have been able to use miniature objects, such as animals, cars, or dolls, appropriately in pretend play. Neither his parents nor the school staff could recall or observe an instance indicative of make-believe play.

In terms of restricted, repetitive, and stereotyped patterns of behavior, interests, and activities, Seth demonstrated only one of the four criteria in this domain (only one was needed to meet the requirement). He showed a persistent preoccupation with parts of objects; his play consisted primarily of touching (rubbing with his fingers, sometimes licking) and banging toy cars and blocks together. Unlike some children with ASD, he did not have an intense, preoccupying interest or stereotyped movements, such as hand flapping or toe walking, and he did not adhere inflexibly to nonfunctional routines or rituals. In other words, he could easily make transitions from one activity to another, and he tolerated changes in his classroom and routine. His enrollment in a half-day special education preschool since the age of 3 had most likely promoted this flexibility.

The Childhood Autism Rating Scale (CARS; Schopler, Reichler, & Renner, 1988; to be described below) was completed with a high degree of agreement by the speech pathologist, the school psychologist, and Seth's parents. Seth obtained a total score of 38.5, with seven items scored at the "moderately abnormal" to "severely abnormal" level, placing him in the severely autistic range. He was most markedly deviant from normal in terms of his relationships with people, his motoric imitation, his unusual affect, his unusual pattern of auditory representation, his level of verbal communication, his activity level, and general impressions of the raters.

Seth's final diagnosis was very different from the initial formulation of his case as rheumatoid arthritis at age 2. In our experience, it is not uncommon for the initial referral question or diagnosis to differ from the final diagnosis, particularly in children diagnosed at very young ages.

DEFINITIONAL CRITERIA

Despite the fact that autism as a diagnostic group has the highest reliability and validity of any child psychiatric category (Klin, Lang, Cicchetti, & Volkmar, 2000; Rutter &

Schopler, 1987), there are a number of challenges in making a diagnosis. Children with ASD can look very different from one another on the surface (e.g., mute to fluent language, attractive to severely disabled appearance). Moreover, many of the symptoms overlap with those of other developmental disorders, yielding a number of individuals who exhibit some but not all of the symptoms. As Young, Newcorn, and Leven (1989) put it, "the diagnostic category of PDD is clear at its center (autism), unclear but very fuzzy at its margins" (p. 1781). Most of the difficulty involves making judgments at the extremes of the IQ range—especially between Asperger syndrome and autism in high-functioning children, and between autism and mental retardation in low-functioning children (Newsom & Hovanitz, 1997). Professionals become diagnostically confident through extensive contact with children with ASD and through knowledge and consideration of concurrent or alternative diagnoses.

That ASD can be fairly reliably identified is amazing when one considers the range of clinical phenomena that cloud the diagnostic picture (Young et al., 1989). The progression of normal development itself makes diagnosis particularly challenging. Human infants are born with relatively few functional capacities, which make it very difficult to identify specific disorders at early ages. ASD sometimes has a gradual onset, again making it very difficult to identify, especially when a retrospective history is taken from parents a few years later. Finally, the fact that normal development changes both normal abilities and abnormal symptoms also interferes with diagnostic assessments (Young et al., 1989). For example, there is evidence that the stereotyped and repetitive behaviors characteristic of ASD (e.g., hand flapping, sniffing objects) may occur infrequently in children with ASD before age 4 (at least those with mild to moderate mental disabilities as opposed to severe), and that many children with receptive and expressive language disorders and those developing typically display some of the social and language impairments characteristic of ASD at 20 months (e.g., not offering to share, not offering comfort, and nodding) but have outgrown them by 3-6 years of age, while children with ASD have not (Cox et al., 1999).

Qualitative Impairment in Social Interaction

The first criterion for autistic disorder has to do with the qualitative impairment in reciprocal social interaction that occurs between infants/toddlers and their caregivers. Emotional understanding and expression (e.g., smiling in response to a tickle or coo on the part of a parent) play a fundamental role in early communication and in the establishment and regulation of reciprocal relations from the earliest months of life. These "basic building blocks for interpersonal relationships" (Travis & Sigman, 1998, p. 65) are impaired in children with autism. However, social development is also delayed in children with mental retardation independent of autism (their social skills develop at a slower pace, and they tend to be less competent at each age). Thus it is essential to define any delay in social behavior in relation to a child's mental age. To assist evaluators, Table 13.2 shows the developmental progression of social interaction in normally developing children relative to the criteria for autistic disorder.

Recent research on both social development and this aspect of ASD has greatly refined our understanding of the particular social abnormalities that characterize ASD. A qualitative impairment in social interaction is now thought to represent a basic impairment in humans' "predispositions to orient to salient social stimuli, to naturally seek to impose social meaning on what they see and hear, to differentiate what is relevant from what is not, and to be intrinsically motivated to solve a social problem once

TABLE 13.2. Developmentally Oriented DSM-IV-TR Criteria for Autistic Disorder

Note. A diagnosis of autistic disorder requires at least two items from 1, and one each from 2 and 3; at least six overall. (See Table 13.1.)

1. Qualitative impairment in social interaction

a. **Marked impairment in the use of multiple nonverbal behaviors such as eye-to-eye gaze, facial expression, body postures, and gestures to regulate social interaction.**
   Developmental examples:
   - Gives a social smile in response to listening to caregiver (MA[a]: 1–4 mo)
   - Vocalizes in response to social smile and talking (MA: 1–6 mo)
   - Reaches out arms to be picked up (MA: 6–10 mo)
   - Responds to an inhibition on command (MA: 7–17 mo)

b. **Failure to develop peer relationships appropriate to developmental level.**
   Developmental examples:
   - Looks on with notable curiosity about peers (MA: 6–9 mo)
   - Engages in parallel play (MA: 20–24 mo)
   - Engages in associative group play (MA: 36–42 mo)
   - Engages in cooperative play (MA: 42–48 mo)

c. **A lack of spontaneous seeking to share enjoyment, interests, or achievement with other people (e.g., by a lack of showing, bringing, or pointing out objects of interest).**
   Developmental examples:
   - Social reference: Shares pleasure/information (MA: 8–14 mo)

d. **Lack of social or emotional reciprocity.**
   Developmental examples:
   - Shows anticipatory excitement at initiation of care (MA: 1–4 mo)
   - Discriminates between familiar and unfamiliar adults (MA: 3–8 mo)
   - Repeats a performance that is laughed at (MA: 8–17 mo)
   - Exhibits emotional reaction when caregiver is sad/hurt (MA: 24–30 mo)

2. Qualitative impairments in communication

a. **Delay in, or total lack of, the development of spoken language (not accompanied by an attempt to compensate through alternative modes of communication such as gesture or mime).**
   Developmental examples:
   - Listens selectively to familiar words (MA: 5–14 mo)
   - Points/uses gestures to get wants met (MA: 11–19 mo)
   - Labels several familiar objects/pictures (MA: 17–30 mo)

b. **In individuals with adequate speech, marked impairment in the ability to initiate or sustain a conversation with others.**
   Developmental examples:
   - Engages in simple nonverbal interactions (e.g., pat-a-cake) (MA: 5–12 mo)
   - Jabbers expressively, imitates words (verbal MA: 9–18 mo)
   - Uses words to make needs known (verbal MA: 14–27 mo)
   - Relates stories (verbal MA: 48–54 mo)

c. **Stereotyped and repetitive use of language or idiosyncratic language.**
   Developmental examples:
   - Repeatedly babbles consonant–vowel combinations (≤ verbal MA: 18–24 mo)
   - Echoes two or more of last two words heard (≤ verbal MA: 24–30 mo)
   - Refers to self by pronoun (verbal MA: 24–32 mo)

(continued)

TABLE 13.2. *(continued)*

d. **Lack of varied, spontaneous make-believe play or social imitative play appropriate to developmental level.**
   Developmental examples:
   - Carries and hugs a teddy bear or doll (MA: 14–18 mo)
   - Engages in concrete, repetitive play (MA: 24–32 mo)
   - Understands simple fairy tale (MA: 36–42 mo)

3. Restricted repetitive and stereotyped patterns of behavior, interests, and activities

a. **Encompassing preoccupation with one or more stereotyped and restricted patterns of interest that is abnormal either in intensity or focus.**
   Abnormal at any MA; developmental counterexample:
   - Persistently imagines being a fantasy character (e.g., fireman, ballerina) (MA: 36–42 mo)

b. **Apparently inflexible adherence to specific, nonfunctional routines or rituals.**
   Abnormal at any MA; developmental counterexample:
   - Insists on having transitional object along (MA: 18–24 mo)
   - Knows what comes next in bedtime routine (MA: 36–42 mo)

c. **Stereotyped and repetitive motor mannerisms (e.g., hand or finger flapping or twisting, or complex whole-body movements).**
   Developmental examples:
   - Flaps hands/tenses when excited (not > MA: 6–9 mo)
   - Rocks on all fours (just prior to crawling)

d. **Persistent preoccupation with parts of objects.**
   Developmental examples:
   - Puts most objects into mouth (not > MA: 12–16 mo)
   - Shows interest in strongly sensory stimuli (e.g., Pat-the-Bunny) (MA: 12–16 mo)

Note. Material in **boldface** reprinted with permission from the *Diagnostic and Statistical Manual of Mental Disorders*, Fourth Edition, Text Revision. Copyright 2000 American Psychiatric Association. Example adapted from Siegel (1991). Copyright 1991, adapted with permission from Elsevier.
[a] MA, mental age.

it has been identified" (Klin, Jones, Schultz, & Volkmar, 2004, p. 133). Lacking typically developing infants' already developed preferential looking at eyes and hearing of human sounds, and later extensive (by 12–14 months) use of eye tracking that results in joint attention, individuals with ASD prefer inanimate objects to people. The lack of salience of social stimuli impairs the capacity to form relationships, due to a marked lack of either awareness of the existence of feelings of others (Siegel, Vukicevic, & Spitzer, 1990) or understanding of those feelings if they are aware of them (Dissanayake, Sigman, & Kasari, 1996). Without the input and understanding of social stimuli, children with ASD lack the knowledge and motivation to construct a "theory of mind"—an ability to create mental representations of self and others as motivated by beliefs, desires, emotions, and intentions (Klin et al., 2004; Leslie, 1987; Leslie & Roth, 1993). While high-functioning children with ASD can learn and apply social skills in highly structured situations, they cannot apply these skills "on the fly," such as in a fast-moving playground game or in the cafeteria.

Under this general category are several subcategories of related concepts. Children with ASD show the following difficulties in social development:

• Inadequate reading of social or emotional cues (e.g., a mother's frown might be interpreted by a normally developing child as "She doesn't like it that I'm playing near the dirt in my best clothes," whereas it goes unnoticed and is definitely not interpreted by a child with ASD).

• Lack of response to other people's emotional states. These children appear to be unmindful of and uninterested in a familiar person's joy, excitement, or sadness (e.g., "Mom's in a bad mood, so it's probably not a good time to ask her to take me outside").

• Lack of modulation of behavior in accordance to their social context (e.g., they do not hurry through a coloring project when a preschool teacher indicates that very little time is left).

• Weak integration of social, emotional, and communicative behaviors. For instance, unlike a normally developing preschooler, a child with ASD will not act tired and whiny at the end of a long shopping trip to convey effectively to the mother, "I'm tired. We've been doing your stuff long enough. Now take me home and make a fuss over me." This child might throw a tantrum instead.

• Lack of social or emotional reciprocity (Rutter & Schopler, 1987). The affective display of children with ASD is less contingent upon social circumstances than is characteristic of children with other developmental delays. For example, when they laugh or smile, they are just as likely to do it in a random or self-absorbed way as they are when interacting socially (e.g., playing peek-a-boo). These noncontingent affective displays almost never happen with other developmentally delayed children (Snow, Hertzig, & Shapiro, 1987). Furthermore, children with ASD display significantly less positive affect than children in the delayed comparison group do.

As can be seen in these examples, the social behaviors described overlap a great deal with communicative behaviors; reading the social and emotional signals of others involves verbal and nonverbal communication. Thus it is hard to differentiate some features that could be categorized as "social interaction" from those that could fit just as well in the "verbal and nonverbal communication" category. A good example of this would be joint attention (e.g., catching an adult's eye and then looking at a cookie to convey desire) or pointing and other nonverbal gestures (e.g., beckoning) that involve both social interaction and communication. Children with ASD rarely point or use gestures. If they do, it is more likely to be for instrumental purposes (e.g., to get a cookie) than to share interest or get a parent to look at something (called *protodeclarative* pointing). It is as if they have no awareness (part of "theory of mind") that a social partner can understand their intent unless they demonstrate something. Instead of pointing or beckoning a partner to the refrigerator to indicate a desire for food or drink, they might pull a parent to the door of the refrigerator and then bang on the door.

Because children with ASD are seen as having a basic impairment in the ability to form relationships, there has been great interest in whether they form the attachment bonds seen in all children with consistent caregivers. Researchers have now concluded that they behave in ways consistent with the attachment behavior of nonautistic children of similar age and cognitive level. When scoring systems are modified to account for children's autistic behaviors, they show similar patterns and levels of attachment security, and security is related to caregiver sensitivity and responsivity just as it is in normally developing children (Capps, Sigman, & Mundy, 1994). These findings support the anecdotal comments of parents during clinical interviews that their children were "attached in their own way" (Shapiro & Hertzig, 1991).

Other unusual social behaviors include a lack of need for touch or for assistance when sick or upset; a lack of interest in the activities of others, which appears to interfere with their capacity to learn to imitate the behaviors of others (e.g., they frequently do not wave goodbye); a tendency and often a preference, even at fairly young ages, to be satisfied with being isolated and playing with themselves for long periods of time; and (as noted earlier) demonstrating an interest in inanimate objects that is often greater than their interest in people, even people they are quite familiar with (Young et al., 1989). Most children with ASD have no age-appropriate friends. A few make social approaches, but in an odd way (e.g., no eye contact, violating norms for intruding on physical boundaries). There are anecdotal reports by researchers studying peer relationships that higher-functioning children report having friends in childhood and adolescence, but the nature of these friendships is unclear (Travis & Sigman, 1998). Children with ASD, as previously noted, may show isolated and minor aspects of reciprocal social interaction; however, if there were too many such interactions, an ASD diagnosis would be ruled out, as in the following example:

> P. J., a boy age 3-10 years, was referred by his parents for a psychoeducational evaluation because of developmental delays and "unusual behavior." ASD was suspected because of language deviance and delay, variability in his response to people, and hand flapping. P. J. did not speak until the age of 1-6. When seen, he had a language age of 2-5 on the Vineland-II Communication domain; he answered questions and used language pragmatically. However, there were times when he would not engage in conversation at all. Periodically, he demonstrated immediate and delayed echolalia, had atypical sentence formation, and was inconsistent in his use of sounds. He frequently displayed interest and enjoyment when interacting with his parents and siblings, but he often preferred to play alone in his preschool class—where he had yet to establish any friendships, although he did display a keen interest in the other children. With a mental age of 2-8 (IQ = 75), he was in a class of normally developing children, where his language and cognitive impairments placed him at a social disadvantage; he was largely ignored by his classmates. Nevertheless, because of his social and emotional responsivity, spontaneous and emotionally appropriate sharing of enjoyment with his family members, use of gestures to regulate social interaction, and ability to imitate, he was not diagnosed with ASD but with a mixed receptive–expressive language disorder. P. J.'s case is diagnostically problematic, as some clinicians would consider him "on the spectrum" and others would not. Early intervention and close monitoring of his case would clarify the diagnosis over time.

Qualitative Impairments in Communication

The language of children with ASD is clearly *deviant* as opposed to just *delayed*. This can be complex to assess. Preschoolers with ASD can range from being completely mute to being verbally fluent but with deficits in pragmatics (communicating to get their needs met) and comprehension. Their deviance is most clearly seen when these children are compared to typically developing infants and preschool-age children (see Table 13.2). Typically developing infants use sounds and babbling in a reciprocal way to communicate well before they can talk. This is not often the case with infants with ASD. Deaf children who lack speech are able to develop a nonverbal means of communication, while most children with ASD do not (Rutter & Schopler, 1987). Four- and 5-year-old children with ASD do not resemble normal 2- and 3-year-old children, even though their language level may be equivalent. In their early language, children with ASD also tend to echo back very formally what they have just heard, as opposed to normal children. This immediate echolalic speech is a normal part of early language development (ages 18–22 months), just before the onset of phrase speech (Hart & Risley, 1999); however, when immediate echolalic speech occurs after 24 months and is the only form of language used, then this is a sign of abnormality, and a child should be referred. Delayed echolalia shows up in the frequent use of scripts or ritualized phrases from videos, television, commercials, or overheard conversations in the child's speech. Some such phrases become incorporated into appropriate conversational contexts or come to have communicative value. For example, one boy sang, "Mighty Mouse is here to save the day!" whenever he was worried or frightened. Other children show problems with pronouns (e.g., *we*, *she*, *they*) basic relational concepts (i.e., *over*, *above*), and other words that change meaning in context. Normally developing children, especially in their two-word phrases, use telegraphic and creative language thoroughly integrated with gestures and prosody to convey meaning effectively (e.g., "Mommy, hurt!" said with appropriate intonation and imploring facial expression to indicate that the new sandals being forced on were too tight). This is not characteristic of children with ASD (Shapiro & Hertzig, 1991).

It was once thought that this particular set of abnormalities had to do with general speech and language impairment. However, it is now clear that language features more often involve deviance rather than delay, although delay in development is also usual, particularly with individuals of lower intellectual ability (Berument, Rutter, Lord, Pickles, & Bailey, 1999). Morever, the abnormalities in ASD go well beyond speech to many aspects of communication. Studies have shown that often the strictly linguistic features of language, such as grammar, are the least affected in these individuals. Many youngsters with ASD have the sensory–motor capacity to communicate, and when they speak, they may articulate clearly. However, they do not seem to be able to grammatically assemble language or understand requests as automatically as typically developing peers. What appears to be most impaired is *the ability to use language for social communication* (Rutter & Schopler, 1987; Wilkinson, 1998). What is seen in children with both mental retardation and autism is the failure to develop nonverbal or verbal communication skills; only 37%–50% of children with autism develop phrase speech by age 6 (Billstedt, Gillberg, & Gillberg, 2005; Wilkinson, 1998). In children with high-functioning autism or Asperger syndrome, there is language that appears normal on the surface, but has impaired pragmatics (use of language) and prosody of speech (emotional tone and stress patterns).

For example, children with high-functioning autism or Asperger syndrome may *sound* fine, but what they say may be awkward and inappropriate in the conversational context (e.g., talking in a loud voice about cars that have headlights with windshield wipers during a school concert). They may also show a very poor response to what is being communicated to them (e.g., hitting the child sitting next to them on the rug after the preschool teacher reprimands the whole class for talking during story time). Or what they say may have very little communicative intent (e.g., a difficult-to-follow description of an event that occurred at some unknown time in the past) and may be of little or no interest to the listener (e.g., a recitation of the well-known and less familiar holidays occurring during the current month). They may miss the point of questions addressed to them even when the words used are in their vocabulary; this is particularly true if more than a factual reply is expected. Prosody is also affected. The cadence and emphasis in their remarks may be odd, and their speech may lack the emotional tone that conveys so much meaning in normal conversation (e.g., they may speak in a pedantic monotone instead of modifying their intonation when telling a joke).

Finally, the lack of imaginative or social imitative play reflects a real absence of activity and spontaneity in language in children with ASD. Their play often consists of banging, lining things up in rows, opening and closing closet doors, staring at the air conditioner fan or some other object to the exclusion of all else on the playground, or at best rigidly enacting a story that has been repeatedly told to them (such as "Goldilocks and the Three Bears").

Markedly Repetitive and Stereotyped Patterns of Behavior, Interests, and Activities

Repetitive and stereotyped patterns of interests, activities, and behaviors features are among the most striking and noticeable features in individuals with ASD. These features are not exclusively related to ASD, but have been shown by research to occur in other disorders and to be particularly associated with mental retardation, especially the more severe forms (Lewis & Bodfish, 1998). As mentioned earlier, they may not be present in very young children without severe mental retardation (under age 4) who later meet full criteria for autistic disorder (Cox et al., 1999). The symptoms reflecting these very restricted and repetitive patterns include some of those that make children with ASD appear the most bizarre and seem to dominate their activity. They include stereotypic movements (e.g., toe walking, rocking, pacing, hand flapping); preoccupation with objects or parts of objects (e.g., repeating letters of the alphabet and numbers, staring at palms held close to the face as they are moved back and forth to capture reflected light from the window); resisting minor environmental changes (e.g., a piece of meat cut into four rather than the usual three pieces, recess shifted to 15 minutes earlier than usual) and responding to them with unusual distress (e.g., having a major tantrum, angrily refusing a much-wanted ice cream cone unless Dad says, "Ice is nice," before offering it); or having a very narrow interest in only one or a few objects or activities (e.g., examining 250 squares of magazine cuttings, reading the telephone directory). In DSM-IV-TR, one item is required to be present under this last cluster of symptoms to meet criteria for autistic disorder and Asperger's disorder. Such symptoms may or may not be present in PDDNOS.

EPIDEMIOLOGY

The incidence and prevalence of autism in preschool populations in developed countries have risen steadily since an autistic syndrome was first defined by Kanner in the 1940s. Although the incidence of the particular syndrome defined by Kanner—that is, extreme social aloneness, language abnormalities, an obsessive desire for environmental sameness, good cognitive potential seen in splinter skills, and basically normal physical development with better fine than gross motor development (Kanner, 1943; Newsom & Hovanitz, 1997)—does not seem to have changed, that of autistic disorder as defined by DSM-IV-TR and ICD-10 (which includes Kanner syndrome but is less restrictive) has exploded, along with that of PDDNOS and Asperger syndrome. This increase has generated much controversy and raised questions about possible environmental causes, as genes alone could not account for it.

In an excellent analysis of the data, Wing and Potter (2002) explore several reasons why incidence and prevalence rates have risen. They note that the relative rarity of ASD and the lack of easily identifiable biological markers make it difficult to conduct epidemiological studies, given the large samples that are needed for reliable findings. It is also difficult to compare findings across studies, because definitions of ASD (e.g., Kanner's, DSM's, Wing's triad of social impairments, etc.), case-finding methods (e.g., review of records, repeated yearly assessments) and the types of ASD included in the screenings vary. (To date, only the study by Chakrabarti & Fombonne [2001] has included all types of ASD; most exclude Rett's disorder or Asperger syndrome, etc.) Wing and Potter (2002) note that the highest rates are found when studies' case-finding methods include close and repeated involvement in the assessment of children's development over the first 5 years of life (usually smaller samples), and the lowest rates are found when studies have used state records of children known to agencies (usually the largest samples). Although these authors do not rule out the possibility that environmental factors might precipitate ASD in a small number of genetically vulnerable children, they attribute the rise in prevalence to other factors.

The leading environmental hypothesis is that the mercury formerly used as a preservative in the combined measles, mumps, and rubella vaccine is related to the increase in rates. However, Wing and Potter (2002) note that in the four studies of ASD incidence (number of new cases identified each year, as opposed to prevalence, the number of all known cases) examining this hypothesis, the slope in the rise in cases did not change when the vaccine was introduced. This indicates that the vaccine was not a factor in the rise in cases, unless it played a role in such a small number of children that the incidence rate was unaffected. In addition, the one epidemiological study that has held diagnostic criteria and case-finding methods constant while following successive birth cohorts in the same population has not found an increase in rates of autism from 1972 to 1985 (Fombonne, du Mazaubrun, Cans, & Grandjean, 1997), suggesting that a rise in prevalence has not occurred. Finally, a retrospective cohort study of all Danish children born between 1991 and 1998 found no association between receipt of the vaccine and diagnosis with autism or another ASD (Madsen et al., 2002). Because of the size and completeness of the cohort and the meticulous collection of data on Danish children, this last study is particularly compelling. Wing and Potter (2002) conclude, as have others (e.g., Bryson & Smith, 1998; Chakrabarti & Fombonne, 2001; Hyman, Rodier, & Davidson, 2001), that the rising rates are probably due to (1) greater parent and public awareness (e.g., mentally retarded children were often not evaluated for autism in the past; when they are, the rates for autism rise and mental retardation without autism fall—Croen, Grether, Hoogstrate, & Selvin, 2002); (2) broader definitions of ASD (e.g., DSM-IV-TR criteria are less restrictive than Kanner's criteria, Asperger syndrome was virtually unknown until the 1980s); and (3) better measures and training for diagnosis, which increase professionals' willingness to make a diagnosis and reduce the age at which children are identified.

In general, ASD diagnoses are much more common than previously believed. While the prevalence of Kanner syndrome (2–5 per 10,000), CDD, and Rett's disorder (considerably less than 1 per 10,000 each) have not changed, there has been a large increase in the number of identified cases of autistic disorder (now estimated as 17 per 10,000), Asperger syndrome (2–8 per 10,000) and PDDNOS (36 per 10,000), with at least 60 per 10,000 for all ASD (Chakrabarti & Fombonne, 2001, 2005; Fombonne, 1999). Even these figures may be underestimates. Most recently, Baird et al. (2006) conducted a careful prevalence study of all 9- to 10-year-old children in the South Thames region of the United Kingdom who had an ASD diagnosis or were known to have social and communication difficulties. They found a prevalence rate of 38.9 in 10,000 for autism and 77.2 in 10,000 for nonautism ASDs. This gave an overall prevalence, which the authors considered a minimal estimate, of 116 per 10,000 or 1% of the child population.

The presence of ASD is not related to SES (American Psychiatric Association, 2000; Gillberg, 1990) or to ethnic or racial group. All studies have shown a significantly greater number of boys with ASD, with boy–girl ratios averaging 3:1 to 4:1. Ratios have been lowest (2:1) in cases with severe and profound mental retardation (Lord & Schopler, 1985; Ritvo et al., 1990; Wing, 1981b) and greatest in cases of Asperger syndrome (10:1) and Kanner syndrome (Gillberg, 1990; Wing, 1981a). Girls with autism tend to have significantly lower IQs than boys, with one large study finding that all female participants had IQs ranging from 13 to 23 points lower (Ritvo et al., 1990). The prevalence of epilepsy in children with ASD ranges from 5% (Ciadella & Mamelle, 1989) to 40%, with increased prevalence as children move into adolescence and early adult life (Gillberg, 1992; Billstedt et al., 2005).

ETIOLOGY

Autism and other ASDs are now almost universally seen as a "behavioral-defined syndrome of a neurological impairment with a wide variety of underlying medical etiologies" (Gillberg, 1990, p. 106), although the strongest evidence is that the specific brain abnormalities are due to genetic factors that influence brain development very early in life (Szatmari et al., 1998). The evidence for strong genetic factors comes from twin studies, which show high concordance for monozygotic twins (this means that twins sharing 100% of their genetic material are very likely to both have symptoms of autism—about 60% have the full syndrome, and 90% have related social/cognitive symptoms), while dizygotic twins (who share 50% of their unique genes) show low concordance rates (Cook, 1998). Siblings of children with autism have an elevated risk of having the disorder of 4.5% compared to a population risk of 0.05%–0.1%, again indicating a strong genetic influence. Statistical modeling suggests that two to five genes, acting in a multiplicative manner (i.e., mutations must be present at two or more locations to make an individual susceptible) lead to the disorder (Pickles et al., 1995). The lack of full concordance in monozygotic twins suggests (1) that environmental factors, such as infections and teratogens, may play a role in the expression of symptoms of autism in those who are genetically vulnerable (Burger & Warren, 1998; Rodier & Hyman, 1998); and (2) that the alleles or genetic material associated with autism may be fairly common (Rodier & Hyman, 1998). This is an area of intense research effort.

DIFFERENTIAL DIAGNOSIS

Despite the earlier-noted fact that autism, as a diagnosis, has the highest reliability/validity of any child psychiatric category, making a differential diagnosis can be challenging. Many of its symptoms overlap with those of other developmental disorders, resulting in individuals who exhibit some but not all of the symptoms. Again as noted earlier, this is particularly true at the ends of the intellectual continuum. At the lower end of the continuum, autistic disorder must be distinguished from CDD and Rett's disorder, and autism in general must be differentiated from mental retardation without autism, stereotypic movement disorder, and reactive attachment disorder. At the upper end, high-functioning autism or PDDNOS must be distinguished from Asperger syndrome, and all of these must be differentiated from childhood-onset schizophrenia, developmental language disorders, attention-deficit/hyperactivity disorder (ADHD), obsessive–compulsive disorder (OCD), Tourette's disorder, selective mutism, visual impairments, and hearing impairments. To clarify the diagnostic picture, it is very useful to understand differences between ASD and alternative diagnoses. These differences are summarized in the sections that follow.

Mental Retardation

About 25%–40% of children with ASD have mental retardation (IQ < 70; Chakrabarti & Fombonne, 2005), while 25%–40% of children with mental retardation have ASD (Shah, Holmes, & Wing, 1982; Wing & Gould, 1979), including about 10% of children with Down syndrome (Howlin, Wing, & Gould, 1995). Children with autism are generally much more impaired in cognitive and language development than those with Asperger syndrome or PDDNOS (Chakrabarti & Fombonne, 2001). Given the high percentage of children with mental retardation who exhibit behaviors that overlap with autism (echolalia, self-stimulation, self-injurious behavior, attentional deficits), it can be particularly difficult, diagnostically, to distinguish between autism and mental retardation. This difficulty increases with the degree of mental retardation.

A key distinguishing feature is that the majority of children with mental retardation react responsively to the social efforts of others by seeking attention and showing affection. As do normal infants and toddlers, they establish eye contact and respond with pleasure to touch and affection. It takes some time, but they can learn to integrate taught social skills with genuine emotional connection. On the other hand, many infants with autism fail to cuddle, very often show gaze aversion or abnormal gaze, and exhibit apparent dislike of or indifference to physical contact. As they grow older, they exhibit little pleasure or interest in the presence of others and are generally unresponsive socially. Children with high-functioning autism or Asperger syndrome are socially odd, even if they are interested in others, demonstrating very poor reading of social cues. They can be taught social skills prosthetically (e.g., using rules of thumb, social scripts, peer coaches), but they lack the genuine empathetic understanding of others that allows for smooth social interaction and emotional connectedness. A useful guideline is the DSM-III-R axiom that PDD abnormalities are not normal for *any* stage of development, whereas in mental retardation "the person behaves as if he or she were passing through an earlier normal developmental stage" (American Psychiatric Association, 1987, p. 31).

A second distinguishing feature is the evenness of the cognitive deficits in the population with mental retardation as opposed to the scatter or unevenness of skills in the population with ASD. Typically, children with autism show significant scatter across all IQ levels (Freeman, Ritvo, Needleman, & Yokota, 1985; Rutter, 1987). Children with autism tend to do the worst at tasks that involve higher-level verbal skills, problem solving, and social comprehension. They perform significantly better on nonverbal tasks, particularly those involving visual–spatial skills (e.g., Block Design on the WPPSI-III) or rote memory (Freeman et al., 1985; Rutter, 1987). Children with Asperger syndrome often have just the opposite pattern on IQ tests, with higher verbal than performance IQs (Volkmar & Klin, 2000). In rare cases, a child may show isolated exceptional abilities (traditionally known as "idiot savant" characteristics), such as unique skills in memory, mathematics, mechanics, or music (Schreibman, 1988; Wing, 1990). In fact, most savants have autism (Rimland & Fein, 1988). A final area that may distinguish between the two groups is that children with ASD tend to approach normal levels of physical development, while children with mental retardation often show delays. However, a child with ASD may be strong in gross motor skills but weak in fine motor skills, or vice versa (Gillberg, 1992). It is important to note that motor skills are often a *relative* strength for such a child, not necessarily a normative strength relative to same-age peers.

Stereotypic Movement Disorder

Stereotypic movement disorder consists of the repetitive overdoing of nonfunctional behaviors, many of which are quite common in early childhood (e.g., body rocking, skin picking, and head banging). However, the behaviors may be carried out at a level where the child's involvement in them interferes with development in other areas. This disorder is common among moderate or severely mentally retarded children and children who live in institutions or suffer from sensory deprivation, such as a hearing or vision impairment. Typically, children exhibiting this disorder do not meet other criteria for ASD.

Reactive Attachment Disorder of Infancy or Early Childhood

Children with reactive attachment disorder fail to establish normal attachment to a caregiver or exhibit indiscriminate sociability, usually as a result of severe psychosocial deprivation or child abuse. These children often appear listless and unresponsive when attempts are made to engage them. Like children with ASD, they do not make appropriate eye contact, do not express pleasure by smiling, and do not reach out to others as readily as normal children. Often language impairment is present along with other developmental delays, and frequently mental retardation is suspected. In order to give this diagnosis, it must be clear that *grossly* negligent care (e.g., being left in a crib alone virtually all of the time, being fed with a propped-up bottle and rarely held, crying but never being responded to) preceded the onset of the disorder. Often this diagnosis is confirmed when a child shows significant improvement after placement in a responsive, warm, and stimulating environment. These children differ from children with ASD in that they do have the potential for normal development, normal imaginative play, and social responsiveness. Also, they do not have the behavioral and sensory oddities or motor abnormalities of children with ASD, and they typically do not qualify for a diagnosis of mental retardation once given an appropriate environment.

Developmental Language Disorders

Because language difficulties are common to both groups, there is diagnostic confusion at times, between ASD and language disorders. The least diagnostic difficulty occurs when children have an expressive disorder with good comprehension alone. Children who have mixed receptive–expressive language disorder and children with semantic–pragmatic impairments (also called *semantic–pragmatic disorder*; Rabin & Allen, 1998) are the ones who cause the most confusion. Children with these disorders are often unable to understand and process language, leading to difficulties in expression and appropriate social interaction because of their inability to make shared meaning with a social partner (Brook & Bowler, 1992; Rabin & Allen, 1983, 1998). Pragmatic difficulties are common in children with high-functioning autism or Asperger syndrome, as well as in these children with language disorders. All are poor at conversational turn taking and may display echolalia, unusual paucity of vocabulary, problems in structuring conversational content to take into consideration the role or interests of a conversational partner, and superficially complex syntax but odd or inappropriate semantic content (Brook & Bowler, 1992; Howlin & Rutter, 1987; Rabin & Allen, 1987). Some children with semantic–pragmatic disorders have abnormalities in joint referencing behavior, which is a characteristic of ASD, although they are much more likely to grow out of it in the preschool years than those with ASD (Cox et al., 1999). Clearly, there is some overlap between these two diagnostic groups, and this needs to be further examined by researchers. On the whole, children who have developmental language disorders are capable of and do form warm relationships with their caregivers, adults, and peers. They rarely show odd motor behavior and tend not to relate to objects in an idiosyncratic manner (Young et al., 1989).

Childhood-Onset Schizophrenia

Children with schizophrenia and those with ASD share several common features, such as social impairment, resistance to environmental change, and inappropriate affect (Phelps & Grabowski, 1991). However, they differ considerably in terms of typical age of onset, level of intellectual functioning, language impairment, and the presence of hallucinations or delusions. In children with ASD, language may be absent, deficient, deviant, or excessive (Rumsey & Denckla, 1987). ASD is characterized by the failure to develop complex language in younger or more intellectually impaired children, or by odd language with pragmatic deficits in higher-functioning children. In schizophrenia, language acquisition and development are often normal (although sometimes delayed), but as the illness develops language is characterized by illogical thinking, loose associations, and impaired discourse (Caplan, 1994), as in the example below.

> A 6-year-old child with schizophrenia who was seen in our clinic responded as follows to the Children's Apperception Test card showing an older dog spanking a puppy with a toilet in the background: "Sally said, 'Don't you fear me because this is a bathroom is going to be.' Little Matthew said, 'Okay, Sally [mumble]' . . . I really really really love you. And valentine I wish care more. Cause she's . . . By the title was dogs. Two dogs. They were serious. . . . "

Childhood-onset schizophrenia also typically appears after the age of 6, usually at puberty (the child just described was unusual in this respect). Children with schizophrenia often use language to create an involved fantasy life; an absence or impairment of fantasy life is a characteristic of ASD. Newsom and Hovanitz (1997) note that children with schizophrenia also have a narrowing of interests, as well as bizarre somatic complaints, fears that seem irrational or paranoid, and a negative and interpersonally difficult manner.

Attention-Deficit/Hyperactivity Disorder

Many children with ASD have ADHD; however, the converse is not true. One study found that 74% of children with high-functioning autism had been misdiagnosed as having ADHD (Jensen, Larrieu, & Mack, 1997). One of us (M. R. B.) assessed a 7-year-old boy, classified as "developmentally delayed" on his IEP by the referring preschool program, whose classroom behavior was creating a great deal of distress for his competent young special education teacher. Nothing she did engaged him or obtained his compliance; she wondered whether he might have ADHD. He did meet criteria for ADHD, but he also met criteria for autistic disorder—a diagnosis that rules out a further diagnosis of ADHD.

Obsessive–Compulsive Disorder

Like children with OCD, children with ASD may show the combination of persistent, unusual ideas and repetitive behaviors. Although ritualistic behaviors (e.g., rigidly lining up toys in a specified order) and stereotyped behaviors (e.g., head banging, body rocking) are characteristic of children with both ASD and OCD, there is an absence of intrusive thoughts in children with ASD, and these behaviors do not appear to be driven by anxiety. From the little research that we have on OCD in young children, it appears that onset of their symptoms may be more acute rather than insidious, and that the first symptoms may appear at a later age than they do in ASD (usually adolescence and rarely before age 6). Children with ASD often pursue their interests with pleasure and may become frustrated and angry if their repetitive behaviors/thoughts are interrupted. Youngsters with OCD, on the other hand, experience a great deal of internal discomfort and are dismayed by the degree of control that their symptoms have over their lives (Young, Grasic, & Leven, 1990). They are interested in their environment and have normal social and cognitive development (Tsai, 1992). Some children with ASD meet criteria for both disorders as they grow older.

Tourette's Disorder

Tourette's disorder involves involuntary rapid movements (e.g., tongue protrusion) or vocalizations (e.g., throat clearing, grunting) that may on the surface resemble ASD when they manifest themselves in severe or unusual form (e.g., twirling when walking, sniffing objects or materials). Tourette's disorder, however, typically correlates with normal intelligence and normal language and social development, as well as a typical and developmentally appropriate range of interests and activities. Sometimes there is social withdrawal because of embarrassment or social rejection due to the symptoms, but this can be easily differentiated from the extreme social aloofness or socially odd behavior seen in children with ASD. Children with ASD, on the other hand, do not seem to be at all disturbed by their facial or vocal tics; in fact, they may engage in them with satisfaction. Cases of Tourette's disorder can co-occur with ASD, especially Asperger syndrome, however, so that the presence of one does not necessarily rule out the other (Kadesjö & Gillberg, 2000; Young et al., 1989).

Selective Mutism

In selective mutism, children do not speak in some (not necessarily all) of their environments. By definition, there is no speech at school. However, these children may communicate effectively through gestures and short utterances. Although children with ASD may speak more in familiar than in unfamiliar environments, in general they show a pervasive disturbance in language that is apparent in all situations.

Visual Impairments

Visual problems often result in children's being unable to initiate, maintain eye contact, visually imitate, and participate in sighted children's play—all aspects of reciprocal engagement with others facilitated by vision. They may hold their hands or objects in their hands close to their eyes in order to examine them closely. However, differential diagnosis is not difficult in these cases, because these children typically do not show other typical cognitive difficulties and they tend to communicate and relate socially in a sometimes delayed, but normal, manner. This is not to stay that children with visual problems do not have autism; a surprisingly high number of congenitally blind children meet criteria for autism, and even those who do not meet criteria may have autistic features as rated by the CARS (Hobson & Bishop, 2004). Visual acuity and field screening exams can be done to rule out underlying visual difficulties.

Hearing Impairments

With any child for whom language is absent or delayed, hearing needs to be evaluated immediately. The practice parameters for the diagnosis and evaluation of autism that the Child Neurology Society and the American Academy of Neurology have jointly issued (Filipek et al., 1999) specify that a formal hearing evaluation must be conducted by an audiologist who has experience with very young children and difficult-to-test populations, even if the child has passed a neonatal audiology screening. They recommend that the evaluation be comprehensive and include a battery consisting of behavioral audiometric measures, electrophysiological procedures, and an assessment of the functioning of the middle ear (see Filipek et al., 1999, for a detailed description of measures and procedures). Children with ASD are frequently suspected of being deaf, due both to their lack of age-appropriate language development and to their lack of social responsiveness. Some children with hearing impairments do become socially withdrawn and make little effort to communicate. However, the majority show a normal interest in communication and use gestures. Children who have had partial hearing impairment, including severe ear infections, may have atypical language development. They may have difficulty hearing certain sounds, or they may produce certain sounds in an odd manner; they may speak little or in an idiosyncratic fashion (Young et al., 1989). An audiology evaluation and review of medical records should clarify the role of hearing in the language and social symptoms observed.

CONCURRENT MEDICAL CONDITIONS

Clear concurrent medical conditions are present in 10%–37% of children with ASD (Chakrabarti & Fombonne, 2001; Gillberg, 1990), with higher rates associated with more thorough evaluations and greater severity of mental retardation. Accordingly, there is a strong argument to be made for having any child suspected of ASD receive a comprehensive medical evaluation and regular medical evaluations on a continuing basis. The practice parameters of the Child Neurology Society and the American Academy of Neurology (Filipek et al., 1999) recommend that physicians should search for acquired brain injury or other comorbid conditions, as well as difficulties that are relatively common in ASD. These include gathering information on "pregnancy, delivery, perinatal history, developmental history including milestones, regression in early childhood or later in life, encephalopathic events, Attention Deficit Disorder, Seizure Disorder (absence or generalized), depression or mania, troublesome behaviors such as irritability, self-injury, sleep, and eating disturbances, and pica for possible lead exposure" (p. 470). They also recommend that the physician question the parents or other caregivers about autism, mental retardation, fragile X syndrome, and tuberous sclerosis complex in the extended family, and recommend chromosomal or genetic evaluation if any of these disorders are present. Finally, they recommend physical and neurological examinations that include assessments of the following: (1) head circumference; (2) unusual features of the face, limbs, or stature that might suggest a need for genetic evaluation; (3) neurocutaneous abnormalities (using an ultraviolet Wood's lamp); and (4) gait, muscle tone, reflexes, and cranial nerves (see Filipek et al., 1999, for an extended discussion of medical considerations relevant to ASD).

DEVELOPMENTAL PROGRESSION AND LONG-TERM PROGNOSIS

It is difficult to make a confident diagnosis of any ASD prior to the age of 2–3 years. Support for early diagnosis comes from professional observations and studies of the home movies taken by families of children later diagnosed with ASD. Some children with ASD exhibit typical characteristics of such a disorder from the beginning (Adrien et al., 1991, 1992; Baranak, 1999; Werner et al., 2000). These include unusual ways of looking (or not looking) at the caregiver's face, which in some cases are present at birth; deficits in anticipating a reaction during the first few months of life; and the development of other deviant behaviors, such as stereotyped movements, refusal of or withdrawal from body contact, a lack of exploration of the environment, a lack of initiative, and noted passivity. Fewer social smiles and a lack of response to one's name being called have also been noted (Frith, 2003). Deviant patterns of babbling, speech, and early language have not emerged as typical features among young children with ASD even when language development has been specifically examined. This suggests that the focus of early identification should be shifted from speech and language problems to abnormal perceptual responses and the social dysfunctions noted above.

Some infants show normal development but then regress (called "autistic regression") between 15 and 24 months in age, losing initial language development and social behaviors. Early versus late onset of symptoms, and regression versus no regression, are not related to intellectual ability or symptom severity (Werner, Dawson, Munson, & Osterling, 2005).

Frith (1991, 2003) describes the preschool years of a child with ASD and the child's family as being very troublesome. It is during this stage that ASD begins to produce a very recognizable pattern of behavior that can be reliably identified by professionals and is clearly deviant to most parents. Although children with ASD show enormous individual variation in behavior, parents usually begin to become concerned about severe language delay or complete absence of language; their children may have some language, but appear not to comprehend what others are saying to them or even what is going on around them. Frequently deafness is suspected and evaluated before being ruled out, as it should be for differential diagnosis. The interpersonal skills and the social interaction of these children are both very limited and often deviant, and imaginative behavior and pretend play are absent. Children seem isolated from others—looking through people, or not even glancing at others' faces. They are unmotivated by wanting to please parents; social praise doesn't work; and finding anything that motivates them can be difficult. Play routines and general behavior are often focused on a very narrow set of activities, and these children may make their family life very difficult by their lack of tolerance for any change in routine. Higher-functioning children, particularly those with nonautism ASD, may be diagnosed with ADHD or an anxiety disorder (e.g., OCD) in the preschool years, with the diagnosis becoming clarified after formal schooling begins. Asperger syndrome is rarely diagnosed before children start formal schooling (Gillberg, 2002).

As children with ASD move into early school age (between 5 and 10 years of age), children who have shown very little language may demonstrate considerable improvement, especially if they have received early intervention. With development of language frequently comes an increased ability for the child to get his or her needs met, and for parents and school professionals to communicate their interests to the child. The level of language development, in terms of ability to communicate, and general intellectual ability are the most important prognostic indicators of how well a child will do both in school and in the future. Some children with severe mental retardation may not develop any language or develop only minimal language, either of which indicates a poor prognosis. On the other hand, brighter and more language-competent children may show a very rapid improvement in both their social and communicative behavior around this age, which bodes fairly well for their long-term development. These children fall into the group with high-functioning autism, Asperger syndrome, or PDDNOS. They tend to have very fluent, well-developed language by the age of 5 or 6, even though their language and social interactional style are remarkably odd. This may occur even if their language was severely delayed at first.

Some of these high-functioning children may become more interested in others as they grow older, although their social ineptness remains. Anxiety is often a co-occurring problem, especially separation anxiety or OCD (Gillot, Furniss, & Walter, 2001). When they move into adolescence, they often begin to realize that they are very different from their peers, and they may become depressed as a result. Some high-functioning individuals may go on to complete undergraduate or graduate education; they may be able to live independently and have meaningful jobs or careers, as long as their work does not require a high level of interpersonal skill. They tend to lead fairly restricted social lives, although some do marry and have families (Frith, 1991; Howlin, 2000). As these individuals move into adulthood, characteristics initially contributing to the diagnosis of ASD persist. Most of them will continue to meet criteria for a diagnosis of ASD, although some will move in and out of the diagnosis. It should be noted that some adults with ASD develop concurrent psychiatric disorders.

Adults with autism and mental retardation resemble other adults who have mental retardation. They leave home for group care in adolescence or young adulthood and have a higher rate of mortality than their age group. The most comprehensive study to date is the population-based study by Billstedt et al. (2005) of 120 individuals diagnosed with autism or atypical autism in childhood. Both initial and follow-up evaluations used state-of-the-art assessment criteria and measures for the time. On initial assessment 46% were found to have severe mental retardation, 33% mild mental retardation, 15% borderline or low-average IQs, and 5% average IQs. At follow-up 13–22 years later, when the participants were 17–40 years of age, 5% had died; four individuals led independent but severely isolated lives; and 78% had poor or very poor functioning, defined as severe obvious disabilities, inability to lead independent lives, and either few or no clear verbal or nonverbal communicative skills. Forty percent had epilepsy; 50% had engaged in moderate to severe self-injurious behavior; 32% had been prescribed neuroleptic medications by independent psychiatrists to control major behavior problems; and 49% had major medical problems needing medical attention. Higher childhood IQ level and some communicative phrase speech at age 6 were correlated with better adult outcomes. There was no difference in functioning between those diagnosed in childhood with autism and those diagnosed with atypical autism. These outcomes were much worse than predicted by the authors. They caution against generalizing these results to children currently diagnosed with high-functioning autism or Asperger syndrome.

ASSESSMENT

Given the breadth of developmental domains in which children with ASD show delay or deviance, a very strong case can be made for having multidisciplinary teams conduct the assessments of these children. Siegel, Plinar, Eschler, and Elliott (1988) found that parents most often expressed their initial concerns to their pediatrician when their child was from 1 to 6 years of age. An early and accurate diagnosis was most likely to be made if the pediatrician referred the child to a multidisciplinary team than if the child was sent on serial visits to single examiners. It appears that the multidisciplinary team was better able to pull single-discipline assessments together into a diagnosis, which may relate to their shared sense of responsibility in making a definitive diagnosis. Although seeing a series of examiners was better than seeing a single professional, the process and stress of going to a series of appointments to have conditions ruled out was confusing to parents.

We recommend that, if possible, any assessment of a child suspected of having ASD be conducted following a thorough hearing evaluation, not a screening. At a minimum, the assessment team should consist of a psychologist, a speech–language specialist, and an appropriate physician (child psychiatrist, neurologist, pediatrician) or pediatric nurse who coordinates the medical component of the evaluation. If the evaluation includes the development of an IEP, which is generally the case, then an early childhood special educator is an essential member of the team.

Essential Features of the Assessment

The assessment of a child suspected of having ASD should begin with the administration of at least one screening measure. If a screening measure indicates valid reasons for concern, the next step should be establishing the child's mental age and developmental level for diagnostic purposes; this would include the administration of an individualized intelligence test, if possible, and an adaptive behavior measure. Diagnostic assessment should also include structured observation of the child's interaction with his or her caregiver and another adult in a play situation, as well as a structured parental interview. Assessment for curricular/intervention planning should include measures of self-help skills, language competencies, social competencies, and any behavior problems that may interfere with instruction and management. Finally, the child should receive a medical examination to identify concurrent medical conditions and/or alternative diagnostic possibilities. The sections that follow describe procedures and measures for all these aspects of assessment except the medical exam.

Screening for ASD

As noted earlier, the Child Neurology Society and the American Academy of Neurology have published practice parameters for the diagnosis and evaluation of autism (Filipek et al., 1999). These recommendations were developed by a distinguished multidisciplinary panel after a systematic examination of the problem. Although the recommendations focus primarily on physical examinations done by pediatricians seeing young children, many of them are also useful for mental health and educational professionals who see very young children. Specifically, it is recommended that all children be referred to the local educational agency or public health authority responsible for young children with disabilities if the following are seen:

- No babbling by 12 months.
- No pointing or other gestures by 12 months.
- No single words by 16 months.
- No two-word spontaneous (not echolalic) phrases by 24 months.
- Any loss of any language or social skills by any age.

Filipek et al. (1999) also recommend that if pica (the eating of nonfood substances, such as feces, dirt, paint chips, etc.) is identified, a child should be referred for a lead screening by a pediatrician. The presence of any of these signs is not necessarily indicative of ASD per se, but can suggest language or more general developmental delays as well. We recommend that educational or health agencies receiving referrals for children who exhibit some of these symptoms of developmental delay be explicitly screened for ASD prior to a more detailed evaluation.

Several very quick and valid screening measures for ASD have been developed for very young children. They vary in terms of the ages for which they are most appropriate, the source of information used to derive scores, and (to a minimal extent) the time involved in administering them. Some of them have acceptable reliability and validity to screen for ASD in children under the age of 3, the youngest age focused on in this book. We include such measures because preschool assessors are increasingly being asked to assess very young children with suspected ASD, given the promise of improved outcomes with early, intensive intervention. The measures presented are not exhaustive. We have been selective in choosing measures to highlight in this chapter; others are reviewed in Appendix 13.1.

Checklist for Autism in Toddlers

The Checklist for Autism in Toddlers (CHAT; Baron-Cohen, Allen, & Gillberg, 1992) includes a 10- to 15-minute interview with a parent or other caregiver, and observation of the child's response to an interviewer's questions and behaviors. It can easily be incorporated into a screening of toddlers by mental health, educational, or physical health professionals (Baron-Cohen et al., 1996, 2000). It was developed for screening by general practitioners or health visitors with a large general population of children at 18 months of age (excluding children already identified as developmentally delayed). The CHAT is presented in Figure 13.1. A parent is asked nine straightforward questions (section A) that screen for either ASD or developmental delay without autism. In addition, a professional observing the child has to answer five questions based on his or her observations (section B). Children who receive "no" responses to items A5, A7, Bii, Biii, and Biv are considered to be at high risk for ASD; children who receive "no" responses to items A7 and Biii, and/or items A5 and Biii, are considered to be at high risk for non-ASD developmental delay. Normally developing children are expected to receive "yes" responses to all five of the ASD risk items.

The diagnostic and predictive validity of the CHAT was examined in an English population of over 16,000 children evaluated at 18 months of age, rescreened at 3 and 5 years, and followed up at 7 years (Baird et al., 2000). The CHAT was found to have excellent specificity, in that if a child passed, there was little chance that he or she had ASD (98% specificity on one administration, 100% if rescreened 1 month later). However, sensitivity (percentage of children with the disorder who are accurately identified) was only 38% on the initial screen and dropped to 20% if a 1-month rescreening occurred. Still, the false positives (children falsely identified by the CHAT as having ASD) almost all had another developmental disorder (language disorders, general developmental delay, cerebral palsy, attention deficit disorder, etc.), indicating that the CHAT is a highly accurate and efficient screening measure for ASD and developmental delay in toddlers without severe developmental disabilities. Scambler, Rogers, and Wehner (2001) further explored the ability of the CHAT to differentiate autism from other severe developmental disorders using a rigorously diagnosed sample of 44 children (26 with autism)

Child's name:

Date of birth:

Age:

Child's address:

Phone number:

Section A. Ask parent:

1.	Does your child enjoy being swung, bounced on your knee, etc.?	Yes	No
2.	Does your child take an interest in other children?	Yes	No
3.	Does your child like climbing on things, such as up stairs?	Yes	No
4.	Does your child enjoy playing peek-a-boo/hide-and-seek?	Yes	No
5.	Does your child ever pretend, for example, to make a cup of tea using a toy cup and teapot, or pretend other things?	Yes	No
6.	Does your child ever use his/her index finger to point, to ask for something?	Yes	No
7.	Does your child ever use his/her index finger to point, to indicate interest in something?	Yes	No
8.	Can your child play properly with small toys (e.g., cars or bricks) without just mouthing, fiddling, or dropping them?	Yes	No
9.	Does your child ever bring objects over to you (parent), to show you something?	Yes	No

Section B. General practitioner's or health visitor's observation:

i.	During the appointment, has the child made eye contact with you?	Yes	No
ii.	Get child's attention, then point across the room at an interesting object and say, "Oh look! There's a [name a toy]!" Watch child's face. Does the child look across to see what you are pointing at?[a]	Yes	No
iii.	Get the child's attention, then give child a miniature toy cup and teapot and say, "Can you make a cup of tea?" Does the child pretend to pour out tea, drink it, etc.?[b]	Yes	No
iv.	Say to the child, "Where's the light?" or "Show me the light." Does the child point with his/her index finger at the light?[c]	Yes	No
v.	Can the child build a tower of bricks?	Yes	No
	If so, how many? Number of bricks:	______	

[a]To record yes on this item, ensure the child has not simply looked at your hand, but has actually looked at the object you are pointing at.

[b]If you can elicit an example of pretending in some other game, score a yes on this item.

[c]Repeat this with "Where's the teddy?" or some other unreachable object, if child does not understand the word "light." To record yes on this item, the child must have looked up at your face around the time of pointing.

FIGURE 13.1. The Checklist for Autism in Toddlers (CHAT). To be used by general practitioners or health visitors during the 18-month developmental check-up. From Baron-Cohen, Allen, and Gillberg (1992). Copyright 1992 by the Royal College of Psychiatrists. Reprinted by permission.

ages 2–3 years. The sensitivity and specificity of the CHAT was 65% and 100%, respectively, with no false positive and 35% false negatives, using the original authors' medium-risk criteria. These criteria were that the child must fail the protodeclarative pointing items by both observer and parent, A7 and Biv, but may pass one or more of the items A5, Bii, and Biii regarding pretend play or gaze monitoring. Sensitivity rose to 85% while maintaining specificity of 100% in the Scambler et al. sample, when the minor modification of considering children to meet criteria for risk of autism if a parent answered yes to either A5 on pretend play or A7 on protodeclarative pointing rather than answering yes to both items. These findings reinforce the utility of this measure for front-line screening of young children for autism.

Screening Tool for Autism in Two-Year-Olds

The Screening Tool for Autism in Two-Year-Olds (STAT; Stone, Coonrod, & Ousley, 2000) is a promising measure for children 24–35 months of age. Unlike the CHAT, which is a combination of parent report and direct observation, the STAT consists of 12 items administered within a play-like interaction that takes 15–20 minutes. Included are 2 play items, 4 imitation items, 4 directing-attention items, and 2 items involving response to requests (these 2 are included to facilitate interaction, but are not included in the score). An example of an imitation item is the examiner's rolling a toy car and saying to the child, "Do this." An example of a directing-attention item is the examiner's inflating a balloon and then letting it go so it flies across the room. The child passes or fails the item depending on whether he or she directs attention to the balloon or not.

Because of the developmentally sensitive nature of the items, the STAT is likely to be helpful only as an initial screening tool for young children within its age range. It is particularly useful in that it covers the age ranges when children with ASD are most likely to be referred for professional evaluation, and it is brief and easy to administer. More research is needed on its predictive and concurrent validity with standardized diagnostic measures.

In addition to the CHAT and the STAT, which include an observational component, there are five teacher/parent rating scales (requiring 5–10 minutes each to complete) that could easily be administered as part of an evaluation in order to screen out ASD. However, two of these measures—the Autism Behavior Checklist (ABC), which is part of the Autism Screening Instrument for Educational Planning—Second Edition (ASIEP-2; Krug, Arick, & Almond, 1993), and the Gilliam Autism Rating Scale—Second Edition (GARS-2; Gilliam, 2005)—have serious problems with false negatives (i.e., they sometimes identify children as not having autism when they do). The ABC and GARS are not recommended, but are reviewed in Appendix 13.1.

Modified Checklist for Autism in Toddlers

The CHAT was modified into the Modified Checklist for Autism in Toddlers (M-CHAT; Robbins et al., 2001) for ages 16–30 months, after it became clear that the CHAT's focus on autism missed children with PDDNOS and those who went through an "autistic regression" after 18 months; as noted earlier, such a regression most often occurs between 15 and 24 months (Robbins et al., 2001). The M-CHAT is a 23-item, yes–no parent report screening measure that builds on the parent report section of the CHAT. A child fails the initial screening if he or she fails any 3 of the 23 items or 2 of 6 critical items. The most discriminating item is 7. "Does your child ever use his/her index finger to point, to indicate interest in something?" The M-CHAT has excellent psychometric characteristics and is recommended for this age range. Recently Wong et al. (2004) have developed the Checklist for Autism in Toddlers-23 (CHAT-23) for the identification of ASD in Chinese children. The CHAT-23 is a combination of the 23 M-CHAT parent-rated items (with a 4-point Likert scale rather than yes–no format) and the five CHAT observation items. The authors recommend the parent-rated items for stage 1 screening followed by observation for stage 2 if the child screens positive for an ASD. The CHAT-

23 has promising psychometric characteristics and a wider age range, 13–86 months, than the M-CHAT.

Pervasive Developmental Disorders Screening Test—Second Edition

The Pervasive Developmental Disorders Screening Test—Second Edition (PDDST-II; Siegel, 2004) is the first clinical screening tool for all types of PDD or ASD in children 12–48 months old. It is also the first screening measure to be standardized with large groups of children with other types of neurodevelopmental disorders, so that ASD can be differentiated from nonspecific developmental delays, mental retardation, language disorders, infant psychiatric disorders, and typical development. It consists of three forms designed to be used in three different clinical settings: stage 1, the Primary Care Screener (pediatrics and family practice settings, 22 items); stage 2, the Developmental Clinic Screener (special education, department of developmental services, Early Start, or child-finding settings, 14 items); and stage 3, the Autism Clinic Severity Screener (clinics for autism-specific assessment, 12 items). The forms for stages 1 and 2 are used primarily to differentiate children with a high likelihood of ASD from those with mild or transient developmental concerns and from those with related non-ASD developmental disorders, respectively; the stage 3 form is primarily utilized to differentiate autism from other PDD. There are also 41 supplemental items that may be used to elicit further information on history or other diagnostic signs.

The PDDST-II has excellent sensitivity and specificity for stage 1, but not for stages 2 and 3. No screening measure is good at distinguishing autism from other types of ASD, the goal of stage 3. The M-CHAT is more accurate in differentiating ASD from other developmental disorders. The ease of administration and the detailed probes provided in the manual make the PDDST-II a user-friendly screening tool. It has the largest age range of any of the screening measures for young children.

Social Communication Questionnaire

The Social Communication Questionnaire (SCQ; Rutter, Bailey, & Lord, 2003) is a 40-item, parent report screening measure originally designed to serve as a companion screening measure for the Autism Diagnostic Interview—Revised (ADI-R, discussed later). The items chosen for the SCQ tap into symptoms of ASD and match items on the ADI-R found to have discriminative diagnostic validity. This screening measure is applicable to subjects of any chronological age above age 4-0 years, provided that their mental age is at least 2-0 years.

The SCQ has a Lifetime form that is completed with reference to an individual's entire developmental history, and a Current form that is completed with reference to the individual's behavior during the most recent 3-month period. According to the authors, the Lifetime form produces results that are relevant for a referral for a more complete diagnostic assessment, while the Current form produces results that are pertinent to understanding everyday living experiences and to evaluating treatment and educational plans over time.

The SCQ is very good at discriminating children with autism from mental retardation and children with ASD from those with other diagnoses clinically determined after administration of the ADI-R and the Autism Diagnostic Observation Scale (ADOS, also discussed later). Scores from the SCQ agree with those on the ADI-R at the total score level and the domain level. Level of agreement is not affected by age, gender, language ability, or Performance IQ. The SCQ is easy to administer and score, and closely matches current research criteria for autism. Further research is needed to determine how the SCQ would fare as a screening instrument in the general population, since all the findings thus far concern children who have come to clinical notice for one reason or another.

Diagnosis of ASD

Once a child meets criteria for cutoffs on a screening measure for ASD, professionals need to obtain a mental age so that they can effectively make a diagnosis using DSM-IV-TR criteria. This is particularly important with young children, who may not have reached a developmental level where certain DSM-IV-TR criteria come into play. Three of the DSM-IV-TR criteria are likely to be irrelevant for a substantial number of young children: poor peer relationships, limited conversational skills, and stereotyped language. It is impossible to judge the quality of peer relationships in children who have mental ages below 24 months, and one cannot evaluate the language delay or abnormalities of children who haven't yet acquired spoken language (Stone et al., 1999). The DSM-IV-TR criteria most likely to be met in young children are lack of nonverbal social communicative behaviors, lack of social or emotional reciprocity, and delayed acquisition of spoken language. In addition, several studies of preschool children with autism have shown that the domain of repetitive patterns of behavior, interests, and activities is highly variable and is not seen in a number of cases. Some researchers speculate that adherence to routines or rituals, endorsed infrequently for young children, may emerge later (i.e., at ages 4–6) in children with autism (Lord, 1995; Lord, Storoschuk, Rutter, & Pickles, 1999; Stone et al., 1999).

The best indicators of prognosis for an individual with ASD are IQ and the presence or absence of spoken language by age 6 (Billstedt et al., 2005). Wing's model (Wing & Gould, 1979) suggests that nonverbal or Performance IQ should be measured separately and should be used as the assessment of the child's overall intellectual competence. Second, the triad of social impairments that characterize ASD should then be evaluated, to see whether they reflect delay in development beyond the nonverbal mental age. A child's communicative competence can be better evaluated if measures of both verbal and nonverbal intelligence are used, since children with autism by definition have deficits in the verbal domain, and verbal competence is what distinguishes autistic disorder from Asperger syndrome. Verbal IQ should also be assessed because it and other measures of language functioning are powerful predictors of long-term outcomes, such as adaptive functioning and academic achievement (Venter, Lord, & Schopler, 1992). Chapters 11 and 12 provide guidance on selecting an appropriate measure of intelligence and organizing observations as a check on the validity of the IQ score obtained.

Normal developmental milestones can be used as benchmarks for assessing whether a child's behavior actually meets DSM-IV-TR criteria. Table 13.2 displays the mental ages at which developmental milestones are typically achieved, relative to the DSM-IV-TR criteria for autistic disorder. It is an updated version of a table developed by Siegel (1991) using DSM-III-R criteria. These milestones, and the child's development relative to them, can be used to determine how delayed a child is, how much the child has lost if there has been regression, or whether there has been little or no development in those areas. Siegel (1991) recommends that the "50% rule" (i.e., the child is functioning at a level half or less of what is expected for a child his or her age) be used in order to determine whether a particular behavior is sufficiently delayed to be judged as atypical.

Establishing a mental age for children suspected of ASD at the initial assessment can be difficult to do. With 25%–40% of children with ASD having comorbid mental retardation, professionals are often faced with a limited number of tests that are both appropriately normed for a child's chronological age and adequate for assessing children with very limited mental ability. In addition, many preschool children suspected of ASD lack test-taking skills (e.g., sitting still, attending to the examiner's directions, and responding appropriately to simple verbal prompts) which are necessary in order to participate in an assessment process. As a result, quite a few young children with autism are untestable with individually administered intelligence tests until they have learned these skills in an early intervention program. Examiners are forced then to rely upon mental ages obtained from adaptive behavior scales administered to the primary caregiver and, if possible, a teacher or daycare worker who sees the child on a regular basis. This is less of a problem with children suspected of nonautism ASD.

We recommend that evaluators administer an adaptive behavior rating scale to the primary caregiver first, to obtain some idea of a child's mental age in the domains of communication, daily living skills, socioemotional, and motor functioning. If a child has been previously evaluated by a speech–language pathologist, physical therapist, or occupational therapist, estimates of mental age in the areas of language, fine motor, and gross motor functioning are likely to be available. These can be then cross-checked with what has been reported by the primary caregiver. Not only does adaptive behavior provide a starting point for estimating what tests might be appropriate to assess intellectual ability, or what module to use to assess ASD with the ADOS (see below), but it provides useful information for diagnosis and educational planning as well. We return to this topic later.

Procedures for Preparing to Administer Cognitive Measures to Children Suspected of Having ASD

Prior to testing a young child suspected of having ASD (or any young child, for that matter), the professional should assess the child's (1) test-taking skills, (2) reinforcement preferences, and (3) knowledge of any basic concepts being used on the measure selected for administration.

Test-taking skills involve being able to look at the examiner's face (except in cases where this is culturally inappropriate); sit still with hands in the lap while giving the examiner visual attention; and respond to simple verbal prompts and queries, such as "Look at me," "Point to _____," and "Give me ______." If the child is being seen in an educational setting, the child's test-taking skills can be observed in the classroom, or the teacher or daycare worker can provide reliable information on whether these skills are present. Intervention programs target these skills, as they are essential for instruction. If the child is being seen for the first time out of his or her usual educational setting, the ASIEP-2 (discussed in detail later) has a subtest that systematically evaluates a child's ability to imitate and respond to adult prompts and instructions. It has a straightforward, standardized format and provides information on test-taking skills as well as diagnostically useful information relative to a diagnosis of autism. As indicated earlier in the chapter, children with ASD tend to have a very difficult time with imitation—a skill assessed by this subtest. The subtest also assesses receptive language (by noting whether a child responds appropriately to adult direction) and expressive language; these two areas are also often delayed or deviant in ASD, although they are also problematic for individuals with developmental delays or language disorders. If a child does not have test-taking skills, assessors may want to wait until they are acquired, or an attempt has been made to teach them, before giving an intelligence test. Another option is to give a measure like the Griffiths Mental Development Scales (which includes observation, parent report, and direct assessment) to obtain an estimated IQ, and then to retest (or recommend retesting) later after a child has entered an instructional program and acquired test-taking skills (see Chapter 11).

It is very important to select powerful reinforcers when one is evaluating children suspected of having ASD. Individuals with ASD are often not motivated by the same things that motivate typical children or even children with mental retardation (e.g., social reinforcement). Teachers and parents tend to be very good sources of information on reinforcers for assessment. Many intervention programs have taken to assessing preferences empirically by recording the child's approach to stimuli presented singly or concurrently with other stimuli (known as *multiple stimuli without replacement*; DeLeon & Itawa, 1966). A variation on this procedure is to record duration of engagement with stimuli. Hagopian, Long, and Rush (2004) review preference assessment procedures for children with developmental disabilities. Examples of effective reinforcers include the following: giving a child a favorite food or snacks, a "high five," tickles, or time to play with a puzzle; letting the child look into a closed jar for candy tokens (if these have been used in an educational program), play with push-button or jack-in-the–box cause-and-effect toys, or read books (e.g., phone books, dictionaries, baseball cards, books about animated characters like Thomas the Tank Engine); or allowing the child to have a minute or so of nondestructive self-stimulatory behavior (e.g., lining up certain objects or toys).

Finally, as mentioned before, most measures of cognitive functioning, emergent literacy, or language involve instructions that include basic concepts (e.g., *after*, *different*). It is very important to assess children's knowledge of basic concepts prior to administering such tests. If children fail a subtest that involves the use of instructions they do not understand, one cannot conclude that they could not do the subtest if they understood the basic concept. For example, one boy, age 4-11 years, received 0 points on the Numbers Reversed subtest of the Woodcock–Johnson III Tests of Cognitive Abilities because he did not know the concept *backward*. He repeated the digits forward as they had been read to him, and appeared indignant when the examiner kept repeating the instruction to "Say the numbers *backward*." When the subtest was readministered to him a week later, after he had been taught the concept, he received a subtest score that placed him in the low-average range; this raised his General Intellectual Ability score into the borderline range from the mildly mentally retarded range. We recommend that the Boehm Test of Basic Concepts—Third Edition: Preschool Version (Boehm, 2001) be administered prior to the administration of any intelligence test, and that those concepts that are essential for instructions be taught (or an attempt at instruction be made) to a child prior to administering the intelligence battery. Another good source of information on basic concept knowledge for a child enrolled in an educational program may be his or her program book, which sometimes includes concepts mastered and those being taught. Parents, teachers, nannies, and speech pathologists are other good sources of information on concept knowledge. Strategies for teaching each basic concept are included in the *Boehm Resource Guide of Basic Concept Teaching* (Boehm, 1976).

Once test-taking skills are assessed and judged to be minimally adequate, effective reinforcers are identified, and knowledge of basic concepts is sufficient, then the evaluator can proceed with the administration of the selected battery. Research shows that the IQs of children with ASD are clearly stable past infancy (Lord & Schopler, 1989) and are the best predictors of academic success (Rutter, 1983; Venter et al., 1992), while measures of adaptive behavior are the best predictors of independent functioning. In order to obtain the most valid assessments, some experts recommend that intelligence testing wait until children have had time to adjust to the testing location or center. Other frequently used adaptations are administering the test in the presence of a child's mother or another familiar adult who can help maintain the child's attention, and administering the tests in short chunks of time (e.g., several subtests at a time; Harris & Handleman, 2000; Koegel, Koegel, & Smith, 1997). Research shows that attending carefully to factors that will promote the motivation and increase the attention of children with ASD is likely to result in significantly higher IQs that are consistent over time (Koegel et al., 1997) than when motivational factors are not attended to. All adaptations used during testing should be described in the report.

Assessment of Adaptive Behavior

Adaptive behavior is important to assess in any child referred for a suspected disabling condition. Standardized assessment of adaptive behavior is part of a diagnosis of mental retardation. It can also inform the diagnosis of ASD, in that these children tend to have a very typical pattern of adaptive behaviors; it's useful in identifying strengths and weaknesses for educational and treatment planning; it can document progress over time in important adaptive behaviors; and it can be used for program evaluation (Carter et al., 1998). Although there are a number of very good adaptive behavior scales (see Chapter 12), some of which have been recently normed, the focus here is on the Vineland Adaptive Behavior Scales, Second Edition (Vineland-II) because of the extensive use of the original Vineland in research on ASD, its demonstrated usefulness in case identification, and its supplementary norms for individuals with ASD (Carter et al., 1998).

The Vineland-II (Sparrow, Cicchetti, & Balla, 2005), which has norms for individuals from birth to 90 years of age, assesses daily living skills, communication, socialization, motor skills (optional above age 6), and minor and significant maladaptive behavior. Children with ASD show a unique pattern of scores across the different dimensions of adaptive behavior in relation to peers matched for both chronological and mental age. When compared to children with mental retardation, who have relatively flat and low profiles across adaptive behavior areas, children with ASD tend to show significant impairments in the Socialization domain of the original Vineland and the Vineland-II (particularly on the Interpersonal Relationships subscale), relative strengths in Daily Living Skills, and an intermediate score in Communication (Carter et al., 1998; Kraijer, 2000; Loveland & Kelly, 1991; Sparrow, Cichetti, & Balla, 2005; Volkmar et al., 1987). The Vineland-II profile comparisons were developed because of this unique pattern. The authors developed profiles for two groups of individuals with ASD, defined according to chronological age and verbal skills: individuals between ages 2 and 10 who used fewer than five words purposefully and meaningfully each day, and individuals between ages 3 and 19 who used more than five words purposefully and meaningfully each day.

The Vineland-II profiles were based on norms from a sample of 77 individuals with ASD who had been diagnosed with either the ADI-R (Rutter, LeCouteur, & Lord, 2003), the ADOS (Lord et al., 2002), or the original GARS (Gilliam, 1995), along with data on intellectual functioning. Of this sample, the majority were male (67 cases), ranging in age from 3 to 18, largely verbal (60%), and mostly European American; over 68% of their mothers had at least some college education.

The authors recommend comparing an individual's level and pattern of performance to those of individuals in particular diagnostic groups when one is conducting a psychological assessment. They provide examiners with profiles related to (1) high-functioning autism and Asperger syndrome, and (2) autism and mental retardation. While the standard scores are useful for evaluating an individual's overall adaptive functioning and strengths and weaknesses, the profile comparisons provide evidence for differential diagnosis. However, the authors caution against using the profiles alone as diagnostic evidence. A more detailed description of the Vineland-II is provided in Chapter 12.

Observational Measures for Diagnosis

Once a mental age is obtained, assessors are in a position to determine whether a child meets criteria for ASD, given his or her developmental level. They then need to gather information on the child's behavior relative to criteria for these disorders. This is typically done through the use of structured observation measures and parent interviews.

CHILDHOOD AUTISM RATING SCALE

The CARS (Schopler et al., 1988) is a diagnostic instrument designed to discriminate children with autism from those with other developmental disorders. It can be used with children age 2 and up. Although the CARS is designed as an observational instrument, information obtained from records, parent, or other professionals' reports (e.g., the speech pathologist) can be incorporated into the rating system as well, making it very flexible. The CARS has 15 subscales on which a child's behavior is rated on a continuum ranging from 1 ("within normal limits") to 4 ("severely abnormal"), relative to the child's chronological age. Since half-point values are allowed, this is in essence a 7-point, behaviorally anchored scale. The 15 behavioral subscales include Relating to People; Imitation; Emotional Response; Body Use; Object Use; Adaptation to Change; Visual Response; Listening Response; Taste–Smell–Touch Response and Use; Fear or Nervousness; Verbal Communication; Nonverbal Communication; Activity Level; Level and Consistency of Intellectual Response; and General Impressions.

The manual provides detailed behavioral descriptions for each domain to guide professionals in the ratings of the behavior, taking the peculiarity, frequency, intensity, and duration of each behavior into account. Total scores can range from 15 to 60 and result in a classification of either no autism, mild to moderate autism, or severe autism. Excellent training tapes are available from the authors showing a skilled examiner administering the Psychoeducational Profile—Revised (PEP-R; Schopler, Reichler, Bashford, Lansing, & Marcus, 1990), a measure widely used for treatment programming, which is excellent for eliciting behavior relevant to scoring the CARS. (The PEP-3 is discussed later in the chapter.) The first tape illustrates each subscale on the CARS and the types of information that would result in different ratings of the subscale items, while the second tape provides an opportunity for professionals learning the CARS to rate items themselves and receive feedback on their responses.

There is a wealth of reliability and validity data supporting interrater agreement, test–retest reliability, and concurrent validity with other diagnostic systems (Pilowsky, Yirmiya, Shulman, & Dover, 1998). The CARS is as accurate in diagnosing children with autism as any other measure, including the ADI-R, which is often considered the "gold standard" of diagnostic measures of autism (Pilowsky et al., 1998). In addition to its psychometric qualities, the strengths of the CARS are that it has a very flexible format and can be easily used by professionals from different backgrounds who have just learned to work with autistic children. Observations can be made in classrooms, clinics, or other settings, and this information can be combined with information from parent interviews and records. And it is not tied to any diagnostic system, but was based on a comprehensive review of a wide variety of classification systems and theoretical perspectives. Its weaknesses are that it is not based on the most recent and widely used diagnostic system, DSM-IV-TR/ICD-10. As such, it includes domains that are no longer considered essential criteria for a diagnosis of autism (e.g., the subscales on Taste–Smell–Touch Response and Use, Activity Level, and Fear or Nervousness). Some have suggested that the CARS would be better if the severity rating gave greater weight to social relatedness and social communication, as opposed to unusual responses to the environment (Prizant, 1990). It has also been criticized because it assumes that the user will understand what developmentally appropriate behavior is across the domains assessed. However, this is a criticism that can be fairly applied to all of the diagnostic systems in use: They all assume some knowledge of what is appropriate behavior for a given chronological or mental age.

Given the excellent psychometric characteristics of the CARS, its tremendous flexibility, the relatively short amount of time needed to administer it (30–45 minutes), and the availability of excellent training tapes, we think it is a very good measure for clinicians to use in diagnosing preschool children with ASD.

AUTISM DIAGNOSTIC OBSERVATION SCALE

The other observation measure with excellent psychometric properties is the ADOS, which is a "semistructured, standardized assessment of communication, social interaction, and play or imaginative use of materials for individuals who have been referred because of possible autism or other pervasive developmental disorders" (Lord et al., 2002, p. 1). It was developed to be used in conjunction with the original Autism Diagnostic Interview (ADI; LeCouteur et al., 1989), a caregiver interview, the revised version of which is described later. The instrument was developed for research on autism and other ASD, with a particular focus on disentangling expressive language levels from the severity of the autism/ASD.

The ADOS consists of four modules, 30 minutes in length, only one of which is given to an individual. Module 1 is designed for preverbal children who, at most, have single words and do not use spontaneous speech consistently. Module 2 is designed for children who have some flexible phrase speech but who are not verbally fluent (an age equivalent of at least 30 months is required on the original Vineland expressive language subdomain). Module 3 is for children and adolescents with fluent speech, while module 4 is for adolescents and adults with fluent speech (an age equivalent of at least 48 months on the original Vineland expressive language subdomain is required for both modules).

Modules 1–3 consist of 10–14 activities with accompanying ratings. Modules 1 and 2 are conducted while examinees are moving around a room and engaging in activities that would be of interest to young children with no or limited language. Children are rated on their use of gestures, unusual eye contact, quality of social overtures, response to joint attention, and so forth, while engaged in free play, a snack, a birthday party activity, bubble play, and the like. Module 3, to be used with verbally fluent young children, requires a greater ability to sit still and a higher language level than module 2, but two-thirds of the activities overlap. The examiner takes notes during specific tasks, but scoring for each item is based on the entire observational setting.

The ADOS uses algorithms (a set of rules) to determine whether an individual meets criterion for autism or for nonautism ASD in two of the three domains used to diagnose autism: (1) Social Interaction, and (2) Communication. A child needs to exceed the threshold or cutoff score on each of these domains, as well as on a combined Social

Interaction–Communication score, in order to meet criteria for autism or nonautism ASD. These two domains are focused on because the test developers found that it was very difficult in 30 minutes to consistently obtain information relevant to the third diagnostic domain of restricted and repetitive patterns of behavior, activities, and interests. Scores can be given for behaviors in this domain if they are displayed during the observation.

One of the great advantages of using the ADOS is that it takes only 30 minutes for a skilled examiner to administer it. It also has excellent psychometric characteristics. The ADOS is very accurate at discriminating autism from non-ASD and at discriminating PDDNOS from non-ASD, but is not as accurate at differentiating autism from other ASD diagnoses (Mahoney et al., 1998). Its most outstanding feature is that it controls for the role of language in the criteria for ASD. An individual who exceeds the cutoff for autism on one of the modules is being compared to individuals with comparable levels of expressive language. Relative to those individuals, the child is judged to be deviant or not in his or her use of speech and gesture as part of social interaction. This alone, of course, is insufficient for a diagnosis of autism. To meet criteria, a child must also display evidence of restricted and repetitive patterns (which can be demonstrated during the ADOS or in another context) and meet criteria for age of onset of the first symptoms. The ADOS does provide some information for treatment planning, in that there are opportunities for children to make requests for action, food, or objects; this provides an opportunity to observe how they make requests and in what circumstances they are able to communicate interest or needs.

The drawbacks of the ADOS include the amount of training, supervision, and practice needed to master its use. Competent use requires broad experience with both normally and abnormally developing young children, a sophisticated understanding of ASD and language development, and complete knowledge of a complex instrument. There are also some problems with the test stimuli. There are a great number of highly attractive toys (the authors worked hard to make the items motivating for children with ASD), but some are flimsily constructed (e.g., feather, eyeglasses), and many are unwashable—a major problem for clinics that see young children with health problems. Test stimuli fragility is a problem for any test, but is particularly troublesome for a measure designed for use with developmentally disabled preschoolers. Finally, all of the human figures (those depicted in books, dolls) are white and middle-class. Given the relative insensitivity of children with ASD to social cues, this is unlikely to influence a child's performance; however, it sends an unnecessarily noninclusive message to observing parents and professionals.

We think the ADOS is a very good measure for children with chronological ages of 15 months or more and with nonverbal mental ages of 20 months or more. We particularly recommend its use by clinicians who see many cases of autism, if these clinicians can put in the extra time to become and stay reliable on the measure. Its clinical use may be restricted to settings that specialize in ASD, unless research demonstrates enough added value in diagnostic accuracy to make it compelling for clinicians to be trained in it.

Structured Parent/Caregiver Interviews

A structured interview with a parent or caregiver is an essential part of the comprehensive evaluation of any child with ASD. An interview with both parents is ideal, but at the very least, the primary caregiver (usually the mother) should be interviewed. Nannies or other regular caregivers such as grandmothers should also be interviewed if they spend a great deal of time with the child. Included in the interview should be an exploration of the following: any prenatal or perinatal difficulties; the acquisition of developmental milestones; the extent to which the child was responsive to cuddling and human contact in infancy; the child's responsiveness as a toddler and preschooler to social interactions with family members and peers; the child's speech–language development and current abilities; the presence of any self-stimulating or self-injurious behaviors; the degree to which the child tolerates a change in routine; and the degree to which the child's emotions are appropriate to the social environment and circumstances (Schreibman, 1988). Two structured interviews have been developed by research teams in order to obtain information from parents in a standardized fashion.

AUTISM DIAGNOSTIC INTERVIEW—REVISED

The ADI-R (Rutter, Le Couteur, & Lord, 2003) was designed as a structured interview to be used with a child's primary caregiver and to accompany a structured observation scale (the ADOS). It can obtain information that is not likely to appear during the relatively short period of time of a typical observation, and it takes into account a child's lifetime behaviors, which are essential in diagnosing ASD. Like the ADOS, it includes a focus on trying to disentangle expressive language level from ASD severity in children with ASD. The ADI-R consists of 93 items applicable to any person with a mental age of 2 and above, and its three main areas are related to current diagnostic criteria for autism. These are (1) qualities of reciprocal social interaction, including such things as greeting behavior, offering and seeking comfort, emotional sharing, and the development of intense friendships; (2) communication and language, with a particular focus on social usage, syncretic and stereotyped language, and type of conversational interaction; and (3) restricted, repetitive, and stereotyped behaviors and interests, such as unusual preoccupations, rituals, unusual sensory interests, and abnormal attachments. In addition, behaviors that frequently occur in developmental disorders and are relevant to treatment planning, although not as diagnostically important, are assessed; these include self-injury, pica, aggression, and overactivity. The ADI-R requires a highly skilled and experienced interviewer who has received specific training in the instrument's use.

The great advantages of the ADI-R are that it was designed in line with a great deal of cognitive and social-psychological research on how to structure interviews and enhance memory; its algorithms have been scientifically derived and repeatedly tested; many different samples have been evaluated with the ADI-R; and very sophisticated psychometric research has been done with it. Clinicians can use the ADI-R with great confidence for children ages 42 months and older, as long as they do not use it as the sole measure for diagnosis; few children with nonautism ASD (i.e., PDDNOS, Asperger syndrome) met ADI-R thresholds on all three dimensions at the 42-month time point (Cox et al., 1999). It can also be used as a good structured interview for parents of children as young as 20 months—again, as long as professionals are aware that it does a better job of deciding that children do not have ASD than of identifying children who do have ASD. Administration time is long (up to 3 hours), and professionals need extensive training in administration in order to give it reliably. Clinicians using the ADI-R should also keep in mind the emotional toll that it can take on parents, due to its time length and nature of questions. Evaluators should make sure to provide ample time for breaks and give parents a chance to discuss their child's strengths as well as weaknesses. Due to the extensive length of time needed for administration, it may not be practical for use in all settings (it may be better suited for clinical rather than school settings).

PARENT INTERVIEW FOR AUTISM

Parent Interview for Autism (PIA; Stone & Hogan, 1993a) was developed to obtain diagnostic information relative to ASD from parents. It consists of 118 questions about children's behavior in the areas of social relating, affective responses, peer interactions, motor imitation, communication, nonverbal communication, language understanding, object play, imaginative play, sensory responses, motoric behaviors, and need for sameness. Parents are asked to rate on a 5-point scale their child's current behavior, with responses ranging from 1 ("almost never, less than 10% of the time") to 5 ("almost always, over 90% of the time"). For example, in the area of social relating, parents are told, "The first questions are about ___________'s social behavior. Tell me about how ___________ interacts with others: Does ___________ enjoy interacting with familiar adults?" Administration time is approximately 30–45 minutes. The PIA does not have an algorithm or cutoff score for the diagnosis of autism, so it is primarily useful in eliciting information from parents relevant to a diagnosis of autism. It is easy to administer, does not require extra training, takes about 15–20 minutes (depending on how much follow-up questioning is done), and provides relevant information for treatment. It does not have the psychometric characteristics or detailed interviewer guidance available for the ADI-R. The PIA's psychometric characteristics are promising, but it is clearly in need of further work before it can be used as a diagnostic instrument.

Assessment for Curricular/Intervention Planning

Psychoeducational Profile—Third Edition

The PEP-3 (Schopler et al., 2005) was developed by Division TEACCH (Treatment and Education of Autistic and Related Communication Handicapped Children) in North Carolina to assess treatment-relevant strengths and weaknesses in children between the ages of 2 years and 7-6 years, or children 21 years of age and under with developmental delays and to assist in the diagnosis of children with ASD. The authors of the PEP-3 updated an instrument that provides important developmental information, and yet is highly flexible and able to get around the peculiarities of children with autism. There are 10 Performance Scale subtests that involve direct observation and testing of the child, which were standardized and normed on typically developing children ages 2–6 years and those with ASD ages 2–21 years. Six subtests assess communication (Cognitive Verbal–Preverbal, Expressive Language, Receptive Language) and motor skills (Fine Motor, Gross Motor, Visual–Motor Imitation) and four assess maladaptive behavior common in children with ASD (Affective Expression, Social Reciprocity, Characteristic Motor Behaviors, Characteristic Verbal Behaviors), yielding composite scores in these three areas. A Caregiver Report Form has three subscales (Problem Behaviors, Personal Self-Care Skills, and Adaptive Abilities).

The PEP-3 has a number of attractive features that may make it useful in the evaluation of children with ASD. These include administrative flexibility, untimed items, limited dependence on language (the only items that require language are the language items), and the items' developmental range (allowing every child to have some success). It does a good job of eliciting behavior for diagnosis, is a useful screening measure for treatment planning, has a very low floor, is easy to administer, moves at a fast pace, and uses appealing tasks that maximize the limited motivation and attention of impaired young children. The PEP-3 manual encourages an examiner to use the session to evaluate a child's awareness of the examiner's feelings by using exaggerated affect and varied intonation and volume, and observing the child's reaction. Effective ways of motivating the child can also be assessed by trying different types of rewards and observing the frequencies and patterns of reinforcement that are most successful in maintaining attention and interest in items. The examiner can also evaluate the child's competence in responding to directions by following a hierarchy of administrative prompts in giving directions—from simple verbal directions, to gesture, to demonstration, to physical guidance. The PEP-3 combines all of these attractive clinical features with very good psychometric properties, making it a useful measure for educational programming and diagnosing young children with ASD, especially those who are lower functioning.

Autism Screening Instrument for Educational Planning—Second Edition

The ASIEP-2 (Krug et al., 1993) is a collection of five measures useful for evaluating low-functioning children with ASD, including diagnosis, curricular placement, and treatment planning. The teacher/parent rating form, the ABC, has been mentioned earlier in the chapter. The other four measures are designed for children whose language and social ages are between 3 months and 49 months of age.

The Educational Assessment measure, also mentioned previously, evaluates a child's test-taking competencies and readiness to learn. It covers the child's ability to stay in his or her seat, understand adult directions (e.g., "Come here"), respond to questions (e.g., "What is your name?"), understand body concepts (e.g., ears), and imitate speech (e.g., "cookie"). To complete this measure successfully, a child must be able to stay seated with hands in lap and look at specified objects. The child also must not have any disruptive behaviors that are incompatible with test taking or instruction. Scores are interpreted by comparing a child's score with the means for children with autism and for children with severe, nonautism disabilities on each subscale. Percentile scores for these two groups are provided as well. This is a useful measure for assessing where to begin with educational interventions.

The Interaction Assessment subtest elicits a child's social responses in a controlled play setting where test stimuli are presented in a structured fashion. It measures both spontaneous social responses (child-initiated contact) and reactions to requests (e.g., "Give me . . . "). This subtest was designed primarily for differential diagnosis, but it can also provide a baseline description of social interaction with an adult. Administration requires two adults who are thoroughly familiar with the procedure. A training videotape is available for this purpose. One adult interacts with the child, while the other codes the behaviors observed during a 12-minute session, using time sampling, anecdotal recording, and frequency counts. There are three adult presentation conditions that are prompted by an audiotape: active modeling, passive/no initiation, and direct cues. Child behavior is coded as interaction, constructive independent play, no response, and aggressive negative. A child's score is interpreted by comparing his or her performance in each of the four areas to those for children in the normative sample with autism and for children with mental retardation without autism, to see which the better fit is. An autistic interaction score can also be obtained, with percentile scores available for children with autism (ABC score > 68) and for children with severe disabilities but no autism (ABC score < 67). Anecdotal information can be used to design educational interventions.

The Sample of Vocal Behavior subtest evaluates expressive speech at both the preverbal and emerging language levels. Designed for use by special educators and speech–language pathologists, the object of this subtest is to elicit from the child the best sample of vocal behavior that he or she can produce. Even cries, coughs, laughs, or giggles are scored. Administered in an unstructured setting, such as a play area, a free-time area, or an activity table, a verbatim record is made of all the child's utterances (use of a tape recorder is recommended to ensure accuracy). Picture books, toys, bubble play, or musical instruments are all suggested as activities to elicit a verbal response. If they do not work, then physical stimulation, such as bouncing, tickling, or hugging, is recommended to elicit a response. If these are not successful, the evaluator is to identify a part of a child's day when he or she typically vocalizes (e.g., toileting or self-stimulation). The goal is to obtain 50 vocalizations. In order to maximally discriminate the speech of children with autism from that of very low-functioning children with mental retardation, subtest scoring focuses on four areas identified by research as typical of the speech of children with autism (Krug et al., 1993). That is, speech is scored as repetitive (to assess stereotypy), noncommunicative (to assess social relating), unintelligible (to assess language delay or deviance), and babbling (to assess nonmeaningful vocalizations). The number of words used (i.e., length of utterances) is also scored. Three scores are produced: mean length of response, language age, and autistic speech characteristics. Information from this measure can be used to determine which module to use with the ADOS.

Finally, there is the Prognosis of Learning Rate subtest. To take this subtest, a child must be able to physically pick up (or to attempt to pick up) a plastic chip. The child's learning rate is assessed by the number of trials it takes to learn a rule. This measure is designed to assess stimulus oversensitivity—a characteristic often seen in children with ASD, who may be so selective in their attention that they have trouble responding to stimuli in context (this is a problem for children with severe mental retardation as well). Total responses to criteria for required learning steps and continued learning steps are scored. Again, percentile scores are available for children with autism and those with severe, nonautism disabilities.

All five measures are reasonably reliable, and validity data are based on the fact that children with autism (as determined by ABC scores) have profiles on these measures differing from those of children with other severe disabilities. The ABC serves its purpose of using educators' ratings to screen for autism among young, severely delayed children; it is less sensitive in identifying children of higher ability and those who are older (Volkmar et al., 1988; Yirmiya, Sigman, & Freeman, 1994). Because of this high false-negative rate for one segment of children with ASD it is not recommended for general screening. The Sample of Vocal Behavior and Educational Assessment subtests have additional construct validity, based on moderate to high correlations with the Sequenced Inventory of Communication Development (Hedrick, Prather, & Tobin, 1975). The ASIEP-2 is a useful set of measures for children with autism and mental retardation that can serve as baseline measures of social functioning with adults, receptive and expressive speech and language, test taking and basic instructional competencies, and rate of response to new learning. One of the advantages of the ASIEP-2 is that it was designed for use by school personnel and, with some practice, is user-friendly.

The Assessment Feedback Session with Parents

Parenting a preschool child with ASD is very demanding. Parents are usually the first to realize that there is something unusual about or wrong with their child, and yet it may take some time and considerable persistence on their part before they obtain a confirmed diagnosis that seems to make sense. Even when they have wanted to understand what is wrong with their child, it still may be very difficult to accept a diagnosis that implies lifelong developmental disabilities in a significant majority of individuals. Some young children with ASD do improve dramatically over the course of the preschool years. Further complicating the situation is that a very small number of children diagnosed with ASD do eventually, after intensive treatment, display typical development. Thus some parents are given a very dire diagnosis, and yet at the same time hold out hope for dramatic recovery. This situation can create a very complex set of emotions in parents, including tremendous sadness and disappointment that their child has such a significant problem; frustration over the differing diagnostic opinions they may receive; frustration over the difficulty of finding appropriate services for their child; and anger at professionals who either may be insisting that their child has ASD when they're not yet ready to accept that diagnosis, or may be deferring a diagnosis when the parents believe there's clearly something wrong.

Our most stressful and unpredictable assessment feedback sessions are with parents of preschool children suspected of having ASD. The diagnosis of any ASD is a powerful one, and it evokes a wide range of responses from parents; these range from accepting the information presented to rejecting it forcefully or even threatening the assessor. An example of an accepting response came from the father of Seth (a child described earlier in the chapter), who interrupted our tactful presentation of findings with "You don't have to pussyfoot around with us, Doc. We already know he's pretty weird." A rejecting response came from a mother of a 5-year-old who screamed "No!" and threw the report on the floor when she heard us recommend that a previous diagnosis of PDDNOS at age 3 be changed to one of autistic disorder. Another parent, seeking a third opinion from our clinic, was threatening and made repeated efforts to get us to omit our diagnosis from our report, including having an attorney call and imply that we could be harmed by a complaint filed with the president of the university or a lawsuit. This happened in the context of a university clinic, where parents have the option of never sharing the report with anyone if they don't like the findings. Sometimes parents are disappointed when an ASD is *not* diagnosed. One couple was upset when we found no supporting evidence in our evaluation of a 4-year-old boy for a previous PDDNOS diagnosis at age 2, perhaps because of the excellent early intervention program he had attended. We instead gave a diagnosis of mild mental retardation. They felt that this changed their son from a potentially normal, although eccentric, individual to "damaged goods." They later made several phone calls to us to discuss both their sadness and their anger over our findings and their son's continuing difficulties.

Many parents accept the diagnosis but struggle with what an ASD is. They ask themselves, "What does it mean?", "Why did it happen?", or "What did I do wrong for my child to have this?" We often see self-blame and blaming others; a parent may displace anger on a spouse/partner and/or other supports (the therapists, teachers, other professionals, the theoretical approach of the child's program, etc.). Similarly, early childhood professionals are often critical of families for not following through with staff suggestions, forgetting how hard parenting a child with ASD can be.

Judging from the copies of previous evaluations that we have received for children who are evaluated by our clinic, and our past experiences on preschool committees for children with disabilities, many schools and clinics delay giving firm diagnoses until children enter elementary school and parents "figure it out for themselves," as one preschool speech pathologist put it. This is particularly likely if a child with ASD has an accompanying diagnosis of mental retardation. We see many children ages 4 and 5 who carry a PDDNOS diagnosis, but meet clear criteria for autism and moderate to profound mental retardation. Assessors are often quite reluctant to tell parents what they believe the real diagnoses are, even when they have compelling evidence to support their opinion. We believe that much of this is driven by the very real unpleasantness of giving parents information that they often find difficult to accept. Research suggests that parents and professionals are most likely to disagree on a child level of functioning when a child scores very poorly on standardized measures (Geiger, Smith, & Creaghead, 2002). The authors speculate that this may occur because parents see behaviors that professionals do not, because parents may overemphasize splinter skills in their assessment of global functioning, or because parents may interpret a child's not performing a requested behavior as willful while a professional will interpret it as evidence of an inability to do it. It is also the case that preschool children can receive services with a label of "developmental delay" (depending on the state) or a PDDNOS diagnosis alone under IDEA, making a comprehensive diagnosis unnecessary for placement and treatment in many cases. Chapter 8 offers recommendations on presenting assessment findings to parents in a therapeutic manner.

Family Assessment Issues

In addition to all the stressors of having a preschool child with ASD, family life itself has its own demands. Parents may be single parents; they may be in unsupportive or unhappy marriages/relationships; and/or they may have other children. Professionals should remember that each child's family is unique and must be addressed with that uniqueness in mind. Nonetheless, all families should be assessed for their needs in four areas: (1) their need for information (e.g., about ASD, genetics testing, IDEA eligibility categories, community support groups); (2) their need for stress reduction and/or support to help them cope with the tensions and/or disappointments of raising a child with ASD (including its impact on marital/couple and sibling relationships), as well as their need for respite care, appropriate schools, transportation, or other services; (3) the social and financial resources available to help them meet their needs, particularly those they prioritize as most important; and, in some cases, (4) the parents' interest and ability to participate effectively in a home-based intervention in conjunction with their child's educational program.

In regard to information, most states have developed a guide for parents whose children are judged to have a disabling condition under the IDEA. At a minimum, parents should be given a copy of this guide; the name of their child's school's parent advocate for parents of disabled children; a two- to three-page description of ASD in preschool children; and some resources for further reading on ASD, as well as on basic child development. To give parents a comprehensive overview of ASD, we have found the books *Autism: Explaining the Enigma* (Frith, 2003) and *Helping Children with Autism Learn: Treatment Approaches for Parents and Professionals* (Siegel, 2003) to be particularly useful. *Caring for a Child with Autism: A Practical Guide for Parents* (Ives & Munro, 2002) is another good book. We also recommend the Division TEACCH book for parents, *Parent Survival Manual: A Guide to Crisis Resolution in Autism and Related Developmental Disorders* (Schopler, 1995). This book is packed with practical solutions to common, everyday problems faced by parents of a child with ASD. Although each child is unique, there are so many ideas offered for common problems that some are bound to be useful for parents working with their own child.

Assessment for stress and mental health problems, adequate resources, and interest and ability to participate in a home-based intervention program are covered in Chapter 8.

CHARACTERISTICS OF PROGRAMS WITH DEMONSTRATED EFFICACY

As the recent report *Educating Children with Autism* (National Research Council, 2001) has stated, the goals for educational services for children with ASD should be the same as those for other children—that is, to promote personal independence and social responsibility. The report notes that these goals "imply progress in social and cognitive abilities, verbal and non-verbal communication skills, and adaptive skills; reduction of behavioral difficulties; and generalization of abilities across multiple environments" (p. ES-4). Several very thorough reviews of preschool programs for children with ASD have found empirical support for the following characteristics of learning environments that are related to optimal outcomes:

- early entry into an intervention program;
- active engagement in intensive instructional programming or the equivalent of a full school day, including services that may be offered in different sites, for a minimum of five days a week with full year programming;
- use of planned teaching opportunities, organized around relatively brief periods of time for the youngest children (e.g., 15–20 minute intervals); and
- sufficient amounts of adult attention in 1:1 or very small group instruction to meet individualized goals. (National Research Council, 2001, p. ES-5; see also Dawson & Osterling, 1997)

The National Research Council report notes that many intensive intervention programs (ones that have been evaluated and shown to be promising, as well as ones based on those models but not directly evaluated) have real differences in their philosophy and practice, even though the programs have many things in common. This means that parents and school systems can consider a variety of approaches. However, the report notes that the keys to a child's education are the IEP, the IFSP, and the ways in which these plans are implemented. It therefore recommends that appropriate educational objectives for children with ASD (and all children) should be observable and measurable behaviors and skills. It also recommends that objectives should be developed that can be accomplished within 1 year, and that these should place a priority on increasing a child's ability to participate in education, the community, and family life. Specifically, the National Research Council recommends the following:

- social skills to enhance participation in family, school, and community activities (e.g., imitation, social initiations, and response to adults and peers, parallel and interactive play with peers and siblings);
- expressive verbal language, receptive language, and non-verbal communication skills;
- a functional, symbolic communication system;
- increased engagement, flexibility, and developmentally appropriate tasks and play including the ability to attend to the environment and respond to an appropriate motivational system;
- fine and gross motor skills used for age appropriate functional activities as needed;
- cognitive skills, including symbolic play and basic concepts, as well as academic skills;
- replacement of problem behaviors with more conventional and appropriate behaviors;
- independent organizational skills and other behaviors that underlie success in regular educational classrooms (e.g., completing a task independently, following instructions in a group, asking for help). (2001, p. ES-6)

The National Research Council report argues that six kinds of interventions for preschool children with ASD should take priority over others. First, functional, spontaneous communication should be promoted vigorously, on the assumption that most children can learn to speak. Chapter 5 of the report provides an outstanding review of the literature on the use of alternative modes of functional communication and their relationship to the development of sign and verbal language. Second, social instruction should be delivered in all of a child's settings throughout the day, using interventions that are age-appropriate. These can range from family "floor time" for a mother and toddler (where the mother tries to elicit a response to maternal imitation of the child's behavior) to getting a preschool child to participate in cooperative activities with peers. Third, the report recommends the explicit teaching of play skills, including appropriate use of toys and other materials, as well as strategies for play with peers. Fourth, it recommends the promotion of cognitive development through focusing on skills in the context in which they are expected to be used, with explicit attempts to teach generalization and maintenance in natural contexts. Fifth, it recommends that interventions designed to decrease problem behaviors should attend to the context in which these behaviors occur, and that a positive and proactive approach should be used along with research-supported techniques, such as functional assessment and reinforcement of alternative behaviors. Finally, it recommends that functional academic skills be taught when these are appropriate for the abilities and needs of an individual child.

The New York State Department of Education has published a guide to evaluating the quality of programs for children ages 3–21 with ASD (Crimmins, Durand, Theurer-Kaufman, & Everett, 2001; see Appendix 13.2). Prepared by well-known experts in the field, this guide can be used by parents to identify preferred educational placements and by professionals to evaluate the quality of the services they are providing. The authors caution that it is unlikely that any program will have all of the indicators, given the variety of educational practices and the age range covered.

As one can see from this comprehensive description of the goals, priorities, and characteristics of learning environments that provide optimal outcomes, assessment of children with suspected ASD requires a competent, interdisciplinary team of professionals who are familiar with early child development, ASD, mental retardation, other frequently co-occurring or alternative diagnoses, and evidence-based instruction and treatment methods.

Children with ASD are among the most diverse and interesting young clients who present for assessment. Researchers have learned a great deal about how best to assess and treat this group of disorders, but much is still unknown. Because of the wealth of first-rate applied and basic research being done, examiners need to keep up with the research literature and the latest educational developments in this area, in order to provide the best services for young children with ASD and their families.

APPENDIX 13.1. Review of Measures

Measure	**Aberrant Behavior Checklist (ABC). Aman and Singh (1986).**
Purpose	Rating inappropriate and maladaptive behavior of individuals with mental retardation living in residential settings.
Areas	Irritability, Lethargy, Stereotypy, Hyperactivity, Inappropriate Speech.
Format	58 items rated 0–3.
Scores	Raw scores.
Age group	5–51 years.
Time	5 minutes.
Users	Direct caregivers or other staff members familiar with individual.
Norms	Data collected on 754 New Zealanders ages 5–51+ years, and 508 individuals from United States ages 7–51+ years. Subjects were living in residential facilities, had moderate to profound metal retardation, and were 60% male/ 40% female. Excluded were nonambulatory and blind individuals. Norms more inclusive of younger population were released after test publication (666 students ages 6–21 years enrolled in special classes).
Reliability	Internal Consistency, .86–.95; test–retest (4 weeks), .96–.99; interrater, .55–.69.
Validity	Content, supported.
Comments	Crucial information pertaining to empirical data is not provided in manual, but must be obtained from external sources. There is limited evidence of sensitivity to pharmaceutical treatment effects. Measure is best suited as a research instrument and as a measure of severity of symptoms. Low interrater reliabilities raise concern.
References consulted	Gaddis (1995); Grill (1995). See book's References list.

Measure	**Asperger Syndrome Diagnostic Scale (ASDS). Myles, Bock, and Simpson (2001).**
Purpose	Assessing the manifestation of Asperger syndrome in individuals.
Areas	Language, Social, Maladaptive, Cognitive, Sensorimotor.
Format	Parent/teacher screening rating scale; 50 items rated as observed/not observed. Also, Asperger Syndrome Questionnaire (likelihood of Asperger syndrome).
Scores	Percentiles, standard scores, total score.
Age group	5–18 years.
Time	10–15 minutes.
Users	Professionals and/or persons who have had close contact for 2 weeks with participant.
Norms	Data collected on 115 individuals without independently confirmed diagnoses; authors collected sample by contacting professionals and asking them to complete questions on children they knew with Asperger syndrome, also parents; all items rated.
Reliability	Internal consistency, .64–.83; test–retest, not reported; interrater (small sample of parents and teachers), .93. No interscale reliability; no positive or negative predictive power reported.

Validity	Content, no steps to rule out autism first or establish language competence (as required by DSM-IV-TR); criterion-related, none.
Comments	Not recommended, as there was no independent clinical assessment of criterion groups with Asperger syndrome or with autism. Relevant characteristics of criterion groups are unknown.
References consulted	Blair (2001); Goldstein (2002); Mirenda (2001). See book's References list. www.proedinc.com

Measure	**Autism Diagnostic Interview—Revised (ADI-R). Rutter, Le Couteur, and Lord (2003).**
Purpose	Providing a lifetime assessment of the behaviors of a child with autism or another PDD.
Areas	Communication; Social Development and Play; Repetitive and Restricted Behaviors; General Behavior.
Format	93-item, semistructured parent/caregiver interview; items are rated on a 0–3 scale (scores of 2 and 3 are weighed the same).
Scores	Uses an empirically derived algorithm to derive diagnoses.
Age group	A mental age of 18 months or higher.
Time	1½ hours or longer; 2½ hours or longer for older children (4+ years).
Users	Interviewers who have received training specific to ADI-R.
Norms	Reliability study: Data collected on 10 children with autism (8 male, 2 female) and 10 children with mental disabilities or language impairments from clinical and local preschool programs in Canada. All children had shown significant language delays by 36 months. Children performing below the 12-month level overall were omitted. Age range, 36–59 months; mean nonverbal IQ/DQ, 64.12 for group with autism and 63.80 for group with other disabilities; mental age range, 21–74 months. Validity study: In addition to reliability group, data collected on 30 children (15 with and 15 without autism). Criteria same as reliability study, with inclusion of participants from Greensboro, North Carolina, and surrounding areas: 12% African American and West Indian; 82% European American; 6% Asian, Hispanic, and Native American. Mean nonverbal IQ/DQ, 71.88 for group with autism and 71.48 for group without; mean mental age, 34 months (autism) and 32 months (no autism).
Reliability	Internal consistency, .69–.95; test–retest (2–3 months), .83–.91; interrater, .62–.89.
Validity	Criterion-related, supported. Effective at diagnosing ASD in individuals who have mental ages above 18 months of age, but over- and underdiagnosis of autism in children with lower mental ages (Lord, 1995; Lord, Storoschuk, Rutter, & Pickles, 1993; Pilowsky, Yirmiya, Shulman, & Dover, 1998). Diagnoses are also stable from 2 to 3 years of age if the match of any ASD diagnosis to another is the measure of accuracy, rather than exact diagnosis within the ASD group (e.g., if PDDNOS to autism is considered reliable, rather than requiring PDDNOS to PDDNOS to consider the diagnosis accurate; Stone et al., 1999). Lord (1995) found that the ADI-R was most likely to underdiagnose children who had IQs in the mildly mentally retarded range. Overdiagnosis occurred in the more severely impaired 2-year-old children (those with IQs in the moderately to severely retarded range). In another study, with a

	very large sample, the ADI-R demonstrated high specificity but poor sensitivity for identifying autism at 20 months. Sensitivity increased at age 42 months (Cox et al., 1999).
Comments	Appropriate for use with caregivers of children and adults with autism or other ASD/PDD. Linked to ICD-10 and DSM-IV-TR criteria; it is the instrument most consistent with current diagnostic criteria. Effective for diagnosing individuals with mental ages over 18 months. Designed in line with much cognitive and social-psychological research on how to structure interviews and enhance memory. Algorithms have been scientifically derived and repeatedly tested. The ADI-R has been used to evaluate a wide range of samples and to conduct very sophisticated psychometric research. However, administration time is long, and professionals need extensive training in order to give it reliably. Training tapes and workshops are offered by the publisher. Measure is worthwhile for professionals who specialize in autism, but too long for routine clinical practice, and often emotionally draining for parents.
References consulted	Lord (1995); Lord, Rutter, and Le Couteur (1994); Lord, Storoschuk, Rutter, and Pickles (1999); Pilowsky, Yirmiya, Shulman, and Dover (1998); Lord et al. (1997); Stone et al. (1999). See book's References list. www.wpspublish.com

Measure	**Autism Diagnostic Observation Scale (ADOS). Lord, Rutter, DiLavore, and Risi (2002).**
Purpose	To provide an assessment of the behaviors of a child with autism or another ASD. Designed to be used in conjunction with the original ADI and now the ADI-R.
Areas	Communication; Social Interaction.
Format	Semistructured observation of child interacting with observer. Four modules; selection of module to be administered depends on child's verbal skills and chronological age.
Scores	Uses empirically derived algorithms to derive diagnoses.
Age group	A chronological age of 15 months or higher, and a mental age of 20 months or higher.
Time	30 minutes.
Users	Interviewers who have received training specific to ADOS.
Norms	Not normed per se. Criterion groups of children clinically diagnosed with autism, PDDNOS, and nonautism developmental disorders used to establish discriminant validity.
Reliability	Test–retest (n = 27, 2–3 months), .78 for Social Interaction, .73 for Communication, .82 for Total Social Interaction–Communication. Interrater (mean percentage of exact agreement across items), 91.5% for module 1, 89% for module 2, and 88.2% for module 3. All items 80% exact agreement or better across raters for modules 1–3 except for one. Interclass correlation for domain scores, .80–.92 (n = 62) for live–live ratings.
Validity	Criterion-related, supported. Classified 95% of those clinically diagnosed with autism, 92% of those outside the spectrum. Not effective at distinguishing children with PDDNOS from those with autism (33% of those with PDDNOS were diagnosed as having nonautism ASD and 53% as having autism).

Comments	Appropriate for use with children and adolescents with autism or other ASD. Linked to ICD-10 and DSM-IV-TR criteria. Effective for diagnosing individuals with mental age over 20 months. Algorithms have been scientifically derived and repeatedly tested. Wide-ranging samples have been evaluated. Disentangles language ability from symptoms of autism/ASD. Professionals need extensive training in administration in order to give ADOS reliably. Training tapes and workshops are offered by the publisher. Measure is worthwhile for professionals who specialize in autism.
References consulted	Brassard review.

Measure	**Autism Screening Instrument for Educational Planning—Second Edition (ASIEP-2). Krug, Arick, and Almond (1993).**
Purpose	Aiding professionals in the identification of autism, and providing information for educational plans.
Areas	Subtests: Autism Behavior Checklist (ABC), Sample of Vocal Behavior (SVB), Interaction Assessment (IA), Educational Assessment (EA), and Prognosis of Learning Rate (PLR).
Format	ABC is a 57-item checklist, used as a diagnostic tool. For format of other subtests, see text.
Scores	ABC: Subscales are profiles and total score has cutoff. SVB: Mean length of response, language age, and a percentile score for autistic speech characteristics. IA, EA, and PLR: Percentile rank.
Age group	1-6 years to adult.
Time	1½–2½ hours.
Users	School psychologists or experienced educators of children with ASD.
Norms	Data collected on three samples: (1) 1,049 individuals, 172 of whom were previously diagnosed with autism; (2) 62 individuals, all of whom were previously diagnosed with autism; and (3) 953 individuals, 95% of whom were diagnosed with severe mental retardation.
Reliability	For ABC: Interrater, .95; split-half, .87. Reviewers also report psychometric support for the SVB, IA, EA, and PLR.
Validity	Based on the fact that children with ASD have different profiles on the subscales than children with other severe disabilities in theoretically meaningful ways. The sample of Vocal Behavior and the Educational Assessment subscales have moderate to high correlations with the SICD and the ABC with other measures of autism. (As one of the oldest measures it has been used in validity studies of most other measures of autism—e.g., the Teacher total scale has moderate to high correlations with all but one subscale of the PEP-3.)
Comments	As an educational programming tool, there are alternative developmental instruments that are stronger, but the ASIEP-2 has user-friendly components that can be used efficiently in schools. The ABC can be used alone and is the most widely used component. It is an effective screening tool for educators who are identifying autism in severely delayed young children. It has a high false-negative rate with children who are older and/or higher functioning with ASD and thus is not recommended as a general screening measure. Questions have been raised about the use of parent ratings.
References consulted	Olmi (1998); Oswald (1998a). See book's References list. www.proedinc.com

Measure	Checklist on Autism in Toddlers (CHAT). Baron-Cohen, Allen, and Gillberg (1992).
Purpose	Screening by general practitioners or health visitors with a large general population of children at 18 months of age (excluding children already identified as developmentally delayed).
Areas	Gaze Monitoring, Pretend Play, Protodeclarative Pointing.
Format	Nine yes–no questions answered by parent, and five yes–no questions answered by examiner after brief interactions with child.
Scores	Failure of certain items suggests possible ASD; failure of subsets of these items suggests developmental delay.
Age group	18 months (with later rescreenings as necessary).
Time	10 minutes.
Users	Professionals.
Norms	Data collected on over 16,000 English children age 18 months, who were rescreened at 3 and 5 years and followed up at 7 years.
Reliability	Not reported.
Validity	Predictive, strongly supported. Excellent specificity; sensitivity is low, although false positives have developmental problems.
Comments	The CHAT is an accurate and efficient screening measure for deciding who does not have ASD and/or a developmental delay in toddlers without severe developmental disabilities; it should not be used as the sole screening measure.
References consulted	Dumont-Mathieu and Fein (2005). See book's References list.

Measure	Checklist for Autism in Toddlers-23 (CHAT-23). Wong, Hui, Lee, Leung, Ho, Lau, Fung, and Chung (2004).
Purpose	Screening tool for Chinese children with autism.
Areas	Gaze monitoring, pretend play, protodeclarative pointing.
Format	Part A, a 23-item graded response (i.e., never, seldom, usually, often) questionnaire answered by parent; part B, a 5-item examiner-graded response questionnaire based on child–examiner interactions.
Scores	Answering "seldom" or "never" to any 2 of 7 key questions or any 6 of all 23 questions was defined as positive for autism. In part B, not passing at least 2 of the first 4 items is indicative of autism.
Age group	Children with mental ages 18–24 months.
Time	10 minutes.
Users	Professionals.
Norms	Data was collected on 276 13- to 86-month-old children (mental ages 18–24 months), which included 87 children with autistic disorder (*n* = 53) or PDD (*n* = 33) and 120 children without ASD.
Reliability	None reported.

Validity	Part A, failing any 6 of the 23 items had a sensitivity of .84 and specificity of .85; part B, failing any 2 of 4 items had a sensitivity of .74 and a specificity of .91 and a positive predictive value of 85%. False positives were low. The psychometric properties of the CHAT-23 with Chinese children are very similar to those of the M-CHAT for North American children, supporting external validity.
Comments	The CHAT-23 is a combination of the observation section of the CHAT and 23 questions of the M-CHAT designed to screen Chinese children with autism. The test authors indicate that CHAT-23 could be used as a two-part screening measure, with part A's questionnaire serving as the first stage and part B's behavior observations serving as a second step for those children who scored positive for autism in part A. More research is needed on the CHAT-23's efficacy with children whose mental ages are lower or higher than 18–24 months.
References consulted	Brock, Jimerson, and Hansen (2006); Dumont-Mathieu and Fein (2005). See book's References list.

Measure	**Childhood Autism Rating Scale (CARS). Schopler, Reichler, and Renner (1988).**
Purpose	Identifying children with autism, distinguishing children with autism from children without autism, and distinguishing levels of severity of ASD.
Areas	Relating to People; Imitation; Emotional Response; Body Use; Object Use; Adaptation to Change; Visual Response; Listening Response; Taste–Smell–Touch Response and Use; Fear or Nervousness; Verbal Communication; Nonverbal Communication; Activity Level; Level and Consistency of Intellectual Response; General Impressions.
Format	Observational instrument with flexibility when examiners are provided with records, parental report, or other professionals' report; items on 15 subscales are rated on a 4-point scale (or 7-point scale if half-points are used).
Scores	Cutoff scores.
Age group	2 years and older.
Time	30–45 minutes.
Users	Professionals, but can be completed by a variety of individuals familiar with the child and does not require a structured observation period.
Norms	Developed over 15 years, using data from approximately 1,600 cases in Division TEACCH program (75% male, 67% white, ages 6 and above).
Reliability	Internal consistency, .94; test–retest (over 1 year), .88; interrater, .71.
Validity	Criterion-related, .84 with clinical ratings, .80 with expert clinical judgments.
Comments	Revision of the Childhood Psychosis Rating Scale. Excellent training tapes are available from the authors (see text for descriptions). Classification rates for diagnosis are as strong as those for the ADI-R. No strong bias toward any diagnostic framework. Scores place child on a continuum rather than making a yes–no diagnostic decision. Requires familiarity with age-appropriate functioning across domains assessed. Reliability and validity data from 1980 are dated but have been used in many research studies since then.
References consulted	Prizant (1992); Welsh (1992). See book's References list. www.wpspublish.com

Measure	Gilliam Autism Rating Scale—Second Edition (GARS-2). Gilliam (2005).
Purpose	Assisting in the diagnosis of autism among individuals.
Areas	Subscales: Stereotyped Behaviors, Communication, Social Interaction.
Format	Behavioral checklist of 42 items grouped into three subscales and a structured parent interview form. Items on the GARS-2 are based on the definitions of autism adopted by the Autism Society of America and DSM-IV-TR.
Scores	Standard scores, Autism Index (AI). Subtest standard scores of 8 and above and AIs of 90 and above are associated with higher probabilities of the subject being a person with autism.
Age group	3–22 years.
Time	5–10 minutes.
Users	Designed to be completed by a parent, teacher, or other caregiver who knows the individual well. No special training is required to administer and score.
Norms	Data for the GARS-2 was collected on a sample of 1,107 persons whom their parents, teachers, school psychologists, or educational diagnosticians identified as having autism from 48 states within the United States. There was no independent verification of the diagnosis.
Reliability	Coefficients of reliability (internal consistency and test–retest) for the subscales and entire test are all large to very large in magnitude.
Validity	Documented through instrument's ability to discriminate between individuals with autism and those with severe behavior disorders based on standard scores.
Comments	The second edition of the GARS provides a separate chapter in the test manual that list multiple discreet target behaviors for each item, which are operationally defined and include specific examples. A separate booklet, *Instructional Objectives for Children Who Have Autism*, is included in the test kit to assist in the formulation of instructional goals and objectives based on GARS-2 results. In this way, instruction can be directly related to assessment results from GARS-2. The major weakness of the original GARS was the unknown accuracy of the autism diagnoses and its high under identification of strictly diagnosed children as having autism. South et al. (2002) found that the GARS falsely identified as not having autism 52% of children independently diagnosed as having autism by expert clinicians using the ADOS and the ADI-R. Because the second edition does not address these issues satisfactorily, the test should be used with caution.
References consulted	Brock, Jimerson, and Hansen (2006); South et al. (2002). See book's References list.

Measure	Modified Checklist for Autism in Toddlers (M-CHAT). Robbins, Fein, Barton, and Green (2001).
Purpose	Screening by general practitioners or health visitors with a large general population of children (excluding children already identified as developmentally delayed).
Areas	Protodeclarative Pointing, Gaze Monitoring, Pretend Play.
Format	23-item, yes–no parent report questionnaire.
Scores	Child fails test if 3 of 23 items failed or if 2 of 6 critical items are failed.
Age group	16–30 months.
Time	5 minutes.

Users	Professionals.
Norms	Data collected on two groups: (1) 1,122 children (570 male, 531 female, 21 unreported) screened during well-baby checkups at 18 or 24 months; (2) 171 children (123 male, 46 female, 2 not reported) between 18 and 30 months without a previously diagnosed DSM-IV disorder, screened via early intervention service providers. Children were excluded if they had either (a) a total lack of expressive language or functional communication system, or (2) severe motor deficiencies that prohibited meaningful responses.
Reliability	Internal consistency, .85.
Validity	Predictive, .80; negative predictive, .99; sensitivity, .87; specificity, .99.
Comments	The M-CHAT is an extension of the CHAT. It was modified to make it more sensitive to nonautism ASD, and the age was moved up to 30 months because autistic regression is unlikely after that time. Psychometric characteristics are excellent.
References consulted	Dumont-Mathieu and Fein (2005); Robbins, Fein, Barton, and Green (2001). See book's References list.

Measure	**Parent Interview for Autism (PIA). Stone and Hogan (1993a).**
Purpose	Gathering diagnostic information from parents of children suspected of having autism.
Areas	Social Relating, Affective Responses, Peer Interactions, Motor Imitation, Communication, Nonverbal Communication, Language Understanding, Object Play, Imaginative Play, Sensory Responses, Motoric Behavior, Need for Sameness.
Format	118-item, 5-point scale administered orally to the parent so that questions and answers can be clarified.
Scores	Total and domain raw scores.
Age group	Preschool level and below.
Time	30–45 minutes.
Users	Professionals.
Norms	165 children under 6 years of age whose parents served as respondents. Children were not previously diagnosed with autism, preventing skewed responses by parents.
Reliability	Internal consistency, .94; test–retest (2 weeks), .93 on 29 subjects.
Validity	Concurrent: Supported by –.42 correlation between PIA and CARS total scores, and –.49 with number of DSM-III-R criteria met independently of the parent interview. Discriminant: The total PIA score and 6 of 11 dimensions discriminated a group of children with autism from a group with mental retardation.
Comments	Allows examiners to gain perspective across time and different contexts of child's life. Altogether, the PIA is a promising measure in need of further development: It is easy to administer, does not require extra training, takes about 15–20 minutes (depending on how much follow-up questioning is done), and provides relevant information for treatment. It does not have the psychometric characteristics or detailed interviewer guidance available for the ADI-R.
References consulted	Stone and Hogan (1993b). See book's References list.

Measure	**Pervasive Developmental Disorders Screening Test—Second Edition (PDDST-II). Siegel (2004).**
Purpose	Designed as a clinical screening tool for all types of PDD or ASD.
Areas	Behaviors characteristic of young children with ASD.
Format	Three forms: stage 1, Primary Care Screener (PCS, 22 items); stage 2, Developmental Clinic Screener (DCS, 14 items); and stage 3, Autism Clinic Severity Screener (ACSS, 12 items). Also includes a set of 41 supplemental items. Yes–no format.
Scores	Cutoff scores.
Age group	12–48 months.
Time	Approximately 15 minutes.
Users	Nonspecialist clinicians.
Norms	Standardization sample consisted of 410 children with autistic disorder, 108 children with other types of ASD, 89 children with a language disorder, 36 children with another neuropsychiatric disorder, 44 children diagnosed with mental retardation alone, and a comparison group of 256 very-low-birth-weight preterm infants with a history of intraventricular hemorrhage. Sample included children ages 19 months to over 48 months, with more males than females.
Reliability	Not reported.
Validity	Sensitivity and specificity were reported for each of the three forms: Stage 1 (PCS): 92% sensitivity and 91% specificity. Stage 2 (DCS): 73% sensitivity and 49% specificity. Stage 3 (ACSS): 58% sensitivity and 60% specificity.
Comments	The PDDST-II is a reliable and valid screening tool for distinguishing young children in need of a full evaluation for suspected ASD. It is less good at differentiating ASD from other developmental disorders or distinguishing nonautism ASD from autism. It is user-friendly and has a wide age range. It provides an efficient use of diagnostic procedures, while still allowing for examiner clarification in order to assure accuracy. No sensitivity or specificity data available for screening of large unselected sample.
References consulted	Dumont-Mathieu and Fein (2005). See book's References list.

Measure	**Psychoeducational Profile: TEACCH Individualized Psychoeducational Assessment for Children with Autistic Spectrum Disorders—Third Edition (PEP-3). Schopler, Lansing, Reichler, and Marcus (2005).**
Purpose	Assisting in the educational planning and diagnosis of children with ASD.
Areas	Performance Scales and Caregiver Report.
Format	Performance section is made up of 10 subtests (6 measuring developmental abilities and 4 measuring maladaptive behaviors that frequently occur in children with ASD) individually administered to the child. Caregiver Report is comprised of two sections and three subtests (Problem Behaviors, Personal Self-care Skills, and Adaptive Abilities).

Scores	Performance subtests combine into three composite scores: Communication, Motor, and Maladaptive Behaviors. Items on Performance Scale are scored as Passing (2 points), Emerging (1 point), and Failing (0 points). The three subtests from the Caregiver Report can be scored for normative purposes as well. Raw scores are converted into developmental ages based on typically developing sample (with some extrapolation for ages below 2 and above 7) and percentile ranks based on autism comparison sample. Developmental–adaptive levels are also included, ranging from adequate to severe.
Age group	Ages 2–7-6 years, or older children functioning with this age range.
Time	45–90 minutes.
Users	Trained professionals.
Norms	Data collected on a generally representative national sample consisting of 407 children with ASD (95% with autistic disorder) and a comparison group of 148 typically developing children assessed by professionals at TEACCH centers or those who had purchased and used the PEP-R within the last two years. There was no independent verification of ASD diagnoses. This is of less concern in regard to the TEACCH professionals as they are likely to be experts in the diagnosis of children with ASD. However, the purchasers of the PEP-R who agreed to collect data have an unknown level of expertise. Most of the children with ASD were between the ages of 3 to 6 but ranged in age from 2 to 21 years of age; normally developing children were ages 2 through 6 years. Children were disproportionately from the southern United States but region was not related to scores on the PEP-3.
Reliability	Internal consistency, high with average Cronbach's alphas of .90–.97 on the Performance Scales and .84–.90 on the Caregiver Report subscales. Composite alphas are .99 Communication, .97 Motor, and .97 Maladaptive. No differences by gender, race, ethnicity, or income but alphas are lower on the Maladaptive Scales for the normally developing group; test–retest: 33 children with ASD ages 4–14 years retested within two weeks and the Performance Scales were .95–.99 and Caregiver Report .98–.99; interrater reliability for Caregiver Report using both parents for 40 children ages 2-1–7-6 years in 7 states (31 with ASD) found a mean of .85 for Problem Behavior, .78 for Adaptive Behavior, and .90 for Self-Care.
Validity	Content: Based on over 20 years of use in North Carolina to program children with ASD. Item discrimination and difficulty statistics also support content validity. Construct: Supported with moderate to high mean correlations in the predicted direction with the CARS, the original Vineland, the ABC-2, and the Brief Ability Rating Scale. Median percentile scores for normally developing children were at the 92–99 percentile, nonimpaired range, while all the children with ASD were in the impaired range with median percentile ranks of 38–56. Confirmatory factor analysis revealed a good fit for the three Performance Scale composites. The developmental scales are correlated with age while the nondevelopmental scales are not.
Comments	The PEP-3 provides a profile of a student's development in a variety of domains relevant to educational programming for low-functioning children and those displaying autistic behaviors. Its long history of educational use and good psychometric properties make it highly recommended for educational planning. It is also useful for diagnosis as it does a good job of eliciting relevant behaviors and it is highly correlated with total scores on the CARS

	(.78). The PEP-3 now contains all of the toys and materials needed to administer the test (except food, drink, and a light switch) not included in previous versions of the test. It continues to have a very low floor, is easy to administer, moves at a fast pace, and includes appealing tasks that maximize the limited motivation and attention of young children suspected of ASD.
References consulted	Brock, Jimerson, and Hansen (2006). See book's References list.

Measure	**Screening Tool for Autism in Two-Year-Olds (STAT). Stone, Coonrod, and Ousley (2000).**
Purpose	Identifying children in need of further, specialized diagnostic evaluation for autism.
Areas	Play, imitation, directing attention, and (not scored) response to requests.
Format	12 items administered in play-like interaction.
Scores	Cutoff score for each of the first three areas; cutoff on total scale is failing any two of these three areas.
Age group	24–35 months.
Time	15–20 minutes.
Users	Healthcare workers and other service providers.
Norms	Data collected on developmental sample of 40 children (age 2 years) with either autism (*n* = 3), or nonautism developmental delays (*n* = 33), and on validation sample of 33 children (12 with autism and 21 without autism, as rated by the CARS and DSM-IV).
Reliability	Not reported.
Validity	Sensitivity, .83; specificity, .86.
Comments	Because of the developmentally sensitive nature of the items, the STAT is likely to be useful only as an initial screening tool for young children within its age range. It is particularly useful in that it covers the age ranges when children with ASD are most likely to be referred for professional evaluation. It is brief and easy to administer. More research is needed on its predictive and concurrent validity with standardized diagnostic measures.
References consulted	Dumont-Mathieu and Fein (2005); Stone, Coonrod, and Ousley (2000); Stone et al. (2004). See book's References list.

Measure	**Social Communication Questionnaire (SCQ). Rutter, Bailey, and Lord (2003).**
Purpose	Providing a screening measure for referral for a complete diagnostic evaluation for children suspected of ASD.
Areas	Three subscores that correlate with Social Development and Play, Communication, and Repetitive and Restricted Behaviors domains on the ADI-R.
Format	40-item, yes–no parent report questionnaire. Two versions, Lifetime and Current.
Scores	Three subscores and total score. Total score is compared to a cutoff of 15.
Age group	Over 4-0 years; minimum mental age of 2-0 years.
Time	10 minutes.

Users	Clinicians and educators.
Norms	Standardization sample consisted of 160 individuals with ASD and 40 individuals with non-ASD diagnoses who had participated in previous studies of ASD, including a family genetic study of autism; a study of adolescents with clinically diagnosed Asperger syndrome or conduct disorder; a study of individuals with Rett syndrome; and a study of the diagnosis of autism in young children presenting with developmental problems. Sociodemographic information about the standardization sample is not included in the SCQ manual, making it difficult to assess the validity of the SCQ with various socioeconomic and ethnic groups.
Reliability	Internal consistency, .90.
Validity	Construct, supported, as it is based on the ADI-R; discriminant, supported. Is able to separate ASD from non-ASD diagnoses at all IQ levels. The scale does not do a good job of differentiating between autism and other types of ASD, which is also true of the best diagnostic instruments.
Comments	Items are based on ADI-R, but modified for easy understanding and focused on deviance rather than developmental delay. It is easy to administer and score, making it an efficient screening instrument. Psychometric characteristics are excellent for a screening measure. Formerly the Autism Screening Questionnaire. German version available.
References consulted	Brassard review. www.wpspublish.com

APPENDIX 13.2. Autism Program Quality Indicators

Score	Description
NA	Not applicable. The program is not responsible for this area.
0	There is no evidence of this indicator.
1	There is minimal evidence of this indicator, but clear evidence exists that the program is in the process of planning for implementation and/or staff development.
2	There is some evidence of this indicator *or* there is clear evidence of the indicator for only a portion of students with autism.
3	This quality indicator is clearly evident for all students with autism.

	INDIVIDUAL EVALUATION: Thorough diagnostic, developmental, and educational assessments using a comprehensive, multidisciplinary approach are used to identify students' strengths and needs.	Score	Comments
1)	Evaluations are conducted by multidisciplinary teams made up of qualified personnel who are familiar with the characteristics and response patterns of students with autism.		
2)	The medical and developmental history review factors specific to autism.		
3)	Evaluations include the examination of the individual skills and strengths of students with autism, as well as their needs.		
4)	Evaluations use a variety of measures and sources of information, including: a) appropriate standardized, developmental, and observational methods, b) autism-specific measures, c) parent and family input, d) review of recent progress and functional level.		
5)	For both verbal and nonverbal students, speech and language evaluations use standardized measures, parental report, observation, and spontaneous language samples to assess: a) receptive language, b) expressive language, c) speech production, d) communicative intent, e) pragmatics.		
6)	Evaluation reports integrate results from all areas in ways that lead directly to programmatic recommendations for instruction.		
7)	Evaluation reports are written in a meaningful, understandable manner.		
8)	Evaluation reports are shared with the student (if appropriate), parents, educators, and other professionals who work collaboratively with the family.		
	Summary Rating for Individual Evaluation		

DEVELOPMENT OF THE INDIVIDUALIZED EDUCATION PROGRAM: The Committee on Preschool Special Education (CPSE) and the Committee on Special Education (CSE) use evaluation results, parent and family concerns, and present levels of performance in developing individualized education programs (IEPs) to meet students' needs.		Score	Comments
1)	The IEP identifies developmental, health, social-emotional, and behavioral needs.		
2)	While the IEP addresses a broad range of developmental and educational needs, it specifically includes the areas of: a) communication, b) social interaction, c) behavior and emotional development, d) play and use of leisure time.		
3)	Goals and objectives: a) relate directly to the student's present level of performance and identified needs, b) reflect parental input and family concerns, c) are observable and measurable, relate to long-term outcomes, d) are selected to achieve long-term outcomes.		
4)	The IEP identifies program modifications, including environmental and instructional adaptations and accommodations that are needed to support the student.		
5)	"Parent counseling and training" is indicated as a related service as appropriate.		
6)	Augmentative and alternative communication systems are considered for students with limited verbal abilities.		
7)	Opportunities for interaction with nondisabled peers are provided as appropriate.		
Summary Rating for Development of the IEP			

CURRICULUM: The program uses a curriculum that addresses the significant skill deficits of students with autism and relates to the New York State Learning Standards.		Score	Comments
1)	The curriculum contains a written statement of goals and philosophy from which instructional objectives, methods, and activities proceed.		
2)	The curriculum focuses on maximizing independent functioning in home, school, vocational, and community settings.		
3)	The curriculum is adapted to the different ages, abilities, and learning styles of students with autism.		
4)	The curriculum emphasizes the development of: a) attention to social stimuli, b) imitation skills, c) communication and language, d) social relationships, e) symbolic play, imagination, and creativity, f) self-regulation, g) skills to meet the learning standards, h) vocational skills.		
5)	With respect to communication, the curriculum emphasizes the development of a functional communication system for both verbal and nonverbal students with autism.		

6)	With respect to social relationships, the curriculum emphasizes the development of social interaction skills with adults and peers for a range of occasions and environments.		
7)	The curriculum focuses on the maintenance and generalization of learned skills to more complex environments.		
Summary Rating for Curriculum			

INSTRUCTIONAL ACTIVITIES: The program provides a variety of developmentally and functionally appropriate activities, experiences, and materials that engage students in meaningful learning.		Score	Comments
1)	Instructional activities: a) enhance response opportunities, b) are appealing and interesting, c) promote active engagement of the student, d) focus on basic skills before more complex skills, e) provide multiple opportunities for practicing skills identified on the IEP, f) are (whenever possible) embedded within ongoing and natural routines of home, school, vocational, and community settings.		
2)	Activities use a variety of instructional formats—one-to-one instruction, small group instruction, student-initiated interactions, teacher-directed interactions, play, peer-mediated instruction—based upon the skill to be taught and the individual needs of the student.		
3)	IEP goals and instructional methods are compatible and complementary when the program uses components of different intervention approaches.		
4)	Instructional activities are adapted to the range of ages, abilities, and learning styles of students with autism.		
5)	Daily instruction is provided to meet the individual communication needs of students with autism.		
Summary Rating for Instructional Activities			

INSTRUCTIONAL METHODS: Teaching methods reflect the unique needs of students with autism and are varied depending on developmental appropriateness and individual strengths and needs.		Score	Comments
1)	Instructional methods are adapted to the range of ages, abilities, and learning styles of students with autism.		
2)	Instructional methods reflect empirically validated practices or solid evidence that demonstrates effectiveness over time.		
3)	The degree of structure and intensity of teaching are geared to the functional abilities of the student.		
4)	Instructional methods: a) emphasize the use of naturally occurring reinforcers, b) promote high rates of successful performance, c) encourage communication and social interaction, d) encourage the spontaneous use of learned skills in different settings.		
5)	As instruction proceeds, an effort is made to teach students to cope with the distractions and disruptions that are an inevitable part of daily living.		
6)	There is a clear plan showing methods for systematically promoting the maintenance and generalization of learned skills to new and different environments.		

Summary Rating for Instructional Methods			

INSTRUCTIONAL ENVIRONMENTS: Educational environments provide a structure that builds on a student's strengths while minimizing those factors that most interfere with learning.		Score	Comments
1)	Environments are initially simplified to help students recognize relevant information.		
2)	When needed (particularly for younger students), classrooms have defined areas that provide clear visual boundaries for specific activities.		
3)	Environmental supports (e.g., the use of visual schedules) are available that facilitate the student's ability to: a) predict events and activities, b) anticipate change, c) understand expectations.		
4)	Communication toward and with students: a) is geared to their language abilities, b) is clear and relevant, c) encourages dialogue (when appropriate), rather than being largely directive.		
Summary Rating for Instructional Environments			

REVIEW AND MONITORING OF PROGRESS AND OUTCOMES: The program uses a collaborative, ongoing, systematic process for assessing student progress.		Score	Comments
1)	The program provides regular and ongoing assessment of each student's progress on his/her specific IEP goals and objectives.		
2)	Student progress is summarized and reviewed by an educational team.		
3)	Students are assessed and the instructional program is refined when: a) target objectives have been achieved, b) progress is not observed after an appropriate trial period, c) target objectives have not been achieved after an appropriate trial period, d) there is an unexpected change in a student's behavior or health status, e) significant changes occur in the home, school, vocational, or community setting.		
4)	The program routinely reports to the CPSE or CSE when there is a need to consider modifications to the IEP.		
Summary Rating for Review and Monitoring of Progress			

FAMILY INVOLVEMENT AND SUPPORT: Parents are recognized and valued as full partners in the development and implementation of their child's IEP.		Score	Comments
1)	Parents and family members are supported as active participants in all aspects of their child's ongoing evaluation and education to the extent of their interests, resources, and abilities.		
2)	Parents are informed about the range of educational and service options.		
3)	The program demonstrates an awareness and respect for the culture, language, values, and parenting styles of the families it serves.		
4)	The program makes available "parent counseling and training" services, which:		

		Score	Comments
	a) provide parents with information about child development, b) assist parents to understand the needs of their child, c) foster coordination of efforts between school and home, d) support the family in behavior management, e) enable parents to acquire skills to support the implementation of their child's IEP.		
5)	Parents are provided with opportunities to meet regularly with other parents and professionals in support groups.		
6)	Parents receive regular communication from the program regarding their child's progress.		
7)	Parents are assisted in accessing services from other agencies (when available and as appropriate), such as respite, in-home behavior support, home health care, transportation, etc.		
Summary Rating for Family Involvement and Support			

INCLUSION: Opportunities for interaction with nondisabled peers are incorporated into the program.		Score	Comments
1)	The program offers opportunities for interaction with nondisabled peers in both informal and planned interactions.		
2)	In their contact with nondisabled peers, students are provided with instruction and support to maximize successful interactions.		
3)	The program provides nondisabled peers with knowledge and support (e.g., peer training) to facilitate and encourage spontaneous and meaningful interactions.		
4)	Training and ongoing support are provided to the general education teachers and staff.		
Summary Rating for Inclusion			

PLANNING THE MOVE FROM ONE SETTING TO ANOTHER: Parents and professionals work collaboratively in planning transitions from one classroom, program, or service delivery system to another.		Score	Comments
1)	All aspects of planning include the student (whenever appropriate), parents and other family members, current and receiving professionals, and other relevant individuals.		
2)	Transitional support services are provided by a special education teacher with a background in teaching students with autism.		
3)	Transition planning: a) begins while the student is in the current placement, b) provides the student and family with the opportunity to visit the new setting (i.e., meet teachers, view classrooms).		
4)	Planning integrates considerations of future placements (i.e., skills needed in the next classroom or school setting) with the student's current program.		
5)	Planning includes teacher preparation and other supports to ensure success of the student in the new classroom, school, or work site.		
Summary Rating for Planning the Move from One Setting to Another			

CHALLENGING BEHAVIOR: Positive behavior supports, based on a functional behavioral assessment (FBA), are used to address challenging behavior.		Score	Comments
1)	The program has a school-wide behavioral system that: a) defines expectations for appropriate behavior in all instructional settings, b) uses proactive approaches to managing behavior, c) has established strategies for crisis intervention, d) provides training for staff in recommended behavioral strategies.		
2)	A FBA is used to direct intervention planning for persistent challenging behaviors.		
3)	Multiple methods (e.g., direct observations, functional analysis, rating scales, and interviews) are used in conducting the FBA.		
4)	The FBA identifies both immediate (e.g., request to perform a task) and more distant (e.g., poor sleeping habits) factors that increase challenging behaviors.		
5)	The FBA identifies one or more functions for the challenging behaviors.		
6)	Environmental accommodations and adaptations are used to prevent or minimize occurrences of the problem behavior.		
7)	Instruction in alternative, appropriate skills (e.g., communication, social, or self-regulatory skills) is routinely incorporated into behavior intervention plans.		
8)	Behavior interventions are based on positive supports and strategies.		
9)	Behavior intervention plans focus on long-terms outcomes (e.g., making new friends, participating in extracurricular activities).		
Summary Rating for Challenging Behavior			

COMMUNITY COLLABORATION: The program links with community agencies to assist families in accessing supports and services needed by students with autism.		Score	Comments
1)	The program develops links with different community agencies that provide the comprehensive services often needed by students with autism.		
2)	The program assists parents in defining their child's outside-of-school needs, such as respite, in-home behavior support, home health care, transportation, etc.		
3)	Parents are assisted in accessing services from community agencies.		
Summary Rating for Community Collaboration			

PERSONNEL: Teachers, teacher aides and assistants, related service providers, school psychologists, administrators, and support staff are knowledgeable and skilled related to the education of students with autism.		Score	Comments
1)	Staff [members] are knowledgeable and skilled in the areas of expertise specific to autism, including: a) characteristics of autism, b) familiarity with assessment methods, c) developing IEPs to meet the unique needs of each student, d) curriculum, environmental adaptations and accommodations, and instructional methods, e) strategies to improve communication and social interaction skills, f) classroom and individual behavior management techniques.		
2)	Staff [members] participate in continuing professional development (e.g., consultation, workshops, conferences) designed to further develop their knowledge and skills.		

3)	Staff [members] are available in a ratio sufficient to provide the support necessary to accomplish IEP goals.		
4)	Teachers and related service providers have access to students' IEPs and are informed of their responsibilities for implementation.		
5)	Paraprofessionals receive specific and direct instruction and supervision regarding their IEP responsibilities to the student.		
6)	Ongoing support and technical assistance are available to resolve concerns related to learning and behavior.		
Summary Rating for Personnel			

PROGRAM EVALUATION: Systematic examination of program implementation and impact is conducted, including the aggregation of individual student outcomes and consumer satisfaction.		Score	Comments
1)	The program incorporates evaluation systems that assess program-wide effectiveness in the areas of: a) students' progress toward mastery of IEP goals, b) student performance on state- and district-wide tests (including, as appropriate, student performance on the State Alternate Assessment), c) students' generalization of skills, d) student progress toward long-term outcomes.		
2)	The program evaluates short-term (e.g., weekly or biweekly), intermediate (e.g., quarterly), and long-term (e.g., yearly) changes in student progress.		
3)	Parents regularly receive feedback on their child's progress toward meeting IEP goals and objectives.		
4)	Program evaluation includes measures of consumer satisfaction with services.		
5)	Information obtained from program evaluation is used for program improvement.		
Summary Rating for Program Evaluation			

	Summary Rating
Individual Evaluation	
Development of the Individualized Education Program	
Curriculum	
Instructional Activities	
Instructional Methods	
Instructional Environments	
Review and Monitoring of Progress and Outcomes	
Family Involvement and Support	
Inclusion	
Community Collaboration	
Planning the Move from One Setting to Another	
Challenging Behavior	
Personnel	
Program Evaluation	

Chapter 14

Assessment of Emotional Development and Behavior Problems

Until very recently, few screening or diagnostic measures existed to assess social and emotional competence and problems in young children. Typically, screening measures would have one or two items often asked of parents during a brief interview as part of 1-day screening events, such as preschool or kindergarten roundups; these measures would then be omitted from the cutoff score for determining whether a child would be referred for further evaluation. The first diagnostic measures that were developed (e.g., Child Behavior Checklist/2–3 [CBCL/2–3]; Achenbach, 1992) asked parents or teachers/caregivers about behavior that was clearly pathological. Such questions made respondents reluctant to answer honestly, fearing stigmatization of the children (Fantuzzo, Blue-Sky, McDermott, Muscat, & Lutz, 2003). Recently, however, this situation has begun to change. The change has been influenced by (1) the successful development of early and effective diagnostic measures and interventions for autistic spectrum disorders (ASD), a group of a conditions with the most severe form of social and emotional impairment (see Chapter 13); (2) a growing recognition, as a result of longitudinal and intervention studies, that emotional and behavioral problems appear very early in life, and can quickly become entrenched and difficult to remediate if professional involvement is delayed until children start formal schooling (U.S. DHHS, 1999); (3) a recognition that emotional development is as important as cognitive development in later academic success of young children, and thus should be routinely assessed for progress in early childhood programs (Raver, 2003); and (4) the realization that emotional development is the pathway to social competence (Denham et al., 2003).

Emotional skills and regulation play a key role in the development of children's interpersonal relationships, problem behaviors, and readiness to learn. We begin this chapter by reviewing the research on emotional development in early childhood, including milestones in emotional development from birth through age 5 in typical children; key aspects of emotional competence for preschoolers; the constitutional and environmental factors that influence emotional competence; and the relevance of this information for early childhood assessors and educators. Next, we discuss the frameworks used to diagnose preschool children's emotional and behavior problems, as well as the degree to which these frameworks are truly applicable to the problems most often present in early childhood. We then describe all the steps, procedures, and methods used to screen children for emotional development and behavior problems. Children who are developing problems need early identification for purposes of intervention, and an assessment of all children's emotional skills can be used for curriculum development and instruction to promote emotional and social competence. Finally, we present the steps and methods of diagnosing preschool children for internalizing and externalizing problems and identifying appropriate treatments, along with two case studies.

We make the assumption in this chapter that a mental health professional (school or child clinical psychologist, social worker, or child psychiatrist) experienced in working with young children will play a central role in the screening and/or diagnostic evaluation of any suspected emotional or behavior problem. The prevention and intervention programs described below give teachers and early childhood special educators the lead role in the implementation of classroom-based programs designed to promote emotional development.

REVIEW OF RESEARCH ON EMOTIONAL DEVELOPMENT IN EARLY CHILDHOOD

An *emotion* is "a subjective reaction to a salient event, characterized by physiological, experiential, and overt behavioral change" (Sroufe, 1996, p. 15). Emotions are subjective, in that "the same event may elicit different emotional reactions (or none) in different people or even in the same person across time or context" (p. 15). Emotions also have cognitive and evaluative components—how a person perceives, interprets, and responds to an event determines the particular emotion experienced—although these components can be quite primitive in early infancy.

Emotions are assumed to have evolved across species to promote safety, mastery of the environment, and reproductive success for the animals possessing them. Human emotions are built on this "old vertebrate brain," with a core set of emotions identified as culturally universal and emerging very early in childhood. These include interest, joy, sadness, and anger, which have been shown to account for more than 95% of facial expressions shown by infants (Izard et al., 1995). Also among core emotions are startle/surprise, disgust/revulsion, contempt/scorn, fear/terror, shame/shyness/humiliation, and guilt/remorse. Emotions are particularly important in humans, because infants do not have instincts to guide their behavior (unlike, say, ducklings following their mother soon after birth). The few reflexes that human infants possess have limited value in terms of promoting survival and adaptation. Emotions fulfill the functions of instincts and reflexes, in that they allow infants and young children to "signal their needs, desires, and distress through affective channels, and, thereby, elicit effective care from their caregivers" (Abe & Izard, 1999, p. 527).

Throughout the life span, emotions communicate internal states (vital information for our highly social species), promote competence in exploring and mastering the environment, and prepare individuals to respond appropriately to emergency situations.

Emotions are vital to achieving individual goals, which for infants can include resisting restraint or indicating extreme distress in order to mobilize a rapid parental response. As children grow older, fear can mobilize an escape from danger; anger can help someone overcome an obstacle; and interest and joy promote and maintain a relationship (Abe & Izard, 1999). However, as Sroufe (1996) notes, although "emotionally guided behavior is more flexible and modifiable," in humans it "represents a major vulnerability" because it makes them "susceptible to enumerable patterns of distortion" (p. 17). An example of this vulnerability is an infant's cutting off awareness of anger at maternal rebuffs when the child is in need of comfort, in order to prevent the display of angry feelings and further rejection by the mother. Over time such a process can lead to a lack of awareness of anger, which "leaks" out nonetheless, straining relationships.

Milestones in Emotion Development, with an Emphasis on Attachment

The major theorists/researchers in the area of emotional development use different concepts, and time periods to denote stages of emotional development. Yet there is a great deal of agreement on important milestones that occur from infancy to the preschool years in typically developing children. Table 14.1 draws on the work of Sroufe and colleagues (Sroufe, 1996; Sroufe, Egeland, Carlson, & Collins, 2005), Greenspan and colleagues (Greenspan, DeGangi, & Wieder, 2001), and Izard and colleagues (Abe & Izard, 1999; Izard et al., 1995) in describing these milestones and achievements. All three groups of theoreticians integrate emotional experience with cognitive and social development. Greenspan et al. and Izard et al. see emotions in a driving role, while Sroufe et al. describe all three as reciprocally influential. Because of its central importance in emotional development, attachment is described in some detail below.

Attachment is a biologically based predisposition on the part of an infant to develop a preference for a regularly present and effectively involved caregiver (usually the mother, but sometimes other caregivers). Greenspan et al. (2001) see attachment as beginning to develop in the 2nd to the 7th months of life, when the infant is very involved in forming a relationship with the primary caregiver—beginning to smile preferentially at her, mastering her smell, and attending deeply to her face and voice. Sroufe (1996) also sees attachment as an important developmental task but places it at the 9th–12th months, when the infant, now beginning to crawl, can play an active role in maintaining proximity to the caregiver and begins to show stranger anxiety and distress at the caregiver's absence. Sroufe believes that the infant develops an internal working model of the relationship based on the history of experience with the caregiver, and acts according to expectations of how the caregiver will behave. The attachment relationship promotes physical proximity between the infant and caregiver, thus protecting the infant from predators and other dangers in the environment. When the caregiver is present, attachment provides a secure base from which the infant can explore and begin to master the environment. The infant's (and later the child's) degree of exploration increases as physical proximity becomes less important for security.

By 12 months of age this working model of the relationship with the caregiver, known as an *attachment style*, can be reliably assessed with the Ainsworth Strange Situation procedure (Ainsworth, Blehar, Waters, & Wall, 1978)—a standardized set of separation and reunion experiences in the laboratory with caregiver and infant. The early style is unique to each caregiver relationship and can change over time. This is a rich, complex area of research with important implications for emotional and social development. The following is a brief synopsis of each attachment style as it relates to socioemotional func-

TABLE 14.1. Milestones in Typical Emotional Development

Age	Behaviors
0–3 months	Homeostasis • Stimulus barrier in first months protects child, but then gives way to stimulus vulnerability and need for caregiver to modulate stimulation. • Forming of sleep–wake, feeding, alertness cycles. • First social smiles.
3–10 months	Dyadic interaction/two-way communication • Transition from infant's following lead of caregiver to infant's taking turn in synchronized interactions; caregiver uses emotional expression of infant to guide level of stimulation. • Infants with sensitive caregivers become increasingly able to maintain positive affect, promoting positive engagement with caregivers and world; infants of depressed caregivers lack this support, making them prone to irritability, listlessness, and withdrawal. • Initiative develops around 7–9 months, along with joy at success and anger at failure or interference. • Infant begins to communicate purposefully and flexibly, using all emotions and senses.
2–12 months	Attachment • Biologically based predisposition on part of infant to develop preference for regularly present, affectively involved caregiver (see text for more detail).
10–12 months	Social referencing • Infant uses adult facial expressions to interpret ambiguous situations (is a stranger scary or safe?) and monitor adult emotions and behavior (e.g., Dad's good mood indicates receptivity for play or other demands; Mom's lack of attention indicates a need to move closer). Major milestone, as this is a foundation for a theory of mind and for moral development, as infants see which behaviors are parentally disapproved.
18–24 months	Sense of self • Increasing behavioral organization and problem solving lead to sense of self as independent of caregiver. • Child becomes more defiant, shows a conflict in wills, is able to be affectionate, makes independent decisions, and shows first signs of shame and positive self-evaluation.
18–48 months	Sense of others • Deeper understanding of others leads to first signs of empathy, learning emotion words, curiosity about others' feelings. • Child uses talk about emotions to get help, make excuses, and get others to do his or her bidding. • By age 4 years, child understands that people respond emotionally in different ways to the same event.
2–5 years	Representation of thoughts and feelings in play and fantasy
2–5 years	Moral standards. • Moral standards are developed and internalized as the child watches how parents respond to rule violations and tantrums, making clear the limits before consequences ensue; adults are still needed for support. • Pride, shame, and guilt develop, making moral events salient.

Note. Data from Abe and Izard (1999); Greenspan, DeGangi, and Wieder (2001); Izard et al. (1995); and Sroufe (1996).

tioning through the preschool years; these descriptions are based largely on the research of Sroufe et al. (2005).

Children with a *secure* attachment style have reliable and responsive caregivers who give their infants confidence that they will have proximity when they need it and in the way they need it. Play ratings at 18 months show them to be more highly invested in fantasy play than children who are insecurely attached to their primary caregivers, as well as more socially flexible with play partners, more advanced in play verbalizations, more people-oriented and balanced, and more likely to develop positive resolutions to negative themes of conflict and sadness. Preschool peer group ratings of secure children show them to be more actively involved, more affectively positive, less affectively negative, and more popular than children with insecure attachment styles. Teachers find them warm and straightforward in their engagement, hold them to age-appropriate standards, and expect them to be compliant and follow directions.

Children who have an *anxious/ambivalent* style maximize the expression of attachment behaviors in order to keep their undependable caregivers nearby. These children act as if they believe that they must cling as hard as they can to attachment figures, because these figures are likely to abandon them unless they are constantly vigilant. They tend to be overwhelmed by attachment issues and are often in a chronic state of arousal, which limits their perspective taking and exploration. Their fantasy play ratings at 18 months incorporate relationship themes and negative themes related to environmental danger. Their preschool teachers are unduly nurturing and caretaking, treating them as if they were a year or two younger than their actual age; the teachers are quite tolerant of minor violations of classroom rules and expect less compliance.

Children with an *anxious/avoidant* style have caregivers who are rejecting when they are fussy, dependent, or upset. These children learn to pretend that they are not needy by distracting themselves when upset and minimizing attachment behaviors. Their strategy leaves them without help in regulating their emotions, but it keeps them in proximity to their caregivers, so that help can be provided in dangerous circumstances. Over time these children lose the ability to know how they are feeling in situations when they are angry or needy. Their lack of comfort with emotions and closeness often leaves them on the periphery of groups. At 18 months their fantasy play ratings show less positive themes than those of securely attached children, and they are less concerned with interpersonal relationships. Aggression is prevalent, and emotions are rarely attributed to characters or action. Preschool peer group ratings show them to be less empathetic, more likely to show antiempathetic behavior (i.e., to act in ways that make the distress worse), and more likely to engage in behaviors that make teacher or other children angry (e.g., hostile, defiant) than children with the other attachment styles. Friendships are less deep between avoidant children and other children, in terms of less mutuality, responsiveness, and affective involvement. Their teachers' relationships with them are controlling and at times angry.

Finally, there is a *disorganized or fearful* attachment style. These children have difficulty organizing a strategy for maintaining proximity to their caregivers, who either are incoherent in their behavior or are actual sources of threat. These children have trouble developing an integrated sense of self, have impulse control problems, and are most at risk for global psychopathology.

In addition to the milestones described in Table 14.1, there are three important components of emotional development during the toddler/preschool years (ages 2–5): emotional knowledge or understanding, emotional expressiveness, and emotional regulation. The three components are critical features of emotional competence, which predicts both preschool and kindergarten social competence (Denham et al., 2003).

Key Aspects of Emotional Competence for Preschoolers

Emotional Knowledge or Understanding

As they approach age 2, most children have developed an emotion vocabulary (e.g., sad, thirst) that allows them to identify emotions in themselves and others, using situational behavior and facial expressions as cues (Fabes, Eisenberg, Nyman, & Michealieu, 1991). This knowledge becomes an ever-growing database that a child uses to encode and interpret social cues (Izard, 2002). Children use this information to interpret emotional signals in themselves and in others, as well as to interpret the role of context in those emotions. Preschoolers who understand emotions react more appropriately to others, are better liked by peers, and are rated as more socially competent by teachers (Denham, McKinley, Couchoud, & Holt, 1990). Emotional knowledge makes it easier for children to be socially competent because it increases their ability to perceive social cues accurately, to respond appropriately to what's going on, and to regulate their own emotional reactions. Higher verbal ability is related to greater use of emotion vocabulary, the ability to discuss emotions, and the ability to handle negative emotions effectively (Cook, Greenberg, & Kusche, 1994; Cutting & Dunn, 1999). Girls are more skilled in more aspects of emotional knowledge than boys are (Schultz, Izard, & Ackerman, 2000), and they are more likely to behave prosocially than boys; in particular, they are kinder and more considerate (Eisenberg & Fabes, 1998). (See "Gender," below.)

Emotional Expressiveness

Clear expression of the full range of emotion is a key component of emotional competence, because of the important role that it plays in understanding the self and other human beings. Emotional expressiveness is also important in initiating and maintaining relationships. In particular, children who demonstrate more positive than negative affect are rated by teachers as more competent and friendly and as less aggressive or sad. They are more likely to respond prosocially to the emotions of peers and are better liked by peers (Denham et al., 2003). Positive emotions usually recruit relationships, while a preponderance of negative emotions can drive them away.

Emotional Regulation

Regulation, the third component of emotional competence, is clearly the most complex. It is defined by Thompson (1994) as consisting "of the extrinsic and intrinsic processes responsible for monitoring, evaluating, and modifying emotional reactions, especially their intensive and temporal features, to accomplish one's goals" (p. 28).

Infants develop the ability to shift attention voluntarily between 3 and 6 months of age. Prior to that, they have obligatory attention; that is, they cannot disengage visually from emotionally arousing events. Once the ability to shift attention is developed, parents can use visual distraction to regulate infants' emotions, and the infants become easier to soothe as a result (Rothbart, Ziaie, & O'Boyle, 1992). As children grow older, they learn to regulate their emotions themselves. Early attentional strategies may include covering their eyes or ears, removing emotionally evocative stimuli, or leaving the situation. Later, children become able to redirect their attention internally, by thinking pleasant thoughts during distressing events or talking to themselves and focusing on positive events or outcomes. Children who become aware of how strongly they feel about a situation can decrease their reaction over time as they stop thinking about things that upset them and do something else to take their mind off the situation (Thompson, 1994). As preschoolers, they become aware of the fact that they can feel both sad and mad or sad and happy. Individuals who do not develop awareness that mixed emotions are accepted and common are described as "splitting." (This is most often seen in individuals with borderline personality disorder, who may have trouble integrating the fact that one individual, such as their mother, can be both good and bad; instead, they alternate between seeing her as all good or all bad.) Children also realize that they can manipulate the intensity with which they express their feelings in order to create the social response they want (Thompson, 1994). By age 6, most children know that they can exaggerate or diminish their emotional expressions in order to mislead others about how distressed they are.

Competent children develop a variety of coping strategies and use these across the life span to regulate emotions. Increasing the availability of external support is a popular strategy; children or adults may turn to friends or family when feeling worried, sad, or angry. They may also use other things that help themselves calm down, such as snuggling under a favorite blanket, reading stories, eating special foods, playing, or exercising. Parents often establish caregiving routines in order to selectively reduce or expand emotional arousal. For example, giving a child a snack in the afternoon or the late afternoon, or maintaining a regular afternoon naptime, ensures a more pleasant, less cranky child at dinner. Intense roughhousing after dinner creates a very pleasant emotional high, with enough time for a bath to calm the child down and become relaxed and ready for storybook reading prior to bedtime. By preschool age, children can regulate emotional arousal themselves. A preschooler who is anxious and timid in highly competitive games may choose to play alone or with quieter, less competitive peers, for example.

Finally, children learn to regulate emotions by selecting different response alternatives (Thompson, 1994). Until children learn to talk, they only have crying to exhibit distress or displeasure. With the advent of language, crying drops off dramatically, and children begin to say "No" and express dislike or disapproval of what parents are proposing. As situations become more socially complex (e.g., when children begin attending preschool, where there are peers and teachers), selecting the best way of expressing emotion in a specific situation can become complicated. The best choice depends on the child's goals and on how social partners are likely to respond. Dealing with such challenges promotes social cognition and competence.

Research on emotion regulation indicates the following key findings:

- *Whether emotion is regulated or dysregulated is determined to a large extent by context.* Dysregulation occurs when individuals have trouble managing their emotional expression in ways that are appropriate to the context, and/or when the level of emotional arousal that they experience disorganizes their own thinking or behavior in their interactions with others. This becomes a problem when individuals develop stable styles of managing emotions that are clearly dysfunctional, such as attacking first when angry or withdrawing/avoiding new situations and people (Thompson, 1994).
- *Emotionally regulated individuals have access to the full range of emotions* (Cole, Michel, & Teti, 1994). It is very adaptive when individuals can feel fear when they are threatened, sadness when they are bereaved, and angry when their goals have been blocked. It is a sign of difficulty either (1) when individuals do not report or experience an emotion that is typical in a particular situation (e.g., laughing when someone has hurt them), or (2) when their emotional style is dominated by a particular emotional experience, such as anger or sadness, to the extent that they seem to have a great deal of difficulty experiencing or expressing any other emotion.
- *Emotionally regulated children can move fluidly and smoothly from one emotional state to another, in a way that is flexible and coherent.* Dysregulation is seen in

abrupt, unexpected, and dramatic changes in emotion and mood. As children grow older, they become less emotionally labile. For example, a crying baby might be distracted by a parent showing a novel toy, creating a rapid move from crying into delight; a preschooler would not make such a rapid shift. Extreme lability, in the absence of a major change in immediate circumstances, signals a significant problem. Children with good emotional regulation display emotions in ways that fit with the rules of the culture, whereas violation of these rules is often a sign of difficulty.

• *Being able to think and talk about emotions is an important part of self-regulation* (Cole et al., 1994). Growing language competence allows children to label, describe, conceptualize, and understand their own feelings and that of others. Children can then learn to talk about being angry rather than to act it out behaviorally; they also become better able to delay in making decisions about how to respond emotionally, and to reflect later on what worked or did not work in terms of responding emotionally to a situation with a parent, a teacher, or a peer. These developing skills allow them to change their behavior in ways that will enable them to meet their goals.

Factors That Influence Emotional Competence

Temperament

Temperament has been defined as "psychological qualities that display considerable variation among infants and young children, and, in addition, have a relatively, but not indefinitely, stable physiological basis that derives from the individual's genetic constitution" (Kagan, 1994, p. 16). These psychological qualities for young children include fearful distress, irritable distress, positive affect, agreeableness/adaptability, effortful control/task persistence, and activity level (Rothbart & Bates, 1998). While temperament researchers focus on the constitutional aspects of such behavior, they acknowledge that experience always influences how these psychological qualities influence behavior.

Some of the best-known work in the area of temperament is that of Kagan and his colleagues, who have identified behavioral inhibition and disinhibition in unfamiliar situations in about 40% of the 1- to 2-year-old children they have studied (Kagan, 1994). Inhibited children (15% of the group), when presented with unfamiliar people and events in an unfamiliar laboratory situation, become very quiet, highly alert, very restrained in their movements, and avoidant of novel people or events. Uninhibited children (25% of the group) are minimally fearful and display vigorous motor activity with minimal crying. Neuropsychological measures suggest that the uninhibited children are much more likely to experience joy or happiness, while the inhibited children experience greater fear, anxiety, or uncertainty. Kagan (1994) concludes that the development of "a stable inhibited behavioral style requires a combination of a low threshold of reactivity in the limbic sites, the temperamental component, and a social environment that either encourages or fails to discourage timidity" (p. 21). Children with a stable inhibited style are more likely to experience internalizing problems, and uninhibited children are more likely to have externalizing problems, than children who fall at neither extreme (Biederman et al., 1990; Fox, Henderson, Rubin, Calkins, & Schmidt, 2001).

Greenspan et al. (2001) conceptualize temperament more broadly as including constitutional-maturation characteristics that contribute to infants' and children's regulatory capacities. These include the following:

- Sensory reactivity, including hypo- and hyperreactivity in each sensory modality (tactile, auditory, visual, vestibular, olfactory). For example, children with ASD are noted for their underreactivity to human sounds and their hyperreactivity to tactile sensations such as labels in clothing.

- Sensory processing in each sensory modality (e.g., the capacity to decode sequences, configurations, or abstract patterns). For example, children with ASD are typically better at detecting visual abstract patterns than decoding auditory sequences found in language.
- Sensory affective reactivity and processing in each modality (e.g., the ability to process and react to degrees of affective intensity in a stable manner). For example, children of depressed parents are highly reactive to sadness in these parents.
- Muscle tone and motor planning and sequencing. For example, some children with speech problems have trouble with articulation and drooling related to motor-planning difficulties.

Neither the extreme forms of the sensory capacities described above, nor difficult temperamental characteristics alone, necessarily predict psychopathology; a sensitive and responsive caregiver can influence these characteristics in a more positive developmental direction (Greenspan et al., 2001; Kagan, 1994). However, both sets of qualities make children much more developmentally vulnerable. These children have greater difficulty developing emotional competence, and their unique characteristics make it much more difficult for caregivers (no matter how competent) to provide care.

Several measures assess temperamental characteristics in young children. Although such measures are not a focus of this chapter, information on temperament is relevant to helping parents, and later teachers, respond optimally to a child's temperamental style. The Temperament and Atypical Behavior Scale for children ages 11–71 months (Bagnato, Neisworth, Salvia, & Hunt, 1999) addresses temperament, attention and activity, attachment and social behavior, neurobehavioral state, play, vocal and oral behavior, senses and movement, self-stimulation/injury, and misbehavior. It yields a profile of atypical behavior in the areas of Detached, Hypersensitive–Active, Underactive, and Dysregulated. The Temperament Assessment Battery for Children—Revised (Martin & Bridger, 1999) is a parent and teacher/caregiver rating form that assesses Activity Level, Adaptability, Approach/Withdrawal, Emotional Intensity, Distractibility, and Task Persistence in children ages 2–7. The goal of the measure is to categorize children into one of seven temperamental styles: typical, reticent, inhibited, impulsive, highly emotional, uninhibited, or passive. This information is used to guide parenting and teaching strategies.

Developmental Disabilities

INTELLECTUAL DELAYS

Intellectual delays have a significant impact on children's (1) experience of emotion, (2) ability to perceive and interpret the emotional expressions of others, and (3) ability to produce recognizable emotional expressions. Developmentally delayed infants and young children may have limitations in "the ability to remember and to associate events that have emotional content, what is painful or not, and to remember who is familiar or strange" (Lewis & Sullivan, 1996, p. viii); such limitations may dampen any emotional reaction. Toddlers with mental retardation are much more likely to respond similarly to different people, and to need more levels of stimulation to elicit a response such as laughter (Cicchetti & Sroufe, 1978; Greenberg & Field, 1982). Children with Down syndrome have difficulty detecting and understanding emotional signals, which makes it harder for parents and other caregivers to provide an appropriate response; their caregivers take longer to respond and respond with less confidence, both of which make it less likely that the children will understand their response, even if it is appropriate (Walden & Knipes, 1996). Children with severe mental retardation are mostly passive, tend to be emotionally unresponsive, and cry only occasionally (Field, 1996). Typically developing toddlers, in comparison, are much more intense in their responses to hunger, exposure to new food and strangers, and daily routines (such as diaper changes and baths).

As a result of these emotional limitations, parents, teachers, and peers who interact with intellectually delayed children may find them unreadable, unresponsive, and unpredictable, making them frustrating social partners. For parents, this can reduce their sense of efficacy and place attachment security at risk, given the major role that maternal sensitivity plays. Child neglect is more likely. Peers may be less likely to engage or continue to engage with these children. Children with intellectual delays are likely to develop inappropriate social behavior or behavior that is poorly matched to situational requirements (Walden & Knipes, 1996).

AUTISTIC SPECTRUM DISORDERS

Children with ASD are delayed in achieving, and some may never achieve, the emotional milestones described earlier. They are typically poor at reading their own and others' emotions, producing emotional expressions that others can read and interpret, and (in particular) responding to the emotional signals of others. In terms of producing emotions, children with ASD are much more likely to display facial expressions that do not match any discrete identifiable emotion or combine more than one emotion—including incongruent blends such as joy and sadness, which are never seen in typical children (Kasari & Sigman, 1996). This makes their facial expressions harder to read and, when coupled with their ambiguous emotional vocalizations, makes reading many of their emotional expressions challenging, although parents and researchers are frequently able to identify their emotional expressions (Travis & Sigman, 1998). This unique emotional style poses significant problems for both the parent–child relationship and relationships with peers. As with other children with developmental disabilities, if parents have trouble reading children's emotional signals, it is hard for them to be responsive to the children's needs. Similarly, if children with ASD express little positive affect to peers and fail to respond to negative emotions in others, they may appear (and may actually be) socially uninterested, self-absorbed, or indifferent (Travis & Sigman, 1998).

Gender

Girls mature earlier than boys do, to the point that by school entry, girls tend to be about 1 year ahead of boys in emotional as well as physical and social development (Emde, 1992). In particular, girls develop earlier language competence; this allows them to communicate their needs more clearly and gives them more control of their own environment. Their parents may feel more efficacious, since they have a better sense of how to respond to their daughters' needs, increasing communication and the likelihood of positive parent–child interaction. Parents also use much more emotion language and spend more time discussing emotional reactions and behaviors with their daughters than they do with their sons. This is thought to influence the higher frequency of prosocial behavior and empathetic responding in young girls than in young boys (Keenan & Shaw, 1997).

Whereas there are few sex differences in temperament or in the rate or frequency and severity of behavioral problems through age 3, sex differences emerge at about 4 years of age. Keenan and Shaw (1997), in their review of the literature, attribute this to the more rapid development of adaptive behavior in girls because of their earlier biological maturation, making the developmental challenges of the preschool years a better match for their abilities than they are for boys. Socialization by parents also appears to "channel" any early problems that exist in girls into more of an internalizing style (socially withdrawn, worried), as opposed to the more externalizing style (aggressive, undercontrolled) that becomes more characteristic of boys by age 4.

Socialization

As Sroufe (1996) so eloquently states,

> The most fundamental aspects of emotional development occur in the context of the caregiver–infant relationship. The general course of emotional development may be described as movement *from dyadic regulation to self-regulation* of emotion. Moreover, dyadic regulation represents a prototype for self-regulation; the roots of individual differences in the self-regulation of emotion lie within the distinctive patterns of dyadic regulation. (p. 151; emphasis in original)

Although it is clear that constitutional factors, such as temperament, developmental disabilities, and gender, influence emotional development and functioning, there is also robust evidence that socialization—particularly by parents, but also by siblings, peers, and teachers—is extremely influential in children's development of emotional understanding, emotional expressiveness, and emotional regulation.

DENHAM'S MECHANISMS OF SOCIALIZATION

Denham (1998) believes that children learn about the nature of emotions and their expressions and acceptability in intimate interactions with others, including parents, peers, siblings, and other adults. Using Halberstadt's (1991) model, Denham notes that children are socialized in emotions through three mechanisms of social learning: modeling, coaching, and contingency. *Modeling* refers to how socializing agents such as parents and teachers express their own emotions; *coaching* refers to how these agents teach children (or not) about emotions; and *contingency* is defined as how agents react to the emotions of others.

Parents influence children's expression of emotion in four ways (Barrett & Campos, 1991; Denham, 1998). First, they unconsciously teach children about emotions—which emotions are acceptable in the family, and which emotions are appropriate for what circumstances. For example, a little girl might learn that her mother withdraws when she acts angry at her mother; this teaches the child that expressions of anger lead to social isolation. Second, parents model how specific emotions are displayed. Third, they demonstrate the action tendencies that are associated with certain emotions. For example, a parent may express anger directly but in a controlled manner (e.g., saying "I am very mad at you for breaking my new lamp"), while another might scream at a child, making derogatory remarks. Fourth, parents create an affective environment within the home, projecting an emotional world view. This general emotional tone may reflect a fairly positive, calm, happy atmosphere; a conflictual, hostile atmosphere; or a bleak, uninvolved atmosphere.

Research suggests that children's emotional expressiveness reflects their mothers' predominant mood, as well as the patterns with which they experience happiness, sadness, or anger, with the expressive patterns of toddlers and mothers becoming more similar over time (Malatesta, Culver, Tesman, & Shepard, 1989). In general, happy mothers have happy children, sad mothers have sad children, and angry mothers have tense and sad children. Much less is known about fathers' influence on children's emotions, but paternal depression in a child's early life seems to have persisting negative effects on the child's development (Ramchandani et al., 2005). Gottman, Katz, and Hooven (1997) found that in the nonclinical two-parent families they studied, fathers' emotions and parenting behavior were more influential than those of mothers—perhaps because there was less variability among mothers in the quality of parenting than there was among fathers. Some fathers had a very negative impact on their preschoolers, and some had a very positive impact. Denham (1998) found that coaching (defined as parents' talking about emotions and fostering children's ability to do so, as noted above) increased children's knowledge of their own and others' feelings and allowed them to share their emotional experiences with parents in a way that allowed them to discuss, anticipate, and set goals. Mothers who discussed and explained emotions in laboratory simulations had children who were happier, less sad, and less angry in preschool, while mothers who "wallowed" in sadness and anger in their discussions had children who seemed to find this punishing and debilitating (Denham, 1998). They were more sad, angry, and tense, and less happy, in situations without their mothers.

In regard to contingency, or others' reactions to children's emotions, Denham (1998) discovered that children did better when parents responded in certain ways to their emotions. Matching angry responses with anger led to angry and noncompliant behavior in children; a calm, neutral, or cheerful response had better outcomes. Children did well with mothers who were affectively balanced—demonstrating much more positive than negative emotion, but exhibiting enough negative emotion that children gained experience in understanding sad and angry feelings and learned to tolerate them. Children with such experience were more likely to be empathetic and sympathetic to others in preschool.

Children who were exposed to intense parental anger or sadness that was not explained to them, and was left unresolved, became very distressed and found such displays incapacitating. These children seemed to pull back from the emotionally upsetting events and to focus on their own feelings, limiting their ability to learn from the situation and about emotions in general (Denham, 1998). They were much less likely to respond prosocially to peers' emotions in preschool.

FAMILY META-EMOTIONS

Gottman et al. (1997) proposed that meta-emotions, or parents' feelings about feelings, are "the very fabric of the emotional life of the family" (p. 190). The authors define *meta-emotions* as "parents' awareness of specific emotions, their awareness of these emotions in their child, and their coaching of the emotions in the child" (p. 6). By studying intact families with 4- to 5-year-olds in the context of their ongoing and highly sophisticated study of marriage and its effects on child development, Gottman and colleagues were able to identify three types of families with respect to how parents responded to children's sadness or anger. The first type they described was dismissing or disapproving of children's emotions. These families were uncomfortable with their children's sadness or anger. The parents might interpret sadness as a demand to solve a problem, and thus respond to it with annoyance or criticism. Or sadness might be interpreted as an attempt to manipulate them, and they subsequently might ignore or minimize the sadness as much as possible, seeing it as something that they might be forced to confront, but something that they were not interested in or did not warrant attention. They might describe it as something they wanted to "get over, ride out, look beyond, or not dwell on" (p. 51). During periods of sadness, these parents often used distractions to move the children along; if they used comfort, it was within specified time limits. "They prefer a happy child, and often do not present a clear or insightful description of their child's emotion experience" (p. 51). A few parents in this group moved beyond dismissing and disapproving into ridiculing or making fun of a child's anger or sadness.

The second type of family was a "coaching family," described as actively involved in how children were feeling and regarding children's emotions as opportunities for teaching and intimacy. Parents who provided emotional coaching (1) were aware of children's emotions, even low-intensity emotions (e.g., sadness as opposed to weeping); (2) saw the children's emotions as opportunities for intimacy or teaching and would connect with their children while they were in the early stages of an emotional reaction, rather than waiting until it escalated to a high level of intensity; (3) helped the children directly label the emotions they were having, which could involve either the use of standard labels or putting feelings into words, such as "you felt that the way the teacher treated you was unfair"; (4) empathized with or validated the children's emotions (communicated that they genuinely understood why the children might feel this way at this time); and (5) helped the children with problem solving, which might involve setting limits, as well as helping the children figure out what their goals were for the situation and what might work to accomplish those.

The third type of family was accepting of negative emotions, but low in coaching. They did not set limits (e.g., prevent attacking a younger brother when angry) or solve problems when it came to emotions; they just allowed their children to experience them. They had "a 'hands-off' philosophy about their children's anger" (p. 77) and/or sadness. Many of these parents appeared to think that their children should freely express emotions so that they were released, but did not see a need to be involved with the children, help the children cope, or discuss how anger or sadness might be dealt with and what it might mean.

Gottman et al. (1997) found that parents' awareness of their own anger or sadness and their comfort with those emotions were related to their response to their children's emotions. Children of emotionally coaching parents at ages 4–5 were rated as socially competent by teachers at age 8 and behaved very competently with their best friends in a play situation at age 8. They also did better academically, even after IQ was controlled for. A physiological measure of coping (vagal tone) was related to the parents' use of emotional coaching, suggesting that such coaching may actually change a child's physiological response in stressful situations. The coaching approach to parenting involved what would typically be called authoritative and responsive parenting practices, such as warmth, limit setting, structuring, and praise to inform the children about what they were doing right. It also involved an absence of insulting children, calling them names, making fun of them, or taking over their work in a teaching task in a way implying that the children were incompetent to do it.

Gottman has produced two videotapes to be used in interventions to help parents become emotional coaches: *The Heart of Parenting: Raising an Emotionally Intelligent Child* (Gottman, 1996) and *Raising an Emotionally Intelligent Child: The Heart of Parenting* (Gottman, 1999). Both can be obtained from his website (www.gottman.com). The work of Haim Ginott heavily influenced Gottman's work in this area. The book and training materials by two of Ginott's other students, Faber and Mazlish (1980), titled *How to Talk so Kids Will Listen and Listen so Kids Will Talk*, cover many of the same concepts. Both sets of materials are recommended for all parents and preschool programs.

Implications of Research on Emotional Development for Assessment

The review of the literature on emotional development above has clear implications for curriculum-related assessment in preschool classrooms, for screening and assessment for emotional disorders, and for intervention planning. First, emotional competence is directly linked to competent social functioning. Promoting emotional competence is an important component of an early childhood curriculum, and all preschool children in daycare or preschool should be screened for delays or deviancies in emotional milestones and skills. Interventions are relatively easy to implement with young children and their families; efficient means of doing this are described below.

Second, if there are problems in emotional development, examiners should consider the role of age, gender, temperament, developmental disabilities, and socialization. These factors may suggest different intervention approaches in different cases. In regard to age, oppositional and defiant behavior is so common in 3-year-olds that very high levels are not necessarily prognostic of future problems; however, a large percentage of such children continue to have problems, so they should not be ignored. In regard to temperament, children and parents may need support in coping with enduring personality traits, such as social timidity or high emotionality. In regard to developmental disabilities, mental age is a key variable. A 5-year-old child with a mental age of 2 cannot be held to the same emotional and behavioral standards as a 5-year-old with a mental age of 5. Once an evaluator has established that a child does have a significant emotional delay or problem relative to peers, it must be determined whether the behavior is *developmentally* inappropriate, given his or her mental age. Mental age can be assessed with either an individual intelligence test (see Chapter 11), a measure of adaptive behavior like the Vineland Adaptive Behavior Scales, Second Edition (Vineland-II; see Chapter 12), or both. In regard to socialization, when a significant problem has been identified, the evaluator needs to consider the extent to which the problem represents a parent–child relationship problem, a child constitutional problem, or an interaction of both. Parent–child observation measures and parent interviews are useful for this purpose (see discussion below).

Third, since current emotional competence is built on earlier competence, examiners may want to assess not only current functioning but milestones expected at earlier ages, to have a complete understanding of a child's functioning and areas in need of support. Greenspan et al. (2001) have developed the Functional Emotional Assessment Scales (FEAS; described later) to be used for this purpose. The emotional milestones presented in Table 14.1 and the discussion of key emotion skills are also helpful for this purpose.

Fourth, examiners should consider whether the emotional or behavioral problems identified are consistent with another type of disability. For example, it is not uncommon for children with ASD to show significant elevations on anxiety scales or measures of attention-deficit/hyperactivity disorder (ADHD), because attentional problems and obsessive–compulsive behavior are characteristic of these disorders. Only a few screening and diagnostic rating scales have items designed to flag symptoms of ASD—for example, the Ages and Stages Questionnaires: Social-Emotional (ASQ:SE; Squires, Bricker, & Twombly, 2002) and the Achenbach System of Empirically Based Assessment (ASEBA; Achenbach & Rescorla, 2000a)—so examiners should be aware of what behaviors the screening or diagnostic measures they use are covering. To take another example, children referred for suspected externalizing disorders with extreme levels of hostile, defiant, destructive, moody behavior may be demonstrating early symptoms of a prepubertal bipolar disorder (commonly known as manic–depressive disorder; see Case 2 later in this chapter).

DIAGNOSTIC CLASSIFICATION SYSTEMS FOR EMOTIONAL AND BEHAVIOR PROBLEMS

Assessment for possible diagnosis of an emotional or behavioral problem, using clinical or educational criteria, generally occurs as the result of either a screening that indicates a problem or a referral by a caregiver, teacher, parent, or physician. If measures of social and emotional competence and/or behavior problems indicate that there is a clinically significant problem, the examiner then has to determine whether it is occurring at a level that requires professional intervention and/or meets criteria for a disorder. There are three diagnostic systems in use for young children; however, none of them have been tailored for or validated with the preschool population as part of their development. Recent efforts by professional organizations and investigators have identified areas where modifications are warranted in diagnostic criteria for two of these systems and where further research is needed.

Professionals working in clinics, hospitals, and other mental health settings use either the *Diagnostic and Statistical Manual of Mental Disorders*, fourth edition, text revision (DSM-IV-TR; American Psychiatric Association, 2000) or, to a much lesser extent, the *Diagnostic Classification of Mental Health and Developmental Disorders of Infancy and Early Childhood: Revised Edition* (DC:0–3R; Zero to Three, 2005) for children from birth to 3 years of age. DC:0–3R was, in its revision, informed by the *Research Diagnostic Criteria—Preschool Age* (RDC-PA; see Task Force on Research Diagnostic Criteria: Infancy and Preschool, 2003), a document produced by a task force of investigators informally sponsored by the American Psychiatric Association and the American Academy of Child and Adolescent Psychiatry to review the research evidence on the usefulness of DSM-IV-TR criteria for young children. This group recommended modifications to some DSM-IV-TR criteria for young children, as we discuss below.

School-based professionals are required to use criteria from IDEA (the latest version of which is IDEA 2004), which defines *emotional disturbance* as follows in the federal regulations implementing this law (Assistance to States for the Education of Children with Disabilities, 2000):

> The term means a condition exhibiting one or more of the following characteristics over a long period of time and to a marked degree that adversely affects a child's educational performance:
>
> (A) An inability to learn that cannot be explained by intellectual, sensory, or health factors.
> (B) An inability to build or maintain satisfactory interpersonal relationships with peers and teachers.
> (C) Inappropriate types of behaviors or feelings under normal circumstances.
> (D) A general pervasive mood of unhappiness or depression.
> (E) A tendency to develop physical symptoms or fears associated with personal or school problems. (Section 300.7(c)(4)(i))

The term *emotional disturbance* as defined by the IDEA is broad, probably covering much of what is included in DSM-IV-TR that would relate to children or adolescents, but the exact relationship between the regulations and DSM-IV-TR is unclear. This creates a tension between the systems used by school personnel and by other mental health professionals (Kamphaus & Frick, 2002). The IDEA regulations were also not developed with preschool children in mind, limiting their sensitivity to the manifestation of emotional and behavior problems at this age.

With both the IDEA regulations and the DSM-IV-TR criteria, the process involves determining whether a primary disorder exists and identifying co-occurring medical disorders or conditions. Use of the DSM-IV-TR five-axis system also requires assessing significant stressors and assessing highest level of functioning both currently and within the past year; this is a more appropriate model for older children and adolescents than for preschoolers, given the rapid developmental change during the preschool period and thus the lack of a static reference point for comparison.

As noted above, the RDC-PA was published in 2003. In developing this set of criteria, the Task Force on Research Diagnostic Criteria: Infancy and Preschool (2003) reviewed all of the available empirical studies on disorders in infancy and the preschool years, and evaluated the degree to which these studies supported the application of DSM-IV-TR criteria to this age group. The RDC-PA covers 19 disorders, 13 of which come directly from DSM-IV-TR and 6 of which are proposed expanded classifications involving feeding and sleeping disorders. Most DSM-IV-TR symptoms and algorithms were not changed (e.g., for ADHD, oppositional defiant disorder [ODD]); a few symptoms were modified to be developmentally appropriate without changing the meaning of the symptoms (e.g., major depressive disorder, separation anxiety disorder [SAD]); and a very few were completely revised because they were developmentally inappropriate (e.g., for posttraumatic stress disorder [PTSD]). DSM-IV-TR remains the system of choice for diagnosis of preschool children unless working within a school system requires use of the IDEA criteria.

Externalizing Disorders

Only a few disorders occur with enough frequency in preschool children that they merit a detailed presentation here. In the area of externalizing behavior, ODD and ADHD occur with sufficient frequency as syndromes during the preschool years that assessors should be familiar with their presentation and assessment.

Oppositional Defiant Disorder

The DSM-IV-TR diagnostic criteria for ODD define it as "a pattern of negativistic, hostile defiant behavior lasting at least six months, during which four (or more)" symptoms are present (see Table 14.2 for the full list of diagnostic criteria). To qualify for a diagnosis, the behavior also has to occur more frequently than in other individuals who are the same age and developmental level and it must include clinically significant impairment in social or academic functioning. Because ODD is frequently a precursor for conduct disorder (CD) and because effective interventions for it are available, families of children exhibiting this syndrome should be offered treatment even if a clinician is conservative in offering this diagnosis.

Lavigne et al. (1998a, 1998b), in a longitudinal study designed to identify the prevalence of DSM diagnoses in unreferred preschool children, found that ODD was the most common diagnosis in children attending regular pediatric practices; 16.8% of children met the criteria for ODD, with 8.1% showing severe symptoms. Twice as many boys were identified as girls. However, the diagnosis peaked at age 3 and had leveled off by age

TABLE 14.2. DSM-IV-TR Criteria for Oppositional Defiant Disorder (ODD)

A. A pattern of negativistic, hostile, and defiant behavior lasting at least 6 months, during which four (or more) of the following are present:

(1) often loses temper
(2) often argues with adults
(3) often actively defies or refuses to comply with adults' requests or rules
(4) often deliberately annoys people
(5) often blames others for his or her mistakes or misbehavior
(6) is often touchy or easily annoyed by others
(7) is often angry and resentful
(8) is often spiteful or vindictive

Note: Consider a criterion met only if the behavior occurs more frequently than is typically observed in individuals of comparable age and developmental level.

B. The disturbance in behavior causes clinically significant impairment in social, academic, or occupational functioning.

C. The behaviors do not occur exclusively during the course of a Psychotic or Mood Disorder.

D. Criteria are not met for Conduct Disorder, and, if the individual is 18 years or older, criteria are not met for Antisocial Personality Disorder.

Note. Reprinted with permission from the *Diagnostic and Statistical Manual of Mental Disorders*, Fourth Edition, Text Revision.

5. Follow-up showed that about 50% of the children with an externalizing diagnosis at intake between the ages of 2 and 5 continued to have this diagnosis when reassessed 1–3 years later. The younger the children were at the initial assessment, the more likely they were to outgrow their problems. The high rate of ODD at age 3 co-occurs with children's development of autonomy and self-regulation, which may make their parents more likely to see them as defiant and uncooperative. Using a 12-month rather than a 6-month duration criterion for children under age 4, as recommended by Barkley (1997a), or restricting this diagnosis until children are age 4 would make it easier to separate age-appropriate difficulties with defiance and emotional regulation from more significant problems (American Psychiatric Association, 2000; Campbell, 2002). However, some children present with such severity of impairment in their functioning that a diagnosis is warranted at age 3 or after a 6-month duration.

ODD is most common in children whose parents and/or other close relatives are diagnosed with a disruptive behavior disorder, a mood or anxiety disorder, or a substance use disorder. Although ODD is a precursor of almost all cases of CD (over 90%), it does not typically lead to CD (only in about 25% of ODD cases; Loeber, Keenan, Lahey, Green, & Thomas, 1993). It can be an extreme form of normal development, an outgrowth of difficult temperament, or a transitory response to family conflict and coercive parenting. Research also shows that ODD often co-occurs with ADHD, and that it is almost always a precursor or comorbid diagnosis of childhood-onset bipolar disorder, also called prepubertal mania (Wozniak & Biederman, 1995). ODD that does lead to CD has been linked to multifaceted and transactional causal factors, which include male gender, genetic risk, discordant or maltreating parent–child interactions, lower Verbal IQ, and co-occurring ADHD (Hinshaw & Anderson, 1996).

Attention-Deficit/Hyperactivity Disorder

ADHD is the only externalizing diagnosis other than ODD that occurs with any frequency in preschool children (Lavigne et al., 1996); it is found in only 2% of these children and, like ODD, is more common in boys. It typically co-occurs with ODD (Lavigne et al., 1996; Keenan & Shaw, 1997). Indeed, very few preschool children are identified as having ADHD without comorbid ODD. In addition to ODD, where the comorbidity is about 65%, preschool children with ADHD have very high rates of comorbidity with other psychiatric disorders. In a sample of almost 2,000 unselected clinic referrals, Wilens et al. (2002) identified 165 4- to 6-year-old children with ADHD (78% male) and compared them with 381 7- to 9-year-old children with ADHD (76% male) on symptom patterns, comorbidity, and adaptive functioning. They found that 74% of the preschoolers had another diagnosis as did 79% of the older children. Both groups had an average of 1.4 additional diagnoses. About half of both age groups had a mood disorder: 42% Major Depression and 26% Bipolar disorder among the preschoolers and 47% Major Depression and 18% Bipolar disorder among the older children. Multiple anxiety disorders were high in both groups as well: 28% among the preschoolers and 33% among the older children. For the preschoolers the mean age of onset was very early: non-comorbid ADHD 2.2 (SD 1.3), ADHD and ODD 3.1 (SD 1.3), ADHD and Major Depression 3.1 (SD 1.6), ADHD and Bipolar disorder 2.6 (SD 1.4), and ADHD and anxiety disorders 2.6 (SD 1.5). Both age groups showed significant school, social, and behavioral impairments and were positive for the same number of symptoms for ADHD.

When preschool children meet the criteria for ADHD, it is usually for the hyperactive–impulsive type, as the inattentive type consists of demands that are made on children once they begin attending school and are not necessarily observed at an earlier developmental stage. However, DSM-IV-TR notes that most 2- and 3-year-olds can sit attentively for storybook reading with parents, while a child with ADHD would have trouble focusing in this or other similar situations.

To meet criteria for ADHD, children must have six or more symptoms of either an inattentive or a hyperactive–impulsive nature, which have persisted at least 6 months to a degree that is both maladaptive and inconsistent with developmental level (see Table 14.3 for the full diagnostic criteria). In addition, the symptoms must cause some clinically significant impairment in two or more settings, such as home and childcare. Because many preschool children are not in childcare or preschool, the cross-setting requirement is often waived; use of parents as the sole source of information leads to an increased rate of diagnosis than when teacher reports are also obtained (Pineda et al., 1999). As examiners familiar with the behavior of preschool children can attest, ADHD symptoms are commonly observed behaviors in preschool children. DSM-IV-TR is aware of this and cautions the clinician, "It is difficult to establish this diagnosis in children younger than age 4 or 5 years, because their characteristic behavior is much more variable than that of older children and may include features that are similar to [ADHD]" (American Psychiatric Association, 2000, p. 89). Due to the commonness of these behaviors in 2- to 3-year-olds and the fact that the DSM-IV field trials were conducted only with children ages 4–16, Barkley (1997a) recommends that clinicians use a higher threshold of symptoms for children under 4. He also recommends that the duration criteria be extended from 6 months to 12 months, as young children whose symptoms persist for a year are much more likely to have significant symptoms in elementary school (Campbell & Ewing, 1990).

Like ODD, ADHD is more common in children whose parents and other close relatives are diagnosed with a disruptive behavior disorder, a mood or anxiety disorder, or a substance use disorder, with higher rates of these problems in cases of pure ODD than of

TABLE 14.3. DSM-IV-TR Criteria for Attention-Deficit/Hyperactivity Disorder (ADHD)

A. Either (1) or (2):

(1) six (or more) of the following symptoms of **inattention** have persisted for at least 6 months to a degree that is maladaptive and inconsistent with developmental level:

Inattention

(a) often fails to give close attention to details or makes careless mistakes in schoolwork, work, or other activities
(b) often has difficulty sustaining attention in tasks or play activities
(c) often does not seem to listen when spoken to directly
(d) often does not follow through on instructions and fails to finish schoolwork, chores, or duties in the workplace (not due to oppositional behavior or failure to understand instructions)
(e) often has difficulty organizing tasks and activities
(f) often avoids, dislikes, or is reluctant to engage in tasks that require sustained mental effort (such as schoolwork or homework)
(g) often loses things necessary for tasks or activities (e.g., toys, school assignments, pencils, books, or tools)
(h) is often easily distracted by extraneous stimuli
(i) is often forgetful in daily activities

(2) six (or more) of the following symptoms of **hyperactivity–impulsivity** have persisted for at least 6 months to a degree that is maladaptive and inconsistent with developmental level:

Hyperactivity

(a) often fidgets with hands or feet or squirms in seat
(b) often leaves seat in classroom or in other situations in which remaining seated is expected
(c) often runs about or climbs excessively in situations in which it is inappropriate (in adolescents or adults, may be limited to subjective feelings of restlessness)
(d) often has difficulty playing or engaging in leisure activities quietly
(e) is often "on the go" or often acts as if "driven by a motor"
(f) often talks excessively

Impulsivity

(g) often blurts out answers before questions have been completed
(h) often has difficulty awaiting turn
(i) often interrupts or intrudes on others (e.g., butts into conversations or games)

B. Some hyperactive–impulsive or inattentive symptoms that caused impairment were present before age 7 years.

C. Some impairment from the symptoms is present in two or more settings (e.g., at school [or work] and at home).

D. There must be clear evidence of clinically significant impairment in social, academic, or occupational functioning.

E. The symptoms do not occur exclusively during the course of a Pervasive Developmental Disorder, Schizophrenia, or other Psychotic Disorder and are not better accounted for by another mental disorder (e.g., Mood Disorder, Anxiety Disorder, Dissociative Disorder, or a Personality Disorder).

(continued)

TABLE 14.3. *(continued)*

Code based on type:

314.01 Attention-Deficit/Hyperactivity Disorder, Combined Type: if both Criteria A1 and A2 are met for the past 6 months

314.00 Attention-Deficit/Hyperactivity Disorder, Predominantly Inattentive Type: if Criterion A1 is met but Criterion A2 is not met for the past 6 months

314.01 Attention-Deficit/Hyperactivity Disorder, Predominantly Hyperactive–Impulsive Type: if Criterion A2 is met but Criterion A1 is not met for the past 6 months

Coding note: For individuals (especially adolescents and adults) who currently have symptoms that no longer meet full criteria, "In Partial Remission" should be specified.

Note. Reprinted with permission from the *Diagnostic and Statistical Manual of Mental Disorders*, Fourth Edition, Text Revision. Copyright 2000 American Psychiatric Association.

pure ADHD. Twin and adoption studies show a high degree of heritability for ADHD, especially in more symptomatic cases (Samudra & Cantwell, 1999). Because of the high degree of co-occurrence between ODD and ADHD in preschool children, and the similarity of family and classroom interventions that have been shown to be effective with these disorders at this age, children exhibiting these symptoms (whether they rise to a diagnostic level or not) merit very similar approaches to assessment and intervention.

An evaluation for a suspected externalizing problem should begin when behavior rating scales administered to parents and caregivers/teachers show increased elevations (borderline or clinical range) on the externalizing scale or subscales. If the respondents agree that there is a problem, the evaluator asks parents to complete a questionnaire that asks for information on the family situation; developmental, educational, and medical history; problematic times at home; and disruptive behavior. A parent interview then follows. If the problem is occurring at home but not at childcare/preschool, then there may be a parent–child relationship problem that needs to be addressed. If the problem is occurring only at childcare/preschool, then a classroom observation should clarify whether there are setting or management problems that might be contributing to the problem. If the observation suggests a supportive and appropriately structured setting, then it is possible that the child has a significant problem but that the parents have a limited awareness of normal development and thus do not consider their child's behavior abnormal. This can be assessed through interview and parent–child observation. The recommended steps in a diagnostic assessment are described (and summarized in Table 14.6) later in this chapter.

Treatment of Externalizing Disorders

As we have noted in Chapter 8, there are three commercially available parenting programs with demonstrated effectiveness in treating children with ODD: (1) Helping the Noncompliant Child (Forehand & McMahon, 1981; McMahon & Forehand, 2003); (2) Parent–Child Interaction Therapy (Eyberg & Boggs, 1998; Hembree-Kigin & McNeil, 1995); and (3) The Incredible Years (Webster-Stratton, 1999, 2000). Barkley's Defiant Children program (Barkley, 1997a) is similar in content but has not been evaluated as thoroughly. It is the only program specifically adapted for children with ODD and ADHD. All four programs are based on social learning principles and were heavily influenced by the clinical work and supervision of Constance Hanf (1969, 1970). A fuller description of their similarities and differences is provided in Chapter 8.

Internalizing Disorders

Internalizing disorders are challenging to identify in young children. As the authors of the RDC-PA (Task Force on Research Diagnostic Criteria: Infancy and Preschool, 2003) note, the fact that language and cognitive abilities are emerging and evolving at these ages makes if difficult to tell whether a child has the developmental capacity for certain symptoms, such as sadness and worries. Moreover, internalizing symptoms manifest differently at different ages; language and cognitive capacities may limit children's ability to report symptoms; and caregivers and researchers probably underestimate the degree of psychopathology, because children with these disorders can be more easily managed, and adults may thus dismiss their problems as normative developmental disruptions that will subside. This area is the focus of an intense research effort, and our knowledge of young children's experience of anxiety and mood disorders should grow dramatically over the next decade.

Separation Anxiety Disorder

Only SAD appears to occur with sufficient frequency in preschoolers to be addressed here (Campbell, 2002). Symptoms of anxiety, fearfulness, social withdrawal, or sadness are fairly frequent in young children. Besides being common, they are often transient to the point that children have to show a fairly high degree of sadness or withdrawal before it can be identified as a clear syndrome requiring treatment. Lavigne et al. (1996) found very low levels of internalizing/emotional disorders in their sample. Unless this type of symptomatic behavior occurs over a fairly long period of time and really begins to impair a child's developmental progress (including peer functioning), it is hard to justify a diagnosis of depression or anxiety other than SAD (Campbell, 2002). Even SAD, specific to childhood, often occurs in response to significant life stressors (e.g., death of a family member or pet, major changes in household membership, or illness). Thus clinging to a caregiver and demonstrating anxiety may be developmentally appropriate during times of stress, rather than signs of pathology (Campbell, 2002). Even when a parent denies any major event in a young child's life that may have been a precipitant for the development of SAD, the parent may be unaware of the importance of a specific event (e.g., the death of a beloved grandmother may have created fears that the mother will suddenly leave the child as well); may project his or her own fear of separation onto the child; or may deny a major family problem (such as domestic violence) that may be terrifying a child, as in the case described below.

> Ahmed, age 4, was referred for suspected SAD. His mother reported that he followed her constantly around the house as she did her chores, into the bathroom when she bathed or used the toilet, and into the yard when she did gardening; he also always ended up in her bed at night. Ahmed would only cooperate with his mother's leaving him when he was dropped at his maternal grandmother's house while the mother went to her job. He would then scream and have tantrums when his mother would try to get him into the house at the end of the day. Often neighbors would have to help get Ahmed into the house, where again he would never leave his mother's side. From an analysis of his responses to the MacArthur Story Stem Battery (MSSB; Emde, Wolf, & Oppenheim, 2003; see below), followed by a further interview with his mother, it became clear that Ahmed was terrified that his mother was going to be hurt or killed by her boyfriend. His symptoms abated after his mother terminated the relationship.

SAD is defined as "developmentally inappropriate and excessive anxiety concerning separation from home or from those to whom the individual is attached" (American Psychiatric Association, 2000, p. 125). Children must exhibit three or more symptoms for at least 4 weeks, and the symptoms must result in clinically significant distress that impairs social or academic functioning. Table 14.4 presents the DSM-IV-TR diagnostic criteria for SAD. In regard to the criterion A anxiety symptoms, the RDC-PA recommends that symptom 4 ("persistent reluctance or refusal to go to school or elsewhere because of separation") include a note that in young children this might appear as fear or distress of leaving home for daycare or school; anticipatory fear or distress related to a daycare or school situation; or the child's staying out of daycare or school because of fear, distress, or emotional disturbance. The RDC-PA also recommends that symptom 7 ("repeated nightmares involving the theme of separation") include a note that in preverbal or barely verbal children, frightening dreams that have no identifiable context can be considered as

TABLE 14.4. DSM-IV-TR Criteria for Separation Anxiety Disorder (SAD)

A. Developmentally inappropriate and excessive anxiety concerning separation from home or from those to whom the individual is attached, as evidenced by three (or more) of the following:

   (1) recurrent excessive distress when separation from home or major attachment figures occurs or is anticipated
   (2) persistent and excessive worry about losing, or about possible harm befalling, major attachment figures
   (3) persistent and excessive worry that an untoward event will lead to separation from a major attachment (e.g., getting lost or being kidnapped)
   (4) persistent reluctance or refusal to go to school or elsewhere because of fear of separation
   (5) persistently and excessively fearful or reluctant to be alone or without major attachment figures at home or without significant adults in other settings
   (6) persistent reluctance or refusal to go to sleep without being near a major attachment figure or to sleep away from home
   (7) repeated nightmares involving the theme of separation
   (8) repeated complaints of physical symptoms (such as headaches, stomachaches, nausea, or vomiting) when separation from major attachment figures occurs or is anticipated

B. The duration of the disturbance is at least 4 weeks.

C. The onset is before age 18 years.

D. The disturbance causes clinically significant distress or impairment in social, academic (occupational), or other important areas of functioning.

E. The disturbance does not occur exclusively during the course of a Pervasive Developmental Disorder, Schizophrenia, or other Psychotic Disorder and, in adolescents and adults, is not better accounted for by Panic Disorder With Agoraphobia.

Specify if:
Early Onset: if onset occurs before age 6 years.

Note. Reprinted with permission from the *Diagnostic and Statistical Manual of Mental Disorders*, Fourth Edition, Text Revision. Copyright 2000 American Psychiatric Association.

meeting this criterion. Furthermore, the RDC-PA proposes adding a symptom 9 to the criterion A list: a persistent preoccupation or worry about the whereabouts of attachment figures, such as might be seen in looking out of a window or stopping play. Finally, under D, the impairment criterion, the RDC-PA proposes adding a note that in a young child the disorder may cause parents to modify their behavior in order to modify their child's behavior.

Anxiety disorders have strong heritability. A very high percentage of children with anxiety disorders have mothers with a concurrent anxiety disorder or a lifetime diagnosis of such a disorder (Frick et al., 1994; Last, Hersen, Kazdin, Francis, & Grubb, 1987). Infant temperament, derived in part from inherited characteristics, has also been identified as a risk factor for internalizing disorders. Children with behavioral inhibition (Biederman, Rosenbaum, Chaloff, & Kagan, 1995; Schwartz, Snidman, & Kagan, 1999) or a difficult temperament (e.g., negative emotionality; Keenan, Shaw, Delliquadri, Giovannelli, & Walsh, 1998) are at higher risk for internalizing problems and are significantly more likely to have parents and siblings with an anxiety disorder than are either uninhibited children or those who are neither inhibited or uninhibited (Rosenbaum et al., 1991). Although these findings suggest that children may inherit a vulnerability to anxiety, other factors must play a role in its occurrence; behavioral inhibition in the absence of parental disorders does not predict a later anxiety disorder. The environmental factors of early experience with uncontrollability, particularly in the caregiver–child relationship, and high levels of negative life changes and parental conflict have been implicated in the development of internalizing problems (Albano, Chorpita, & Barlow, 1996; Shaw, Keenan, Vondra, Delliquadri, & Giovannelli, 1997). Infants with insecure attachment styles, especially anxious/ambivalent and disorganized or fearful attachment, are most at risk for the development of internalizing problems (Shaw et al., 1997; Sroufe et al., 2005; Warren, Huston, Egeland, & Sroufe, 1997). Both of these attachment styles are characterized by caregivers' unpredictable (and thus uncontrollable) behavior and by children's fears of abandonment.

SAD will appear as elevated scores on the internalizing domain and subscales of parent and teacher rating scales (e.g., BASC-2). Extreme and persistent separation protests with babysitters or at daycare/preschool will make the problem apparent. Examiners can use a structured interview or DSM-IV-TR criteria in the form of questions to assess for the diagnosis. A parent interview that includes information on family history for psychopathology, as well as recent life events (especially traumatic events, such as deaths, car accidents, or family violence) can help clarify the situation and the diagnosis (see Chapter 8). If the child is at least age 3 and verbal, the MSSB may reveal a refusal to separate when the story calls for it and other story features characteristic of children with internalizing disorders, particularly anxiety (Warren, 2003; see Table 14.7, below). Assessment of social behavior in the childcare center/preschool classroom should clarify whether the child has general problems with social withdrawal.

Treatment of Internalizing Disorders

If a child does meet criteria for SAD, an evidence-based treatment plan can be developed by using Gimpel and Holland's (2003) book, *Emotional and Behavioral Problems of Young Children*. This book is also useful for treating young children with internalizing problems that are distressing but do not meet the criteria for a disorder. Behavioral approaches have proven efficacy in reducing symptoms, even if they may not completely eliminate the tendency to be inhibited, to be shy, to worry, or to be prone to sadness.

Because of the high degree of co-occurrence of parent and child anxiety disorders, many interventions involve parents actively in treatment. The Primary Mental Health Project (Cowen et al., 1996) is a school-based program for grades pre-K–4 that is effective with internalizing problems. A carefully selected and supervised paraprofessional meets once or twice a week individually or in a small group with a child or children identified by teacher ratings as having adjustment difficulties. The intervention consists of building a trusting, supportive paraprofessional–child relationship, with the adult following the child's lead during the session and encouraging expressive play.

Parent–Child Relationship Problems

Parent–child relationship problems are diagnosed when "the focus of clinical attention is a pattern of interaction between parent and child (e.g., impaired communication, overprotection, inadequate discipline) that is associated with clinically significant impairment in individual or family functioning or the development of clinically significant symptoms in parent or child" (American Psychiatric Association, 2000, p. 737). As Campbell (2002) notes, parent–child relationship problems as defined in DSM-IV were the second most frequent classification in Lavigne et al.'s (1996) study. It occurred in 4.6% of the unreferred population, second only to ODD and twice as often as ADHD. It was present in 9.2% of 2-year-olds and 2.8% of 4-year-olds, but in only one child at age 5. Because of the substantial evidence implicating parenting practices in the development of emotional and behavioral problems in children, this classification category is an extremely important one for examiners working with young children. Observation of the parent–child relationship in the clinic with the FEA-S (Greenspan et al. 2001) or the Parent–Child Game (Forehand & McMahon, 1981), or in the home with the home adaptation of the Parent–Child Game or the HOME (Caldwell & Bradley, 2003) will help determine whether there is a problem and the degree to which intervention is warranted. See Chapter 8 for detailed information on the assessment of problematic parent–child and family relationships and evidence-based interventions.

SCREENING PROCEDURES AND SELECTED INSTRUMENTS

The purposes of screening for emotional development and behavior problems are (1) to accurately, and inexpensively (in terms of time and money), identify young children in need of a more comprehensive evaluation and/or (b) to assess children's knowledge of curricular relevant material in order to design instruction. Ideally, all children under the age of 5 should be routinely screened and monitored for developmental competence, including emotional competence. Table 14.5 presents recommended steps in the screening process.

In this section, we review three parent and teacher rating scales that can be used effectively for screening for behavior problems. The first two also screen for socio-emotional competence. All of them take approximately 5–10 minutes to administer, are very easy to score and interpret, and have acceptable reliability and validity. The first two measures ask about behavior in a nonpathologizing way, while the third uses a mix of measures that assess competence and maladaptive behavior in the context of a "child-finding" process with teachers. (Appendix 14.1 contains descriptions and reviews of the psychometric characteristics of all measures described in this section and later in this chapter, as well as similar measures that are not covered in the text.) The section then

TABLE 14.5. Screening for Emotional Development and Behavior Problems

- Step 1: Annually, administer a screening measure to all parents (e.g., ASQ:SE, PKBS-2) to assess for appropriate and problematic behavior.
- Step 2: Annually or semiannually, administer a screening measure to teachers/caregivers to assess for problematic behavior (e.g., ESP, PKBS-2) and emotional competence (e.g., SCBE).
- Step 3: Screen all children for emotional milestones and skills.
- Step 4: Implement a center/school curriculum for emotional development.
- Step 5: Offer parents organized programs (e.g., The Incredible Years), as well as videos and books from a lending library to promote children's emotional and social competence (e.g., *The Heart of Parenting, How to Talk so Kids Will Listen and Listen so Kids Will Talk*).
- Step 6: Perform diagnostic assessments for children identified in screening as having delayed emotional development and/or behavior problems who have not benefited from intervention or for whom more services may be needed to promote emotional and behavioral competence.

describes how teachers/caregivers and other early childhood specialists can easily screen for competence in emotional expressiveness, understanding, and regulation, and use this information to plan instruction.

Step 1: Annual Screening of All Parents to Assess Child Development

In our opinion, emotional and social development is as important as language and cognitive development. We would like all agencies and schools that have contact with children from birth to age 5 to engage in screening and monitoring of children's development, including socioemotional development. Parents are the best source of information on their child. We are impressed with the Ages and Stages Questionnaires (ASQ; Bricker, Squires, & Mounts, 1995; Bricker & Squires, 1999) as a screening measure for child development in general (see Chapter 6 for other measures), and we particularly like the new expansion of the socioemotional section, the ASQ:SE (Squires et al., 2002). For preschoolers, the Preschool and Kindergarten Behavior Scales—Second Edition (PKBS-2; Merrell, 2002) is a good screening measure for social skills and behavior problems with parallel forms for home and school. The Early Screening Project (ESP; Walker, Severson, & Field, 1995) is an efficient system for preschools to use for identifying children at risk for socioemotional problems.

Ages and Stages Questionnaires: Social–Emotional

The ASQ:SE (Squires et al., 2002) is a parent report measure written at a fifth- to sixth-grade reading level, with illustrations to assist in understanding items. It has eight questionnaires for ages 6, 12, 18, 24, 30, 36, 48, and 60 months. The authors have designed the questionnaire so that it can be used within 3 months of each target age. The number of questions per questionnaire ranges from 19 at 6 months, to 33 at 48 and 60 months. There is a Spanish version.

The ASQ:SE was designed around two conceptual frameworks. The first ensures that items are sensitive to the setting or time in which the behavior occurs, the child's developmental level, the child's health status, and family or cultural factors that might be potentially associated with the behavior. The authors believe that these variables have a large influence on children's socioemotional functioning and need to be taken into consideration in deciding whether or not a child has a problem that needs further evaluation. The authors recommend that evaluators keep these areas in mind when interpreting parents' responses. For example, evaluators should ask themselves whether behavior occurs both at home and at school, since parents and school staff may play a role in reinforcing or deterring its occurrence. They also recommend first ruling out a possible developmental delay as an important first step in interpreting young children's socioemotional competence. Health factors are also important, because chronic illnesses such as otitis media can play a large role in children's socioemotional functioning, as can more transient health concerns (e.g., little sleep the night before and living in a home environment where there is insufficient food). Finally, the authors note that children's socioemotional behaviors are influenced greatly by family values and culture, as well as by unique family dynamics (such as family violence).

The second conceptual framework used by the authors consists of seven behavioral areas that their review of the literature identified as important aspects of socioemotional functioning:

1. Self-Regulation (e.g., "can calm down").
2. Compliance (e.g., "follows simple direction/routine").
3. Communication (e.g., "lets you know/uses words when hungry, sick, tired").
4. Adaptive Functioning (e.g., "stays away from danger").
5. Autonomy (e.g., "checks in when exploring").
6. Affect (e.g., "is interested in things around him/her").
7. Interaction with People (both parents and other adults—e.g., "other children like to play with your child").

The authors have developed an excellent test manual that instructs the reader in how to set up a child-monitoring system for socioemotional behaviors as part of a Head Start program or other outreach/home visiting/early intervention program. In the manual, they provide many useful clinical examples of how a program can be developed and implemented to be as useful and as least burdensome as possible for program staff.

In summary, the ASQ:SE has many advantages as a screening measure for socioemotional functioning in young children. The questionnaires are readable, age-appropriate, nonpathologizing for parents, and easy to score and use for early intervention program staff. The authors went through an extensive process to ensure content validity, discriminant validity, and utility. For a screening measure, the ASQ:SE is adequately reliable and valid. We recommend its use as a front-line measure to monitor the achievement of socioemotional milestones, and to identify children who may be in need of further evaluation.

Step 2: Annual or Semiannual Screening of Teachers/Caregivers

Preschool and Kindergarten Behavior Scales—Second Edition

The PKBS-2 (Merrell, 2002) is a screening measure for parents and teachers, designed to identify preschool and kindergarten-age children (ages 3–6) who may be at risk for social skills deficits or behavioral problems. It avoids the use of items that represent more extreme psychopathology, minimizing language that would confuse or offend parents or teachers. The measure consists of the Social Skills Scale and the Behavior Problem Scale, which were conormed with a nationally standardized and somewhat representative population. Supplemental Problems Scales are available for exploration of the reasons for significant elevations on the Behavior Problems Scale. There are three supplemental scales for exploring externalizing problems (Self-Centered/Explosive, Attention Problems/Overactive, Antisocial/Aggressive) and two for internalizing problems (Social Withdrawal, Anxiety/Somatic Problems). The measure is available in both Spanish and English. The PKBS-2 appears to have excellent psychometric characteristics for a brief screening measure. Although the normative sample included ages 3–6, a small sample size for age 3 suggested that the measure is best used with children ages 4–6. The ease of administration and scoring, presence of separate norms for home and school raters, and good convergent and divergent validity with other widely used measures of social skills and behavior problems, as well as the test's ability to discriminate children not at risk from those at risk or with possible delays, suggests that it is reliable and accurate in identifying children who merit a comprehensive evaluation for problems in this area. It has been criticized as being a psychometrically weaker version of the CBCL/2-3 (Achenbach, 1992) and the Social Skills Rating Scales (SSRS; Gresham & Elliott, 1990). The PKBS-2's major scales are highly correlated with these two measures, which have better norms and a wealth of established predictive and criterion validity data. If a child's behavior is clearly of concern, the use of a screening measure like the PKBS-2 is not indicated. An examiner would use diagnostic-quality measures (such as the current age-appropriate version of the CBCL) from the beginning. However, if routine screening of all children is the purpose of the assessment or if an examiner is interested in ruling out other potential problems for a child referred for other reasons, the nonpathologizing PKBS-2, which screens for both behavior problems and social skills, is a good choice.

Early Screening Project

The ESP (Walker et al., 1995) is a multistep child-finding process, designed to efficiently identify children ages 3–6 who are at risk for internalizing and externalizing behavior problems. The test is a downward extension of the Systematic Screening for Behavior Disorders (Walker & Severson, 1990) and was designed to meet the child-finding requirement of IDEA.

During stage 1, teachers evaluate students in the fall and the spring. The teachers are given definitions of externalizing and internalizing behavior, and are asked to list the five most internalizing (withdrawn, socially isolated) and the five most externalizing (acting-out, disruptive) children in their class. They are then asked to rank them in the order in which they display these behaviors. No child can be listed on both scales. The three highest-ranking children in each group are then rescreened by their teachers as part of stage 2.

In stage 2, these six children are evaluated with the Critical Events Index (e.g., "sets fires"), the Adaptive Behavior Scale, the Maladaptive Behavior Scale, and either the Aggressive Behavior Scale (externalizing children) or the Social Interaction Scale (internalizing children). Teachers use separate normative tables for boys and girls, resulting in critical scores by level of risk: "at risk" (1 *SD* above or below the mean), "high risk" (1.5 *SD*), and "extreme risk" (2 *SD*). Only children who are normatively at risk are evaluated at stage 3 and considered for referral to the school's or school district's committee on special education or intervention.

In stage 3, a parent questionnaire and a direct Social Behavior Observation (SBO) of each referred child are used. The parent measure is short and simply designed to assess the degree to which the parent concurs with teacher ratings and observations through the use of items that overlap with other information.

An excellent training tape and detailed scoring examples in the manual are provided to facilitate coding of observed behaviors on the SBO. The SBO is easy to use, as it is simply a measure of duration—specifically, the percentage of time a child either is not interacting with others socially or is interacting in an antisocial manner out of the total time observed. Because of its simplicity, an examiner can take anecdotal notes on what transpires during the observation. After the observation is completed, the examiner is encouraged to ask a teacher or aide whether the child's observed behavior is typical. Users should be aware that research distinguishes between anxious, reticent, uninvolved children who hover on the edges of play groups observing without involvement, and children who play alone in constructive, object-related play. The former are likely to be socially isolated, distressed, and rejected by peers, while the latter are not (Rubin, 1993).

In summary, the ESP is an easy-to-use child-finding process that requires minimal teacher time, does not overidentify children, has strong psychometric characteristics, and has an outstanding manual with very clear instructions for teachers and other mental health professionals. It is better at discriminating children with externalizing problems from normal children than it is at discriminating children with internalizing problems. This finding is not a negative reflection on the ESP; rather, it reflects robust research findings showing that children with undercontrolled or externalizing behavior are relatively easy to distinguish from normal children, but overcontrolled or internalizing behavior differ less significantly from normally developing children (Hart, Atkins, & Fegley, 2003). We particularly like the SBO, which is remarkably easy to use and yet provides very useful information on the social behavior of both acting-out and socially isolated children. Although the authors do not require this, it seems that a mental health professional knowledgeable about both externalizing and internalizing disorders should actively be involved in the process, so that children do not become inappropriately labeled (Knoff, 2001a). The ESP is an efficient way to identify children with emotional or behavior problems as part of a child-finding process initiated by the school. If a school or daycare center does not use the ASQ:SE or PKBS-2 on a routine basis, we recommend that the ESP be used.

Step 3: Screening All Children for Emotional Milestones and Skills

Emotional Understanding

Emotional understanding has typically been assessed by asking preschool children to (1) recognize and label emotional expressions representing happiness, sadness, anger, and fear; and (2) interpret emotional situations enacted by puppets. Assessing whether children can recognize and label the four basic emotions has been done with actual pictures of emotional expression (Field & Walden, 1982) or with faces of pure expressions depicted on felt circles (Dunn & Hughes, 1998). Denham and Couchard (1990) argue that the pictures on felt circles are easier for very young children to identify than pictures of actual children. In their procedure, an examiner lays out four faces made of felt. Children are first asked to name the four faces in response to the question "What is this face feeling?" Then they are required to point to each expression in response to the question "Where is the '____________' face?" Faces are randomly shuffled and laid on the table before each pair of questions. All four faces are on the table for the pointing task. Children get 1 point correct for naming and 1 for pointing at each expression, for a possible total score of 4 on the naming measure and 4 on the recognition measure. Cronbach's alphas were .73 for both measures with 2-, 3-, and 4-year-old children. The book *Dina*

Dinosaur's Classroom-Based Social Skills, Problem-Solving, and Anger Management Curriculum (Webster-Stratton, 2001) also has materials that can be used to assess and teach emotional knowledge (see below).

To assess how children interpret emotional situations, Denham and Couchard (1990) developed a procedure that has been used in a number of studies. Using family puppets made of cloth, they had the examiner enact eight vignettes modeled on those of Borke (1971). The puppets were used because they were seen as more engaging to children and lessened the cognitive demands of the task. The brief vignettes were enacted by both the puppet and the examiner; vocal tone, the examiner's facial expression, and the body language of the puppet were used to convey an emotional experience (see Denham & Couchard, 1990). For example, to illustrate "happy," the puppet (same sex as the child) had an ice cream cone, spread its arms, and bounced along. A broad smile was demonstrated by the puppeteer, who used relaxed, cheerful vocal tones to convey happiness. There were two vignettes for each emotion for the four basic emotions. After each vignette, the child was asked, "How does the puppet feel?" The child was then asked to affix the proper face from the four faces identified in the previous task onto the puppet; this minimized the verbal demands of the task. Cronbach's alpha for the measure was .82. In line with others' findings using similar tasks, there were no gender differences. The children most easily identified happiness, followed by sadness, then anger, and then fear. They clearly understood the difference between pleasant and unpleasant emotions, and rarely confused happiness with any of the negative emotions, although the negative ones were often confused with one another. The confusion of sadness and anger seems to make sense, since in many situations either emotion may be predominant and may be appropriate.

Emotional Expressiveness

Assessing the degree to which young children are able to access and clearly express a full range of emotions is best assessed through observation. If the examiner has the time, this can be done in a daycare or preschool classroom over several days. As part of a play evaluation session, the examiner attempts to see the degree to which a child can demonstrate closeness or dependency, pleasure and excitement, assertiveness and exploration, cautious or fearful behavior, anger, limit setting on the self, and separation and loss. These affects can be observed either in direct displays of emotions or in themes carried out in play or commentary on play. For example, Greenspan and Wieder (2001) give the example for cautious or fearful behavior of "pretend drama in which baby doll is scared of loud noise," and the example for anger of "soldiers shoot ten guns at one another" (p. 97).

Emotional Regulation

Emotional regulation is best assessed by observing a child over time in the daycare/classroom setting and by asking teachers or caregivers about children's emotional expression and regulation (see Figure 14.1, below). The Social Competence and Behavior Evaluation, Preschool Edition (SCBE; LaFreniere & Dumas, 1995), a rating scale completed by teachers or caregivers and described below, is also a good measure of emotional regulation. The key component here is to understand what are the strategies the child uses to "up-regulate" or "down-regulate" and whether these strategies are adaptive in this setting. If a problem is identified and a child is at least 3 years of age and verbal, the MSSB, also described below, provides useful information on both the child's emotional regulation and the supportive and dysregulating influences in the social environment.

Step 4: Implementing a Center/School Curriculum for Emotional Development

A number of social and emotional learning (SEL) prevention/intervention programs have developed curricula for which there is evidence supporting its efficacy, with preschoolers (for reviews, see Joseph & Strain, 2004; Denham & Burton, 2003). Joseph and Strain ranked the Incredible Years program and the First Step to Success Program (Walker et al., 1998) as having the highest level of empirical support. Denham and Burton based their reviews on the theoretical and developmental soundness of the curricula on a skill-by-skill basis as well as the degree of empirical support. They give the highest ratings to the Preschool PATHS program (Domitrovitch, Cortes, & Greenberg, 2002), Incredible Years Program, and their own Social–Emotional Intervention for 4-Year-Olds at Risk (Denham & Burton, 1996) in terms of empirical support, but preferred the theoretical and developmental focus of their program and PATHS to the behavioral approach of Incredible Years.

As mentioned previously, the Incredible Years program (Webster-Stratton, 2000) has a teacher training component, the Teacher Classroom Management Series; this has been shown to improve the emotional and behavioral functioning of young, unreferred, but at-risk Head Start children. It is designed as a group skills training program delivered in 14 sessions lasting 2 hours each, or over 4 intensive days. Research showed that after this component was implemented, teachers were less harsh and critical, had improved relationships with parents, and used more praise and proactive discipline. Their students were more positive and cooperative in their relationships with teachers. The students had better peer relationships, greater engagement in school tasks, and better school readiness (Webster-Stratton & Reid, 2004; Webster-Stratton et al., 2004). As part of this program, Webster-Stratton (1999) has written an excellent book for teachers, *How to Promote Children's Social and Emotional Competence.* This volume integrates most of the research on positive teacher–student relationships, proactive teaching, motivational systems, managing misbehavior, promoting peer relationships and problem solving, and helping children manage their emotions. Webster-Stratton (2001) has also developed Dina Dinosaur, a social curriculum to be used with young children ages 4–8 in the classroom as a prevention program or in small-group treatment of highly aggressive children. It covers understanding and communicating feelings, anger management, friendship and conversational skills, appropriate classroom behavior, and problem-solving strategies. Two randomized clinical trials showed that it increased children's cognitive problem-solving strategies, prosocial conflict management strategies, social competence, and appropriate play skills, and reduced conduct problems at home and school.

The First Step to Success Program is a behavioral intervention that starts with the use of the Early Screening Project described previously. For those high-risk children who make it to the third stage of evaluation there is a targeted school intervention involving the teacher, peers, and the target child as well as a parent/caregiving training component to help the parent(s) support the child's school adjustment. The Preschool PATHS Program and the Social–Emotional Intervention for 4-Year-Olds at Risk both have a strong emphasis on emotional understanding and regulation, social competence, building relationships, and interpersonal problem solving. They are designed to be integrated fully into a preschool curriculum and taught over most of the school year. Joseph and Strain

(2004), Denham and Burton (2003), and Chesebrough, King, Gullota, and Bloom (2004) are good resources for selecting SEL curricula for preschool children.

Step 5: Offering Parent Programs and a Lending Library to Promote Children's Socioemotional Competence

Preschools should be proactive in offering support to parents in ways that parents find helpful. One way of doing this is to conduct a needs assessment to identify topics of interest to parents and the ways in which they would most like to receive information or support. Some parents would like an organized series of short courses on child development, behavior management, toilet training, sleep problems, or the like. Others are interested in a support group to help them cope with noncompliant children, children with disabilities, or just the normal stresses of raising typical children. Still others are interested in videos and books that they can borrow on similar topics. A needs assessment can be as simple as sending out a questionnaire, or it can elicit more nuanced information by inviting 8–10 parents to participate in a focus group. The staff member conducting a focus group uses a small-group format and a moderator's guide (prepared questions that structure the discussion) to ask about sensitive issues (Basch, 1997). The questions could include what challenges parents face in parenting, what they would find helpful from a preschool program, how they would prefer to receive the help, and how they evaluate the acceptability of some alternatives.

Step 6: Referring Children for Diagnostic Assessment

Some families and children are unresponsive to a curriculum designed to improve functioning in all children, or have problems so severe that a comprehensive evaluation is needed to examine all possible causes of the problems and identify the most promising approaches to intervention. Young children who have problem behaviors at a level meriting referral need to be carefully screened for developmental problems in all areas, to ensure that no co-occurring or contributory factor is overlooked. An efficient means of doing this is to administer the Vineland-II (Sparrow et al., 2005; see Chapters 12 and 13) or the full ASQ to parents. Doing so would make it likely that the assessment team has the full complement of appropriate professionals needed to identify the problem accurately and suggest effective interventions.

ASSESSMENT OF EMOTIONAL AND BEHAVIOR PROBLEMS: STEPS AND SELECTED MEASURES

In this section, we describe the steps in a comprehensive psychoeducational diagnostic assessment of a preschool-age child referred for emotional and behavior problems. Table 14.6 provides an outline of the steps.

Step 1: Broad-Band, Normative Assessment of Problems

The initial referral interview provides information on the nature of the referring party's concerns, enabling us to develop an initial assessment battery. We recommend that the examiner begin by collecting multi-informant, cross-setting data on a child's functioning in order to gain a clear sense of where the problem is exhibited, how serious it is relative

TABLE 14.6. Diagnostic Assessment for Emotional and Behavior Problems

- Step 1: Broad-band, normative assessment of problems.
  - Administer rating scales to multiple informants (e.g., Mom and Dad, two caregivers), across settings if possible (e.g., CBCL/1½–5; C-TRF).
- Step 2: Parent/family assessment (see Chapter 8).
  - Obtain a developmental, health, and educational history of the child.
  - Assess family history and current functioning.
  - Screen parents for depression, anxiety, ODD, ADHD, stress, marital/couple problems, and social support.
  - Obtain description of problematic behavior and its context.
  - Review symptoms and severity for diagnoses being considered.
  - Assess adaptive behavior across developmental domains (e.g., Vineland-II).
  - Observe parent–child interaction (e.g., Parent–Child Game, FEAS, HOME).
- Step 3: Teacher/caregiver interview, if child is in childcare/preschool.
  - Obtain description of problematic behavior and its context.
  - Review symptoms and severity for diagnoses being considered.
  - Assess socioemotional development via interview (Figure 14.1) or rating scale (e.g., SCBE).
  - Review records, examine portfolios.
- Step 4: Observation/assessment of social and classroom behavior, if child is in daycare/preschool.
  - Observe social behavior in unstructured (play) setting (e.g., SBO).
  - If considering a diagnosis of ADHD, observe behavior in structured setting (e.g., DOF).
  - Assess quality of peer relationships (e.g., SSRS).
  - Assess quality of care/instruction being offered (see Chapter 5).
- Step 5: Assessment of the child.
  - If child is verbal, administer story stem to obtain child's representation of his or her social world, emotional development (e.g., MSSB).
  - If child is not verbal, assess cognitive ability (see Chapter 11) and language (see Chapter 10); assess emotional development through play (e.g., FEAS, measures covered in Chapter 4).
- Step 6: Case formulation.
  - Identify clinically significant findings.
  - Look for convergence across informants, settings, and measures.
  - Make sense out of discrepant findings.
  - Identify any missing information needed for case formulation or treatment planning, and obtain it.
  - Create a framework for explaining the problem.
  - Identify appropriate and accessible interventions.
- Step 7: Therapeutic presentation of findings and recommendations.
  - Present findings in straightforward, jargon-free, empathetic manner.
  - Support what parents are doing right.
  - Offer realistic hope and encouragement; motivate parents for treatment.
  - Minimize shame.
  - Offer to facilitate referrals, if relevant.

to similar age and gendered peers, and whether it suggests the development of a particular syndrome of behavior. Typically, after obtaining formal consent, a copy of the CBCL/1½–5 (Achenbach & Rescorla, 2000b) or the Behavior Assessment Scale for Children, Second Edition (BASC-2; Reynolds & Kamphaus, 2004) is sent to the parent(s), requesting that the adults involved in care (e.g., mother, father, grandmother, stepfather, and nanny) complete the form and mail it back prior to our first session. If applicable, we also request that one or more childcare providers or preschool teachers also complete the form with parental consent, prior to the first assessment with the family. If the referral comes from a systematic screening process at a center or school, such as the ESP, this may already have been done with teachers; in this case, they should not be burdened with the completion of an additional form unless there is a compelling reason. Scoring these forms provides some information on the degree to which one or more adults see the child as having problems that are significant in comparison with peers, and the degree to which these problems are cross-situational and are observed by two or more adults in the same situation.

Achenbach System of Empirically Based Assessment: Preschool Forms and Profiles

The original CBCL, a parent rating form for ages 4–16 (Achenbach & Edelbrock, 1983), and later the original Teacher Report Form (TRF) for children ages 6–16 (Edelbrock & Achenbach, 1984), transformed the assessment of socioemotional and behavior problems by demonstrating the usefulness of an empirically driven approach that identifies problems as they cluster within actual children. This is in contrast to the top-down approach used by classification systems such as the DSM-IV-TR (APA, 2000), which is clinician/expert-driven. The Preschool Forms currently included in Achenbach's ASEBA battery include the Caregiver–Teacher Report Form (Achenbach, 1997) for daycare providers and preschool teachers of children ages 2–5 (C-TRF), and the CBCL for Ages 1½ to 5 (CBCL/1½–5; Achenbach & Rescorla, 2000b), with an accompanying Language Development Survey (LDS). The ASEBA is designed to be an integrated system of multi-informant assessment. The authors state that the CBCL/1½–5 and the C-TRF, if applicable, should be completed by at least two adults in each of two settings: home and childcare/preschool. Because children with emotional and behavior problems often have language delays, the coadministration of the LDS allows an evaluator to immediately assess the hypothesis that language delays may play a role in such problems observed.

The CBCL/1½–5 and the C-TRF are designed to assess emotional and behavior problems in young children and to identify empirically based syndromes of problems that occur together, as well as to profile the degree to which children's symptoms resemble certain DSM-IV-TR diagnostic categories. Parents and caregivers are asked to rate each item on a list of 100 behavior problems for the degree to which the item "now or within the past two months" describes the child's behavior. Items are rated 0, "not true (as far as you know)"; 1, "somewhat or sometimes true"; or 2, – "very true or often true." The items are behavioral descriptions of easily observed behavior, such as "cruel to animals," "hits others," and "rapid shifts between sadness and excitement."

In addition, the respondent is asked whether the child has any illnesses or disabilities and, if so, to describe them. If the child being rated has a disability, raters are instructed to base their ratings on what would be typical for a normally developing peer of the same age. This can be difficult for parents or professionals who have limited experience with normally developing children (parents who have only one disabled child, or teachers who work exclusively with special education populations). Adults can develop skewed internal norms of what is appropriate for each age if they lack contact with normally developing children. Examiners should be aware of this possibility when interpreting all behavior rating scales.

The C-TRF asks the staff members who know the child best, and have known the child for at least 2 months, to complete the form. Responses are based on the child's behavior in the last 2 months. In order to help interpreters use the information obtained, the C-TRF asks about each respondent's training and experience with the child, including the size of the facility and how many hours per week the child attends.

Scores obtained on both the CBCL/1½–5 and the C-TRF include a Total Problem Behavior score, which includes items from all seven subscales, as well as 33 items that do not cluster uniquely on any one scale, but are problematic and are included in the Total Behavior Problems Scale. Two domain scores, Internalizing and Externalizing, are also obtained, and they each have two or more subscales. For Internalizing, these include Emotionally Reactive, Anxious/Depressed, Somatic Complaints, and Withdrawn; for Externalizing, these include Attention Problems and Aggressive Behavior. One subscale is not correlated with the Internalizing or the Externalizing factors, Sleep Problems, and it has a scale of its own.

A new feature of the ASEBA Preschool Forms is the DSM-oriented scales. Since past research has shown a significant relationship between certain DSM diagnoses and CBCL and TRF scores, the scale authors developed scales that were consistent with the criteria for five DSM-IV-TR categories. These categories are Affective Problems, Anxiety Problems, Pervasive Developmental Problems, Attention-Deficit/Hyperactivity Problems, and Oppositional Defiant Problems. The authors caution examiners that the DSM-oriented scales are not directly equivalent to the corresponding DSM-IV-TR diagnoses, for the same reasons that the empirically derived scales are not. Specifically, (1) the items do not have precise correspondence to the DSM diagnoses, as items were not specifically written to match criteria, but rather come from a pool of empirically derived items; (2) the items are scored based on children's behavior of the past 2 months, which does not necessarily correspond to the age of onset or duration of problem criteria for the DSM-IV-TR; (3) the 0–2 scoring system is different from the DSM-IV-TR criteria, which are simply judged as present or absent; and (4) the scales are normative, in that the child is compared to a national sample of same-age and (in most cases) same-gender peers rated by the same types of respondents, whereas the DSM-IV-TR criteria are the same for all ages, genders, and sources of data relevant to diagnostic criteria.

In summary, the ASEBA Preschool Forms are excellent rating scales of emotional and behavior problems for young children. They cover a large age range; have a nationally representative sample; are translated (and in some cases normed) in many languages (e.g., Zulu, Samoan, Norwegian); have excellent cross-informant, cross-setting, and stability coefficients for this type of measure; and have very strong content, discriminant, concurrent, and predictive validity data, with new studies being completed all the time. Written at a fifth-grade reading level and taking very little time to complete, the measures can be used repeatedly, making them very useful for initial evaluation as well as follow-up to address treatment effectiveness and program evaluation. Computer scoring minimizes errors and scoring time, and facilitates the comparison of ratings across informants and settings. The LDS provides an initial screen for language delays. The only drawback of the ASEBA Preschool Forms is the absence of any assessment of socioemotional competence. The authors of the Infant–Toddler Social–Emotional Assessment (Carter & Briggs-Gowan, 2000) and the BASC-2 (Reynolds & Kamphaus, 2004) have demonstrated how scales assessing adaptive behavior could be successfully added to a battery such as the ASEBA—allowing an examiner to assess the degree to which positive development is not occurring, as well as the degree to which problems are present.

Behavior Assessment System for Children, Second Edition

The BASC-2 (Reynolds & Kamphaus, 2004) is a popular and well-respected assessment battery that includes five components for integrated multimodal evaluation of individuals 2–5 years of age at the preschool level (the upper age limit for the battery as a whole is 21). It was designed to "facilitate the differential diagnosis and educational classification of a variety of emotional and behavioral disorders of children and to aid in the design of treatment plans." The BASC-2 has five parts: Teacher Rating Scales (TRS), Parent Rating Scales (PRS), Self-Report Personality Scales (SRP) for children 8 and older, a Structured Developmental History form (SDH), and a Student Observation System (SOS). The BASC-2 also has a Spanish version available.

The preschool versions of the TRS (TRS-P) and PRS (PRS-P) measure observable behaviors in the classroom and in the home, respectively. Each has four composite scores and 18 subscales: Externalizing Problems (Aggression, Hyperactivity), Internalizing Problems (Anxiety, Depression, Somatization), Adaptive Skills (Adaptability, Social Skills), School Problems (attitudes to school and teachers), and a Behavior Symptoms Index (overall level of problem behaviors). The Adaptive Skills composite on the preschool versions consists of items in the domains of adaptability, social skills (e.g., "says please and thank you"), functional communication (e.g., "provides full name when asked"), and activities of daily living on the PRS-P (e.g., "needs help putting on clothes"). The SDH form provides a format to elicit an extensive historical survey of a child's physical and psychosocial development. Finally, the SOS provides assessors with an observation tool for recording frequency and disruptiveness of behavior in school. The SOS can be used at the preschool level for 4- and 5-year-olds in regular and special education classrooms, but there are no norms. The manual also describes the use of SOS computer software on a laptop or personal digital assistant; this software provides cues for recording behaviors and automatically scores observations. Because it assesses adaptive behavior, many assessors prefer it to the ASEBA Preschool Forms and Profiles as a diagnostic quality behavior rating system.

Overall, the BASC-2 provides a multimethod and multidimensional measure of a child's social, emotional, and adaptive functioning, with ample norm samples for the preschool level at all ages and sound psychometric properties. The multimodal and integrated nature of the battery makes it an efficient and comprehensive assessment tool. However, it should be noted that it does not discriminate different clinical subgroups in the 2- to 3-year-old range. Because it assesses adaptive behavior, many assessors prefer it to the ASEBA Preschool Forms and Profiles as a diagnostic quality behavior rating system.

Step 2: Parent/Family Assessment

If parents or other caregivers see a child as having significant problems in related areas, this indicates that there is a behavior problem at home. We organize our interview according to Barkley's (1997a) Clinical Interview—Parent Report Form, because it asks for detailed information about parental concerns that have led to a referral; reviews criteria for childhood disorders that may be alternative diagnoses or comorbid diagnoses (e.g., ODD, ADHD, CD, anxiety, and depression); and gathers information on parents' child management strategies, the child's past evaluation and treatment history, educational history, strengths, and family psychiatric history.

We also give a measure of adaptive behavior, such as the Vineland-II (Sparrow et al., 2005). The Vineland, reviewed in Chapters 12 and 13, is widely used for developmental assessments in referred children ages 0–5, as well as older individuals with mental retardation, autism, and dementia. The Socialization domain assesses the development of interest in others, emotional responsivity, emotional expression, emotional understanding, and success in making friends. The absence of these skills, when expected based on either age or mental age, would alert the evaluator that a more extensive assessment of emotional and social functioning may be appropriate. The Interpersonal Relationships subscale is particularly sensitive in identifying children with ASD. If adaptive behavior is low across the board or in the domains of Communication or Daily Living Skills, administration of an individually administered intelligence test and collection of a language sample (see Chapter 10) may be appropriate. If the Motor Skills score is low, assessment by a physical or occupational therapist may be in order.

Direct observations of parent–child interaction are very useful for both diagnosis and treatment planning. Because of the training involved in mastering structured systems and maintaining interrater agreement many examiners either omit direct observation or do it informally (see Chapter 4). There are three observation measures that we recommend spending the time to master, depending on the types and numbers of clients seen. If a child is referred for disruptive, noncompliant behavior, we recommend the Parent–Child Game developed by Forehand and McMahon (1981). If a child is referred for delays in emotional milestones, we recommend the HOME (Caldwell & Bradley, 2003; see Chapter 8) or the FEAS.

Parent–Child Game

The Parent–Child Game (Forehand & McMahon, 1981; McMahon & Forehand, 2003) was designed to assess parent–child interaction when a child has been referred for defiant or other acting-out behavior, with a particular focus on the parent's commands, the child's compliance, and the parent's ability to follow a child's lead. Parent and child are observed in a clinic playroom, which is equipped with a one-way mirror and is wired for sound. Age-appropriate toys are provided and might include such things as crayons and paper for drawing; toy trucks and cars; dolls; building materials, such as Legos; and puzzles. An assessor codes the interaction while observing from the observation room through the one-way mirror. Two different games are played. In the Child's Game, the parent is asked to participate in whichever activity the child chooses and to allow the child to be the leader (i.e., determining what will be done and what the rules of the interaction will be), creating a free-play situation. In the Parent's Game, the parent chooses the activities and rules and tells the child what they are going to do, creating a directed situation. Each game lasts for 5 minutes, during which time six parent behaviors (rewards, such as praise or positive physical attention; attending to the child, which can include describing the child's behavior; questions that are asked; any commands that are given; warnings; and time outs) and three child behaviors (compliance; noncompliance; and any inappropriate behavior, such as whining, crying, or being aggressive) are coded by the observer. The Child's Game assesses the parent's competence at supporting the child's autonomy and demonstrating interest in the child, while the Parent's Game assesses the parent's use of appropriate or alpha commands and the child's compliance. All of these are targets of intervention in the Helping the Noncompliant Child program (see Chapter 8).

One of the advantages of the Parent–Child Game is that it takes only 10 minutes to stage, and thus can be used repeatedly during ongoing treatment. It has adequate interrater agreement and test–retest reliability. The interactions of parents and children not undergoing treatment tend to be very stable, while the measure is sensitive to significant treatment affects in the clinic and at home. It has been used successfully in many research studies. Its disadvantages are that it requires training to code (about 25 hours) and ongoing maintenance of interrater reliability—a commitment that only clinics conducting treatment research have typically been willing to make.

Functional Emotional Assessment Scale

Greenspan has, over the past 20+ years, been a leading theoretician and researcher in the area of emotional development. The FEAS (Greenspan, DeGangi, & Wieder, 2001) is a clinical assessment model that operationalizes much of his thinking and research in this area (Greenspan, 1992). The FEAS also fits neatly with the DC:0–3R (Zero to Three, 2005). Clinicians wanting to use Greenspan's assessment model will want to be thoroughly familiar with the manual for the FEAS, the DC:0–3R, and his book *Infancy and Early Childhood: The Practice of Clinical Assessments and Intervention with Emotional and Developmental Challenges* (Greenspan, 1992). In addition, annual workshops involving this assessment model and interventions related to emotional development are offered regularly by the Interdisciplinary Council on Developmental and Learning Disorders in Bethesda, Maryland. The Council maintains a website (www.icdl.com) where materials and training tapes can be purchased.

The purpose of the FEAS is to understand an infant's or young child's "emotional and social functioning in the context of relationships with his or her caregivers or family. The emotional capacities of the infant and young child relate to the infant's ability to deal with his or her real world" (Greenspan & Wieder, 2001, pp. 75–76). The FEAS is a semiformal structured clinical observation form. The foundation of the evaluation consists of interactions between a child and a caregiver (mother, father, nanny, or grandparent) and between the child and the examiner for about 15 minutes each over at least two separate sessions in the home or office, as well as interviewing of the caregiver. Formal tests are then used selectively to answer any questions that cannot be addressed in a clinical assessment. While the FEAS itself focuses on emotional and social capacities at each of six stages, the manual also covers important progressions in motor, sensory, language, and cognitive development that accompany and support the essential emotional and social capacities. General regulatory patterns can be assessed at any age; these include the child's comfort with being touched, movement in space, maintenance of motor tone, enactment of motor-planning sequences, and so forth.

Caregiver patterns are evaluated by history and/or direct observation. Patterns assessed include the caregiver's abilities to comfort the child, especially when the child is upset; to interact at appropriate levels of stimulation that keep the child comfortably involved; to respond to the child's emotional signals; to encourage the child to move forward developmentally, rather than infantilizing the child or being punitive or chaotic; and to engage the child pleasurably in a relationship, as opposed to either ignoring or mistreating the child.

The results of the FEAS are used to (1) generate clinical hypotheses that can be explored further; (2) design interventions to address developmental or regulatory problems, and/or caregiver–child interaction problems; and (3) formulate a clinical diagnosis using DC:0–3R or DSM-IV-TR in conjunction with interview data, parent report measures, review of records, and other formal testing.

In summary, the FEAS has many strengths and is quite promising, but still needs more work before it can be used as a tool on its own with confidence. Its strengths are that it is an observational tool that assesses aspects of emotional functioning in both children and their caregivers from infancy into the middle preschool years. It is theoretically driven and assesses many subtle aspects of socioemotional functioning that are hard to assess in other ways. Interrater agreement is quite high for an observational measure, but its discrimination is good for only certain disorders and problems in certain age ranges (i.e., regulatory disorders from 7 to 24 months, pervasive developmental disorders from 2 to 4 years, and multiple problems in families from 13 to 18 months). Its specificity is weak, as it is not strong in detecting which children are exhibiting typical, as opposed to atypical, socioemotional development. There are no data on its use with children who have anxiety, mood disorders, or ODD. More research is needed in terms of concurrent validity with other measures of emotional and behavioral problems, more ethnically diverse populations, and other child problem samples. Finally, a major time commitment is required to learn the measure and the theory that supports it.

Step 3: Teacher/Caregiver Interview

If a child is in a childcare/preschool setting, we visit the setting with parental consent to interview caregivers/teachers about the child's functioning, review symptoms and severity for diagnoses being considered, review records, examine portfolios, and observe the child and the environment. If the teacher also has concerns about the child and has the time to discuss these issues, we also try to obtain a description of problematic behavior and when it is most likely to occur. In addition, we ask the teacher about the child's emotional development (see Figure 14.1) and/or administer a rating scale. If the child attends childcare or preschool in a highly stressful environment (as sometimes occurs in urban settings), we might speak to the caregiver or teacher briefly to gain some sense of how the child relates to the teacher, to peers, and to the curriculum, and whether the caregiver/teacher has any concerns. We might then only ask him or her to respond to symptoms and criteria for diagnosis, and to tell us what has worked in getting the most competent behavior from the child.

Step 4: Observation/Assessment of Social and Classroom Behavior

As we have stressed throughout this chapter, emotional competence is the most important factor contributing to children's social competence. Social competence with peers is among the most important developmental tasks faced by preschool children. Being able to understand emotions; to express a range of emotions appropriately, depending on the setting and circumstances; and to cope with one's own and others' emotions largely determines how one is received by adults and peers (see Denham, 1998, for a comprehensive review). Having poor peer relationships is a robust and sensitive predictor of current and future maladjustment. It is listed as a diagnostic criterion for many DSM-IV-TR disorders that first appear in childhood, and is an associated feature in many other disorders (Bierman & Welsh, 1997).

Peer interactions during the preschool years are organized around play, particularly fantasy play. To be successful in this type of play, children need to be able to attend to the play task, willingly incorporate their playmates' ideas and additions into the play sequence, and display generally positive emotions (Bierman & Walsh, 1997). Play interactions often last only for short periods of time, and it may be important to learn how to keep other children who want to join out of the play sequence without offending them (Denham, 1998). Children also have to be able to regulate their emotions, because conflicts are frequent and friendships are unstable (Hartup, 1983). Children's play groups are

Emotional Understanding

Child can point to face showing:		Child uses emotion language:	
Happy	______	Happy	______
Sad	______	Sad	______
Mad	______	Mad	______
Scared	______	Scared	______
		Hurt	______
		Hungry	______
		Thirsty	______

Emotional Expressiveness

Child demonstrates:

Pleasure/excitement during play, stories, etc. ______

Anger when goals are blocked ______

Sadness when facing loss ______

Need for comfort when upset, hurt, or sick ______

Fear when feeling threatened ______

Interest and exploration of new toys, people, places ______

How would you describe this child's predominant mood?

Emotional Regulation

- Tell me what you observed about how this child plays.
- How does this child react to frustration?
- Describe for me some typical ways this child might respond if asked to share a toy, or was bumped or hit.
- How does this child approach others to join play?
- How might this child respond if another child approached and joined the play?
- What makes this child angry?
- What makes this child happy?
- How does this child respond when angry or happy?
- Describe circumstances in which this child was aggressive.
- Describe circumstances in which this child was helpful to others.
- Describe circumstances in which this child empathized with another's feelings.

FIGURE 14.1. Teacher interview for emotional development. Questions under "Emotional Regulation" are based in part on Denham and Burton (1996, pp. 22–24).

also very influenced by a child's age, gender, and developmental status or mental age. Cultural and subcultural influences can also play a very large role in influencing the social behaviors that are acceptable and valued; examiners therefore need to be familiar with the culture or subculture of the children whose play they are evaluating (Bierman & Welsh, 1997).

In this section, we review measures that can be used to examine a child's social competence and provide information for diagnosis and intervention planning. The list of measures is purposely limited to save space. Teacher or both teacher and parent rating scales are an efficient means of obtaining information. Observation of children in unstructured play with peers provides an independent source of information and one that is highly desirable for diagnosis. The SBO portion of the ESP, described earlier, contains normative information for both socially withdrawn and antisocial behavior. Additional play measures, such as the Penn Peer Play Scale, are presented in Chapter 4. If the referral issue is an attention problem, and thus a classroom observation in structured settings is important, the ASEBA Direct Observation Form (DOF; Achenbach & Rescorla, 2001) for ages 5 and up is useful.

Social Skills Rating System

The SSRS (Gresham & Elliott, 1990) is a teacher and parent rating scale designed to screen and classify children who are suspected of having social behavior problems and to assist in designing social skills interventions. It is normed for ages 3-0 through 4-11 years and for grades K–12. It takes 15–20 minutes for either a teacher or parent to complete. At the Preschool level, the Teacher form has domain scores for Cooperation (e.g., "waits turn when playing a game"), Assertion (e.g., "initiates conversations with peers"), and Self-Control (e.g., "controls temper in conflict situations with peers"), as well as ratings of academic performance. The Parent form has scores for the same domains plus Responsibility (e.g., "keeps room clean and neat without being reminded"). Teachers rate students' behaviors on frequency (0 = "never true" to 2 = "very often true") and importance (0 = "not important for success in my classroom" to 2 = "critical for success in my classroom"). Parents rate behaviors on frequency and importance for the child's development.

One of the strengths of the SSRS is the Assessment–Intervention Record, which (1) summarizes information from all sources; (2) structures an analysis of the referred child's strengths and weaknesses, such that social skills deficits are highlighted; and then (3) funnels this information into a model for developing an intervention to address either acquisition deficits (frequency = 0, importance = 1 or 2) or performance deficits (frequency = 1, importance = 2). The short Problem Behaviors scale, like the Academic Competence scale, is used to screen for behaviors that may require further assessment because they either overshadow competent social skills (Externalizing Problems, Hyperactivity) or pose a barrier to the development or performance of competent behavior (Internalizing Problems).

The SSRS has been praised for its multidomain assessment of social skills, use of multiple informants, and integrated approach to assessment and intervention (Kamphaus & Frick, 2002). It has good interrater reliability and is easy to use. It has been criticized for inadequately described normative samples that are not representative of the U.S. national population, drawing heavily from the South and North Central regions and underrepresenting Hispanics. There is poor criterion validity for the Internalizing Problems scale. Nevertheless, we think it is a useful tool for identifying and developing interventions to improve social competence.

Social Competence and Behavior Evaluation, Preschool Edition

The SCBE (LaFreniere & Dumas, 1995) is an 80-item teacher rating scale designed to "assess patterns of social competence, affective expression, and adjustment difficulties in children 30 months to 78 months" (p. 1). It is intended to produce information important for the socialization and education of children in classrooms by promoting strengths as well as addressing weaknesses, as opposed to measures that strictly provide diagnostic classifications. It was developed from an ethological and adaptationist theoretical perspective that emphasizes the role of affect exchange in social regulation. The authors chose items to assess emotional expression in social interactions with peers and adults, and characteristic emotions in nonsocial situations. It describes behavior in context (e.g., "is involved when other children are having fun") to facilitate understanding of child–context interaction and to identify points of intervention. It was formerly known as the Preschool Socio-Affective Profile.

The SCBE consists of eight subscales organized into three clusters: Emotional Adjustment (Depressive–Joyful, Anxious–Secure, Angry–Tolerant); Social Interaction with Peers (Isolated–Integrated, Aggressive–Calm, Egotistical–Prosocial); and Social Interactions with Adults (Oppositional–Cooperative, Dependent–Autonomous). The higher the score on these scales, the better the adjustment. There are three summary scales as well: Social Competence represents all of the eight positive poles (e.g., Joyful, Integrated); Internalizing four of the negative poles (Depressed, Anxious, Isolated, and Dependent); and Externalizing the other four negative poles (Oppositional, Aggressive, Angry, Egotistical).

In summary, the SCBE is a brief teacher rating scale that does a good job of capturing emotional adjustment and social relationship competencies that are of key developmental importance during the preschool years. Theoretically motivated, the measure has good psychometric characteristics (despite limited norms), and it provides practical information that can assist teachers and other school personnel in designing classroom-based interventions to support healthy development.

Devereux Early Childhood Assessment

The DECA (LeBuffe & Naglieri, 1999) is based on a review of literature on resiliency and child-protective factors and provides the first standardized norm-referenced behavior rating scale of within-child protective factors. A parent and teacher rating scale, it focuses on a child's strengths as well as weaknesses, and provides information on the areas of social and emotional functioning in which the child has difficulty as well as about attributes within the child that act as protective factors and can be used to bolster intervention strategies. The total protective factors score is comprised of three scales: Initiative, Self-Control, and Attachment. There is also a Behavioral Concerns Scale. The DECA is one part of a comprehensive model that focuses on prevention and intervention strategies through partnerships between families and preschool professionals. It can also be used to make comparisons within or among children over time, across environments, and after interventions. Items are clearly written at a sixth-grade reading level. Low interrater reliability for parent forms should be noted but other psychometric characteristics are adequate for a screening measure, including the representativeness of the normative samples. Exposure to the resiliency literature and knowledge of strength-based interventions is recommended prior to using the DECA so that users can adequately interpret/apply the information from a child's profile.

Social Behavior Observation of the Early Screening Project

The SBO (Walker et al., 1995) was described earlier. It is a simple-to-use duration measure that records the percentage of time (out of total time observed) that a child engages in socially isolated and/or antisocial behavior. Because of the simple recording procedure, an observer can easily take anecdotal notes of a child's behavior. Times are then compared with normative data. Because of the SBO's good psychometric characteristics, ease of use, and ability to gather information on the social behavior of both withdrawn and antisocial behavior, we recommend its use.

Direct Observation Form of the ASEBA

There are no easy-to-use, clinician-friendly observation measures of ADHD or other emotional or behavior problems with good normative data (Barkley, 1997b). Although it was not developed for preschool children, the DOF (Achenbach & Rescorla, 2001) represents a reasonable approach to gathering information on the behavior in structured situations of children age 5 and older suspected of having ADHD. An observer visits a child's classroom and observes for 10 minutes, scoring on-task behavior at 1-minute intervals and writing a narrative. After the observation, the problem behaviors (which are similar to those on the CBCL) are scored for frequency. Comparison observations of two control children in the target child's class are recommended. Limited norms exist for ages 5–14, based on 212 referred children and 287 nonreferred children selected as classroom controls for the referred children.

Step 5: Assessment of the Child

We think that it is very important for the examiner to assess a child's emotional development directly. If a child is at least 3 and is verbal, we recommend the MSSB. This measure provides a view of how the child conceives his or her social world and is able to cope constructively in an age-appropriate manner with various conflictual situations, as opposed to demonstrating impulsivity and aggression. If a child is too young or not verbal enough to take this measure, we recommend a play assessment of the child with one or more caregivers and with the examiner, using the FEAS or other play measures (see Chapter 4).

MacArthur Story Stem Battery

The MSSB (Bretherton et al., 1990; Emde et al., 2003) is a clinical tool developed by researchers to gain access to young children's "representational worlds, to what they understand, to their inner feelings" (Emde, 2003, p. 3). It uses a story stem technique along with human and animal figures, such as those by Duplo, to encourage a child to complete a story based on his or her personal experience and internal representation of the child's social world. Designed to be used with verbal children from ages 3–4 up to 7 (age 3 is the lower limit for most middle-class children, 4 for high-risk samples), the technique has been used to assess attachment, moral development, family relationship conflict, empathy, prosocial orientation, dissociation in maltreated children, and propensity for behavioral problems and emotional stress.

The MSSB can be administered in a child's home or in a clinic setting. The child's performance is videotaped with a camera that can produce an audible soundtrack. The examiner begins with the simple instructions, "Now we are going to tell stories together. I will begin each story; then you will finish it." The examiner introduces the doll family, consisting of a mother, father, and two siblings (same sex as the child being assessed), and models actions and emotional expression with the dolls to suggest that it is okay to express thoughts and feelings openly. A birthday story is used to provide a warm-up and to establish the limits of appropriate action and story length (Bretherton & Oppenheim, 2003).

The 14 story stems are deliberately designed to tap various themes (including attachment, response to authority, response to family conflict, response to getting caught during a transgression, and separation anxiety). For example, in the first story, entitled "Spill Juice," one of the children accidentally spills a pitcher of juice at the dinner table. The participants include two siblings, a mother, and a father, and the issues presented include the parents as attachment and/or authority figures and issues of repairing damage.

Several coding systems have been developed for use with the MSSB. The most widely used system (the MacArthur Narrative Coding System; Robinson, Mantz-Simmons, MacFie, & the MacArthur Narrative Working Group, 1992) assesses two broad domains: the content or themes of stories, and the performance features or manner in which the stories are communicated. The nine themes include interpersonal conflict, such as physical aggression, verbal aggression, and personal injury; response to moral dilemmas; and attachment issues. Performance codes include the intensity of specific emotions portrayed in the narratives, inclusion of parental characters, the child's response to the examiner, denial of the story conflict in the story response, and the child's attempts to control the story stem by requesting additional figures or interrupting the examiner.

Most of the validity data for the MSSB are derived from studies with risk and clinical populations (Emde et al., 2003). Table 14.7 presents a summary (based on the work of Warren, 2003) of the research findings on the stories of young children with internalizing disorders, externalizing disorders, or substantiated maltreatment. The MSSB has also been used to assess treatment outcomes in a nurse home visitor program over the first 2 years of children's lives. Mothers with low levels of psychological resources who used a nurse home visitor had children who had reduced themes of dysregulated aggression and reliance on adults for help in conflict resolution (Robinson, Holmberg, Corbitt-Price, & Wiener, 2002). These are just a few of the studies demonstrating the validity of a measure that is being used by researchers around the world.

The MSSB can provide rich information on how children conceptualize or represent important relationships in their life, their emotional understanding of these relationships, and their ability to regulate their emotions, as well as providing some idea of how they might actually behave in interactions with important others. It can identify significant clinical issues such as externalizing behavior, anxiety, and dissociation, and aspects of the child's social world that may be contributing to them (see Table 14.7). Interobserver reliabilities, internal consistency, and stability are good. The research data support construct, discriminant, predictive, and treatment validity. Major limitations are the lack of national norms (all research findings are based on research and clinical samples); the lack of a standardized training module to ensure consistency of administration and accuracy of scoring; and the limitation of the measure to children who are verbal.

Step 6: Case Formulation

After the scoring of protocols has been doublechecked for accuracy, the first step in case formulation is to identify clinically significant findings. Across measures, what scales fall in the borderline or clinical range? What behaviors occur at a sufficient level of intensity or frequency that diagnostic criteria might be met for a disorder? What evidence indicates that a child has a functional impairment as a result of the symptoms? The next task is to look for convergence across informants, settings, and measures. Do all raters and the examiner agree in their observations of a child as noncompliant, or does the child exhibit markedly different behavior across settings? Convergence of findings facilitates a coherent explanation of the problem, a diagnosis if warranted, and the beginning of a treatment plan. Discrepant findings suggest further investigation.

Why might a child be seen as having a problem in one setting but not another, or by one rater but not another? Sometimes there is intentional bias in reporting. Parents seeking a settlement for medical errors with a child may describe a child on the Vineland-II in

TABLE 14.7. MSSB Themes Identified by Researchers as More Characteristic of Children with Internalizing Disorders, Externalizing Disorders, or Substantiated Maltreatment

Internalizing disorders
- Portrayal of child doll as not competent.
- Not having the child doll go to the parent doll for help in stressful situations.
- Having the child doll assume the parental role or responsibilities.
- Troubles with separation, but denying associated negative feelings.
- Ending the stories negatively.
- Restricted or conflicted father–child relationship.

Externalizing disorders
- Less compliance, fewer verbal reparative responses, more anger.
- More aggressive themes.
- More distress, avoidance, and emotional dysregulation.
- More preoccupation with eating.
- Portrayal of the child doll as a superhero, yet unable to resolve problems competently.
- Negative representations of parent dolls.

Substantiated maltreatment
- Physical or sexual abuse or neglect as a story theme.
- Child doll not being helped by other dolls; fewer child doll and parent doll behaviors to relieve distress, but more participant child behaviors to relieve distress.
- Negative portrayal of child doll.
- Negative portrayals of parent dolls.
- Portrayal of child doll as acting like a parent in relations to parent dolls.
- Fewer moral-affiliative themes and prosocial doll behaviors.
- More conflictual, aggressive, disobedience themes.
- More sexual themes.
- Controlling and/or nonresponsive behavior by child to examiner.

Note. The table is based on material from Warren (2003).

a manner that reduces developmental ages by over a year, compared with specialist evaluations in the child's preschool file. A parent may rate a child as having few problems, while making enormous accommodations in his or her behavior in order to prop up the child's functioning. Preschool or daycare staff members may exaggerate a child's behavior problems when they want the child to leave the school or center. Sometimes situational variables make performances atypically poor as in the example below.

> Mrs. K. had spent her school years miserable in special education, graduating with a special education diploma. She did not bring her immature and impulsive daughter in for the child-finding screening, out of fear that her daughter would be sentenced to the same unfortunate experience. As Mrs. K. was registering her daughter for kindergarten in the late summer, the lack of screening was spotted, and an evaluation was mandated. When the mother and daughter appeared for the evaluation, both were in a highly anxious and defiant state. The girl presented to the screening team as having borderline cognitive ability at best and possibly in need of a full-time aide to manage her behavior. However, a trial in a regular kindergarten class pending a full evaluation revealed a sweet, somewhat impulsive little girl of low-average ability and few readiness skills. She blossomed in the regular classroom with 40 minutes a day of emergent literacy activities with an older peer tutor under the supervision of the reading teacher.

Most often, children's behavior is different in different situations. The reasons for these differences can be very helpful in identifying causes of a problem and potential solutions.

In an excellent chapter on interpreting and integrating assessment information, Kamphaus and Frick (2002) describe how complicated it can be to integrate information from a comprehensive assessment that involves many areas of functioning, multiple techniques, and multiple sources of information. There is a low rate of agreement on children's behavior across settings. A meta-analysis of 119 studies revealed mean correlations of .28 between parents and teachers, and .60 within pairs of parents or pairs of teachers (Achenbach, McConaughy, & Howell, 1987). This finding seems to reflect real differences in how children behave in each setting. They note that there tends to be greater agreement at an aggregate or diagnostic level, and less agreement on individual behaviors. Part of this is due to the use of different techniques to gather information from informants. Low correlations may occur by virtue of how information is being measured, such as when the parents are interviewed, the teacher completes a rating scale, and the individual child is given a story stem. Finally, situational demands in homes, classrooms, testing situations, and playgrounds do result in different behavior. Assessors should therefore try to examine the degree to which discrepant information can be attributed to varying situational demands, to the level of analysis, or to the assessment format.

Once information is collected, there is the issue of how to weigh sources of information. Should each source be weighed equally or differently? Kamphaus and Frick (2002), in reviewing the evidence, suggest that it may make sense to weigh information differently by the source, depending upon the type of the problem and the age of the child. Specifically, research shows that the common clinical practice of giving more weight to teachers' reports of inattentive/hyperactive behaviors than to parents' reports results in better prediction of impairment 1 year later, whereas giving preferential weighting to parents' reports of conduct problems is more predictive of later impairment than is teachers' (although teachers' and children's information is also useful).

The next step is to identify any missing information needed for case formulation or treatment planning, and then obtain it. We frequently find that we need more information before we can finalize a case formulation. This is because we try to work efficiently, tailoring our evaluation to the referral question while screening for other problems and alternative explanations for the behaviors of concern. An in-depth evaluation is not done in every area. We also find that parents are more forthcoming as they gain more trust in the examiner or assessment team over time. For example, a parent might mention late in the evaluation that a child has experienced a potentially traumatizing event such as sexual abuse or family violence, which might explain the behavior of concern. On intake, the parent might have denied that the child had these experiences. We also find that children referred for one reason, such as attentional and oppositional behaviors, may present with symptoms of an alternative or comorbid disorder, such as prepubertal mania or SAD (see Case 2 below), which must be considered after the test data is reviewed.

After all relevant information is collected, the assessor needs to create a framework for explaining the problem to the referral source. We do this by answering the referral question(s). Generally such questions are in the form of "Why does ___ behave the way he [or she] does? Should we be worried about it? What can be done about it?" To answer these questions, the findings have to be coherently organized. One method is to identify the primary problem or diagnosis based on the severity of symptoms, the degree to which the behavior is cross-situational, and the degree to which it interferes with functioning (Kamphaus & Frick, 2002). For example, the DC:0–3R and the RDC-PA argue that PTSD should always be given priority for treatment because of its known devastating effects on development in young children. Primacy of onset of symptoms might also play a role in deciding which problem (or disorder) is primary. The primary problem should receive most of the focus in the framework.

We remind the referral source of the question we were asked to address, describe what we have done to answer the question, and then present our findings organized around what we think is the best explanation of the behavior(s) of concern. We then check for understanding of our explanation, determine the degree to which parents believe the explanation fits, and respond to questions or concerns. Finally, we identify appropriate and accessible interventions to address the problem, and we ask parents what they think would work and what resources they would find helpful or worth trying; these are the first steps in working toward a collaborative treatment plan.

Step 7: Therapeutic Presentation of Findings and Recommendations

A tremendous amount of stigma is associated with emotional and behavior problems at any age. Professionals and families particularly recoil from early diagnosis of young children, often hoping or believing that problems will go away. Sometimes they do, as with less severe oppositional behavior problems at ages 2–3, and with sadness, worries, and fears that are transient during the preschool years. When problems are severe or are highly stable, they are unlikely to go away without treatment, especially if they co-occur with other family problems and/or environmental risk factors. The familial nature of emotional and behavior problems makes it much more likely that early child problems will co-occur with other family problems and risk factors. As aforementioned, children with anxiety problems are likely to have parents with anxiety problems, children with attention problems are likely to have parents with attention problems, and so on. Although the co-occurrence of a disorder in a parent and child often complicates treatment, because it can make it harder for the family to follow through and may increase the likelihood of marital/couple conflict or instability, it can give the affected parent empathy and insight into what may help the child.

Parents often bring a child with ODD and ADHD in for evaluation and treatment after a history of (1) confusing messages from professionals (e.g., "He'll grow out of it" vs. "You have to be the one in charge; you can't have a 2-year-old running the house"); (2) rejection of their child by church nurseries, daycare centers, peers, and neighbors' families; and (3) blaming of the parents by family members, other parents, and school personnel for the child's poor behavior. To add to the sense of failure, stigma, and isolation, assessors often assume that if parents could improve their parenting, the child's behavior would improve. Constitutional factors in the child (e.g., temperament, vulnerability to emotional or behavioral disorders), and the interaction between these factors and parenting behavior in making the child a challenge to rear, are often minimized. To make matters worse, professionals often convey this judgment in a manner that increases a sense of shame and failure, making it less likely that a family will follow through on treatment recommendations and referrals. What parents are looking for from professionals are (1) optimism based on expertise; and (2) a sincere, collegial effort to understand the family's straits and offer practical, effective help that is uniquely tailored to the family's situation.

Webster-Stratton and Herbert's (1994) book, *Troubled Families—Problem Children*, is one of the few writings we have seen on the perspectives of parents seeking treatment for their young children with conduct problems. They conduct qualitative interviews with parents and use session-by-session videotaping during the course of treatment. The parental quotes they provide vividly illustrate where parents are coming from, and they describe therapist interventions that help parents overcome resistance to change and to the hard work that brings change about. We highly recommend this book to assessors and clinicians who work with such families.

Families with a history of anxiety and/or depression may also suffer from stigma or shame. Agoraphobia, panic disorder, or social phobia may have severely restricted the family's activities and one parent's ability to work or function in the outside world. Families with a history of mood disorders may feel tremendous shame because of a family suicide or the bizarre public behaviors of family members prior to hospitalizations. Seeing similar symptoms in a young child may increase the sense of helplessness and collective shame. On the other hand, if family members are given effective treatment, they may be in a good position to support a child in facing and coping with worries and sadness.

To work effectively with families of young children with emotional and behavior problems, clinicians need to be knowledgeable and comfortable in dealing with these problems. They need to respect the challenges faced by families with mental health and behavioral/criminal problems, and to acknowledge the courage and discipline it can take to keep trying to make things work on a daily basis, without resorting to pity or patronization of their clients. If assessors lack personal experience with these types of problems they may want to attend meetings of groups such as the National Alliance on Mental Illness (NAMI), Al-Anon (an anonymous group for family and friends of individuals with alcoholism), or Children and Adults with Attention-Deficit/Hyperactivity Disorder (CHADD). These organizations provide support for individuals with a disorder, for their relatives and friends, or for both.

CASE STUDIES

The two case studies that follow describe a multidisciplinary assessment of two preschool children with emotional and/or behavioral problems; one has relatively mild difficulties and a good prognosis and the other very severe difficulties and a guarded prognosis. Both cases illustrate the integration of multiple sources of information—history, observation, behavior ratings, family and child assessment—into a case formulation and treatment plan.

Case Study I

Olivia, age 5-2 years, was seen for a reevaluation when she was enrolled full-time in a public preschool program for children with disabilities. A year before, she had been diagnosed as having ADHD and developmental language disorder in another preschool center. At that time her Full Scale IQ was average (100), and both her gross and fine motor development were age-appropriate. The school district's committee for students with disabilities had recommended speech and language therapy twice a week, referred her to a physician for medication, and recommended therapeutic preschool and parental counseling. She was placed on Ritalin. Over the summer, her parents had separated, and her mother moved to the catchment area of the preschool in which she was seen. Because of her diagnoses, she was provided with a full-day therapeutic preschool program, including push-in speech and language services. She was reevaluated in the late spring as she was preparing to enter kindergarten in the fall, and the receiving district wanted to know what her classification (if any) should be and what program would be most appropriate for her.

Olivia's mother completed the CBCL/1½–5, the Conners' Parent Rating Scale—Revised, and the Barkley History Forms, and was interviewed with Barkley's Clinical Interview—Parent Report Form. Then Olivia was observed in her classroom with the DOF on two occasions for 20 minutes each. She was also observed once during playtime with the SBO portion of the ESF. Her teacher completed the C-TRF, the Conners' Teacher Rating Scale—Revised, and the SCBE. The speech pathologist who had been treating her summarized her session notes over the year and administered some formal measures.

Olivia's mother reported that she was a strong-willed child who did not respond to the word "No." She had a tendency to keep pushing against her mother's restrictions until she got spanked, but then she would quickly forget the punishment. For example, she wandered off in the mall and was punished as a result, but this punishment did not result in her transferring her experience there to other situations, and she continued to wander off.

Until Olivia was 2, her mother didn't feel that she could take her to anyone else's house because of her hyperactivity and impulsiveness. She now took her to the homes of Olivia's maternal grandmother and aunt, but had to monitor her behavior closely and contend with her relatives' critical remarks about Olivia's behavior and her mothering. On the positive side, Olivia's mother reported that she was very loving to her younger sister and the family's pets, and that she liked to have fun. She shared with friends and had a good sense of humor.

In describing the family background, Olivia's mother reported that she herself had also had attentional problems and had been diagnosed with learning disabilities in school. She had dropped out of high school at the end of 10th grade and now made her living cleaning houses. She reported that Olivia's father had a problem with a high activity level. She noticed that Olivia's behavior had gotten worse during the initial separation from her husband, but that it improved as they settled into a new home and school, near Olivia's mother's family. Olivia had regular visits with her father. Olivia's mother denied any problems with depression, anxiety, antisocial behavior, family violence, or substance abuse in the family. She reported that her husband had been paying child support, and that the presence of her sister in the area had provided emotional and practical support, as well as helping her in finding work and meeting new friends through the church.

On the CBCL/1½–5, Olivia's mother's ratings placed her in the average range on the Total Behavior Problems and Internalizing scales, and the borderline range on the Externalizing scale. She was in the borderline range on the Withdrawn subscale, and the clinical range on Attention Problems and the DSM-IV Attention-Deficit/Hyperactivity Problems subscales. On the CPRS-R, Olivia fell in the moderately atypical range on the ADHD Index and the DSM-IV scales.

Olivia was an attractive girl with shoulder-length dark hair, creamy skin, and pierced ears. She was tall for her age and did not wear glasses. On both occasions when an assessor used the DOF to observe her in the classroom, she was on task only about half of the time—first during the group work in a circle, and then during seatwork. She did not seem significantly less attentive than other children in the special class, but would have been quite inattentive relative to children in a regular class. The observation confirmed her mother's and teacher's descriptions of her as being of average ability, but prone to a high level of impulsive activity and self-absorption, which kept her from responding quickly and appropriately to adult requests. For example, during the first observation period, she was able to answer all the questions the teacher put to her during the group session, which included naming shapes, numbers, and colors. She was the first child to leave the group to do the seatwork art project, wherein children were to assemble leaves on a construction paper tree. She performed this task immediately and then proceeded to disassemble and reassemble the tree while waiting for the other children to come over to the table one by one. During this time, she restlessly made humming noises, put her head on the table, made sounds such as "pick pick pick pick pick," whipped the tree around in the air, and lolled about in her chair. These behaviors fit with the DSM-IV-TR criterion of "often fidgets with hands or feet or squirms in seat." Her tendency to leave her seat in the classroom in other situations where remaining seated was expected (behavior that was reported at significant levels by both mother and teacher), was seen during circle time: In the middle of a calendar activity, she announced that she had to go to the potty, and immediately leaped to her feet and ran at full speed to the bathroom in the back of the class. She came back with her pants unzipped and her hand on the zipper. Her teacher said to her, "Remember to flush and wash your hands." She twirled about to do this and, again, running, returned to her place.

Olivia's tendency not to listen when spoken to directly (one of the DSM-IV-TR criteria for inattentive behavior) was seen in an exchange with her teacher during circle time. She was called upon by her teacher to identify the number 3 and place it up on the board underneath her name. She placed it up in reverse order so that it looked like an "E." She named the number correctly and then announced, "I am making it smooth," and proceeded to pat it down on the flannel board. The teacher stated, "It is fine," but Olivia continued to pat the number. The teacher touched her and gestured her back to her place. She did not move, but continued smoothing the letter. Finally the teacher said, "Goodbye, Olivia," and in one move Olivia returned to her spot, where she began rocking back and forth and rolled herself into a turtle ball.

The same self-absorption that contributed to Olivia's difficulty with following through on instructions and failing to finish assignments, as well as seeming not to listen when directly spoken to, was seen in the project that involved gluing leaves onto the tree. When the teacher came over to her with the glue and sat next to her, Olivia immediately became focused and calm. She quickly reassembled her tree and answered, "I am," when the teacher asked, "Whose turn is it next?" She put glue on one of her leaves and then sat there with the glue drying while she proceeded to pick glue off her fingers. At a prompt from the teacher, she then glued her leaf on. The teacher said, "I have one left," and looked at Olivia; Olivia said, "I want it." The teacher then gave her the additional leaf, and she then sat and picked glue off her fingers while waiting for the glue. When the teacher brought her the glue, she put the glue onto the shape, and again left it to dry while she started to pick off the glue. The teacher said to her, "You can start spreading this around." Olivia kept picking the glue off her fingers. The teacher then said, "What are you supposed to be doing?" Olivia answered, "Spreading," and kept picking at the glue on her fingers. After another prompt, she spread the glue around on her leaf, but did not glue it on. She clapped her hands quietly and then resumed picking at the glue. The teacher then said to her, "You need . . ., " stopped, and then said, "Look at me." Olivia looked at her and resumed picking at the glue. The teacher then took each of Olivia's hands and placed them on the table under her hands and said to Olivia, "You need to glue." Olivia looked at her teacher and then started gluing. She did a good job, successfully glued the leaf on, and then returned to picking the glue off her hands, totally absorbed.

Olivia's teacher reported that she motivated the child by having her work for playtime and getting her to say what she should be doing. She found that clear reinforcers and prompts to help Olivia orient to the task at hand were effective at keeping her on task. The teacher reported that when Olivia came into the program, she was on Ritalin and then went off it for a while. As no difference was noted in her behavior on or off the medicine, the mother, in consultation with the school nurse and the teacher, stopped the medication.

On the C-TRF, Olivia obtained a clinically significant score only on the Attention Problems scale, but borderline scores on the Attention Deficit/Hyperactivity Problems and Withdrawn subscales. On the Conners' Teacher Rating Scale—Revised, she obtained clinical range scores on Cognitive Problems/Inattention, Hyperactivity, Social Problems, the ADHD Index, the Global Index for Restless–Impulsive, the Conners' Global Index Total, the DSM-IV Inattentive, the DSM-IV Hyperactive–Impulsive, and the DSM-IV total scales. She was in the borderline range on the Oppositional scale. On the SCBE, all of her scores fell in the average range—further confirming that except for her attentional problems, her emotional adjustment and social interactions with peers and her teacher were within the normal range. She fell at the lower end of the average range only on the Oppositional–Cooperative scale, reflecting her slow response to teacher directions and her tendency to do what she wanted to do regardless of what was being asked of her.

Olivia was given the diagnosis of ADHD, predominantly hyperactive—impulsive type; she met the criteria for six of the items, according to at least two out of three observers/raters (i.e., the mother, the teacher, and the observing clinician). She also met the criteria for two inattentive symptoms—"often does not seem to listen when spoken to directly" and "often does not follow through on instruction and fails to finish schoolwork, chores, or duties in the workplace." Her difficulty with following through on instructions or tasks did not seem to be due to oppositional behavior or failure to understand instructions. She met the impairment criterion because of her special class placement, her probable need for significant supports when mainstreamed in a regular kindergarten class, and her need for significant supervision by her mother at home and in the community. She scored in the at-risk range on the SBO because of somewhat socially isolated behavior, and was in the borderline range on the Withdrawn subscale of the CBCL/1½–5 and the C-TRF. However, the social isolation problem seemed as if it might be due to her school placement and to her recent move. First, she was the least impaired student in a class of 12 children with mild disabilities, which might have limited her desire to interact socially with her classmates. Second, in moving from her father's home, she had left behind some friends that she played with well and regularly. The recent move had left her mostly with her younger sister and an older cousin as playmates. On the other hand, Olivia seemed to be underreactive to auditory input from adults and peers and very reactive to tactile stimuli (e.g., glue, felt). These observations suggested some sensory differences that might affect her social relationships by giving her an air of being in her own world, and thus withdrawn, even though she was not socially anxious or avoidant.

Because of the good progress Olivia had made in the area of language, the developmental language disorder classification was dropped. However, because of the agreement among her mother, her teacher, and the observer that she had significant hyperactive and impulsive symptoms, the ADHD classification was retained. It was recommended that she be placed in a regular kindergarten classroom, although great care should be taken to match her with a warm but firm teacher who had both the time and interest in working with her to help her modify her impulsive behavior and increase her attentiveness in the classroom, so that she could take advantage of her average intellectual abilities and do well in school. Finally, recommendations were made to her mother and receiving teacher to support her social development with peers.

Case Study 2

Sally, age 2-7 years, was seen for a developmental screening assessment at a diagnostic preschool after being referred by her physician. Sally had been diagnosed 6 months previously as having ADHD by a psychiatrist who specialized in that diagnosis. He had prescribed her stimulant medication. However, when Sally's mother went to pick up the prescription from the pharmacist, he refused to give it to her, saying that there had been no research done on the effects of the drug on children as young as Sally; he asked her to read the insert that came with the drug. After reading about the possible side effects, the mother called the psychiatrist, who said he still felt confident of his diagnosis, but suggested that she seek a second opinion and referred her to a pediatric neurologist. He also suggested that Sally be seen at the diagnostic preschool for an evaluation.

Sally was her parents' second child; her elementary-school-age brother had been diagnosed with a reading disability. He was described as a well-behaved, quiet child who presented no behavior problems, but wore large, thick glasses and had minimal reading ability. An interview with Sally's mother, and later with her father by telephone, indicated that Sally's father also had reading difficulties; he was employed as a truck driver, a position that did not require a high level of reading. His wife described him as "hyper." Sally's mother, a secretary, had no academic difficulties, but did have a family history of mood disorders. She had a sister with a bipolar disorder, a mother with mood swings, a maternal grandmother who was highly anxious, and a maternal grandfather with a history of depression. On Sally's father's side, there was a history of substance abuse and possible depression and ADHD.

The parents' marriage seemed to be under some strain. The father's occupation kept him away from home for up to 10 days at a time, and he often drank excessively when he was home. Raising Sally also posed a challenge to the couple. Not only would neither side of the extended family take care of Sally, but Sally's father did not like being left alone with her. Sally's mother said that she loved her daughter very much, but when she came from work, walked up the steps at daycare, and heard Sally whining or screaming, she wished she did not have to go in. Sally's mother reported feeling very discouraged, stressed out, isolated, and socially stigmatized by the difficulties she was having with Sally. Her husband's family was very critical of how she managed her daughter; her own family was more empathetic, but would not babysit; and no children wanted to play with Sally.

The mother reported that Sally had been a difficult child since birth and had never in her life slept through the night. She reported that Sally spent much of her infancy crying and fussing continually, despite excellent health. Sally's mother's complaints were that her daughter was extremely clingy; was almost always in a bad mood; had frequent tantrums; was unable to get along with other children or adults, including babysitters; and, in particular, needed to be watched continually so that she wouldn't hurt herself.

Sally was an attractive girl with blue eyes and light blond hair, which was pulled back in a ponytail that revealed dark circles under her eyes. She was of appropriate height and weight for a child almost 3 years old, and was dressed attractively. She was very slow to warm up to the professionals who were trying to draw her into testing activities; instead, she sat in her mother's lap, continually interrupting her mother in her attempts to talk with the speech pathologist and school psychologist about Sally. Her mother would say a few sentences, and then Sally would interrupt with "Mommy, Mommy," tugging at her mother and calling to her in an increasingly loud voice until her mother finally attended to her and answered her question. She would be quiet again for a moment and then began demanding that her mother take her outside to play on the swings. She indicated her desire to go out by saying "Swing" unintelligibly and pointing toward the swing set out in the yard. Her mother would pause periodically to try to distract her and tell her that she could not go outside until she was done, but this calmed Sally only for a minute. She would then start fussing, in a whiny tone that rapidly escalated to screaming. This pattern repeated itself throughout the interview.

After about 5 minutes, the special education teacher was able to lure Sally to a nearby table about 2 feet from her mother by shaking a plastic see-through bowl with colored cereal in it. Sally went over to the table and tried to open the lid of the plastic bowl, but was unable to. The special educator was then able to get her to take a piece of cereal out and feed it to the baby doll—a process that she cooperated in. However, after a few minutes she started fussing again, went back to her mother's lap, and resumed her demands that her mother take her outside. The speech pathologist was able to distract her before she went into a tantrum and got her looking at pictures on the Preschool Language Scale—Fourth Edition. Sally answered most of the receptive items for her age accurately by pointing, but before her expressive language could be assessed, she began fussing and pulling at her mother again. The speech pathologist offered her a lollipop if she kept working; she said "Lollipop," reached for it, and worked for a while longer before she once again began fussing and getting upset. Her mother told her to sit still and not to interrupt, at which point Sally began screaming, hitting her mother, hitting the book that the speech pathologist was holding, and finally yelling loudly "No!" She started to shake her head furiously back and forth, and then bit her mother. Her mother, with great patience, tried to calm her down without giving in to her demands. Finally, when her mother ignored her and went back to speaking to the speech pathologist, the occupational therapist was able to get Sally involved in some motor tasks, which she seemed to succeed at and enjoy.

After her mother again refused to take her out to the playground, Sally went into another screaming tantrum. She was finally reengaged by the occupational therapist and the speech educator, who took her to the playground. When she entered the playground, she looked frantically around, seemingly overwhelmed by the number of options that she had. She then began to run from one thing to another and was unable to focus on a particular piece of playground equipment.

The parent interview indicated that Sally had always been a very difficult child to manage. Her behavior had dramatically constrained the family's social life. Her mother reported that except for going to work during the day, she never went out at night and rarely went anywhere on the weekend except to visit family members. The mother avoided taking Sally to public places because she would run out of control (a behavior observed by the occupational therapist when Sally bolted into the parking lot and ran loose at a very fast pace); she showed a complete lack of judgment about what was dangerous to do; and she had tantrums when she was not attended to or given what she asked for. These tantrums ranged from fussing to dropping to the floor and banging her head against the concrete in the grocery store. The family activities consisted of everyone going to work or school and Sally to daycare during the day (she had been removed from two daycares before the current one was identified), and everyone staying at home at night.

Because of the child's dangerous behavior, Sally's mother reported that she had to watch her all the time. She gave the example of the night before, when the family had been at her brother's house, enjoying his swimming pool. Sally was sitting quietly next to her mother on the steps leading down to the pool, where they were watching her cousins swimming. Her mother stood up and turned around to answer a question, at which point Sally dashed to the other end of the pool, got onto the diving board, and jumped off into the deep end. Sally's mother said that this was typical behavior for her; if she was not watched continually, she would dash in front of oncoming traffic, jump off high places, climb up to the top of monkey bars, and engage in other dangerous activities. Babysitters had also reported that she successfully opened car doors and tried to leap out of the car while the car was moving. Sleeping was another area of difficulty: Sally had never slept through the night and would not go to sleep unless her mother lay down next to her for 10–15 minutes before she dropped off to sleep. She rarely took a nap and was on the go constantly from the time she got up until she went to bed.

Sally's relationships with others were a further cause for concern. Not only was Sally in a chronically bad mood, which made her unpleasant to be around, but she was not liked by other children or adults. She rejected children loudly on the few occasions when they asked her to go out and play, but they resisted playing with her because she would bite and hit without provocation. The mother reported that thus far Sally had been dropped by six babysitters, as well as her first two daycare centers. At 10 months she had been kicked out of an infant program because of aggressive and mean behavior toward other children. Other problematic behaviors noted were Sally's spitting or hitting if someone told her "No"—behavior we observed as well.

Yet another area of concern was Sally's extreme clinginess. Sally's mother reported that from the time she got up, she wanted to be with her mother. She found Sally in her bed every morning. If the mother was showering, she would bring in a pillow and lie on the floor. On quiet days she would watch her mother apply her makeup, and on other days she would hold onto her mother's leg and demand, "Mommy, get me this, get me that." She followed her mother around when she did housework, including into the basement laundry area, where she insisted on sitting on the dryer and helping her mother fold clothes. This activity would end when she wanted to get down and run at high speed around the basement or up and down the steep stairs, where she might fall.

The assessment battery began with the Vineland-II, where Sally earned the following domain standard scores and age equivalents: Communication, 96, age 2-5; Daily Living Skills, 83, age 2-0; Motor Skills, 94, age 2-5; and Socialization, 80, age 1-8. On the CBCL/1½–5, Sally obtained clinically significant scores on the following scales: the Total Behavior Problems, Internalizing and Externalizing scales; the subscales Emotionally Reactive, Anxious/Depressed, Withdrawn, Attention Problems, and Aggressive Behavior; and the DSM-oriented scales of Affective Problems, Anxiety Problems, Attention-Deficit/Hyperactivity Problems, and Oppositional Defiant Problems. She was in the borderline range on Sleep Problems. Both of her parents endorsed more than the required number of symptoms for ADHD, ODD, and SAD. Because of her uncooperative behavior, she was not administered an intelligence test. She was too young to be given the MSSB.

Sally was observed at her daycare for 30 minutes with the SBO during unstructured time on the playground. She fell in the extreme range for oppositional defiant behavior and social withdrawal, as her only interactions with others seemed to be antisocial. The other children went out of their way to avoid her. On the C-TRF, completed by the director of Sally's daycare center, Sally fell in the clinical range for Total Behavior Problems, Externalizing, Attention Problems, Aggressive Behavior, Affective Problems, Anxious/Depressed, Attention-Deficit/Hyperactivity Problems, and Oppositional Defiant Problems. She was in the borderline range on Internalizing, Anxiety Problems, Emotionally Reactive, and Withdrawn. The head of the daycare center, with a background in early childhood special education, reported that she and her staff worked hard to manage

Sally's difficult and aggressive behavior. So far they had been able to manage Sally and keep her from hurting herself and other children by using applied behavior analysis techniques and very close supervision.

Observation of the mother and child in the Parent–Child Game suggested that Sally's mother was tentative in giving commands and that Sally was highly noncompliant. In the Child's Game, her mother was very good at following Sally's lead and did not ask questions or try to exert control over the play. Sally seemed very fond of her mother, suggesting that they had a close and affectionate bond despite the tremendous challenges that Sally posed.

Sally's case was very interesting diagnostically. She clearly met criteria for ODD, as in the past 6 months she had often lost her temper, often argued with adults, often actively defied or refused to comply with adult requests or rules, was easily touchy or annoyed by others, and was often angry or resentful. It was likely that she was also spiteful or vindictive, but it is difficult to assess this in a child only 2-7 years old. Sally's mother claimed that these behaviors had been going on even prior to 10 months of age, when she was evicted from the infant program. These behaviors clearly created problems for her in her social relationships with others and in her achievement of developmental competence in the areas of expressive language and daily living skills. For a child to meet criteria for the ODD diagnosis, however, an examiner has to rule out the possibility that the behavior might be better explained by a mood disorder. Sally's family had a history of mood disorders, including both depression and bipolar disorder. Although a bipolar disorder is rarely identified before puberty, the research literature suggests that very high levels of irritable mood, along with severely hostile and defiant behavior that includes episodes of physical aggression and destructive behavior, may be early markers for bipolar disorders in children. Oppositional behavior is seen in almost every case of juvenile-onset bipolar disorder (Wozniak & Biederman, 1995). Age 2-0 is the earliest age such a diagnosis has ever been made, but it might explain the very extreme behavior seen in Sally.

Sally also met many criteria for ADHD. She evidenced the inattentive symptoms of often having difficulties sustaining attention in task or play activities, and of being easily distracted by extraneous stimuli (e.g., on the playground). Under the hyperactive–impulsive criteria (see Table 14.3), Sally often left her seat in situations in which seating was expected; she often ran about or climbed excessively in situations that were inappropriate; she was often "on the go" and acted as if "driven by a motor"; she often interrupted or intruded upon others; and she had difficulty in playing or engaging in leisure activities quietly. Again, these behaviors had been occurring for most of her life, and they clearly caused problems for her at home, in daycare, and with babysitters. They had impaired her social relationships with others and her learning. Under exclusion criteria, the question must be raised as to whether such symptoms are better accounted for by another mental disorder, such as a mood disorder. Again, it was possible that Sally had prepubertal mania, but it was early to make that diagnosis. She did clearly meet criteria for ADHD, predominantly hyperactive–impulsive type. Even if she was later diagnosed with a bipolar disorder, it might be comorbid with her ADHD because as both disorders seem to run in her family and Wilens et al. (2002) found high comorbidity in clinic-referred 4- to 6-year-old children.

To meet criteria for a manic episode, a child has to have a distinct period of at least 1 week of abnormally and persistently, elevated, expansive, or irritable mood, or any period of such a mood that results in hospitalization. Weckerly (2002) has a useful list of how manic and depressive symptoms present developmentally. Sally almost always had an abnormally and persistently irritable mood (also a symptom of ODD). In addition to this first criterion, she needed to demonstrate three or more behaviors co-occurring with the abnormal or persistent mood. She was clearly distractible (also a symptom of ADHD); she seemed agitated, overly active, and abnormally restless (also seen in ADHD); she was excessively involved in reckless activities, a number of which were life-threatening. She also had a decreased need for sleep for a child her age, but she dropped off to sleep after 15 minutes and woke only to move to her parents' bed, not to roam around the house at night. Sally thus met only three criteria. The overlap of symptoms with ODD and ADHD would also call into question the specificity of the diagnosis.

Sally's dangerous, life-threatening behavior could be seen as suicidal, suggesting a review of criteria for depression. Although many professionals believe preschool children can't and don't attempt or commit suicide, the fact is that they can and do (Rosenthal & Rosenthal, 1984). If we review the criteria for a major depressive episode (five symptoms are needed during a minimum of a 2-week period, and these have to represent a change in functioning), Sally seemed to meet four or possibly five of the nine criteria: irritable mood most of the day, nearly every day; taking markedly little pleasure in any of her activities; psychomotor agitation; and dangerous behavior that could be seen as suicide attempts. Her needing very little sleep for her age might be seen as insomnia, but this was questionable. However, there had been no change in her functioning; she had been on a chronic course for some time. Her behavior did cause severe impairment in social relationships and in academic activities, and was not due to the effects of other substances.

Sally came close to meeting criteria for both a major depressive episode and a mania episode, which, if she did, would qualify her for a mixed episode. She clearly met criteria for ADHD and ODD. The co-occurrence of these syndromes and symptoms is common in young children who later develop bipolar disorder (Biederman et al., 1996; Carlson, 1984; Carlson et al., 2000; Geller et al., 2000; Wilens et al., 2002; Wozniak et al., 1995). Sally had a strong family history of mood disorders, further suggesting that she was at high risk for one in the future.

Finally, Sally also met criteria for SAD, demonstrating four of the nine criteria (three are required for a diagnosis; see Table 14.4). She showed recurrent excessive distress when separated from her mother, both in and out of the home; she refused to go to sleep without her mother's presence and always ended up in her mother's bed by morning; and she was persistently reluctant to be left at daycare, with babysitters, or with anyone other than her mother.

Despite her young age, the assessment team believed Sally's problems to be so severe and such a threat to her development that they gave her the educational diagnosis of emotional disturbance and, in consultation with the referring physician, the DSM-IV-TR diagnoses of ADHD, ODD, SAD, and bipolar disorder not otherwise specified. Sally was given the diagnoses of ODD and ADHD *and* a mood disorder diagnosis because (1) research shows that these disorders may be especially comorbid in early onset cases; (2) the characteristics of all these disorders seemed to develop together without one predating and thus accounting for the symptoms of the other; and (3) she had a family history for bipolar disorder and likely ADHD. Sally was offered a placement in the special education preschool, which used a developmental intervention model that included applied behavior analysis. Her mother was invited to join a parent support/training group (her father's work schedule prohibited his attendance). Sally was also referred to a regional university child psychiatry clinic, to further clarify the diagnosis and to help her parents make the very difficult decisions regarding medication in a child so young and yet so disturbed.

CONCLUSION

As can be seen from the review of the literature in this chapter, emotional development leads to social competence. The promotion of emotional skills in preschoolers merits equal emphasis with emerging literacy activities, as they are both necessary for later school success. When emotional and behavioral problems occur in young children, they should not be ignored. The severity of impairment in developmentally appropriate functioning is the best predictor that the problem is likely to continue. Assessors should be conservative in giving preschoolers a diagnosis, but very proactive in providing or referring for treatment.

APPENDIX 14.1. Review of Measures

Measure	**ADHD Symptom Checklist–4 (ADHD-SC4). Gadow and Sprafkin (1997).**
Purpose	Screening for behavioral symptoms of ADHD and ODD.
Areas	Peer Conflict, Stimulant Side Effects, ADHD (Inattentive Type, Hyperactive–Impulsive Type, and Combined Type), ODD.
Format	50-item norm-referenced measure, using a 4-point Likert-type scale for each of the four domains (ADHD, ODD, Peer Conflict, and Stimulant Side Effects). Score Summary Record has two parts: Symptom Count and Symptom Criteria Score. Symptom Severity Profiles also available.
Scores	*T*-scores, percentiles, screening cutoff, symptom count, symptom severity.
Age group	3–18 years.
Time	5 minutes.
Users	Parents and/or teachers.
Norms	Data collected on a sample of preschool children (ages 3–5), located through pediatricians' offices, preschools, and daycares. Consistent with 1990 U.S. census data for race/ethnicity, but not nationally representative. Norms from preschools solely from Long Island, NY. A total of 929 preschoolers sampled (531 parents, 398 teachers). (*Note*: Norms were revised in 1999; revision is included as a handout.)
Reliability	Internal consistency, .92–.95 in parent- and teacher-completed disruptive behavior categories. Test–retest (6 weeks), ADHD and ODD above .60 and .70; Peer Conflict, .35. Interrater, .23–.51.
Validity	Content, good (ADHD and ODD subscales akin to DSM-IV classifications). Discriminant, evident for parent checklist Peer Conflict scale between preschoolers receiving special education services and regular preschoolers.
Comments	Reviewers comment on potential strength of test as screening/monitoring agent. Peer Conflict and Stimulant Side Effects scales need more support for validity. More extensive testing is needed to make test representative of national sample.
References consulted	Rohrbeck (2001); Volpe (2001); DiPerna (2001). See book's References list.

Measure	**Ages and Stages Questionnaires: Social–Emotional (ASQ:SE). Squires, Bricker, and Twombly (2002).**
Purpose	Identifying infants and young children with potential development delays as a result of mental or environmental factors.
Areas	Self-Regulation, Compliance, Communication, Adaptive Functioning, Autonomy, Affect, and Interaction with People.
Format	Eight questionnaires (at 6, 12, 18, 24, 30, 36, 48, and 60 months), containing from 19 to 33 questions with three response choices each. Answers are given point values.
Scores	Cutoff scores for level of risk.
Age group	6–60 months.
Time	10–15 minutes.
Users	Parents.
Norms	Data collected on 3,014 preschool-age children and families.

Reliability	Internal consistency, .67–.91; test–retest (1 and 3 weeks), .94.
Validity	Concurrent, .93; sensitivity, .78; specificity, .95.
Comments	Available in Spanish, and male–female pronouns are alternated. The questionnaires are readable, age-appropriate, nonpathologizing for parents, and easy to score and use. Highly recommended as a frontline measure to monitor the achievement of socioemotional milestones and to identify children who may be in need of further evaluation. Authors note that according to parents in the normative sample, the measure took little time to complete and helped them think about social and emotional development in their children.
References consulted	Brassard review.

Measure	**Attention Deficit Disorders Evaluation Scale, Third Edition (ADDES-3). McCarney and Bauer (2004).**
Purpose	Providing a measure of inattention and of hyperactivity–impulsivity.
Areas	ADHD Inattentive Type, ADHD Hyperactive–Impulsive Type, and ADHD Combined Type.
Format	Home version: 46-item frequency-referenced rating scale, using a 5-point Likert-type scale ranging from "absence of activity" to "hourly occurrences." School version: 60-item frequency-referenced rating scale, otherwise similar to Home version.
Scores	Standard; Percentile; Quick-score computer program available.
Age group	Home version, 3–19 years; School version, 4–19 years.
Time	Home version, 12–15 minutes; School version, 15–20 minutes.
Users	Parents and/or teachers.
Norms	Data collected on two normative samples, males and females (ages 4-0–18-0). Samples were reflective of national population demographics in regard to race, sex, residence, geographic area, father's occupation, and mother's occupation. Home version preschool sample (ages 3–5), 189 children and 312 parents. School version preschool sample (ages 4-6 to 5), 610 students and 205 teachers.
Reliability	Internal consistency for ADHD Inattentive Type and ADHD Hyperactive–Impulsive Type (in both Home and School versions), above .90. Test–retest (30 days), Home version, .88–.93; School version, .88–.97. Interrater, Home version (172 pairs of parents), .80–.84; School version (237 teachers rating 1 or more of 462 students), .81–.90.
Validity	Construct, good; face, present when compared against 18 DSM-IV criteria for ADHD (both home and school versions).
Comments	Reviewers comment on ease of use and strong psychometric properties. With minor changes, useful as a screening measure. Users cautioned that diagnosis requires history of 6 months of meeting criteria. Caution should be taken in using the *SEM* procedures provided. Intervention supplements are not age-specific. Scale items do not always come across clearly, or they refer to behaviors common in normal children. Both versions are available in Spanish.
References consulted	Glenn (2001); Klecker (2001). See book's References list.

Measure	**Behavior Assessment Scale for Children, Second Edition (BASC-2). Reynolds and Kamphaus (2004).**
Purpose	Facilitating the differential diagnosis and educational classification of various emotional and behavioral disorders of children, and aiding in the design of treatment plans.
Areas	Externalizing Problems (Aggression, Hyperactivity), Internalizing Problems (Anxiety, Depression, Somatization), Adaptive Skills (Adaptability, Social Skills), School Problems (Attitudes to School and Teachers).
Format	At the preschool level, Teacher Rating Scale (TRS-P), Parent Rating Scale (PRS-P), Structured Developmental History (SDH), and Student Observation System (SOS).
Scores	*T*-scores, percentile ranks, 4 composite scores, and 18 scale scores, and a Behavior Symptoms Index (overall level of problem behaviors).
Age group	2–5 years (preschool level).
Time	TRS-P, 10–20 minutes; PRS-P, 10–20 minutes.
Users	Trained professionals.
Norms	A total of 2,250 children ages 2–5 made up the standardization sample for the TRS-P and PRS-P norms. The sample reflected the 2001 U.S. population closely in terms of parental education, race/ethnicity, geographic region, and special education classification. The general normative sample consisted of an equivalent number of males and females for ages 2–3 and 4–5 on both the TRS-P (400 children ages 2–3 and 650 children ages 4–5) and the PRS-P (500 children ages 2–3 and 700 children ages 4–5). Clinical norms were only provided for individuals ages 4 and above, with roughly 300 children ages 4–5 in both the TRS and PRS samples. The samples consisted of more males than females and were representative of children with a variety of diagnoses (speech/language impairment, mental retardation or developmental delay, ADHD, emotional disturbance/behavior disorder, PDD, specific learning disability, hearing impairment, and a range of physical disabilities). No norms were provided for the SOS.
Reliability	Internal consistency and test–retest, high (above .80) for preschool TRS and PRS norms; interrater both preschool forms, .65–.74 (still higher than that of older samples).
Validity	Construct and content, both supported.
Comments	A Spanish version of the BASC-2 is also available. The battery comes with a computer scoring program. The SOS has optional computer software that can be used during observation and for scoring observations. Measurement of both adaptive and maladaptive behavior is a strength. The multimodal integrated approach, which provides a comprehensive assessment, is also a strength of the BASC-2. Weaknesses include a lack of norms for the SOS and low interrater reliabilities for parent and teacher rating scales.
References consulted	Meisels and Atkins-Burnett (2005); Grill (2001); Knoff (2001). See book's References list.

Measure	**Caregiver–Teacher Report Form (C-TRF). Achenbach (1997).**
Purpose	Assessing behavioral and emotional problems, and identifying syndromes of problems that tend to occur together.

Areas	Anxious, Depressed, Withdrawn, Somatic Complaints, Emotionally Preactive, Attention Problems, Aggressive Behavior, Internalizing, Externalizing. DSM-oriented scales: Affective Problems, Anxiety Problems, Pervasive Developmental Problems, Attention Deficit/Hyperactivity Problems, Oppositional Defiant Problems.
Format	99 items, 3-point rating scale; 100th item is open response.
Scores	*T*-scores, percentiles.
Age group	1-6 to 5-0 years.
Time	15 minutes.
Users	Professionals.
Norms	Data collected on 1,192 children from 12 states and the Netherlands, stratified on SES, ethnicity, geographical region. High-SES children from U.S. Northeast were overrepresented. Normative group expanded in 2000 when CBCL/1½–5 was published.
Reliability	Test–retest (8.7 days), .84; interrater, .66.
Validity	Content, supported; criterion-related, supported.
Comments	Part of a series of landmark instruments used internationally with enormous research support. Established as a research tool; awaits further empirical validity. Computer and hand scoring available.
References consulted	Carey (2001); Furlong (2001); Pavelski (2001). See book's References list.

Measure	**Child Behavior Checklist (CBCL/1½–5). Achenbach and Rescorla (2000b).**
Purpose	Assessing emotional and behavioral problems in young children and identifying empirically based syndromes of problems that occur together and symptoms resembling certain DSM-IV diagnostic categories.
Areas	Internalizing Domain subscales: Emotionally Reactive, Anxious/Depressed, Somatic Complaints, Withdrawn. Externalizing Domain subscales: Attention Problems, Aggressive Behavior. Other: Total Behavior Problems, Sleep Problems.
Format	A list of 100 behavior problems occurring in the past 2 months are rated "0—not true," "1—sometimes true," or —very true or often true" across seven subscales identified above. DSM-IV-oriented scales are also included (Affective Problems, Anxiety Problems, Pervasive Developmental Problems, Attention Deficit/Hyperactivity Problems, and Oppositional Defiant Problems). Parent rating scale.
Scores	*T*-scores, percentiles.
Age group	1-6 to 5-0 years.
Time	15 minutes.
Users	Trained professionals.
Norms	Data collected from a nationally representative sample.
Reliability	It has the best cross-informant, cross-setting, and stability coefficients one could expect for this type of measure.
Validity	Concurrent, content, discriminant, and predictive validity are excellent. New studies are being done all the time.

Comments	The CBCL is an excellent rating scale of emotional and behavior problems in young children. Written at a fifth-grade reading level, the measures are easy to fill out and take very little time to complete. Computer scoring minimizes errors and scoring time and facilitates comparison of ratings across informants and settings. Weaknesses are that teachers and parents can be reluctant to endorse problems because items sound pathologizing and it does not assess adaptive behavior.
References consulted	Flanagan (2005); Watson (2005). See book's References list.

Measure	**Conners' Rating Scales—Revised (CRS-R). Conners (1997).**
Purpose	Assessing psychopathology and problem behaviors.
Areas	Parent Rating Scale, Teacher Rating Scale, Adolescent Self-Report Scale—long and short versions of each (CPRS-R:L or CPRS-R:S; CTRS-R:L or CTRS-R:S); Parent and Teacher subscales: Oppositional, Cognitive Problems/Inattention, Anxious–Shy, Hyperactivity, Social Problems, Perfectionism, Psychosomatic, ADHD Index, DSM-IV symptoms subscales, Conners Global Index.
Format	Checklists. CPRS-R:L, 80 items; CPRS-R:S, 27 items; CTRS-R:L, 59 items; CTRS-R:S, 28 items.
Scores	*T*-scores, percentiles.
Age group	3–17 years.
Time	Short forms, 5–10 minutes; long forms, 15–20 minutes.
Users	Professionals.
Norms	Data collected on over 8,000 children from over 200 schools in the United States and Canada from 1993 to 1996. For CPRS and CTRS, separate norms are available for boys and girls in 3-year age intervals from 3 to 17.
Reliability	Internal consistency: CPRS-R:L, .73–.94; CPRS-R:S, .86–.94; CTRS-R:L, .77–.96; CTRS-R:S, .88–.95. Test–retest (between 6 and 8 weeks): CPRS-R:L, .47–.85, and CPRS-R:S, .62–.85, for a sample of 49 children and adolescents; CTRS-R:L, .47–.88, and CTRS-R:S, .72–.92, for a sample of 50 children and adolescents.
Validity	Factorial validity studies indicate that subscales assess distinct dimensions of problem behavior and psychopathology. Convergent and divergent: CPRS-R:L and CTRS-R:L, .12–.50 for males and .16–.55 for females; CPRS-R:S and CTRS-R:S, .33–.47 for males and .18–.52 for females.
Comments	A prominent test for over 30 years. Long forms are recommended for use when possible.
References consulted	Hess (2001); Knoff (2001b). See book's References list.

Measure	**Devereux Early Childhood Assessment (DECA). LeBuffe and Naglieri (1999).**
Purpose	Evaluating strengths and weaknesses for within-child protective factors in order to aid in identifying appropriate instructional and parental strategies that encourage the child's strengths and support the child's social and emotional growth.
Areas	Total protective factors score comprised of three scales: Initiative, Self-Control, and Attachment. There is a Behavioral Concerns Scale.

Format	27 items evaluating the frequency of positive behaviors and 10 items evaluating behavioral concerns rated on a 5-point scale varying from "never" to "very frequently" during a 4-week period.
Scores	*T*-scores, percentiles.
Age group	2-0 to 5-11 years.
Time	10 minutes.
Users	Professionals. Raters must have sufficient exposure to child within past 4 weeks (2 or more hours per day for at least 2 days per week for 4 weeks) and can be either parent/guardians or teachers.
Norms	Data collected from two nationally representative samples (2,000 and 1,108) ages 2-0 to 5-11 years. Protective factors sample consisted of 2,000 preschool-age children that closely represented the U.S. population with regard to gender, geographic region of residence, race, ethnicity, and socioeconomic status. Teachers provided ratings on 1,017 of these children, while parents rated the remaining 983 children. Second sample consisted of 1,108 children for the behavioral concerns scale. Parents rated 541 children in the sample and teachers rated 567 children. Behavioral Concerns sample also closely represented the U.S. preschool population.
Reliability	Internal reliability ranged from .71–.91 for parents, .80–.94 for teachers across all five scales. Test–retest reliability (24- to 72-hour interval) ranged from .55–.80 for parents, .68–.94 for teachers across the five scales. Interrater reliability ranged from .21–.44 for parent to parent, .57–.77 for teacher to teacher, and .19–.34 for parent to teacher.
Validity	Content and construct-related validity were unable to be measured since the DECA is the first published behavior rating scale of within-child protective factors and there is no other measure for comparison. Criterion-related validity: sensitivity, .67–.78; specificity, .65–.71.
Comments	Developed based on the review of literature on resiliency and child-protective factors, the DECA provides the first standardized norm-referenced behavior rating scale of within-child protective factors. By focusing on a child's strengths as well as weaknesses, the DECA provides information not only about areas of social and emotional functioning that the child has difficulty in, but it also provides information about attributes within the child that act as protective factors and can be used to bolster intervention strategies. The DECA provides a strong link between assessment and instructional and parental planning. It is one part of a comprehensive model that focuses on prevention and intervention strategies through partnerships between families and preschool professionals. The DECA manual provides several examples of various profiles and their related interpretations. Low interrater reliability for parent forms should be noted. Exposure to the resiliency literature and knowledge of strength-based interventions is recommended prior to using the DECA so that users can adequately interpret/apply the information from a child's profile.
References consulted	Denham and Burton (2003); Meisels and Atkins-Burnett (2005). See book's References list.

Measure	**Direct Observation Form (DOF). Achenbach and Rescorla (2001).**
Purpose	Scoring observations over 10-minute periods in classrooms and group activities.
Areas	On-Task, Internalizing, Externalizing.

Format	96 problem items scored on a four-step rating scale; examiner scores target child's behavior over a 10-minute period as on or off task at 1-minute intervals, writes a narrative description of the child's behavior, and then rates problems observed over that period.
Scores	Four scaled scores comparing target child with two observed control children; six computer-scored syndrome scales derived from norms.
Age group	5–14 years.
Time	10–15 minutes.
Users	Trained professionals.
Norms	Data collected on 287 nonreferred children observed as classroom controls for referred children, and 212 referred children ages 5–14.
Reliability	Interrater (averaged across four studies), .90 for Total Problems and .84 for on-task scores.
Validity	Significantly discriminates between referred and nonreferred children observed in the same classroom when observer blind to referral status. Correlation of .51 between DOF and TRF Total Problem scores. DOF significantly discriminates between outcomes for at-risk children who received different school-based interventions.
Comments	Although not developed for preschool children, the DOF represents a reasonable approach to gathering information on the behavior in structured situations of children age 5 and older suspected of having ADHD. Comparison observations of two control children in the target child's class are recommended.
References consulted	Brassard review.

Measure	**Early Screening Project (ESP). Walker, Severson, and Feil (1995).**
Purpose	Identifying children at risk for internalizing and externalizing behavior problems, using a multistep child-finding process.
Areas	Externalizing behaviors (inappropriate behaviors and behavioral excesses); Internalizing behaviors (self-esteem, social avoidance); Social interaction, adaptive behavior, maladaptive behavior, aggressive behavior, critical events, how child plays with other children, how child interacts with caregivers, how the child interacts with materials; self-care, social adjustment.
Format	Stage 1: Teachers are asked to rate students in the fall and spring and list the five most internalizing and five most externalizing children in their classes. The children are ranked and cannot be on both lists. Stage 2: The three-highest rated children on each list are evaluated based on the Critical Events Index, Adaptive Behavior Index, Maladaptive Behavior Scale, Aggressive Behavior Scale (externalizing children), and Social Interaction Scale (internalizing children). Stage 3: Parent questionnaire and Social Behavior Observation (SBO) are completed on each child that exceed the criteria for stage 2.
Scores	Five-point frequency scale used, standard scores.
Age group	3-0–6-11 years.
Time	60 minutes (total group).
Users	Teachers, mental health professionals.

Norms	Data collected from large standardized sample (2,853) from eight states with separate norms provided for males and females. More than one third of sample is from southeastern states, thus the sample is not nationally representative. Low-income and rural children seem to be overrepresented.
Reliability	Interobserver, .42–.70 (teacher rankings for stage 1); .48–.79 (stage 2 scores); .87–.88 (stage 3 observations); test–retest (6 months), .59 (externalizing); .25 (internalizing); .75–.91 (critical events and adaptive and maladaptive behaviors).
Validity	Concurrent, .19–.95 with the Behar and Conner's rating scales; sensitivity, 62–100% true positives; specificity, 94–100% true negatives.
Comments	ESP is a proactive screening to support the child-find requirement in IDEA and prevent long-term negative outcomes associated with poor social and emotional skills. The tool requires minimal teacher time, does not overidentify children, has strong psychometric characteristics, and has an outstanding manual with very clear instructions for professionals and teachers, as well as a training video for observation procedures. Thus, it is an efficient measure at identifying children with emotional and/or behavioral concerns.
References consulted	Meisels and Atkins-Burnett (2005). See book's References list.

Measure	**Functional Emotional Assessment Scale (FEAS). Greenspan, DeGangi, and Wider (2001).**
Purpose	Measuring emotional functioning in children with constitutional and maturation-based problems; children with interactional problems leading to various symptoms (anxiety, impulsivity, depression, etc.); and children with pervasive developmental disorders.
Areas	Emotional Functioning, Motor, Sensory, Language, Cognitive Capacities, General Tendencies, and Caregiver Tendencies.
Format	Observational measure with two forms, supplemented by caregiver interview. Caregiver form, items use a 3-point scale; Child form, items use a 3-point scale for each age grouping (months 7–9, 10–12, 13–18, 19–24, and 25–35; years 3–4).
Scores	Cutoff scores for normal, at-risk, and deficient functioning for Caregiver and Child forms are provided by age of child.
Age group	7 months to 4 years.
Time	15–20 minutes.
Users	Professionals.
Norms	Data collected on 197 normal infants and children, 190 infants and children with regulatory disorders, 41 children with pervasive developmental disorders (PDD), and 40 children with drug exposure *in utero* and multiproblem families. Sample predominantly middle-class and white; black, Hispanic, and Asian children constituted only 6% of the sample population. *Note*: All children fell in normal range on developmental testing, except those with PDD.
Reliability	Interobserver, .89–.91 (Caregiver form), .91–.97 (Child form), .83–.89 (live and videotaped).
Validity	Construct, supported; concurrent, distinct.

Comments	The FEAS should only be used for descriptive purposes, because it has not been used with a large, diverse sample; it lacks sufficient psychometric data to be administered with confidence. The authors state: "FEAS is designed as an observational tool, [and] it is important to note that findings from the FEAS alone do not lead to a formal diagnosis of specific disorders such as autism, anxiety disorder, attachment disorder, or regulatory disorder" (p. 188). However, it has a strong theoretical foundation, provides a useful framework for clinicians, and merits further research.
References consulted	Brassard review

Measure	**Hawaii Early Learning Profiles (HELP), Strands Preschool Version. Vort Corporation (1999).**
Purpose	Aiding families and educators with curriculum planning, identification of strengths and weaknesses, and monitoring of children's progress.
Areas	Attachment/separation/autonomy; development of self; expression of emotions and feelings; learning rules and expectations; social interactions and play; social language; personal welfare/safety.
Format	Criterion-referenced objectives on social–emotional scales that should be completed across several sessions.
Scores	Approximate developmental age levels; qualitative descriptions of social and emotional competence areas.
Age group	3–6 years.
Time	Depends on the number of sections administered.
Users	Professionals, educators.
Norms	Not norm-referenced.
Reliability	Not reported.
Validity	Content validity good.
Comments	This is an ongoing curriculum-based assessment tool that was designed for use with young children who are delayed; however, the adaptability of the scale allows for tracking progress of nonhandicapped preschoolers as well. The instrument requires more specific assessment goals pertaining to emotional expressiveness, emotion knowledge, emotion regulation, social problem solving, and relationship skills. However, the HELP, Strands Preschool Version, provides very good examples of skills within its measured domains. Furthermore, the assessment takes advantage of spontaneous behavior, such as reaction to new people and places, parent–child interactions, and transitions.
References consulted	Denham and Burton (2003). See book's References list.

Measure	**MacArthur Story Stem Battery (MSSB). Emde, Wolf, and Oppenheim (2003).**
Purpose	Assessing attachment, moral development, family relationship conflict, empathy, prosocial orientation, dissociation in maltreated children, and propensity for behavioral problems and emotional stress.
Areas	Attachment, response to authority, response to family conflict, response to getting caught during a transgression, separation anxiety.

Format	Participants are given human figures to act out scenarios as interpreted from their point of view in 14 different story stems.
Scores	The session is videotaped, then scored.
Age group	3–7 years.
Time	30–40 minutes.
Users	Professionals.
Norms	No representative norms. The MSSB has been used with many small clinical and typically developing samples and some large longitudinal studies nationally and internationally.
Reliability	Internal consistency, .69–.87.
Validity	Scores are correlated with parent ratings, teacher ratings, clinical diagnoses, and other developmental measures over time.
Comments	The MSSB provides insight into the perceptions of preschool children; enhancement could come from teacher and peer ratings. Can only be used with a verbal child.
References consulted	Bretherton and Oppenheim (2003). See book's References list.

Measure	**Parent–Child Game. Forehand and McMahon (2003).**
Purpose	Assessing components of parent–child interaction when a child has been referred for defiant or other acting-out behavior.
Areas	Parent's commands, child's compliance, and parent's ability to follow child's lead.
Format	Consists of 5 minutes of the child's game (child chooses activity) and 5 minutes of the parent's game (parent chooses activity). Six parent behaviors (rewards, attending to the child, questions that are asked, commands that are given, warnings, and time outs) and three child behaviors (compliance, noncompliance, and inappropriate behaviors) are coded by the observer.
Scores	Child's game: percentage of intervals of child inappropriate behavior and rates per minute of parent total commands, questions, attends, and rewards; Parent's game: parent rate per minute of total commands, alpha commands, beta commands, warnings, questions, attends, and rewards as well as parent-contingent attention upon child compliance, and total number of time outs.
Age group	Parent and child, 3 to 10 years.
Time	10 minutes.
Users	Trained professionals.
Norms	Clinic families compared to group of well-functioning families.
Reliability	Adequate interrater (above .75) and test–retest reliability.
Validity	The interactions of parents and children not undergoing treatment tend to be very stable, while the measure is sensitive to significant treatment effects in the clinic and home.

Comments	One of the advantages of the Parent–Child Game is that it requires only 10 minutes to stage. It does require extensive training to code (25 hours) and ongoing maintenance of interrater reliability. Age-appropriate toys must be provided during the interactions. These may include crayons and paper, toy cars and trucks, building materials, and puzzles. The results of the measure are useful in designing and evaluating interventions.
References consulted	Brassard review.

Measure	**Preschool and Kindergarten Behavior Scales—Second Edition (PKBS-2). Merrell (2002).**
Purpose	Identifying preschool and kindergarten children who may be at risk for social skills deficits or behavioral problems.
Areas	Social Skills Scale, Behavior Problem Scale, and Supplemental Problem Behavior Scales. The latter include three scales for exploring externalizing problems (Self-Centered/Explosive, Attention Problems/Overactive, Antisocial/Aggressive) and two scales for internalizing problems (Social Withdrawal and Anxiety/Somatic Problems).
Format	76 items, 4-point rating scale.
Scores	Standard scores, percentile ranks, risk levels.
Age group	3–6 years.
Time	8–12 minutes.
Users	Parents and teachers.
Norms	Data collected on 3,313 children (2,855 for PKBS, 458 for PKBS-2). Sample revision was made to be consistent with 2000 U.S. Census data; 18 states represented, with West being overrepresented in ratings (77%); significant effort was made to be representative of gender, age, race, ethnicity, special education, and SES in the U.S. population.
Reliability	Internal consistency, .96; test–retest (3 weeks and 3 months), .58–.69; interrater in preschool setting, .48–.59; interrater in home and school settings, .16–.38.
Validity	Content, supported; convergent, supported.
Comments	The test has the ability to discriminate children not at risk from those who are at risk or may have a delay. If routine screening of all children is the purpose of assessment, or if the examiner is interested in ruling out potential problems for a child referred for other reasons, the PKBS-2 is a good choice.
References consulted	Fairbank (2005); Madle (2005). See book's References list.

Measure	**Social Competence and Behavior Evaluation, Preschool Edition (SCBE). LaFreniere and Dumas (1995).**
Purpose	Accessing patterns of social competence, affective expression, and adjustment difficulties.
Areas	Eight subscales in three clusters: (1) Emotional Adjustment (Depressive–Joyful, Anxious–Secure, Angry–Tolerant); (2) Social Interactions with Peers (Isolated–Integrated, Aggressive–Calm, Egotistical–Prosocial); and (3) Social Interactions

	with Adults (Oppositional–Cooperative; Dependent–Autonomous). Three summary scales: (1) Social Competence (40 items), (2) Internalizing Problems (20 items), and (3) Externalizing Problems (20 items).
Format	80 items, 6-point Likert-type responses.
Scores	*T*-scores, percentile ranks.
Age group	30–76 months.
Time	15 minutes.
Users	Teachers or childcare professionals.
Norms	Test originally normed in Canada. In united States, 1,263 school children at six sites in two states (Indiana and Colorado); 631 girls, 632 boys enrolled in preschool classes. Examination of demographic characteristics of U.S. normative sample shows that children from families with less education and from black families were overrepresented, and that children from Hispanic families and from families with college experience were underrepresented. Children age 3 comprised only 8.3% of those tested.
Reliability	Internal consistency, .80–.89. Test–retest, no U.S. information presented; Canadian information, 2-week reliability at .74–.84 and 6-month reliability at .59–.70 for the eight subscales. Interrater, Indiana sample only, .72–.89 (similar to earlier Canadian results).
Validity	Construct, good; factor analysis supports three primary factors (Social Competence, Externalizing, and Internalizing). Criterion related, good.
Comments	Development is incomplete and should be used as an aid. Authors' intended purpose seems to be the development of a test to describe behavioral tendencies for the purpose of socialization and education rather than classification (i.e., a test that is more of a personality instrument than a typical rating scale). Instructions are clear and math checks are available to aid in precise calculations. Items ask for interpretive responses that are subject to invalidity, depending on when teacher or childcare professional is asked to complete the form. Strong theoretical and developmental framework.
References consulted	Madle (2001); Poteat (2001). See book's References list.

Measure	**Social Skills Rating System (SSRS). Gresham and Elliott (1990).**
Purpose	Screening and classifying children suspected of having social behavior problems; assisting in interventions.
Areas	Social Skills (Cooperation, Assertion, Responsibility, Self-control); Problem Behaviors (Externalizing Problems, Internalizing Problems, Hyperactivity); Academic Competence.
Format	Rating scale (Teacher and Parent forms at Preschool level).
Scores	Standard scores.
Age group	Preschool (3-0 to 4-11 years), and grades K–12. (*Note*: Focus here is on Preschool level.)
Time	15–20 minutes.
Users	Professionals.

Norms	For all forms/levels, data based on 4,170 self-ratings of children and youth, 1,027 parent ratings, and 259 teacher ratings. Same number of male and female students; regular education students, as well as students in both self-contained and mainstreamed special education. Slight overrepresentation of whites and blacks, and underrepresentation of Hispanics. Sample drawn from rural, urban, and suburban communities in 18 states.
Reliability	Internal consistency, .83–.94 for Social Skills, .73–.88 for Problem Behaviors, .95 for Academic Competence. Test–retest (4 weeks), .65–.93.
Validity	Construct for Preschool level, high (Elementary Student level has 10 subscale items with factor loadings below .30.)
Comments	User-friendly manual. Also contains an Assessment–Intervention Record, which integrates data from Parent, Teacher, and Student forms. A related structural intervention program for preschoolers has been developed. Its use is recommended.
References consulted	Benes (1995); Furlong (1995); Kamo (1995). See book's References list.

References

Abbeduto, L., & Nuccio, J. (1989). Evaluating the pragmatic aspects of communication in school-age children and adolescents: Insights from research on atypical development. *School Psychology Review, 18*(4), 502–512.

Abbott, M., & Crane, J. (1977). Assessment of young children. *Journal of School Psychology, 15*, 118–128.

Abbott-Shim, M. (1991). *Quality care: A global assessment.* Unpublished manuscript, Georgia State University.

Abbott-Shim, M., & Sibley, A. (1987). *Assessment Profile for Family Day Care: Manual.* Atlanta, GA: Quality Assist.

Abbott-Shim, M., & Sibley, A. (1992). *Research Version of the Assessment Profile for Childhood Programs.* Atlanta, GA: Quality Assist.

Abbott-Shim, M., Sibley, A., & Neel, J. (1992). *Assessment Profile for Early Childhood Programs: Research manual.* Atlanta, GA: Quality Assist

Abe, J. A., & Izard, C. E. (1999). A longitudinal study of emotion expression and personality relations in early development. *Journal of Personality and Social Psychology, 77*(3), 566–677.

Abell, S. C., Von Briesen, P. D., & Watz, L. S. (1996). Intellectual evaluations of children using human figure drawings: An empirical investigation of two methods. *Journal of Clinical Psychology, 52*(1), 67–74.

Abidin, R. R., PAR staff, & Noriel, O. (1995). *Parenting Stress Index—Third Edition (PSI-3).* Odessa, FL: Psychological Assessment Resources.

Abrams, E. Z., & Goodman, J. F. (1996). Diagnosing developmental problems in children: Parents and professionals negotiate bad news. *Journal of Pediatrics, 23*, 87–98.

Accornero, V., Morrow, C., Bandstra, E., Johnson, A., & Anthony, J. (2002). Behavioral outcome of preschoolers exposed prenatally to cocaine: Role of maternal behavioral health. *Journal of Pediatric Psychology, 27*, 259–269.

Achenbach, T. M. (1986). *The Direct Observation Form of the Child Behavior Checklist* (rev. ed.). Burlington: University of Vermont, Department of Psychiatry.

Achenbach, T. M. (1992). *Manual for the Child Behavior Checklist/2–3 and 1992 Profile.* Burlington: University of Vermont, Department of Psychiatry.

Achenbach, T. M. (1997). *Caregiver–Teacher Report Form (C-TRF).* Burlington: University Medical Education Associates.

Achenbach, T. M., & Edelbrock, C. S. (1983). *Manual for the Child Behavior Checklist and Revised Child Behavior Profile.* Burlington: University of Vermont, Department of Psychiatry.

Achenbach, T. M., McConaughy, S. H., & Howell, C. T. (1987). Child/adolescent behavior and emotional problems: Implications of cross-informant correlations for situational specificity. *Psychological Bulletin, 101*, 213–232.

Achenbach, T. M., & Rescorla, L. A. (2000a). *Manual for the ASEBA Preschool Forms and Profiles.* Burlington: University of Vermont, Research Center for Children, Youth, and Families.

Achenbach, T. M., & Rescorla, L. A. (2000b). *Child Behavior Checklist for Ages: 1½–5 (CBCL/1½–5). Burlington: University of Vermont, Research Center for Children, Youth, and Families.*

Achenbach, T. M., & Rescorla, L. A. (2001). *Manual for the ASEBA School-Age Forms and Profiles*. Burlington: University of Vermont, Research Center for Children, Youth, and Families.

Ackerman, P. L. (1992). Test review of the Stanford Early School Achievement Test-Third Edition (SESAT). From J. J. Kramer & J. C. Conoley (Eds.), *The eleventh mental measurements yearbook* [Electronic version]. Retrieved from web5s.silverplatter.com.arugula.cc.columbia.edu:2048/webspirs/start.ws?customer=waldo&databases=YB

Ackerman P. L. (1995). Test review of the Kaufman Survey of Early Academic and Language Skills (KSEALS). From J. C. Conoley & J. C. Impara (Eds.), *The twelfth mental measurement yearbook* [Electronic version]. Retrieved from http://web5s.silverplatter.com.arugula.cc.columbia.edu:2048/webspirs/start.ws?customer=waldo& databases=YB

Ackerman, R. J. (1987). *Children of alcoholics: A guide for parents, educators and therapists* (2nd ed.). New York: Fireside/Simon & Schuster.

Adams, M. J. (1990). *Beginning to read: Thinking and learning about print*. Cambridge, MA: MIT Press.

Adams, M. J., Foorman, B. R., Lundberg, I., & Beeler, T. D. (1998). *Phonemic awareness in young children: A classroom curriculum*. Baltimore: Brookes.

Adelman, H. S. (1982). Identifying learning problems at an early age: A critical appraisal. *Journal of Clinical Child Psychology, 11*, 255–261.

Adrien, J. L., Barthelemy, C., Perrot, A., Roux, S., Lenoir, P., Hameury, L., et al. (1992). Validity and reliability of the Infant Behavioral Summarized Evaluation (IBSE): A rating scale for the assessment of young children with autism and developmental disorders. *Journal of Autism and Developmental Disorders, 22*(3), 375–394.

Adrien, J. L., Faure, M., Perrot, A., Hameury, L., Garreau, B., Barthelemy, C., et al. (1991). Autism and family home movies: Preliminary findings. *Journal of Autism and Developmental Disorders, 21*(1), 43–49.

Ainsworth, M. D. S., Blehar, M. C., Waters, E., & Wall, S. (1978). *Patterns of attachment: A psychological study of the strange situation*. Hillsdale, NJ: Erlbaum.

Airasian, P. W. (1991). *Classroom assessment*. New York: McGraw-Hill.

Albano, A. M., Chorpita, B. F., & Barlow, D. H. (1996). Childhood anxiety disorders. In E. J. Mash & R. A. Barkley (Eds.), *Child psychopathology* (pp. 196–241). New York: Guilford Press.

Aldridge Smith, J. A., Bidder, R. T., Gardner, S. M., & Gray, O. P. (1980). Griffiths Scales of Mental Development and different users. *Child: Care, Health and Development, 6*(1), 11–16.

Alessi, G. J., & Kaye, J. H. (1983). *Behavior assessment for school psychologists*. Kent, OH: National Association of School Psychologists.

Alexander, J. F., & Parsons, B. V. (1982). *Functional family therapy*. Monterey, CA: Brookes/Cole.

Alexander, K. L., & Entwisle, D. R. (1988). Achievement in the first 2 years of school: Patterns and processes. *Monographs of the Society for Research in Child Development, 53*(2), 157.

Alfonso, V. C., & Flanagan, D. P. (1999). Assessment of cognitive functioning in preschoolers. In E. V. Nuttall, I. Romero, & J. Kalesnik (Eds.), *Assessing and screening preschoolers* (2nd ed., pp. 186–217). Needham Heights, MA: Allyn & Bacon.

Algozzine, R., Schmid, R., & Mercer, C. D. (1981). *Childhood behavior disorders: Applied research and educational practice*. Austin, TX: PRO-ED.

Allen, D. A. (1988). Autistic spectrum disorders: Clinical presentation in preschool children. *Journal of Child Neurology, 3*(Suppl.), 48–56).

Allen, D. A. (1989). Developmental language disorders in preschool children: Clinical subtypes and syndromes. *School Psychology Review, 18*(4), 442–451.

Allison, J. A. (1998). Test review of the Parenting Stress Index—Third Edition (PSI-3). In J. C. Impara & B. S. Plake (Eds.), *The thirteenth mental measurements yearbook* [Electronic version]. Retrieved from web5.silverplatter.com/webspirs/start.ws?customer=waldo&databases=(YB)

Almy, M., & Genishi, C. (1983). *Ways of studying children* (rev. ed.). New York: Teachers College Press.

Alpern, G., Boll, T. & Shearer, M. (1986). *Developmental Profile II (DP-II)*. Los Angeles: Western Psychological Services.

Althen, G. (1988). *American ways: A guide for*

foreigners in the United States. Yarmouth, ME: Intercultural Press.

Aman, M. G., & Singh, N. N. (1986). *Aberrant Behavior Checklist (ABC)*. East Aurora, NY: Slosson.

American Educational Research Association (AERA), American Psychological Association (APA), & National Council on Measurement in Education (NCME). (1999). *Standards for educational and psychological testing*. Washington, DC: American Educational Research Association.

American Psychiatric Association. (1987). *Diagnostic and statistical manual of mental disorders* (3rd ed., rev.). Washington, DC: Author.

American Psychiatric Association. (2000). *Diagnostic and statistical manual of mental disorders* (4th ed., text rev.). Washington, DC: Author.

American Psychological Association. (2002). *Ethical principles of psychologists and code of conduct*. Retrieved from www.apa.org/ethics/code2002.html

American Psychological Association. (2003). Guidelines on multicultural education, training, research, practice, and organizational change for psychologists. *American Psychologist, 58*(5), 377–402.

Ames, N., Gillespie, S., Haines, J., & Ilg, N. (1979). *Gesell Developmental Schedules*. Rosemont, NJ: Programs for Education.

Amoruso, M., Zia-Fiorello, E., Gould E., Cazes, C., Schwartz, L., Maher, C., et al. (2004, November 12). *Hooked on parents: An assessment/observation/outreach program that works*. Presentation at the Observing and Assessing the Preschool Learner workshop, Teachers College, Columbia University.

Anastasi, A. (1988). *Psychological testing* (6th ed.). New York: Macmillan.

Anastasi, A., & Urbina, S. (1997). *Psychological testing* (7th ed.). Upper Saddle River, NJ: Prentice Hall.

Anderson, P., & Fenichel, E. (1989). *Serving culturally diverse families of infants and toddlers with disabilities*. Washington, DC: National Center for Clinical Infant Programs.

Aram, D. M. (1991). Comments on specific language impairment as a clinical category. *Language, Speech and Hearing Services in the Schools*, 22, 84–87.

Aram, D. M., Ekelman, B. L., & Nation, J. E. (1984). Preschoolers with language disorders: 10 years later. *Journal of Speech and Hearing Research, 18*, 229–241.

Aram, D. M., & Hall, N. E. (1989). Longitudinal follow-up of children with preschool communication disorders: Treatment implications. *School Psychology Review, 18*(4), 487–501.

Aram, D. M., & Nation, J. (1980). Preschool language disorders and subsequent language and academic difficulties. *Journal of Communication Disorders, 13*, 159–170.

Arnold, D. H., Fisher, P. H., Doctoroff, G. L., & Dobbs, J. (2002). Accelerating math development in Head Start classrooms. *Journal of Educational Psychology, 94*(4), 762–770.

Assistance to States for the Education of Children with Disabilities, 34 C. F. R. 300 (2000).

Athanasiou-Schicke, M. (2000). Current nonverbal assessment instruments: A comparison of psychometric integrity and test fairness. *Journal of Psychoeducational Assessment, 18*, 211–229.

Atkinson, L., Bevc, I., Dickens, S., & Blackwell, J. (1992). Concurrent validities of the Stanford–Binet Intelligence Scale Fourth Edition, Leiter, and Vineland with developmentally delayed children. *Journal of School Psychology, 30*, 165–173.

Atwater, J. B., Carta, J. J., & Schwartz, I. (1989). *ACCESS Observation System*. Unpublished manuscript, Juniper Gardens Children's Project, University of Kansas, Kansas City, KS.

Aylward, G. P. (2001). Review of the High/Scope Child Observation Record for Ages 2½–6. In J. C. Impara (Ed.), *The fourteenth mental measurements yearbook*. Lincoln, NE: University of Nebraska Press.

Backlund, P. A. (1998). Test Review of the Early Language Milestone Scale. In J. C. Impara & B. S. Plake (Eds.), *The thirteenth mental measurements yearbook* [Electronic version]. Retrieved from the Buros Institute *Test Reviews Online* website: www.unl.edu/Buros

Backlund, P. A. (2001). Test review of the Test of Early Language Development—Third Edition (TELD-3). In J. C. Impara & B. S. Plake (Eds.), *The fourteenth mental measurements yearbook* [Electronic version]. Retrieved from http://web5.silverplatter.com/webspirs/start.ws?customer=waldo&databases=(YB)

Bagnato, S. J. (1984). Team congruence in development and intervention: Comparing clinical judgment and child performance measures. *School Psychology Review, 13*, 7–16.

Bagnato, S. J. (1992). Assessment for early intervention: Best practices with young children and families. *Assessment News, 2*(4), 1, 8–10.

Bagnato, S. J., & Neisworth, J. T. (1991). *Assessment for early intervention: Best practices for professionals*. New York: Guilford Press.

Bagnato, S. J., & Neisworth, J. T. (1994). A national study of the social and treatment "invalidity" of intelligence testing for early intervention. *School Psychology Quarterly, 9*, 81–102.

Bagnato, S. J., Neisworth, J. T., & Munson, S. M. (1989). *Linking developmental assessment and early intervention: Curriculum-based perspectives* (2nd ed.). Rockville, MD: Aspen.

Bagnato, S. J., Neisworth, J. T., & Munson, S. M. (1997). *Linking assessment and early intervention: An authentic curriculum-based approach.* Baltimore: Brookes.

Bagnato, S. J., Neisworth, J. T., Salvia, J., & Hunt, F. M. (1999). *Temperament and Atypical Behavior Scale (TABS).* Baltimore: Brookes.

Bailey, A., LeCouteur, A., Gottesman, I., Bolton, P., Simonoff, E., Yuzda, E., et al. (1995). Autism as a strongly genetic disorder: Evidence from a British twin study. *Psychological Medicine, 25*, 63–77.

Bailey, D. B. (1988). Assessing family stress and needs. In D. B. Bailey & R. Simeonsson (Eds.), *Family assessment in early intervention* (pp. 95–118). Columbus, OH: Merrill.

Bailey, D. B. (1989). Assessing environments. In D. B. Bailey & M. Wolery (Eds.), *Assessing infants and preschoolers with handicaps* (pp. 97–118). Columbus, OH: Merrill.

Bailey, D. B., & Brochin, H. A. (1989). Tests and test development. In D. B. Bailey & M. Wolery (Eds.), *Assessing infants and preschoolers with handicaps* (pp. 22–46). Columbus, OH: Merrill.

Bailey, D. B., Clifford, R. M., & Harms, T. (1982). Comparison of preschool environments for handicapped and non-handicapped children. *Topics in Early Childhood Special Education, 2*(1), 9–20.

Bailey, D. B., & Roberts, J. E. (1987). *Teacher–child Communication Scale.* Chapel Hill: University of North Carolina.

Bailey, D. B., & Rouse, T. L. (1989). Procedural considerations in assessing infants and preschoolers with handicaps. In D. B. Bailey & M. Wolery (Eds.), *Assessing infants and preschoolers with handicaps* (pp. 47–63). Columbus, OH: Merrill.

Bailey, D. B., & Simeonsson, R. (Eds.). (1988). *Family assessment in early intervention.* Columbus, OH: Merrill.

Bailey, D. B., & Simeonsson, R. J. (1990). *Family Needs Survey (FNS).* Chapel Hill: University of North Carolina, Frank Porter Graham Child Development Center.

Bailey, D. B., & Wolery, M. (1992). *Teaching infants and preschoolers with disabilities.* New York: Macmillan.

Bain, S. (2005). Test review: Stanford–Binet Intelligence Scales, Fifth Edition. *Journal of Psychoeducational Assessment, 23*, 87–95.

Bain, S. K. & Hawkins, J. (2005). Review of Boehm Test of Basic Concepts-3. In R. A. Spies & B. S. Plake (Eds.), *The sixteenth mental measurements yearbook* Electronic version]. Retrieved from http://web5s.silverplatter.com.arugula.cc.columbia.edu:2048/webspirs/start.ws?customer=waldo&databases=YB

Baird, G., Charman, T., Baron-Cohen, S., Cox, A., Swettenham, J., Wheelwright, S., et al. (2000). A screening instrument for autism at 18 months of age: A 6-year follow-up study. *Journal of the American Academy of Child and Adolescent Psychiatry, 39*(6), 694–702.

Baird, G., Simonoff, E., Pickles, A., Chandler, S., Loucas, T., Meldrum, D., et al. (2006). Prevalence of disorders of the autism spectrum in a population cohort of child in South Thames: The Special Needs and Autism Project (SNAP). *The Lancet, 368* (9531), 210–215.

Baker, B. L., Blacher, J., Crnic, K. A., & Edelbrock, C. (2002). Behavior problems and parenting stress in families of three-year-old children with and without developmental delays. *American Journal on Mental Retardation, 107*, 433–444.

Baker, S. K., Kameenui, E. J., Simmons, D. C., & Stahl, S. A. (1994). Beginning reading: Educational tools for diverse learners. *School Psychology Review, 23*, 372–391.

Bandura, A. (1978). The self system in reciprocal determinism. *American Psychologist, 33*, 344–358.

Banerji, M. (1992a). Factor structure of the Gesell School Readiness Screening Test. *Journal of Psychoeducational Assessment, 10*(4), 342–354.

Banerji, M. (1992b). An integrated study of the predictive properties of the Gesell School Readiness Test. *Journal of Psychoeducational Assessment, 10*(3), 240–256.

Bankson, N. W. (1990). *Bankson Language Test—Second Edition (BLT-2).* Austin, TX: PRO-ED.

Baranek, G. T. (1999). Autism during infancy: A retrospective video analysis of sensory–motor and social behaviors. *Journal of Autism and Developmental Disorders, 29*, 213–224.

Barenbaum, E., & Newcomer, P. (1996). *Test of Children's Language (TOCL).* Austin, TX: PRO-ED.

Barker, E. H., & Tyne, T. F. (1980). The use of observational procedures in school psychological services. *School Psychology Monograph, 4*(1), 25–44.

Barker, R. G. (1968). *Ecological psychology: Con-*

cepts and methods for studying the environment of human behavior*. Stanford, CA: Stanford University Press.

Barkley, R. A. (1997a). *Defiant children: A clinician's manual for assessment of parent training* (2nd ed.). New York: Guilford Press.

Barkley, R. A. (1997b). Attention deficit/hyperactivity disorder. In E. J. Mash & L. G. Terdal (Eds.), *Assessment of childhood disorders* (3rd ed., pp. 71–129). New York: Guilford Press.

Barnes, L. L. B. (1998). Test review of the Parenting Stress Index—Third Edition (PSI-3). From J. C. Impara & B. S. Plake (Eds.), *The thirteenth mental measurements yearbook* [Electronic version]. Retrieved from http://web5.silverplatter.com/webspirs/start.ws.customer=waldo&databases=(YB)

Barnett, D. W. (1984). An organizational approach to preschool services: Psychological screening, assessment and intervention. In C. Maher, R. Illback, & J. Zins (Eds.), *Organizational psychology in the schools: A handbook for practitioners*. Springfield, IL: Thomas.

Barnett, D. W. (1995). Test review of *AGS Early Screening Profiles* (AGS). From J. C. Conoley & J. C. Impara (Eds.), *The twelfth mental measurements yearbook* [Electronic version]. Retrieved from http://web5s.silverplatter.com.arugula.cc.columbia.edu:2048/webspirs/start.ws?customer=waldo&databases=YB

Barnett, D. W., Bell, S. H., & Carey, K. T. (1999). *Designing preschool interventions: A practitioner's guide*. New York: Guilford Press.

Barnett, D. W., & Carey, K. T. (1991). Intervention design for young children: Assessment concepts and procedures. In B. A. Bracken (Ed.), *The psychoeducational assessment of preschool children* (2nd ed., pp. 529–544). Boston: Allyn & Bacon.

Barnett, D. W., & Carey, K. T. (1992). *Designing interventions for preschool learning and behavior problems*. San Francisco: Jossey-Bass.

Barnett, D. W., Ehrhardt, K. E., Stollar, S. A., & Bauer, A. M. (1994). PASSkey: A model for naturalistic assessment and intervention design. *Topics in Early Childhood Special Education, 14*, 350–357.

Barnett, S. (1989). Working with interpreters. In D. Duncan (Ed.), *Working with bilingual language disability* (pp. 91–112). New York: Chapman & Hall.

Barnett, W. S., & Escobar, C. (1987). The economics of early educational intervention: A review. *Review of Educational Research, 57*, 387–414.

Barnett, W. S., Lamey, C., & Jung, K. (2005). *The effects of state prekindergarten on young children's school readiness in five states*. U.S. Department of Health and Human Services, Administration for Children and Families, National Child Care Information Center. Retrieved from: http://nieer.org?resources/research/multistate/fullreport.pdf

Baroff, G. S. (1999). General learning disorder: A new designation for mental retardation. *Mental Retardation, 37*, 68–70.

Baron-Cohen, S. (1987). Autism and symbolic play. *British Journal of Developmental Psychology, 5*, 139–148.

Baron-Cohen, S., Allen, J., & Gillberg, C. (1992). Can autism be detected at 18 months? The needle, the haystack, and the CHAT. *British Journal of Psychiatry, 161*, 839–843.

Baron-Cohen, S., Cox, A., Baird, G., Swettenham, J., Nightingale, N., Morgan, K., et al. (1996). Psychological markers in the detection of autism in infancy in a large population. *British Journal of Psychiatry, 168*, 158–163.

Baron-Cohen, S., Wheelwright, S., Cox, A., Baird, G., Charman, T., Swettenham, J., et al. (2000). Early identification of autism by the Checklist for Autism in Toddlers (CHAT). *Journal of the Royal Society of Medicine, 93*(10), 521–525.

Barrett, K. C., & Campos, J. J. (1991). A diacritical function approach to emotions and coping. In E. M. Cummings, A. L. Greene, & K. H. Karraker (Eds.), *Life-span developmental psychology: Perspectives on stress and coping* (pp. 21–41). Hillsdale, NJ: Erlbaum.

Basch, C. E. (1997). Focus group interview: An underutilized research technique for improving theory and practice in health education. *Health Education Quarterly, 14*, 411–448.

Bateson, G. (1979). *Mind and nature*. New York: Dutton.

Bateson, G., Jackson, D. D., Haley, J., & Weakland, J. (1956). Toward a theory of schizophrenia. *Behavioral Science, 1*, 251–264.

Bayley, N. (1993). *Bayley Scales of Infant Development—Second Edition (BSID-II)*. San Antonio, TX: Psychological Corporation.

Bayley, N. (2005). *Bayley Scales of Infant and Toddler Development, Third Edition (Bayley-III)*. San Antonio, TX: Psychological Corporation.

Bayley, N. (2006a). *Bayley Scales of Infant and Toddler Development, Third Edition, Administration Manual*. San Antonio, TX: Psychological Corporation.

Bayley, N. (2006b). *Bayley Scales of Infant and Toddler Development, Third Edition, Technical Manual*. San Antonio, TX: Psychological Corporation.

Beauchesne, M. A., Barnes, A., & Patsdaughter, C. (2004). Children with disabilities need a Head

Start too! *Journal of Learning Disabilities*, *8*(1), 41–55.

Beaver, J. (1997). *Developmental reading assessment*. Parsippany, NJ: Celebration Press.

Beck, A. T., Steer, R. A., & Brown, G. K. (1996). *Beck Depression Inventory, Second Edition*. San Antonio, TX: Psychological Corporation.

Beckman, P. (1983). Influence of selected child characteristics on stress in families of handicapped infants. *American Journal of Mental Deficiency*, *88*(2), 150–156.

Beeghley, M., Weiss-Perry, B., & Cicchetti, D. (1989). Affective and structural analysis of symbolic play in children with Down syndrome. *International Journal of Behavioral Development*, *12*, 257–277.

Beery, K. E. (1989). *The VMI Developmental Test of Visual Motor Integration: Administration, scoring, and teaching manual* (rev. ed.). Cleveland, OH: Modern Curriculum Press.

Beery, K. E. (1997). *Developmental Test of Visual–Motor Integration—Third Edition*. Minnetonka, MN: NCS Pearson.

Beery, K. E., Buktencia, N. A., & Beery, N. A. (2004). *Beery–Buktenica Developmental Test of Visual–Motor Integration, Fifth Edition*. Minneapolis, MN: NCS Pearson.

Beller, E. K., Stahnke, M., Butz, P., Stahl, W., & Wessels, H. (1996). Two measures of the quality of group care for infants and toddlers. *European Journal of Psychology of Education*, *11*(2), 151–167.

Belsky, J. (1984). The determinants of parenting: A process model. *Child Development*, *55*, 83–96.

Belsky, J., & Most, R. K. (1981). From exploration to play: A cross-sectional study of infant free play behavior. *Developmental Psychology*, *17*, 630–639.

Belsky, J., & Steinberg, L. (1978). The effects of daycare: A critical review. *Child Development*, *49*, 929–949.

Belsky, J., & Vondra, J. (1989). Lessons from child abuse: The determinants of parenting. In D. Cicchetti & V. Carlson (Eds.), *Child maltreatment: Theory and research on the causes and consequences of child abuse and neglect* (pp. 153–202). New York: Cambridge University Press.

Benard, B. (1995). *Fostering resilience in children*. Retrieved from http://resilnet.uiuc.edu/library/benard95.html

Benedict, M. I., White, R. B., Wulff, L. M., & Hall, B. T. (1990). Reported maltreatment in children with multiple disabilities. *Child Abuse and Neglect*, *14*, 207–217.

Benes, K. M. (1995). Test review of the Social Skills Rating System (SSRS). In J. C. Conoley & J. C. Impara (Eds.), *The twelfth mental measurements yearbook* [Electronic version]. Retrieved from http://web5.silverplatter.com/webspirs/start.ws?customer=waldo&databases=(YB)

Berk, H. (1993). Early intervention and special education. In R. Smith (Ed.), *Children with mental retardation: A parent's guide* (pp. 173–207). Rockville, MD: Woodbine House.

Berk, R. K. (Ed.). (1984). *A guide to criterion-referenced test construction*. Baltimore: Johns Hopkins University Press.

Berk, R. K. (1986). Minimum competency testing: Status and potential. In B. S. Blake & J. C. Witt (Eds.), *The future of testing* (pp. 89–144). Hillsdale, NJ: Erlbaum.

Berls, A. T., & McEwen, I. R. (1999). Battelle Developmental Inventory. *Physical Therapt*, *79*, 776-783. Retrieved from www.ptjournal.org/August99/public/v79n8p776.cfm

Bernheimer, L. P., & Keogh, B. K. (1988). Stability of cognitive performance in children with developmental delays. *American Journal on Mental Retardation*, *92*, 539–542.

Berninger, V. W., Thalberg, S. P., DeBruyn, I., & Smith, R. (1987). Preventing reading disabilities by assessing and remediating phonemic skills. *School Psychology Review*, *16*, 554–565.

Berrueta-Clement, J., Schweinhart, L., Barnett, W., Epstein, A., & Weikart, D. (1984). *Changed lives: The effects of the Perry Preschool Program on youths through age 19*. Ypsilanti, MI: High/Scope Press.

Berument, S. K., Rutter, M., Lord, C., Pickles, A., & Bailey, A. (1999). Autism Screening Questionnaire: Diagnostic validity. *British Journal of Psychiatry*, *175*, 444–451.

Bessai, F. (2001a). Test review of the Expressive Vocabulary Test (EVT). In B. S. Plake & J. C. Impara (Eds.), *The fourteenth mental measurements yearbook* [Electronic version]. Retrieved from the Buros Institute's *Test Reviews Online* website: http://www.unl.edu.buros

Bessai, F. (2001b). Test review of the Peabody Picture Vocabulary Test—III (PPVT-III). In J. C. Impara & B. S. Plake (Eds.), *The fourteenth mental measurements yearbook* [Electronic version]. Retrieved from http://web5.silverplatter.com/webspirs/start.ws?customer-waldo&databases=(YB)

Bialystok, E. (2001). *Bilingualism in development: Language, literacy, and cognition*. New York: Cambridge University Press.

Biederman, J., Faraone, S., Mick, E., Wozniak, J.,

Chen, L., Ouellette, C., et al. (1996). Attention-deficit hyperactivity disorder and juvenile mania: An overlooked comorbidity? *Journal of the American Academy of Child and Adolescent Psychiatry, 35*, 997–1008.

Biederman, J., Rosenbaum, J. F., Chaloff, J., & Kagan, J. (1995). Behavioral inhibition as a risk factor for anxiety disorders. In J. S. March (Ed.), *Anxiety disorders in children and adolescents* (pp. 61–81). New York: Guilford Press.

Biederman, J., Rosenbaum, J. F., Hirshfeld, D. R., Farone, S. V., Bolduc, E. A., Gersten, M., et al. (1990). Psychiatric correlates of behavioral inhibition in young children of parents with and without psychiatric disorders. *Archives of General Psychiatry, 47*, 21–26.

Bierman, K. L., & Welsh, J. A. (1997). Social relationship deficits. In E. J. Mash & L. G. Terdal (Eds.), *Assessment of childhood disorders* (3rd ed., pp. 328–365). New York: Guilford Press.

Billstedt, E., Gillberg, C., & Gillberg, C. (2005). Autism after adolescence: Population-based 13- to 22-year follow-up study of 120 individuals with autism diagnosed in childhood. *Journal of Autism and Developmental Disorders, 35*(3), 351–360.

Bishop, V. E. (1986). Identifying the components of success in mainstreaming. *Journal of Visual Impairment and Blindness, 80*, 939–946.

Bjorkman, S., Poteat, G. M., & Snow, C. W. (1986). Environmental ratings and children's social behavior: Implications for the assessment of daycare quality. *American Journal of Orthopsychiatry, 56*(2), 271–277.

Blair, K. A. (2001). Test review of Asperger Syndrome Diagnostic Scale (ASDS). In B. S. Blake, J. C. Impara, & R. A. Spies (Eds.), *The fifteenth mental measurements yearbook* [Electronic version]. Retrieved from http://web5.silverplatter.com/webspirs/start.ws?customer=waldo&databases=(YB)

Bliss, S. (2006). Test Reviews, *Test of Early Mathematics Ability—Third Edition. Journal of Psychoeducational Assessment, 24*, 85–88.

Bloom, B. (1964). *Stability and change in human characteristics*. New York: Wiley.

Bloom, L. (1970). *Language development: Form and function in emerging grammars*. Cambridge, MA: MIT Press.

Bloom, L. (1974). Talking, understanding and thinking: Developmental relationship between receptive and expressive language. In R. L. Schiefelbush & L. Lloyd (Eds.), *Language perspectives: Acquisition, retardation, and intervention* (pp. 285–312). Baltimore: University Park Press.

Bloom, L. (1991). *Language development from two to three*. New York: Cambridge University Press.

Bloom, L. (1993). *The transition from infancy to language: Acquiring the power of expression.* New York: Cambridge University Press.

Bloom, L., & Lahey, M. (1978). *Language development and language disorders*. New York: Wiley.

Bloom, L., Margulis, C., Tinker, E., & Fujita, N. (1996). Early conversations and word learning: Contributions from child and adult. *Child Development, 67*, 3154–3175.

Boehm, A. E. (1976). *The Boehm resource guide for basic concept teaching*. New York: Psychological Corporation.

Boehm, A. E. (1980). *The Boehm resource guide of basic concept teaching: Teachers manual.* New York: Psychological Corporation.

Boehm, A. E. (1986). *Manual for the Boehm Test of Basic Concepts*. New York: Psychological Corporation.

Boehm, A. E. (1990). Assessment of children's knowledge of basic concepts. In C. R. Reynolds & R. W. Kamphaus (Eds.), *Handbook of psychological and educational assessment of children: Intelligence and achievement* (pp. 654–670). New York: Guilford Press.

Boehm, A. E. (2000a). *Boehm Test of Basic Concepts—Third Edition*. San Antonio, TX: Psychological Corporation.

Boehm, A. E. (2000b). Assessment of basic relational concepts. In B. A. Bracken (Ed.), *The psychoeducational assessment of preschool children* (3rd ed., pp. 186–203). Boston: Allyn & Bacon.

Boehm, A. E. (2001). *Boehm Test of Basic Concepts—Third Edition: Preschool*. San Antonio, TX: Psychological Corporation.

Boehm, A. E., & Sandberg, B. R. (1982). Assessment of the preschool child. In C. R. Reynolds & T. B. Gutkin (Eds.), *The handbook of school psychology* (pp. 81–120). New York: Wiley.

Boehm, A. E., & Weinberg, R. A. (1997). *The classroom observer: Developing observation skills in early childhood settings* (3rd ed.). New York: Teachers College Press.

Bolton, P., MacDonald, H., Pickles, A., Rios, P., Goode, S., Crowson, M., et al. (1994). A case–control family history study of autism. *Journal of Child Psychology and Psychiatry, 35*(5), 877–900.

Bond, L. A., Creasy, G. L., & Abrams, C. L. (1990). Play assessment: Reflecting and promoting cognitive competence. In E. D. Gibbs & D. M. Teti (Eds.), *Interdisciplinary assess-*

ment of infants (pp. 113–128). Baltimore: Brookes.

Bondurant, J. L., Romeo, D. J., & Kretschmer, R. (1983). Language behaviors of mothers of children with normal and delayed language. *Language, Speech, and Hearing Services in Schools*, *14*(4), 233–242.

Borke, H. (1971). Interpersonal perception of young children: Egocentrism or empathy. *Developmental Psychology*, *5*, 263–269.

Bornstein, M. H., & Sigman, M. D. (1986). Continuity in mental development from infancy. *Child Development*, *57*, 251–274.

Bountress, N. G. (1985). Test review of the Lindamood Auditory Conceptualization Test-Revised (LACT). From J. V. Mitchell, Jr. (Ed.), *The ninth mental measurement yearbook* [Electronic version]. Retrieved from http://web5s.silverplatter.com.arugula.cc.columbia.edu:2048/webspirs/start.ws?customer=waldo&databases=YB

Bowen, M. (1978). *Family therapy in clinical practice*. New York: Aronson.

Bowers, P. G., & Swanson, L. B. (1991). Naming speed deficits in reading disability: Multiple measures of a singular process. *Journal of Experimental Child Psychology*, *51*(2), 195–219.

Bowman, B. T. (1992). Who is at risk for what and why. *Journal of Early Intervention*, *16*, 101–108.

Boyce, B. A. (2005). Review of the Ages & Stages Questionnaires, Second Edition. In R. A. Spies & B. S. Plake (Eds.), *The sixteenth mental measurement yearbook* [Electronic version]. Retrieved from http://web5s.silverplatter.com.arugula.cc.columbia.edu:2048/webspirs/start.ws?customer=waldo&databases=YB

Bracken, B. A. (1983). Observing the assessment behavior of preschool children. In K. D. Paget & B. A. Bracken (Eds.), *The psychoeducational assessment of preschool children* (pp. 63–80). New York: Grune & Stratton.

Bracken, B. A. (1984). *Bracken Basic Concept Scale*. Columbus, OH: Merrill.

Bracken, B. A. (1987). Limitations of preschool instruments and standards for minimal levels of technical adequacy. *Journal of Psychoeducational Assessment*, *5*, 313–326.

Bracken, B. A. (1988). Ten psychometric reasons why similar tests produce dissimilar results. *Journal of School Psychology*, *26*(2), 155–166.

Bracken, B. A. (1991a). The assessment of preschool children with the McCarthy Scales of children's abilities. In B. A. Bracken (Ed.), *The psychoeducational assessment of preschool children* (2nd ed., pp. 53–85). Boston: Allyn & Bacon.

Bracken, B. A. (Ed.). (1991b). *The psychoeducational assessment of preschool children* (2nd ed.). Boston: Allyn & Bacon.

Bracken, B. A. (1994). Advocating for effective preschool assessment practices: A comment on Bagnato and Neisworth. *School Psychology Quarterly*, *9*, 103–108.

Bracken, B. A. (1998). *Bracken Basic Concept Scale—Revised*. San Antonio, TX: Psychological Corporation.

Bracken, B. A. (2000). Maximizing construct relevant assessment: The optimal preschool testing situation. In B. A. Bracken (Ed.), *The psychoeducational assessment of preschool children* (3rd ed., pp. 33–44). Boston: Allyn & Bacon.

Bracken, B. A. (2002). *Bracken School Readiness Assessment*. San Antonio, TX: Psychological Corporation.

Bracken, B. A. (Ed.) (2004). *The psychoeducational assessment of preschool children* (3rd ed). Mahwah, NJ: Erlbaum.

Bracken, B. A., Bagnato, S. J., & Barnett, D. (1990). *NASP position statement on early childhood assessment*. Washington, DC: National Association of School Psychologists.

Bracken, B. A., & Walker, K. C. (1997). The utility of intelligence tests for preschool children. In D. P. Flanagan, J. L. Genshaft, & P. L. Harrison (Eds.), *Contemporary intellectual assessment* (pp. 484–502). New York: Guilford Press.

Braden, J. P. (1989). Organizing and monitoring data bases. In S. H. Fradd & M. J. Weismantel (Eds.), *Meeting the needs of culturally and linguistically different students: A handbook for educators* (pp. 14–33). Boston: College-Hill Press.

Braden, J. P., & Plunge, M. (1994). Linking assessment to children's performance. *Communiqué*, 26.

Bradley, L., & Bryant, P. E. (1985). *Rhyme and reason in reading and spelling*. Ann Arbor: University of Michigan Press.

Bradley, R. H. (1985). Review of the Gesell School Readiness Test. In J. V. Mitchell, Jr. (Ed.), *The ninth mental measurements yearbook* (Vol. 1, pp. 609–610). Lincoln, NE: Buros Institute of Mental Measurements.

Bradley, R. H. (1992). Review of the Gesell School Readiness Test. In J. J. Kramer & J. C. Conoley (Eds.), *The eleventh mental measurements yearbook* (pp. 609–610). Lincoln: University of Nebraska Press.

Bradley, R. H. (1994). The HOME Inventory: Review and reflections. In H. W. Reese (Ed.), *Advances in child development and behavior* (Vol. 25, pp. 241–288). Orlando, FL: Academic Press.

Bradley, R. H., & Caldwell, B. M. (1974). *Issues and procedures in testing young children* (ERIC Clearinghouse on Test, Measure and Evaluation, TM Report No. 37). Princeton, NJ: Educational Testing Service.

Bradley, R. H., & Caldwell, B. M. (1976). The relationship of infants' home environment to mental test performance at fifty-four months: A follow-up study. *Child Development, 47,* 1172–1174.

Bradley, R. H., Corwyn, R. F., Burchinal, M., McAdoo, H. P., & García-Coll, C. (2001a). The home environments of children in the United States Part II: Relations with behavioral development through age thirteen. *Child Development, 72,* 1868–1886.

Bradley, R. H., Corwyn, R. F., Burchinal, M., McAdoo, H. P., & García-Coll, C. (2001b). The home environments of children in the United States Part I: Variations in age, ethnicity, and poverty status. *Child Development, 72,* 1844–1867.

Bradley-Johnson, S. (2001). Cognitive assessment for the youngest children: A critical review of tests. *Journal of Psychoeducational Assessment, 19,* 19–44.

Bradley-Johnson, S., & Durmusoglu, G. (2005). Evaluation of floors and item gradients for reading and math tests for young children. *Journal of Psychoeducational Assessment, 23*(3), 262–278.

Bramlett, R. K., & Barnett, D. W. (1993). The development of a direct observation code for use in preschool settings. *School Psychology Review, 22,* 49–62.

Brandt, R. (1972). *Studying behavior in natural settings.* New York: Holt, Rinehart & Winston.

Brassard, M. R. (1986). Family assessment approaches and procedures. In H. Knoff (Ed.), *The assessment of child and adolescent personality* (pp. 399–449). New York: Guilford Press.

Brassard, M. R., & Rivelis, E. (2006). Psychological and physical abuse. In G. Bear & K. Minke (Eds.), *Children's needs III: Understanding and addressing the developmental needs of children* (pp. 799–820). Bethesda, MD: National Association of School Psychologists.

Bray, C., & Wiig, E. (1987). *Let's Talk Inventory for Children.* San Antonio, TX: Psychological Corporation.

Bredekamp, S. (Ed.). (1987). *Developmentally appropriate practice in early childhood programs serving children from birth through age 6* (exp. ed.). Washington, DC: National Association for the Education of Young Children.

Bredekamp, S. (Ed.). (1991). Guidelines for appropriate curriculum content and assessment in programs serving children ages 3 through 8. *Young Children, 46,* 32–34.

Bredekamp, S., & Copple, C. (Eds.). (1997). *Developmentally appropriate practice in early childhood programs* (rev. ed.). Wahington, DC: National Association for the Education of Young Children.

Brennen, R. L., & Johnson, E. G. (1995). Generalizability of performance assessments. *Educational Measurement: Issues and Practice, 14*(4), 9–12.

Bretherton, I., & Oppenheim, D. (2003). The MacArthur Story Stem Battery: Development, administration, reliability, validity, and reflections about meaning. In R. N. Emde, D. P. Wolff, & D. Oppenheim (Eds.), *Revealing the inner worlds of young children* (pp. 55–80). New York: Oxford University Press.

Bretherton, I., Oppenheim, D., Buchsbaum, H., Emde, R. N., & MacArthur Narrative Group. (1990). *MacArthur Story Stem Battery coding manual.* Unpublished manual, University of Wisconsin–Madison.

Bricker, D., & Pretti-Fontczak, K. (1996). *Assessment, Evaluation, and Programming System for infants and adults: Vol. 4. AEPS curriculum for three to six years.* Baltimore: Brookes.

Bricker, D., & Squires, J. (1999). *Ages and Stages Questionnaires (ASQ): A parent-completed, child-monitoring system* (2nd ed.). Baltimore: Brookes.

Bricker, D., Squires, J., & Mounts, L. (1995). *Ages and Stages Questionnaires (ASQ): A parent-completed, child-monitoring system.* Baltimore: Brookes.

Brigance, A. H. (1989a). *Brigance Comprehensive Inventory of Basic Skills.* North Billerica, MA: Curriculum Associates.

Brigance, A. H. (1989b). *Brigance Diagnostic Inventory of Early Development.* North Billerica, MA: Curriculum Associates.

Brigance, A. H. (1997). *Brigance K and 1 Screen for Kindergarten and First Grade—Revised.* North Billerica, MA: Curriculum Associates.

Brigance, A. H. (1999). *Brigance Comprehensive Inventory of Basic Skills—Revised.* North Billerica, MA: Curriculum Associates.

Brigance, A. H. (2004). *Brigance Inventory of Early Development—II.* North Billerica, MA: Curriculum Associates.

Brock, S. E., Jimerson, S. R., & Hansen, R. L. (2006). *Identifying, assessing, and treating autism in school.* New York: Springer.

Brody, G. H., & Flor, D. L. (1997). Maternal psychological functioning, family processes, and child adjustment in rural, single-parent, African American families. *Developmental Psychology, 33*(6), 1000–1011.

Brody, G. H., Flor, D. L., & Gibson, N. M. (1999). Linking maternal efficacy, beliefs, developmental goals, parenting practices, and child competence in rural single-parent African American families. *Child Development, 70*((5), 1197–1208.

Bronfenbrenner, U. (1977). Toward an experimental ecology of human development. *American Psychologist, 32*, 513–531.

Bronfenbrenner, U. (1979). *The ecology of human development: Experiments by nature and design*. Cambridge, MA: Harvard University Press.

Brook, S., & Bowler, D. (1992). Autism by another name? Semantic and pragmatic deficits in children. *Journal of Autism and Developmental Disorders, 22*(1), 61–81.

Brookhart, S. M. (1998). Test review of the Iowa Test of Basic Skills, Forms K, L, M (ITBS). From J. C. Impara & B. S. Plake (Eds.), *The thirteenth mental measurements yearbook* [Electronic version]. Retrieved from http://web5.silverplatter.com/webspirs/start.ws?customer=waldo&databases=(YB)

Brooks-Gunn, J., & Duncan, G. J. (1997). The effects of poverty on children. *The Future of Children, 7*(2), 55–71.

Brown, R. (1973). *A first language: The early stages*. Cambridge, MA: Harvard University Press.

Brown, R., Cazden, C., & Bellugi, U. (1969). The child's grammar from I to III. In J. P. Hill (Ed.), *Minnesota Symposium on Child Psychology* (Vol. 2, pp. 28–73). Minneapolis: University of Minnesota Press.

Brownell, R. (Ed.). (2000a). *Expressive One-Word Picture Vocabulary Test—2000 Edition*. Novato, CA: Academic therapy.

Brownell, R. (Ed.). (2000b). *Receptive One-Word Picture Vocabulary Test—2000 Edition*. Novato, CA: Academic therapy.

Bruner, J. (1960). *The process of education*. Cambridge, MA: Harvard University Press.

Bruner, J. (1983a). *Child's talk: Learning to use language*. New York: Norton.

Bruner, J. (1983b). Interaction, communication, and self. *Journal of the American Academy of Child Psychiatry, 23*(1), 1–7.

Bryan, T. (1986). A review of studies on learning-disabled children's communicative competence. In R. L. Schiefelbusch (Ed.), *Language Competence assessment and intervention* (pp. 227–259). Austin, TX: Pro-Ed.

Bryant, D. M., Clifford, R. M., & Peisner, E. S. (1991). Best practices for beginners: Developmental appropriateness in kindergarten. *American Educational Research Journal, 28*, 783–803.

Bryant, D. M., & Graham, M. A. (Eds.). (1993). *Implementing early intervention*. New York: Guilford Press.

Bryson, S. E., & Smith, I. M. (1998). Epidemiology of autism: Prevalence, associated characteristics, and implications for research and service delivery. *Mental Retardation and Developmental Disabilities Research Reviews, 4*, 97–103.

Buckhalt, J. A. (1991). Test reviews: Wechsler Preschool and Primary Scale of Intelligence—Revised. *Journal of Psychoeducational Assessment, 9*, 271–279.

Bugental, D., Mantyla, S., & Lewis, J. (1989). Parental attributions as moderators of affective communication to children at risk for physical abuse. In D. Cicchetti & V. Carlson (Eds.), *Child maltreatment: Theory and research on the causes and consequences of child abuse and neglect* (pp. 254–279). New York: Cambridge University Press.

Burack, J. A. (1990). Differentiating mental retardation. In R. M. Hodapp, J A. Burack, & E. Zigler (Eds.), *Issues in the developmental approach to mental retardation* (pp. 27–48). New York: Cambridge University Press.

Burchinal, M. R., Peisner-Feinberg, E., Pianta, R., & Howes, C. (2002). Development of academic skills from preschool through second grade: Family and classroom predictors of developmental trajectories. *Journal of School Psychology, 40*, 415–436.

Burchinal, M. R., Roberts, J. E., Riggins, R., Zeisel, S. A., Neebe, E., & Bryant, D. (2000). Relating quality of center-based child care to early cognitive and language development longitudinally. *Child Development, 71*, 338–357.

Burger, R., & Warren, R. (1998). Possible immunogenetic basis for autism. *Mental Retardation and Developmental Disabilities Research Review, 4*, 137–141.

Byrd, R. S., Weitzman, M., & Auinger, P. (1997). Increased behavior problems associated with delayed school entry and delayed school progress. *Pediatrics, 100*(4), 654–661.

Cabrera, N. J., Ryan, R. M., Shannon, J. D., Brooks-Gunn, J., Vogel, C., Raikes, H., et al. (2004). Low-income fathers' involvement in their toddlers' lives: Biological fathers from the Early Head Start Research and Evaluation Study. *Fathering, 2*(1), 5–36.

Cabrera, N. J., Tamis-LeMonda, C. S., Bradley, R.

H., Hofferth, S., & Lamb, M. F. (2000). Fatherhood in the twenty-first century. *Child Development*, *71*, 127–136.

Caldwell, B. (1951). Test behavior observation guide. In R. Watson (Ed.), *The clinical method in psychology* (pp. 67–71). New York: Harper & Brothers.

Caldwell, B., & Bradley, R. (1984). *Home Observation for Measurement of the Environment (HOME)*. Little Rock: University of Arkansas.

Caldwell, B. M., & Bradley, R. H. (2003). *Home Observation for Measurement of the Environment (HOME): Administration manual*. Little Rock: University of Arkansas.

Calfee, R. C., & Hiebert, E. H. (1991). Classroom assessment of literacy. In R. Barr, M. Kamil, P. Mosenthal, & P. D. Pearson (Eds.), *Handbook of research on reading* (Vol. 2, pp. 281–309). New York: Longman.

California Department of Developmental Services. (2002). *Autistic spectrum disorders: Best practice guidelines for screening, diagnosis, and assessment*. Sacramento: Author.

Campbell, S. B. (2002). *Behavior problems in preschool children: Clinical and developmental issues* (2nd ed.). New York: Guilford Press.

Campbell, S. B., & Ewing, L. J. (1990). Follow-up of hard-to-manage preschoolers: Adjustment at age 9 and predictors of continuing symptoms. *Journal of Child Psychology and Psychiatry*, *31*(6), 871–889.

Canada's census information. (n.d.). Retrieved from www.12.sttcan.ca/english/census01

Cantor, A. (1995). Best practices in developing local norms in behavioral assessment. In A. Thomas & J. Grimes (Eds.), *Best practices in school psychology III*. Bethesda, MD: National Association of School Psychologists.

Cantrell, M. L., & Cantrell, R. P. (1985). Assessment of the natural environment. *Education and Treatment of Children*, *8*, 275–295.

Caplan, R. (1994). Communication deficits in childhood schizophrenia spectrum disorders. *Schizophrenia Bulletin*, *20*(4), 671–683.

Capps, L., Sigman, M., & Mundy, P. (1994). Attachment security in children with autism. *Development and Psychopathology*, *6*(2), 249–261.

Capute, A., Derivan, A. J., Chauvel, P., & Rodriguez, A. (1975). Infantile autism: A prospective study of the diagnosis. *Developmental Medicine and Child Neurology*, *17*, 58–63.

Carey, K. T. (2001). Test review of the Caregiver–Teacher Report Form (C-TRF). In B. S. Plake & J. C. Impara (Eds.), *The fourteenth mental measurements yearbook* [Electronic version]. Retrieved from http://web5.silverplatter.com/webspirs/start.ws?customer=waldo&databases=(YB)

Carlson, G. A. (1984). Classification issues of bipolar disorders in childhood. *Psychiatric Developments*, *2*, 273–285.

Carlson, G. A., Loney, J., Salisbury, H., Kramer, J., & Arthur, C. (2000). Stimulant treatment in young boys with symptoms suggesting childhood mania: A report from a longitudinal study. *Journal of Child and Adolescent Psychopharmacology*, *10*, 175–184.

Carlton, M., & Winsler, A. (1999). School readiness: The need for a paradigm shift. *School Psychology Review*, *28*(3), 338–352.

Carnine, D. W., Silbert, J., & Kame'enui, E. J. (1997). *Direct instruction reading* (3rd ed.). Upper Saddle River, NJ: Prentice-Hall.

Carpenter, C. D. (1992). Test review of the Stanford Early School Achievement Test-Third Edition (SESAT). From J. J. Kramer & J. C. Conoley (Eds.), *The eleventh mental measurements yearbook* [Electronic version]. Retrieved from http://web5s.silverplatter.com.arugula.cc.columbia.edu:2048/webspirs/start.ws?customer=waldo&databases=YB

Carr, J. (1988). Six weeks to twenty-one years old: A longitudinal study of children with Down's syndrome and their families. *Journal of Child Psychology and Psychiatry*, *21*, 407–431.

Carroll, J. M., Snowling, M. J., Hulme, C., & Stevenson, J. (2003). The development of phonological awareness in preschool children. *Developmental Psychology*, *39*, 311–335.

Carrow-Woolfolk, E. (1999). *Test of Auditory Comprehension of Language (TACL-3): Examiner's manual*. Austin, TX: PRO-ED.

Carta, J. J., Greenwood, C. R., & Atwater, J. (1985). *Ecobehavioral System for Complex Assessment of the Preschool Environment: ESCAPE*. Kansas City: Juniper Gardens Children's Project, University of Kansas.

Carter, A. S., & Briggs-Gowan, M. J. (2000). *Manual of the Infant–Toddler Social–Emotional Assessment*. New Haven, CT: Yale University.

Carter, A. S., Volkmar, F. R., Sparrow, S. S., Wang, J., Lord, C., Dawson, G., et al. (1998). The Vineland Adaptive Behavior Scales: Supplementary norms for individuals with autism. *Journal of Autism and Developmental Disorders*, *28*(4), 287–302.

Carter, B., & McGoldrick, M. (1989). Overview of the changing family life cycle: A framework for family therapy. In B. Carter & M. McGoldrick (Eds.), *The changing family life cycle: A frame-*

work for family therapy (2nd ed., pp. 3–28). Needham Heights, MA: Allyn & Bacon.

Casby, M. W. (1997). Symbolic play of children with language impairment: A critical review. *Journal of Speech and Hearing Research, 40,* 468–479.

Casey, A., & Howe, K. (2002). Best practices in early literacy skills. In A. Thomas & J. Grimes (Eds.), *Best practices in school psychology IV* (pp. 721–735). Bethesda, MD: National Association of School Psychologists.

Cassidy, D. J., Hestenes, L. L., Hegde, A., Hestenes, S., & Mims, S. (2005). Measurement of quality in preschool child care classrooms: An exploratory and confirmatory factor analysis of the Early Childhood Environment Rating Scale-Revised. *Early Childhood Research Quarterly, 20*(3), 345–360.

Castro, M., Mendez, J. L., & Fantuzzo, J. (2002). A validation study of the Penn Interactive Peer Play Scale with urban Hispanic and African American preschool children. *School Psychology Quarterly, 17*(2), 109–127.

Catts, H. W. (1991). Early identification of dyslexia: Evidence from a follow-up study of speech–language impaired children. *Annals of Dyslexia, 41,* 163–177.

Cazden, C. (1965). *Environmental assistance to the child's acquisition of grammar.* Unpublished doctoral dissertation, Harvard University.

Chafouleas, S. M., & Martens, B. K. (2002). Accuracy-based phonological awareness tasks: Are they reliable, efficient, and sensitive to growth? *School Psychology Quarterly, 17,* 128–147.

Chafouleas, S. M., Lewandowski, L. J., Smith, C. R., & Blachman, B. A. (1997). Phonological awareness skills in children: Examining performance across tasks and ages. *Journal of Psychoeducational Assessment, 15,* 334–347.

Chakrabarti, S., & Fombonne, E. (2001). Pervasive developmental disorders in preschool children. *Journal of the American Medical Association, 285,* 3093–3099.

Chakrabarti, S., & Fombonne, E. (2005). Pervasive developmental disorders in preschool children: Confirmation of high prevalence. *American Journal of Psychiatry, 162,* 1133–1141.

Chan, S., & Lee, E. (2004). Families with Asian roots. In E. W. Lynch & M. J. Hanson (Eds.), *Developing cross-cultural competence: A guide for working with children and their families* (3rd ed., pp. 219–298). Baltimore: Brookes.

Chapman, R. S. (1981). Exploring children's communicative intents. In J. F. Miller (Ed.), *Assessing language production in children* (pp. 111–136). Needham Heights, MA: Allyn & Bacon.

Chesebrough, E., King, P., Gullota, T. P., & Bloom, M. (Eds.). (2004). *A blueprint for the promotion of prosocial behavior in early childhood.* New York: Kluwer Academic/Plenum.

Children's Defense Fund (CDF). (1993). Economic plight crushes young families. *CDF Reports, 13*(6), 1–3.

Children's Defense Fund (CDF). (1994). Living in fear. *CDF Reports, 15*(2), 1,2.

Chittenden, E. (1991). Authentic assessment evaluation and documentation of student performance. In V. Perrone (Ed.), *Expanding student assessment* (pp. 22–31). Alexandria, VA: Association for Supervision and Curriculum Development.

Chittooran, M. M. (2001). Review of the High/Scope Child Observation Record for Ages 2½–6. In J. C. Impara (Ed.), *The fourteenth mental measurements yearbook.* Lincoln, NE: University of Nebraska Press.

Chomsky, N. (1965). *Aspect of the theory of syntax.* Cambridge, MA: MIT Press.

Chomsky, N. (1988). *Language and problems of knowledge.* Cambridge, MA: MIT Press.

Christensen, A., & Margolin, G. (1988). Conflict and alliance in distressed and non-distressed families. In R. Hinde & J. Stevenson-Hinde (Eds.), *Relationships within families: Mutual influences* (pp. 263–282). Oxford: Oxford University Press.

Christenson, S. L., & Ysseldyke, J. E. (1989). Assessing student performance: An important change is needed. *Journal of School Psychology, 27,* 409–425.

Christian, C. W. (1999). Child abuse and neglect. In J. A. Silver, B. J. Amster, & T. Haecker (Eds.), *Young children and foster care* (pp. 195–212). Baltimore: Brookes.

Ciadella, P., & Mamelle, N. (1989). An epidemiological study of infantile autism in a French department (Rhone): A research note. *Journal of Child Psychology and Psychiatry, 30,* 165–175.

Cicchetti, D., & Sroufe, L. A. (1978). An organizational view of affect: Illustration from the study of Down's syndrome infants. In M. Lewis & L. A. Rosenblum (Eds.), *The development of affect* (Vol. 1, pp. 309–350). New York: Plenum Press.

Cicchetti, D., Toth, S. L., & Rogosch, F. A. (1999). The efficacy of toddler—parent psychotherapy to increase attachment security in offspring of depressed mothers. *Attachment and Human Development, 1,* 34–66.

Cisero, C. A., & Royer, J. M. (1995). The development of cross-language transfer of phonological awareness. *Contemporary Educational Psychology*, *20*(3), 275–303.

Cizek, G. J. (2001). Review of the Developmental Indicators for the Assessment of Learning, 3rd ed. In B.S. Plake & J. C. Impara (Eds.) *The Fourteenth mental measurements yearbook*, pp. 394-398. Lincoln, NE: Buros Institute of Mental Measurements.

Cizek, G. J. (2003). Test review of the Woodcock-Johnson Tests of Achievement—Preschool Cluster, Third Edition (WJ-III). From B. S. Plake, J. C. Impara, & R. A. Spies (Eds.), *The fifteenth mental measurements yearbook* [Electronic version]. Retrieved from http://web5s.silverplatter.com.arugula.cc.columbia.edu:2048/webspirs/start.ws?customer=waldo&databases=YB

Clark, D., Cornelius, J., Wood, D., & Vanyukov, M. (2004). Psychopathology risk transmission in children of parents with substance use disorders. *American Journal of Psychiatry*, *161*, 685–691.

Clay, M. M. (1966). *Emergent reading behaviour.* Unpublished doctoral dissertations, University of Auckland, Auckland, New Zealand.

Clay, M. M. (1972). *Concepts about Print Test: Stones.* Exeter, NH: Heinemann.

Clay, M. M. (1979). *The early detection of reading difficulties* (3rd ed.). Portsmouth NH: Heinemann.

Clay, M. M. (2002). *An Observation Survey of Early Literacy Achievement* (2nd ed.). Portsmouth, NH: Heinemann.

Coggins, T., & Carpenter, R. (1981). The Communicative Intention Inventory. *Journal of Applied Psycholinguistics*, *2*, 213–234.

Coggins, T., Olswang, L., & Guthrie, J. (1987). Assessing communicative intents in young children: Low structured observation or elicitation tasks. *Journal of Speech and Hearing Disorders*, *52*(1), 1–25.

Cohen, D., Stern, V., & Balaban, N. (1997). *Observing and recording the behavior of young children* (4th ed.). New York: Teachers College Press.

Cohen, J. (1960). A coefficient of agreement for nominal scales. *Educational and Psychological Measurement*, *20*, 37–46.

Cole, L. (1985). *Nonstandard English: Handbook for assessment and instruction.* Silver Springs, MD: Author.

Cole, P. M., Michel, M. K., & Teti, L. O. (1994). The development of emotion regulation and dysregulation: A clinical perspective. In N. A. Fox (Ed.), The development of emotion regulation: Biological and behavioral considerations. *Monographs of the Society for Research in Child Development*, *59*(2–3, Serial No. 240), 73–100.

Cole, P. R. (1982). *Language disorders in preschool children.* Englewood Cliffs, NJ: Prentice-Hall.

Coleman, J. M., & Dover, G. M. (1989). *Rating Instrument for Screening Kindergarteners.* Austin, TX: PRO-ED.

Coleman, J. M., & Dover, G. M. (1993). The Risk Screening Test: Using kindergarten teachers' ratings to predict future placement in resource classrooms. *Exceptional Children*, *59*, 468–477.

Collier, C. (1988). *Assessing minority students with learning and behavior problems.* Lindale, TX: Hamilton.

Commissioner's Office of Research and Evaluation & Head Start Bureau. (2001a). *Building their futures: How Early Head Start programs are enhancing the lives of infants and toddlers in low-income families.* Washington, DC: U.S. Department of Health and Human Services.

Commissioner's Office of Research and Evaluation & Head Start Bureau. (2001b, January). *Head Start FACES: Longitudinal findings on program performance: Third progress report.* Washington, DC: U.S. Department of Health & Human Services.

Conn, P. (1993). The relations between Griffiths scales assessments in the preschool period and educational outcomes at seven plus years. *Child: Care, Health and Development*, *19*, 275–289.

Connell, C. M., & Prinz, R. J. (2002). The impact of childcare and parent–child interactions on school readiness and social skills development for low-income African American children. *Journal of School Psychology*, *40*, 177–193.

Conners, C. K. (1989). *Conners' Rating Scales.* North Tonawanda, NY: Multi-Health Systems.

Conners, C. K. (1997). *Conners' Rating Scales—Revised.* North Tonawanda, NY: Multi-Health Systems.

Cook, E. H., Jr. (1998). Genetics of autism. *Mental Retardation and Developmental Disabilities Research Reviews*, *4*, 113–120.

Cook, E. T., Greenberg, M. T., & Kusche, C. A. (1994). The relations between emotional understanding, intellectual functioning, and disruptive behavior problems in elementary school-aged children. *Journal of Abnormal Child Psychology*, *22*(2), 205–219.

Coolahan, K., Fantuzzo. J., Mendez, J., & McDermott, P. (2000). Preschool peer interactions and readiness to learn: Relationships between classroom peer play and learning behaviors and conduct. *Journal of Educational Psychology, 92*(3), 458–465.

Coplan, J. (1993). *Early Language Milestone Scale—Second Edition (ELM Scale-2)*. Austin, TX: PRO-ED.

Cost, Quality, and Outcomes Study Team. (1995). *Cost, quality and child outcomes in child care centers*. Denver: University of Colorado.

Costenbader, V., Rohrer, A. M., & Difonzo, N. (2000). Kindergarten screening: A survey of current practice. *Psychology in the Schools, 37*, 323–332.

Cowan, P. A., & Cowan, C. P. (2003). Normative family transitions, normal family processes, and healthy child development. In F. Walsh (Ed.), *Normal family processes* (3rd ed., pp. 424–459). New York: Guilford Press.

Cowen, E. L., Hightower, A. D., Pedro-Carroll, J. L., Work, W. C., Wyman, P. A., & Haffey, W. G. (1996). *School-based prevention for children at risk: The primary mental health project*. Washington, DC: American Psychological Association.

Cox, A., Klein, K., Charman, T., Baird, G., Baron-Cohen, S., Swettenham, J., et al. (1999). Autism spectrum disorders at 20 and 42 months of age: Stability of clinical and ADI-R diagnosis. *Journal of Child Psychology and Psychiatry, 40*, 719–732.

Cox, J. R. (1985). Test review of the Lindamood Auditory Conceptualization Test-Revised (LACT). From J. V. Mitchell, Jr. (Ed.), *The ninth mental measurements yearbook* [Electronic version]. Retrieved from http://web5s.silverplatter.com.arugula.cc.columbia.edu:2048/webspirs/start.ws?customer=waldo&databases=YB

Coyne, M. D., & Harn, B. A. (2006). Promoting beginning reading success through meaningful assessment of early literacy skills. *Psychology in the Schools, 43*, 33–43.

Crais, E. R. (1990). World knowledge to word knowledge. *Topics in Language Disorders, 10*(3), 45–62.

Cravioto, J., & DiLicardie, E. (1972). Environmental correlates of severe clinical malnutrition and language development in survivors of kwashiorkor or marasmus. In *Nutrition: The nervous system and behavior* (Scientific Publication No. 251, pp. 73–94). Washington, DC: Pan-American Health Organization.

Crehan, K. (2005). Review of the Test of Early Mathematics Ability—Third Edition. In R. Spies & B. Plake (Eds.), *The sixteenth mental measurements yearbook*. Retrieved from EBSCO Mental Measurements Yearbook database.

Crespo, D. (1998). Test review of Child Developmental Inventory (CDI). From J. C. Impara & B. S. Plake (Eds.), *The thirteenth mental measurements yearbook* [Electronic version]. Retrieved from http://web5s.silverplatter.com.arugula.cc.columbia.edu:2048/webspirs/start.ws?customer=waldo&databases=YB

Crimmins, D. B., Durand, V. M., Theurer-Kaufman, K., & Everett, J. (2001). *Austism program quality indicators: A self-review and quality improvement guide for schools and programs serving students with autism spectrum disorders*. Albany: New York State Department of Education.

Crittenden, P. M. (1989). Teaching maltreated children in the preschool. *Topics in Early Childhood Education, 9*, 16–32.

Crnic, K. A., Hoffman, C., Gaze, C., & Edelbrock, C. (2004). Understanding the emergence of behavior problems in young children with developmental delays. *Infants and Young Children, 17*, 223–235.

Crnic, K. A., & Leconte, J. M. (1986). Understanding sibling needs and influences. In R. R. Fewell & P. F. Vadasy (Eds.), *Families of handicapped children: Needs and supports across the life span* (pp. 75–98). Austin, TX: PRO-ED.

Crockett, D. (2003). Critical issues children face in the 2000s. *School Psychology Quarterly, 18*, 446–453.

Croen, L., Grether, J., Hoogstrate, J., & Selvin, S (2002). The prevalence of autism: Is it increasing? *Journal of Autism and Developmental Disorders, 32*, 207–215.

Cronbach, L. J. (1951). *Essentials of psychological testing*. New York: Harper & Row.

Cross, L. H. (1998). Test review of the Iowa Test of Basic Skills, Forms K, L, M (ITBS). From J. C. Impara & B. S. Plake (Eds.), *The thirteenth mental measurements yearbook* [Electronic version]. Retrieved from http://web5.silverplatter.com/webspirs/start.ws?customer=waldo&databases=(YB)

Cross, T. G. (1984). Habilitating the language-impaired child: Ideas from studies of parent–child interaction. *Topics in Language Disorders, 4*(4), 1–14.

Cryer, D. (1999). Defining and assessing early childhood program quality. *Annals of the American Academy of Political and Social Science, 563*, 39–55.

Cummings, E. M., Keller, P. S., & Davies, P. T. (2005). Towards a family process model of maternal and paternal depressive symptoms: Exploring multiple relations with child and family functioning. *Journal of Child Psychology and Psychiatry, 46*(5), 479–489.

Cummins, J. (1976). The influence of bilingualism on cognitive growth: A synthesis of research findings and explanatory hypotheses. *Working Papers on Bilingualism, 9*, 1–43.

Cummins, J. (1980). Psychological assessment of immigrant children: Logic or intuition. *Journal of Multilingual and Multicultural Development, 1*, 97–111.

Cummins, J. (1984). *Bilingualism and special education: Issues in assessment and pedagogy.* San Diego, CA: College-Hill Press.

Cummins, J. (2000). *Language, power, and pedagogy: Bilingual children in the crossfire.* Clevendon, England: Multilingual Matters.

Cunningham, C. C., Glen, S. M., Wilkinson, P., & Sloper, P. (1985). Mental ability, symbolic play, and receptive and expressive language of children with Down's syndrome. *Journal of Psychology and Psychiatry, 26*, 255–265.

Cutting, A. L., & Dunn, J. (1999). Theory of mind, emotion understanding, language, and family background: Individual differences and interrelations. *Child Development, 70*(4), 853–865.

Damico, J., & Oller, J. W., Jr. (1980). Pragmatic versus morphological/syntactic criteria for language referrals. *Language, Speech, and Hearing Services in Schools, 11*, 85–93.

Damico, J., Oller, J. W., Jr., & Storey, M. E. (1983). The diagnosis of language disorders in bilingual children: Surface-oriented and pragmatic criteria. *Journal of Speech and Hearing Disorders, 48*, 385–394.

Dauphinais, P., & King, J. (1992). Psychological assessment with American Indian children. *Applied and Preventive Psychology, 1*, 97–110.

Davis, E. A. (1938). Developmental changes in the distribution of parts of speech. *Child Development, 9*, 309–317.

Dawson, G., & Osterling, J. (1997). Early intervention in Autism: Effectiveness and common elements of current approaches. In M. J. Guralnick (Ed.), *The effectiveness of early intervention: Second generation research* (pp. 307–326). Baltimore: Brookes.

Dawson, M., & Knoff, H. M. (1990). Toward improved early childhood education: Perspectives. *Communiqué, 18*, 8–9.

Dayan, J. (1992). Opinion: Spanish version of DBM may resolve inequities in assessment of LEPs. *CASP Today, 42*(22), 23.

Dayan, J. (1993). Spanish curriculum based measurement: A solution to the problem of bias in the academic assessment of limited English proficient students, *NASP Communiqué, 21*(4), 3–4.

Deacon, S. A., & Piercy, F. P. (2001). Qualitative measures in family evaluation: Creative assessment techniques. *American Journal of Family Therapy, 29*, 355–373.

Dearing, E., Taylor, B. A., & McCartney, K. (2004). Implications of family income dynamics for women's depressive symptoms during the first 3 years after childbirth. *American Journal of Public Health, 94*(8), 1372–1377.

Deb, S., & Prasad, K. B. G. (1994). The prevalence of autistic disorder in children with learning disability. *British Journal of Psychiatry, 165*, 395–399.

deFur, S. H. (2001). Test review of the Test of Early Reading Ability, Third Edition (TERA-3). From J. C. Impara, B. S. Plake, & R. A. Spies (Eds.), *The fifteenth mental measurements yearbook* [Electronic version]. Retrieved from http://web5.silverplatter.com/webspirs/start.ws?customer=waldo&databases=(YB)

DeHirsch, K., Jansky, J., & Langford, W. S. (1966). *Predicting reading failure.* New York: Harper & Row.

DeLeon, I. G., & Itawa, B. A. (1996). Evaluation of a multiple-stimulas presentation format for assesing reinforcer preferences. *Journal of Applied Behavior Analysis, 29*, 519–532.

Delugach, R. R. (1991). Test reviews: Wechsler Preschool and Primary Scales of Intelligence—Revised. *Journal of Psychoeducational Assessment, 9*, 280–290.

Demchak, M. A., & Drinkwater, S. (1998). Assessing adaptive behavior. In H. B. Vance (Ed.), *Psychological assessment of children: Best practices for school and clinical settings* (2nd ed., pp. 297–322). New York: Wiley.

Denckla, M. B., & Rudel, R. G. (1976). Rapid "automatized" naming (R. A. N.): Dyslexia differentiated from other learning disabilities. *Neuropsychologia, 14*, 471–479.

Denham, S. A. (1998). *Emotional development in young children.* New York: Guilford Press.

Denham, S. A., Blair, K. A., DeMulder, E., Levitas, J., Sawyer, K., Auerbach-Major, S., et al. (2003). Preschool emotional competence: Pathway to social competence. *Child Development, 74*(1), 238–256.

Denham, S. A., & Burton, R. (1996). A socioemotional intervention program for at risk four-year-olds. *Journal of School Psychology, 34*, 225–245.

Denham, S. A., & Burton, R. (2003). *Social and*

emotional prevention and intervention programming for preschoolers*. New York: Kluwer Academic/Plenum.

Denham, S. A., & Couchoud, E. A. (1990). Young preschoolers' understanding of emotions. *Child Study Journal, 20*, 171–192.

Denham, S. A., McKinley, M., Couchoud, E. A., & Holt, R. (1990). Emotional and behavioral predictors of preschool peer ratings. *Child Development, 61*(4), 1145–1152.

Deno, S. L. (1987). Curriculum based measurement. *Teaching Exceptional Children, 20*(1), 41–42.

Deno, S. L. (1989). Curriculum-based measurement and special education services: A fundamental and direct relationship. In M. R. Shinn (Ed.), *Curriculum-based measurement: Assessing special children* (pp. 1–17). New York: Guilford Press.

de Villiers, J. G., & de Villiers, P. A. (1973). A cross-sectional study of the acquisition of grammatical morphemes in child speech. *Journal of Psycholinguistic Research, 2*, 267–278.

Diamond, L. J., & Jaudes, P. K. (1983). Child abuse in a cerebral-palsied population. *Developmental Medicine and Child Neurology, 25*, 169–174.

Dickenson, D. K., & Snow, C. E. (1987). Interrelationships among prereading and oral language skills in kindergartners from two social classes. *Early Childhood Research Quarterly, 2*(1), 1–25.

Dickenson, D. K., & Tabors, P. O. (1991). Early literacy: Linkages between home, school and literacy achievement at age five. *Journal of Research in Childhood Education, 6*, 30–46.

Dickenson, D. K., & Tabors, P. O. (Eds.). (2001). *Beginning literacy with language: Young children learning at home and school*. Baltimore: Brookes.

Diefendorf, A. O., Kessler, K. S., & Lindskog, R. (1992). Test review of the Test of Auditory Analysis Skills (TAAS). In J. J. Kramer & J. C. Conoley (Eds.), *The elecventh mental measurement yearbook* [Electronic version]. Retrieved from http://web5s.silverplatter.com.arugula.cc.columbia.edu:2048/webspirs/start.ws?customer=waldo&databases=YB

Dietz, K. R., Lavigne, J. V., Arend, R., & Rosenbaum, D. (1997). Relation between intelligence and psychopathology among preschoolers. *Journal of Clinical Psychology, 26*, 99–107.

DiPerna, J. C. (2001). Test review of theADHD Symptom Checklist—Fourth Edition. In B. S. Plake, J. C. Impara, & R. S. Spies (Eds.), *The fifteenth mental measurements yearbook* [Electronic version]. Retrieved from http://web5.silverplatter.com/webspirs/start.ws?customer=waldo&databases=(YB)

DiSimoni, F. (1978). *Token Test for Children*. Allen, TX: DLM Teaching Resources.

Dissanayake, C., Sigman, M., & Kasari, C. (1996). Long-term stability of individual differences in the emotional responsiveness of children with autism. *Journal of Child Psychology and Psychiatry, 37*(4), 461–467.

Dodd, B., Crosbie, S., McIntosh, B., Teitzel, T., & Ozanne, A. (2003). *Pre-Reading Inventory of Phonological Awareness (PIPA)*. San Antonio, TX: Psychological Corporation.

Doll, B., & Bolger, M. (2000). The family with a young child with disabilities. In M. J. Fine & R. L. Simpson (Eds.), *Collaboration with parents and families of children and youth with disabilities* (2nd ed., pp. 237–256). Austin, TX: PRO-ED.

Domitrovitch, C. E., Cortes, R., & Greenberg, M. T. (2002, June). *Preschool PATHS: Promoting social and emotional competence in young children*. Paper presented at the 6th National Head Start Research Conference, Washington, DC.

Downing, J. (1989). Identifying and enhancing the communicative behaviors of students with severe disabilities: The role of the school psychologist. *School Psychology Review, 18*(4), 475–486.

Downs, M., & Blager, F. B. (1982). The otitis prone child. *Journal of Developmental and Behavioral Pediatrics, 3*(2), 106–113.

Dreher, M., Nugent, J. K., & Hudgins, R. (1994). Prenatal marijuana exposure and neonatal outcomes in Jamaica: An ethnographic study. *Pediatrics, 93*, 254–260.

Duhl, F. J. (1981). The use of the chronological chart in general systems family therapy. *Journal of Marital and Family Therapy, 7*, 361–373.

Dulay, H., Hernandez-Chavez, E., & Burt, M. (1978). The process of becoming bilingual. In S. Singh & J. Lynch (Eds.), *Diagnostic procedures in hearing, speech, and language* (pp. 251–303). Baltimore: University Park Press.

Dumont, R., Cruse, C. L., Alfonso, V., & Levine, C. (2000). Basic review: Mullen Scales of Early Learning, AGS Edition. *Journal of Psychoeducational Assessment, 18*(4), 381–389.

Dumont-Mathieu, T., & Fein, D. (2005). Screening for autism in young children: The Modified Checklist for Autism in Toddlers (M-

CHAT) and other measures. *Mental Retardation and Developmental Disabilities Research Reviews*, *11*, 253–262.

Dumtschin, J. U. (1988). Recognizing language development and delay in early childhood. *Young Children*, *43*(3), 16–24.

Duncan, D. (Ed.). (1989). *Working with bilingual language disability.* New York: Chapman & Hall.

Dunn, J., & Hughes, C. (1998). Young children's understanding of emotions within close relationships. *Cognition and Emotion*, *12*(2), 171–190.

Dunn, L. M., & Dunn, L. M. (1997). *Peabody Picture Vocabulary Test—Third Edition.* Circle Pines, MN: American Guidance Service.

Dunst, C. J., Cooper, C. S., Weeldreyer, J. C., Snyder, K. D., & Chase, J. H. (1988). Family Needs Scale. In C. J. Dunst, C. M. Trivette, & A. G. Deal (Eds.), *Enabling and empowering families: Principles and guidelines for practice* (pp. 149–151). Cambridge, MA: Brookline Books.

Dunst, C. J., Jenkins, V., & Trivette, C. (1984). Family Support Scale: Reliability and validity. *Journal of Individual, Family, and Community Wellness*, *1*, 45–52.

Dunst, C. J., & Leet, H. E. (1987a). *Family Resource Scale (FRS).* Unpublished manual.

Dunst, C. J., & Leet, H. E. (1987b). Measuring the adequacy of resources in households with young children. *Child: Care, Health, and Development*, *13*(2), 111–125.

Dunst, C. J., McWilliam, R. A., & Holbert, K. (1986). Assessment of pre-school classroom environments. *Diagnostique*, *11*, 212–232.

Dunst, C. J., Trivette, C. M., & Deal, A. J. (Eds.). (1988). *Enabling and empowering families: Principles and guidelines for practice.* Cambridge, MA: Brookline Books.

Dunst, C. J., Trivette, C., Hamby, D., & Pollack, B. (1990). Family systems correlates of the behavior of young children with handicaps. *Journal of Early Intervention*, *14*, 204–218.

Durkin, M. S., & Stein, Z. A. (1996). Classification of mental retardation. In J. W. Jacobson & J. A. Mulick (Eds.), *Manual of diagnosis and professional practice in mental retardation* (pp. 67–73). Washington, DC: American Psychological Association.

Duvall, E. (1977). *Marriage and family development* (5th ed.). Philadelphia: Lippincott.

Dykens, E. M., Hodapp, R. M., Ort, S. I., & Leckman, J. F. (1993). Trajectory of adaptive behavior in males with fragile X syndrome. *Journal of Autism and Developmental Disorders*, *23*, 135–145.

Dyson, A. H., & Genishi, D. (1993). Visions of children as language users: Language and language education in early childhood. In B. Spodek (Ed.), *Handbook of research on the education of young children* (pp. 122–136). New York: Macmillan.

Easterbrooks, M. A., & Emde, R. N. (1988). Marital and parent–child relationships: The role of affect in the family system. In R. Hinde & J. Stevenson-Hinde (Eds.), *Relationships within families: Mutual influences* (pp. 83–102). Oxford: Oxford University Press.

Eastman Lukin, L. (2001). Test review of the Kindergarten Language Screening Test—Second Edition (KLST-2). In B. S. Plake & J. C. Impara (Eds.), *The fourteenth mental measurements yearbook* [Electronic version]. Retrieved from the Buros Institute's *Test Reviews Online* website: www.unl.edu/buros

Edelbrock, C. S., & Achenbach, T. M. (1984). The teacher version of the Child Behavior Profile: I. Boys aged 6–11. *Journal of Consulting and Clinical Psychology*, *52*(2), 207–217.

Education for All Handicapped Children Act of 1975, Pub. L. No. 94-142, 89 Stat. 773 (1975).

Education of the Handicapped Act Amendments of 1986, Pub. L. No. 99-457, 100 Stat. 1145 (1986).

Edwards, R., & Edwards, J. (1990). Review of The Instructional Environment Scale: A comprehensive methodology for assessing an individual student's environment. *Journal of Psychoeducational Assessment*, *8*, 204–208.

Egeland, B., & Erickson, M. F. (1990). Rising above the past: Strategies for helping new mothers break the cycle of abuse and neglect. *Zero to Three*, *11*(2), 29–35.

Egeland, B., & Farber, E. (1984). Infant–mother attachment: Factors related to development and change over time. *Child Development*, *55*(3), 753–771.

Egeland, B., Jacobvitz, P., & Papatola, K. (1987). Intergenerational continuity of parental abuse. In J. Lancaster & R. Gelles (Eds.), *Biosocial aspects of child abuse* (pp. 255–278). San Francisco: Jossey-Bass.

Eisenberg, N., & Fabes, R. A. (1998). Prosocial development. In W. Damon (Series Ed.) & N. Eisenberg (Vol. Ed.), *Handbook of child psychology: Vol. 3. Social, emotional, and personality development* (5th ed., pp. 701–778). New York: Wiley.

Elardo, R., Bradley, R., & Caldwell, B. M. (1975).

The relation of infants' home environments to mental test performance from 6 to 36 months: A longitudinal analysis. *Child Development*, *46*(1), 71–76.

Elliott, C. D. (1990). The nature and structure of children's abilities: Evidence from the Differential Ability Scales. *Journal of Psychoeducational Assessment*, *8*, 376–390.

Elliott, C. D. (2006). Differential Ability Scales—Second Edition (DAS-II). San Antonio, TX: Psychological Corporation.

Elliott, S. N., Busse, R. T., & Gresham, F. M. (1993). Behavior rating scales: Issues of use and development. *School Psychology Review, 22(2), 313–321.*

Ellis, R. (1981). The role of input in language acquisition: Some implications for second language teaching. *Applied Linguistics*, 2, 70–82.

Emde, R. N. (1992). Intimacy and the early moral self. *Infant Mental Health Journal*, *13*, 34–42.

Emde, R. N. (2003). Early narratives: A window to the child's inner world. In R. N. Emde, D. P. Wolf, & D. Oppenheim (Eds.), *Revealing the inner worlds of young children: The MacArthur Story Stem Battery and parent–child narratives* (pp. 3–26). New York: Oxford University Press.

Emde, R. N., Wolf, D. P., & Oppenheim, D. (2003). (Eds.), *Revealing the inner worlds of young children: The MacArthur Story Stem Battery and parent–child narratives*. New York: Oxford University Press.

Emery, K. E., & Laumann-Billings, L. (1998). An overview of the nature, causes, and consequences of abusive family relationships: Toward differentiating maltreatment and violence. *American Psychologist*, *53*, 121–135.

Emmons, M. R., & Alfonso, V. C. (2005). A critical review of the technical characteristics of current preschool screening batteries. *Journal of Psychoeducational Assessment*, *23*(2), 111–127.

Engfer, A. (1988). The interrelatedness of marriage and the mother–child relationship. In R. A. Hinde & J. Stevenson-Hinde (Eds.), *Relationships within families: Mutual influences* (pp. 104–118). Oxford: Oxford University Press.

Enhancing the outcomes of low-birth-weight, premature infants. A multisite, randomized trial. Infant Health and Development Program (1990). *Journal of the American Medical Association*, *263*(22), 3035–3042.

Erel, O., & Burman, B. (1995). Interrelatedness of marital relations and parent–child relations: A meta-analytic review. *Psychological Bulletin*, *118*, 108–132.

Erickson, D. (1992). Test review of the Questionnaire on Resources and Stress (QRS). In J. J. Kramer & J. C. Conoley (Eds.), *The eleventh mental measurements yearbook* [Electronic version]. Retrieved from http://web5.silverplatter.com/webspirs/start.ws?customer=waldo&databases=(YB)

Erickson, J. G., & Iglesias, A. (1986). Assessment of communication disorders in non-English proficient children. In O. Taylor (Ed.), *Nature of communication disorders in culturally and linguistically diverse populations* (pp. 181–217). San Diego, CA: College-Hill Press.

Erickson, M. T. (1998). Etiological factors. In T. H. Ollendick & M. Hersen (Eds.), *Handbook of child psychopathology* (3rd ed., pp. 37–62). New York: Plenum Press.

Esler, A. N., Godber, Y., & Christenson, S. L. (2002). Best practices in supporting home–school collaboration. In A. Thomas and J. Grimes (Eds.), Best practices in school psychology IV (pp. 389–411). Bethesda, MD: National Association of School Psychologists.

Espinosa, L. M. (2002). High-quality preschool: Why we need it and what it looks like. *NIEER Preschool Policy Matters, 1, 1-11.* Retrieved from http://nieer.org/resources/policy briefs/1.pdf.

Evans-Jones, L. G., & Rosenbloom, L. (1978). Disintegrative psychosis in childhood. *Developmental Medicine and Child Neurology*, *20*, 462–470.

Everston, C. M., & Green, J. L. (1986). Observation as inquiry and method. In M. C. Wittrock (Ed.), *Handbook of research on teaching* (3rd ed., pp. 162–213). New York: Macmillan.

Eyberg, S. M., & Boggs, S. R. (1998). Parent–child interaction therapy: A psychosocial intervention for the treatment of young conduct disordered children. In J. M. Briesmeister & C. S. Schaefer (Eds.), *Handbook of parent training: Parents as co-therapists for children's behavior problems* (2nd ed., pp. 61–97). New York: Wiley.

Faber, A., & Mazlish, E. (1980). *How to talk so kids will listen and listen so kids will talk*. New York: Avon Books.

Fabes, R. A., Eisenberg, N., Nyman, M., & Michealieu, Q. (1991). Young children's appraisals of others' spontaneous emotional reactions. *Developmental Psychology*, *27*(5), 858–866.

Fagan, J., & Iglesias, A. (1999). Father involvement program effects on father, father figures, and their Head Start children: A quasi-experimental study. *Early Childhood Research Quarterly*, *14*(2), 243–269.

Fagan, J., & Stevenson, H. C. (2002). An experimental study of an empowerment-based intervention for African American Head Start fathers. *Family Relations: Journal of Applied Family Studies, 51*(3), 191–198.

Fairbank, D. W. (2001a). Review of the Developmental Indicators for the Assessment of Learning, Third Edition. In B. S. Plake & J. C. Impara (Eds.), *The fourteenth mental measurements yearbook* (pp. 398-400). Lincoln, NE: Buros Institute of Mental Measurements.

Fairbank, D. W. (2001b). Test review of the Receptive One-Word Picture Vocabulary Test 2000 Edition (ROWPVT). In J. C. Impara, B. S. Plake, & R. A. Spies (Eds.), *The fifteenth mental measurements yearbook* [Electronic version]. Retrieved from the Buros Institute's *Test Reviews Online* website: www.unl.edu/buros

Fairbank, D. W. (2005). Test review of the Preschool and Kindergarten Behavior Scales-2 (PKBS-2). In R. A. Spies & B. S. Plake (Eds.), *The sixteenth mental measurements yearbook* [Electronic version]. Retrieved from http://web5.silverplatter.com.arugula.cc.columbia.edu:2048/webspirs/start.ws?customer=waldo&databases=(YB)

Fan, X., & Chen, M. (2001). Parental involvement and student's academic achievement: A meta-analysis. *Educational Psychology Review, 13*, 1–22.

Fantini, A. (1985). *Language acquisition of a bilingual child: A socio-linguistic perspective.* San Diego, CA: College Hill Press.

Fantuzzo, J. W. (1990). Behavioral treatment of the victims of child abuse and neglect. *Behavior Modification, 14*(3), 316–339.

Fantuzzo, J. W., Blue-Sky, R., McDermott, P., Muscat, S., & Lutz, M. N. (2003). A multivariate analysis of emotional and behavioral adjustment in preschool educational outcomes. *School Psychology Review, 32*(2), 185–203.

Fantuzzo, J. W., Coolahan, K. C., & Manz, P. H. (1996). *Penn Interactive Peer Play Scale (PIPPS): A measure for evaluating peer interactions and informing classroom intervention.* Poster presented at the Head Start Third National Research Conference, Washington, DC.

Fantuzzo, J., Coolahan, K., Mendez, J., McDermott, P., & Sutton-Smith, B. (1998). Contextually-relevant validation of peer play constructs with African American Head Start children: Penn Interactive Play Scale. *Early Childhood Research Quarterly, 13*, 411–431.

Fantuzzo, J. W., De Paola, L. M., Lambert, L., Anderson, G., & Sutton, S. (1991). Effects of interparental violence on the psychology of adjustment and competencies of young children. *Journal of Consulting and Clinical Psychology, 59*, 1–8.

Fantuzzo, J. W., & McWayne, C. (2002). The relationship between peer-play interactions in the family context and dimensions of school readiness for low-income preschool children. *Journal of Educational Psychology, 94*, 79–87.

Fantuzzo, J., Mendez, J., & Tighe, E. (1998). Parental assessment of peer play: Development and validation of the parent version of the Penn Interactive Peer Play Scale. *Early Childhood Research Quarterly, 13*, 659-676.

Fantuzzo, J., & Sutton-Smith, B. (1994). *Play buddy project: A preschool-based intervention to improve the social effectiveness of disadvantaged, high-risk children.* Washington, DC: U.S. Department of Health and Human Services.

Fantuzzo, J. W., Sutton-Smith, B., Coolahan, K. C., Manz, P. H., Canning, S., & Debnam, D. (1995). Assessment of preschool play interaction behaviors in young low-income children: Penn Interactive Peer Play Scale. *Early Childhood Research Quarterly, 10*, 105–120.

Fedoruk, G. M., & Norman, C. A. (1991). Kindergarten screening predictive inaccuracy: First-grade variability. *Exceptional Children, 57*, 258–263.

Feldman, R., & Greenbaum, C. W. (1997). Affect regulation and synchrony in mother–infant play as precursors to the development of symbolic competence. *Infant Mental Health Journal, 18*, 4–23.

Felton, R. H. (1992). Early identification of children at risk for reading disabilities. *Topics in Early Childhood Special Education, 12*(2), 212–229.

Felton, R. H., & Pepper, P. P. (1995). Early identification and intervention of phonological deficit in kindergarten and early elementary children at risk for reading disability. *School Psychology Review, 24*, 405–414.

Fenson, L., Dale, P. S., Reznick, J. S., Bates, E., Thal, D. J., & Pethick, S. P. (1994). Variability in early communicative development. *Monographs of the Society for Research in Child Development, 59*(5, 1–189, Serial No. 242).

Fenton, R. (2005). Review of the Test of Phonological Awareness—Second Edition PLUS. In R. A. Spies & B. S. Plake (Eds.), *The sixteenth mental measurements yearbook.* Retrieved from EBSCO Mental Measurements Yearbook database.

Ferrell, K. A., Trief, E., Dietz, S. J., Bonner, M. A., Cruz, D., Ford, E., et al. (1990). Visually Impaired Infants Research Consortium (VIIRC): First-year results. *Journal of Visual Impairment and Blindness, 84*, 404–410.

Feuerstein, R., Feuerstein, R., & Gross, S. (1997). The Learning Potential Assessment Device. In D. P. Flanagan, J. L. Genshaft, & P. L. Harrison (Eds.), *Contemporary intellectual assessment* (pp. 297–313). New York: Guilford Press.

Fewell, R. R. (1984). Assessment of preschool handicapped children. *Educational Psychologist, 19*(3), 172–179.

Fewell, R. R., Ogura, T., Notari-Sylverson, A., & Wheeden, C. A. (1997). The relationship between play and communication skills in young children with Down syndrome. *Topics in Early Childhood Special Education, 17*, 103–118.

Fiedler, D. J., & Hodapp, R. M. (1998). Importance of typologies for science and service in mental retardation. *Mental Retardation, 36*, 489–495.

Field, M., Fox, N., & Radcliffe, J. (1990). Predicting IQ change in preschoolers with developmental delays. *Journal of Developmental and Behavioral Pediatrics, 11*, 184–189.

Field, T. M. (1996). Expressivity in physically and emotionally handicapped children. In M. Lewis & M. W. Sullivan (Eds.), *Emotional development of atypical children* (pp. 1–27). Mahwah, NJ: Erlbaum.

Field, T. M., & Walden, T. A. (1982). Production and discrimination of facial expressions by preschool children. *Child Development, 53*(5), 1299–1311.

Figueroa, R. (1990). Best practices in the assessment of bilingual children. In A. Thomas & J. Grimes (Eds.), *Best practices in school psychology II* (pp. 93–106). Washington, DC: National Association of School Psychologists.

Filipek, P. A., Accardo, P. J., Baranek, G. T., Cook, E. H., Dawson, G., Gordon, B., et al. (1999). The screening and diagnosis of autistic spectrum disorders. *Journal of Autism and Developmental Disorders, 29*(6), 439–484.

Fine, M. J., & Carlson, C. (Eds.). (1992). *The handbook of family–school intervention: A systems perspective*. Needham Heights, MA: Allyn & Bacon.

Fine, M. J., & Nissenbaum, M. S. (2000). The child with disabilities and the family: Implications for professionals. In M. J. Fine & R. L. Simpson (Eds.), *Collaboration with parents and families of children and youth with exceptionalities* (2nd ed., pp. 3–26). Austin, TX: PRO-ED.

Finn, S. E. (1996). *Using the MMPI-2 as a therapeutic intervention*. Minneapolis: University of Minnesota Press.

Finn, S. E., & Tonsager, M. E. (1992). Therapeutic effects of providing MMPI-2 test feedback to college students awaiting psychotherapy. *Psychological Assessment, 3*, 278–287.

Fish, M. (2002). Best practices in collaborating with parents of children with disabilities. In A. Thomas & J. Grimes (Eds.), *Best practices in school psychology IV* (Vol. 1, pp. 363–376) Bethesda, MD: National Association of School Psychologists.

Fivush, R., & Vasudeva, A. (2002). Remembering to relate: Socioemotional correlates of mother–child reminiscing. *Journal of Cognition and Development, 3*(1), 73–90.

Flanagan, D. P. (1995). Test review of the Reynell Developmental Language Scales (RDLS). In J. C. Conoley & J. C. Impara, *The twelfth mental measurements yearbook* [Electronic version]. Retrieved from the Buros Institute's *Test Reviews Online* website: www.unl.edu/buros

Flanagan, D. P., & Alfonso, V. C. (1995). A critical review of the technical characteristics of recently revised intelligence tests for preschool children. *Journal of Psychoeducational Assessment, 13*, 66–90.

Flanagan, D. P., Alfonso, V. C., Kaminer, T., & Rader, D. E. (1995). Incidence of basic concepts in the directions of new and recently revised American intelligence tests for preschoolers. *School Psychology International, 16*, 345–364.

Flanagan, D. P., & Harrison, P. L. (Eds.). (2005). *Contemporary intellectual assessment* (2nd ed.). New York: Guilford Press.

Flanagan, D. P., & McGrew, K. S. (1997). A cross-battery approach to assessing and interpreting cognitive abilities: Narrowing the gap between practice and cognitive science. In D. P. Flanagan, J. L. Genshaft, & P. L. Harrison (Eds.), *Contemporary intellectual assessment* (pp. 314–325). New York: Guilford Press.

Flanagan, R. (2005). Review of the Achenbach System of Empirically Based Assessment (ASEBA). In R. A. Spies & B. S. Plake (Eds.), *The sixteenth mental measurement yearbook* [Electronic version]. Retrieved from http://web5.silverplatter.com.arugula.cc.columbia.edu:2048/webspirs/start.ws?customer=waldo&databases=(YB)

Fleischman, M., Horne, A., & Arthur, J. (1983). *Troubled families: A treatment program*. Champaign, IL: Research Press.

Fletcher, J. M., & Satz, P. (1982). Kindergarten prediction of reading achievement: A seven-year longitudinal follow-up. *Educational and Psychological Measurement, 42*(2), 681–685.

Flowerday, T. (2005). Review of Preschool Language Scale—Fourth Edition (PLS-4). From R. A. Spies & B. S. Plake (Eds.), *The sixteenth mental measurements yearbook* [Electronic version]. Retrieved from http://web4s.silverplatter.com.arugula.cc.columbia.edu:2048/webspirs/start.ws?customer=waldo&databases=YB

Fluharty, N. B. (2001). *Fluharty Preschool Speech and Language Screening Test—Second Edition*. Austin, TX: PRO-ED.

Flynn, J. R. (1984). The mean IQ of Americans: Massive gains 1932–1978. *Psychological Bulletin, 95*, 29–51.

Fombonne, E. (1999). The epidemiology of autism. *Psychological Medicine, 29*, 769–786.

Fombonne, E., du Mazaubrun, C., Cans, C., & Grandjean, H. (1997). Autism and associated medical disorders in a large French epidemiological survey. *Journal of the American Academy of Child and Adolescent Psychiatry, 36*, 1561–1569.

Ford, L. (1995). Test review of the Kaufman Survey of Early Academic and Language Skills (KSEALS). From J. C. Conoley & J. C. Impara (Eds.), *The twelfth mental measurements yearbook* [Electronic version]. Retrieved from http://web5s.silverplatter.com.arugula.cc.columbia.edu:2048/webspirs/start.ws?customer=waldo&databases=YB

Ford, L., & Dahinten, V. S. (2005). Use of intelligence tests in the assessment of preschoolers. In D. P. Flanagan & P. L. Harrison (Eds.), *Contemporary intellectual assessment* (2nd ed., pp. 487–503). New York: Guilford Press.

Forehand, R. L., & McMahon, R. J. (1981). *Helping the noncompliant child: A clinician's guide to parent training*. New York: Guilford Press.

Fox, N. A., Henderson, H. A., Rubin, K. H., Calkins, S. D., & Schmidt, L. A. (2001). Continuity and discontinuity of behavioral inhibition and exuberance: Psychophysiological and behavioral influences across the first four years of life. *Child Development*, 72, 1–21.

Fradd, S. H., & Weismantel, M. J. (Eds.). (1989). *Meeting the needs of culturally and linguistically different students: A handbook for educators*. Boston: College-Hill Press.

Fraiberg, S. (Ed.). (1983). *Clinical studies in infant mental health: The first year of life*. New York: Basic Books.

Frankenburg, W. K., Dodds, J., Archer, P., Bresnick, B., Maschka, P., Edelman, N., et al. (1990). *Denver Developmental Screening Test II*. Denver, CO: Denver Developmental Materials.

Freeman, B., Ritvo, E., Needleham, R., & Yokota, A. (1985). The stability of cognitive and linguistic parameters in autism: A five-year prospective study. *Journal of the American Academy of Child Psychiatry, 24*, 459–464.

Frick, P. J., Lacey, B. B., Applegate, B., Hedrick, L., Ollendick, T., Hynd, G. W., et al. (1994). DSM-IV field trials for the disruptive behavior disorders. *Journal of the American Academy of Child and Adolescent Psychiatry, 33*, 529–539.

Friedrich, W., Greenberg, M., & Crnic, K. (1983). A short form of the Questionnaire on Resources and Stress. *American Journal of Mental Deficiency, 88*(1), 41–48.

Frisby, C. (1987). Alternative assessment committee report: Curriculum-based assessment. *CASP Today, 36*, 1–15.

Frith, U. (1991). Asperger and his syndrome. In U. Frith (Ed.), *Autism and Asperger syndrome* (pp. 1–36). New York: Cambridge University Press.

Frith, U. (2003). *Autism: Explaining the enigma* (2nd ed.). Oxford: Blackwell.

Frith, U., & Baron-Cohen, S. (1987). Perception in autistic children. In D. J. Cohen, A. M. Donnellan, & R. Paul (Eds.). *Handbook of autism and pervasive developmental disorders* (pp. 85–102). New York: Wiley.

Fuchs, L. S., & Fuchs, D. (1986). Linking assessment to instructional intervention. *School Psychology Review, 15*, 318–323.

Furlong, M. (1995). Test review of the Social Skills Rating System (SSRS). From J. C. Conoley & J. C. Impara (Eds.), *The twelfth mental measurements yearbook* [Electronic version]. Retrieved from http://web5.silverplatter.com/webspirs/start.ws?customer=waldo&databases=(YB)

Furlong, M. (2001). Test review of the Caregiver-Teacher Report Form (C-TRF). In B. S. Plake & J. C. Impara (Eds.), *The fourteenth mental measurements yearbook* [Electronic version]. Retrieved from http://web5.silverplatter.com/webspirs/start.ws?customer=waldo&databases=(YB)

Furstenberg, F., Brooks-Gunn, J., & Morgan, S. P. (1987). *Adolescent mothers in later life*. New York: Cambridge University Press.

Gaddis, L. R. (1995). Test review of the Aberrant Behavior Checklist (ABC). In J. C. Conoley & J. C. Impara (Eds.), *The twelfth mental measurements yearbook* [Electronic version]. Retrieved from http://web5.silverplatter.com/webspirs/start.ws?customer=waldo&databases=(YB)

Gadow, K. D., & Sprafkin, J. (1997). *ADHD*

Symptom Checklist–4 (ADHD-SC4). Stony Brook, NY: Checkmate Plus.

Gadsden, V., & Bowman, P. (1999). African American males and the struggle toward responsible fatherhood. In V. Polite & J. Davis (Eds.), *A continuing challenge in times like these: African American males in schools and society.* New York: Teachers College Press.

Gadsden, V., Brooks, W., & Jackson, J. (1997, March). *African American fathers, poverty and learning: Issues in supporting children in and out of school.* Paper presented at the annual meeting of the American Eductional Research Association, Chicago, IL.

Gadsden, V., & Ray, A. (2003). Fathers' role in children's academic achievement and early literacy. *ERIC Digest: ERIC Clearinghouse on Early Education and parenting* (No. ED482051). Retrieved from www.ericdigests.org/2004–3/role.html

Gagné, R. M. (1965). *The condition of learning.* New York: Holt, Rinehart & Winston.

Gagné, R. M. (1978). Educational research and development: Past and future. In R. Glaser (Ed.), *Research and development and school change* (pp. 83–91). Hillsdale, NJ: Erlbaum.

Gagné, R. M. (1987). *Instructional technology: Foundations.* Hillsdale, NJ: Erlbaum.

Gagnon, S. G., & Nagle, R. J. (2004). Relationships between peer interactive play and Social competence in at-risk preschool children. *Psychology in the Schools, 41*, 173–189.

Gallagher, J. (1989). A new policy initiative: Infants and toddlers with handicapping conditions. *American Psychologist, 44*, 387–391.

Gallagher, T. M. (1983). Pre-assessment: A procedure for accommodating language use variability. In T. M. Gallagher & C. Prutting (Eds.), *Pragmatic assessment and intervention issues in language.* San Diego, CA: College-Hill Press.

Gallagher, T. M. (Ed.). (1991). *Pragmatics of language: Clinical practice issues.* San Diego, CA: Singular.

Gallagher, T. M., & Prutting, C. A. (Eds.). (1983). *Pragmatic assessment and intervention issues in language.* San Diego, CA: College-Hill Press.

Gallerani, D., O'Regan, M., & Reinherz, H. (1982). Prekindergarten screening: How well does it predict readiness for first grade? *Psychology in the Schools, 19*, 175–182.

Garcia, E. E. (1993). The education of linguistically and culturally diverse children. In B. Spodek (Ed.), *Handbook of research on the education of young children* (pp. 372–384). New York: Macmillan.

Garcia, G. E., & Pearson, P. D. (1991). The role of assessment in a diverse society. In E. H. Hiebert (Ed.), *Literacy for a diverse society* (pp. 253–278). New York: Teachers College Press.

Garshelis, J. A., & McConnell, S. R. (1993). Comparison of family needs assessed by mothers, individual professionals, and interdisciplinary teams. *Journal of Early Intervention, 17*, 36–49.

Gauthier, S., & Madison, C. (1998). *Kindergarten Language Screening Test—Second Edition (KLST-2).* Austin, TX: PRO-ED.

Geiger, D. M., Smith, D. T., & Creaghead, N. A. (2002). Parent and professional agreement on cognitive level of children with autism. *Journal of Autism and Developmental Disorders, 32*(4), 307–410.

Gelb, S. A. (2002). The dignity of humanity is not a scientific construct. *Mental Retardation, 40*, 55–56.

Geller, B., Bolhofner, K., Craney, J. L., Williams, M., Del Bello, M. P., & Gunderson, K. (2000). Psychosocial functioning in a prepubertal and early adolescent bipolar disorder phenotype. *Journal of the American Academy of Child and Adolescent Psychiatry, 39*(12), 1543–1548.

Genesee, F. (1976). The role of intelligence in second-language learning. *Language Learning, 26*, 267–280.

Genesee, F. (1987). *Learning through two languages: Studies of immersion and bilingual education.* Rowley, MA: Newbury House.

Genesee, F., Paradis, J., & Crago, M. B. (2004). *Dual-language development and disorders: A handbook on bilingualism and second-language learning.* Baltimore: Brookes.

Genishi, C. (Ed.). (1992). *Ways of assessing children and curriculum: Stories of early childhood practice.* New York: Teachers College Press.

German, D. J. (1983). I know it but I can't think of it: Word retrieval difficulties. *Academic Therapy, 18*, 539–545.

German, D. J. (1989). A diagnostic model and a test to assess word-finding skills in children. *British Journal of Disorders of Communication, 24*(1), 21–39.

German, D. J. (1991). *Test of Word Finding in Discourse.* Austin, TX: PRO-ED.

German, D. J. (2000). *Test of Word Finding—Second Edition (TWF-2).* Austin, TX: PRO-ED.

German, D. J., & Simon, E. (1991). Analysis of children's word-finding skills in discourse. *Journal of Speech and Hearing Research, 34*, 309–316.

Gersten, R., & Woodward, J. (1994). The language-minority student and special education: Issues, trends, and paradoxes. *Exceptional Children*, *60*(4), 310–322.

Gesell Institute of Human Development. (1982). *The gift of time: The developmental point of view*. New Haven, CT: Author.

Gilchrist, A., Green, J., Cox, A., Burton, D., Rutter, M., & Le Couteur, A. (2001). Development and current functioning in adolescents with Asperger syndrome: A comparative study. *Journal of Child Psychology and Psychiatry*, *42*(2), 227–240.

Gillberg, C. (1990). Autism and pervasive developmental disorders. *Journal of Child Psychology and Psychiatry, 331(1)*, 99–119.

Gillberg, C. (1992). Autism and autistic-like conditions: Subclasses among disorders of empathy. *Journal of Child Psychology and Psychiatry, 33*(5), 813–842.

Gillberg, C. (2002). *A guide to Asperger syndrome*. Cambridge, England: Cambridge University Press.

Gilliam, J. E. (1995). *Gilliam Autism Rating Scale (GARS)*. Austin, TX: PRO-ED.

Gilliam, J. E. (2005). *Gilliam Autism Rating Scale—Second Edition (GARS-2)*. Austin, TX: PRO-ED.

Gilliam, R. B. (1992). Test review of the Bankson Language Test-2. In J. J. Kramer & J. C. Conoley (Eds.), *The eleventh mental measurements yearbook* [Electronic version]. Retrieved from the Buros Institute *Test Reviews Online* website: www.unl.edu/Buros

Gillot, A., Furniss, F., & Walter, A. (2001). Anxiety in high functioning children with autism. *Autism*, *5*, 277–286.

Gimpel, G. A., & Holland, M. L. (2003). *Emotional and behavioral problems of young children: Effective interventions in the preschool and kindergarten years*. New York: Guilford Press.

Ginsburg, H. P. (1986). The myth of the deprived child: New thoughts on poor children. In U. Neisser (Ed.), *The school achievement of minority children: New perspectives* (pp. 169–189). Hillsdale, NJ: Erlbaum.

Ginsburg, H. P. (1997a). *Entering the child's mind*. New York: Teachers College Press.

Ginsburg, H. P. (1997b). Mathematics learning disabilities: A view from developmental psychology. *Journal of Learning Disabilities*, *30*, 20–33.

Ginsburg, H. P., & Baroody, A. J. (2003). *Test of Early Mathematics Ability—Third Edition*. Austin, TX: PRO-ED.

Gioia, G. A. (1993). Development and mental retardation. In R. Smith (Ed.). *Children with mental retardation: A parent's guide* (pp. 51–878). Rockville, MD: Woodbine House.

Gitlin-Weiner, K., Sandgrund, A., & Schaefer, C. (Eds.) (2000). *Play diagnosis and assessment* (2nd ed.). Hoboken, NJ: John Wiley & Sons.

Glascoe, F. P. (1991). Developmental screening: Rationale, methods, and application. *Infants and Young Children*, *4*(1), 1–10.

Glascoe, F. P. (2002). *Technical report for the Brigance Screens*. North Billerica, MA: Curriculum Associates.

Glascoe, F. P. (2005). *Technical Report for the Brigance Screens*. North Billerica, MA: Curriculum Associates.

Glascoe, F. P., & Byrne, K. E. (1993). The usefulness of the Battelle Developmental Inventory Screening Test. *Clinical Pediatrics, 32*, 273–280.

Glascoe, F. P., Byrne, K. E., Ashford, L. G., Johnson, K. L., Chang, B., & Strickland, B. (1992). Accuracy of the Denver–II in developmental screening. *Pediatrics, 89*, 1221–1225.

Glenn, H. W. (2001). Test review of the Attention Deficit Disorders Evaluation Scale—Second Edition (ADDES). In B. S. Plake & J. C. Impara (Eds.), *The fourteenth mental measurements yearbook* [Electronic version]. Retrieved from http://web5.silverplatter.com/webspirs/start.ws?customer=waldo&databases=(YB)

Glutting, J. J., & McDermott, P. A. (1988). Generality of test-session observations to kindergartners' classroom behavior. *Journal of Abnormal Child Psychology, 16*, 527–537.

Glutting, J. J., Oakland, T., & McDermott, P. A. (1989). Observing child behavior during testing: Constructs, validity, and situational generality. *Journal of School Psychology, 27*, 155–164.

Gnezda, M. T., & Bolig, R. (1988). *A national survey of public school testing of prekindergarten and kindergarten children*. Washington, DC: National Academy of Sciences.

Goldenberg, C. (1996). The education of language-minority students: Where we are, and where do we need to go? *Elementary School Journal*, *36*(4), 715–738.

Goldenberg, C., & Gallimore, R. (1991). Local knowledge, research knowledge, and educational change: A case study of early Spanish reading improvement. *Educational Researcher, 20*(8), 2–14.

Goldson, E., & Hagerman, R. J. (1992). The fragile X syndrome. *Developmental Medicine and Child Neurology*, *34*, 822–832.

Goldstein, S. (2002). Review of the Asperger Syndrome Diagnostic Scale. *Journal of Autism and Developmental Disorders*, *32*(6), 611–614.

Good, R. H., & Kaminski, R. A. (Eds.). (2002). *Dynamic Indicators of Basic Early Literacy Skills (DIBELS)* (6th ed.). Eugene, OR: Institute for the Development of Educational Achievement.

Good, R. H., & Kaminski, R. A. (2003). DIBELS: Dynamic Indicators of Basic Early Literacy Skills (6th ed.). Longmont, CO: Sopris West.

Good, T. L., & Brophy, J. E. (1991). *Looking in classrooms* (5th ed.). New York: HarperCollins.

Goodenough, F. L., & Harris, D. B. (1964). *Goodenough–Harris Drawing Test*. New York: Psychological Corporation.

Goodman, K. S. (Ed.). (2006). *The truth about DIBELS: What it is, what it does*. Portsmouth, NH: Heinemann.

Goodman, Y. M. (1986). Children coming to know literacy. In W. H. Teale & E. Sulzby (Eds.), *Emergent literacy: Writing and reading* (pp. 1–14). Norwood, NJ: Ablex.

Goodman, Y. M., & Altwerger, B. (1981). *Print awareness in preschool children: A study of the development of literacy in preschool children*. (Occasional Paper No. 4). Tuscon: University of Arizona, Program in Language and Literacy, Arizona Center for Research and Development, College of Education.

Gorman-Smith, D., & Tolan, P. H. (2003). Positive adaptation among youth exposed to community violence. In S. S. Luthar (Ed.), *Resilience and vulnerability: Adaptation in the context of childhood adversities* (pp. 392–413). New York: Cambridge University Press.

Goswami, U. (2001). Early phonological development and the acquisition of literacy. In S. B. Neuman & D. K. Dickinson (Eds.), *Handbook of early literacy research* (Vol. 1, pp. 111–125). New York: Guilford Press.

Gottman, J. M. (Producer). (1996). *The heart of parenting: Raising an emotionally intelligent child* [Videotape]. Seattle, WA: Seattle Marriage and Family Institute. (Available from *www.gottman.com)*

Gottman, J. M. (Producer). (1999). *Raising an emotionally intelligent child: The heart of parenting* [Videotape]. Seattle, WA: Seattle Marriage and Family Institute. (Available from www.gottman.com)

Gottman, J. M., Katz, L. F., & Hooven, C. (1997). *Meta-emotion: How families communicate emotionally*. Mahwah, NJ: Erlbaum.

Gowen, J. W., Johnson-Martin, N., Goldman, B. D., & Hussey, B. (1992). Object play and exploration in children with and without disabilities: A longitudinal study. *American Journal on Mental Retardation*, *97*, 21–38.

Graham, K. K. (2005). Test review of the Boehm Test of Basic Concepts—Third Edition: Preschool Version. In R. A. Spies & B. S. Plake (Eds.), *The sixteenth mental measurement yearbook* [Electronic version]. Retrieved from http://web5.silverplatter.com/webspirs/start.ws?customer=waldo&databases=(YB)

Graham, S. (2001). Test review of the Test of Children's Language (TOCL). In B. S. Plake & J. C. Impara (Eds.), *The fourteenth mental measurements yearbook* [Electronic version]. Retrieved from the Buros Institute's *Test Reviews Online* website: http://www.unl.edu.buros

Graue, M. E. (1992). Social interpretations of readiness for kindergarten. *Early Childhood Research Quarterly*, *7*, 225–243.

Graue, M., & DiPerna, J. (2000). Redshirting and early retention: Who gets the "gift of time" and what are the outcomes? *American Educational Research Journal*, *37*(2), 509–534.

Gredler, G. R. (1978). A look at some important factors in assessing readiness for school. *Journal of Learning Disabilities*, *11*, 284-290.

Gredler, G. R. (1980). The birthdate effect: Fact or artifact? *Journal of Learning Disabilities*, *13*, 239–242.

Gredler, G. R. (1987). Special education in the 80's: A critical analysis. *Psychology in the Schools*, *25*, 92–100.

Gredler, G. R. (1992). *School readiness: Assessment and educational issues* Brandon, VT: Clinical Psychology.

Gredler, G. R. (2000). Early childhood screening for developmental and educational problems. In B. A. Bracken (Ed.), *The psychoeducational assessment of preschool children* (3rd ed., pp. 399–411). Boston: Allyn & Bacon.

Green, J. (1982). *Cultural awareness in the human services*. Englewood Cliffs, NJ: Prentice-Hall.

Greenberg, R., & Field, T. (1982). Temperament ratings of handicapped infants during classroom, mother, and teacher interactions. *Journal of Pediatric Psychology*, *7*, 387–405.

Greenspan, S. I. (1992). *Infancy and early childhood: The practice of clinical assessments and intervention with emotional and developmental challenges*. Madison, CT: International Universities Press.

Greenspan, S. I., DeGangi, G., & Wieder, S. (Eds.). (2001). *The Functional Emotional Assessment Scale (FEAS) for infancy and childhood: Clini-*

cal and research applications. Bethesda, MD: Interdisciplinary Council on Developmental and Learning Disorders.

Greenspan, S. I., & Meisels, S. (1996). Toward a new vision for the developmental assessment of infants and young children. In S. Meisels & E. Fenichel (Eds.), *New vision of the developmental assessment of infants and young children* (pp. 11–26). Washington, DC: Zero to Three National Center for Infants, Toddlers, and Families.

Greenspan, S. I., & Wieder, S. (2001). The clinical applications of the FEAS. In S. I. Greenspan, G. DeGangi, & S. Wieder (Eds.), *The Functional Emotional Assessment Scale (FEAS) for infancy and early childhood: Clinical and research applications* (pp. 75–113). Bethesda, MD: Interdisciplinary Council on Developmental and Learning Disorders.

Greenwood, C. R., & Carta, J. J. (1987). An ecobehavioral interaction analysis of instruction within special education. *Focus on Exceptional Children, 19*, 3–13.

Greer, S., Bauchner, H., & Zuckerman, B. (1989). The Denver Developmental Screening Test: How good is its predictive validity? *Developmental Medicine and Child Neurology, 31*, 774–781. Retrieved from http://www.ncbi.nlm.nih.gov/entrez/query.fcg8?cmd=Retrieve&db=PubMed&list_uids=24.

Gresham, F. M., & Elliott, S. N. (1990). *Social Skills Rating System*. Circle Pines, MN: American Guidance Service.

Gresham, F. M., MacMillan, D. L., & Siperstein, G. (1995). Critical analysis of the 1992 AAMR definition: Implications for school psychology. *School Psychology Quarterly, 10*, 1–9.

Griffiths, R. (1970). *Griffiths Mental Development Scales*. Oxford, England: Test Agency.

Grill, J. J. (1995). Test review of the Aberrant Behavior Checklist (ABC). From J. C. Conoley & J. C. Impara (Eds.), *The twelfth mental measurements yearbook* [Electronic version]. Retrieved from http://web5.silverplatter.com/webspirs/start.ws?customer=waldo&databases=(YB)

Grill, J. J. (2001). Review of the Early Screening Project. In B. S. Plake & J. C. Impara (Eds.), *The fourteenth mental measurements yearbook* (pp. 453–454). Lincoln, NE: Buros Institute of Mental Measurements.

Gronlund, G. (2006). *Making early learning standards come alive*. St. Paul, MN: Redleaf Press.

Gronlund, N. E. (1973). *Preparing criterion-referenced tests for classroom instruction*. New York: Macmillan.

Grosjean, F. (1982). *Life with two languages: An introduction to bilingualism*. Cambridge, MA: Harvard University Press.

Grossman, H. J. (1983). *Classification in mental retardation*. Washington, DC: American Association on Mental Deficiency.

Grotevant, H. D., & Carlson, C. I. (1989). *Family assessment: A guide to methods and measures*. New York: Guilford Press.

Guilford, J. P. (1956). *Fundamental statistics in psychology and education*. New York: McGraw-Hill.

Gump, P. (1975). Ecological psychology and children. In E. M. Hetherington (Ed.), *Review of research in child development* (Vol. 5, pp. 75–126). Chicago: University of Chicago Press.

Guralnick, M. J. (Ed.). (1997). *The effectiveness of early intervention*. Baltimore: Brookes.

Gyurke, J. S. (1994). A reply to Bagnato and Neisworth: Intelligent views versus intelligence testing of preschoolers. *School Psychology Quarterly, 9*, 109–112.

Haeussermann, E. (1958). *Developmental potential of preschool children*. New York: Grune & Stratton.

Hagberg, B. (2002). Clinical manifestations and stages of Rett syndrome. *Mental Retardation and Developmental Disabilities Research Review, 8*, 61–65.

Hagerman, R. J. (1996). Biomedical advances in developmental psychology: The case of fragile X syndrome. *Developmental Psychology, 32*(3), 416–424.

Hagopian, L. P., Long, E. S., & Rush, K. S. (2004). Preference assessment porcedures for individuals with developmental disabilities. *Behavior Modification, 28*(5), 668–677.

Hainsworth, P. K., & Hainsworth, M. L. (1974). *Preschool Screening System: Start of a longitudinal–preventive approach*. Pawtucket, RI: Authors.

Hakuta, K., & Feldman Mostafapour, E. (1996). Perspectives from the history and politics of bilingualism and bilingual education in the United States. In I. Parasnis (Ed.), *Cultural and language diversity: Reflections on the deaf experience* (pp. 38–50). New York: Cambridge University Press.

Halberstadt, A. G. (1991). Socialization of expressiveness: Family influences in particular and a model in general. In R. S. Feldman & S. Rime (Eds.), *Fundamentals of emotional expressiveness* (pp. 106–162). Cambridge, UK: Cambridge University Press.

Haley, J. (1973). *The family life cycle: Uncommon therapy*. New York: Norton.

Hall, P. K., & Jordan, L. S. (1987). An assessment of a controlled association task to identify word-finding problems in children. *Language, Speech, and Hearing Services in Schools, 18*(2), 99–111.

Hamilton, W. (2003). Wechsler Preschool and Primary Scale of Intelligence (3rd ed.). *Applied Neuropsychology, 10*(3), 188–190.

Hammill, D., Mather, N., & Roberts, R. (2001). *Illinois Test of Psycholinguistic Abilities—Third Edition (ITPA-3)*. Austin, TX: PRO-ED.

Hampton, V. R. & Fantuzzo, J. W. (2003). The validity of the Penn Interactive Play Scale with urban, low-income kindergarten children. *School Psychology Review, 32*(1), 77–91.

Hamré, B. K., & Pianta, R. C. (2001). Early teacher–child relationships and the trajectory of children's school outcomes through eighth grade. *Child Development, 72*, 625–638.

Hamré, B. K., & Pianta, R. C. (2005). Can instructional and emotional support in the first grade classroom make a difference for children at risk of school failure? *Child Development, 76*(5), 949–967.

Hanf, C. (1969). *A two-stage program for modifying maternal controlling during mother–child (M-C) interaction*. Paper presented at the meeting of the Western Psychological Association, Vancouver, British Columbia, Canada.

Hanf, C. (1970). *Shaping mothers to shape their children's behavior.* Unpublished manuscript, University of Oregon Medical School.

Hanley, B., Tassé, M. J., Aman, M. G., & Pace, P. (1998). Psychometric properties of the Family Support Scale with Head Start families. *Journal of Child and Family Studies, 7*(1), 69–77.

Hanson, M. J., & Lynch, E. W. (2004). *Understanding families: Approaches to diversity, disability, and risk*. Baltimore: Brookes.

Hanson, R. (1982). Item reliability for the Griffiths Scales of Mental Development. *Child: Care, Health and Development, 8*, 151–161.

Hanson, R., & Aldridge Smith, J. (1987). Achievements of young children on items of the Griffiths Scales: 1980 compared with 1960. *Child: Care, Health and Development, 13*, 181–195.

Harcourt Brace Educational Measurement (1996). *Stanford Early School Achievement Test.* San Antonio, TX: Psychological Corporation.

Harms, T., & Clifford, R. M. (1983). Assessing pre-school environments with the Early Childhood Environment Rating Scale. *Studies in Educational Evaluation, 8*, 261–269.

Harms, T., & Clifford, R. M. (1989a). *Family Day Care Rating Scale.* New York: Teachers College Press.

Harms, T. & Clifford, R. M. (1989b). Family Day Care Rating Scale score sheet [Electronic version]. Retrieved from www.fpg.unc.edu/~ecers

Harms, T., & Clifford, R. M. (1993). Studying educational settings. In B. Spodek (Ed.), *Handbook of research on the education of young children* (pp. 477–492). New York: Macmillan.

Harms, T., Clifford, R. M., & Cryer, D. (1998). *Early Childhood Environment Rating Scale—Revised Edition.* New York: Teachers College Press.

Harms, T., Clifford, R. M., & Cryer, D. (2002). *Escala de Calificacion del Ambiente de la Infancia Temprana—edicion revisada.* New York: Teachers College Press.

Harms, T., Clifford, R. M., & Cryer, D. (2005). *Early Childhood Environment Rating Scale—Revised Edition, updated.* New York: Teachers College Press.

Harms, T., Cryer, D., & Clifford, R. M. (2002). *Infant/Toddler Environment Rating Scale—Revised Edition.* New York: Teachers College Press.

Harms, T., Jacobs, E. V., & White, D. R. (1996). *School-Age Care Environment Rating Scale.* New York: Teachers College Press.

Harms, T., Jacobs, E. V., & White, D. R. (2000). Score sheet School-Age Care Environment Rating Scale [Electronic version]. Retrieved from www.fpg.unc.edu/~ecers/

Harris, S. L., & Handleman, J. S. (2000). Age and IQ at intake as predictors of placement for young children with autism: A four- to six-year follow-up. *Journal of Autism and Developmental Disorders, 30*(2), 137–142.

Harrison, P. L. (1992). Planning and evaluating preschool screening and assessment programs. *Child Assessment News, 2*(3), 1, 8–12.

Harrison, P. L., & Boan, C. H. (2000). Assessment of adaptive behavior. In B. A. Bracken (Ed.), *The psychoeducational assessment of preschool children* (3rd ed., pp. 124–144). Boston: Allyn & Bacon.

Harrison, P. L., Kaufman, A. S., Kaufman, N. L., Bruininks, R. H., Rynders, J., Ilmer, S., et al. (1990). *American Guidance Service (AGS) Early Screening Profiles (ESP).* Circle Pines, MN: American Guidance Service.

Harrower, J. K., & Dunlap, G. (2001). Including children with autism in general education classrooms: A review of effective strategies. *Behavior Modification, 25*, 762–784.

Harry, B. (1992). Developing cultural self-awareness: The first step in values clarification for early interventionists. *Topics in Early Childhood Special Education, 12*(3), 333–350.

Hart, B., & Risley, T. R. (1975). Incidental teaching of language in the preschool. *Journal of Applied Behavior Analysis*, *8*, 411–420.

Hart, B., & Risley, T. R. (1995). *Meaningful differences in the everyday experience of young American children*. Baltimore: Brookes.

Hart, B., & Risley, T. R. (1999). *The social world of children learning to talk*. Baltimore: Brookes.

Hart, D., Atkins, R., & Fegley, S. (2003). Personality and development in childhood: A person centered approach. *Monographs of the Society for Research and Child Development*, *68*(1), vii–109.

Hartman, A. (1979). *Finding families: An ecological approach to family assessment in adoption*. Beverly Hills, CA: Sage.

Hartmann, D. P. (1982). Assessing the dependability of observational data. In D. P. Hartmann (Ed.), *Using observers to study behavior* (pp. 51–65). San Francisco: Jossey-Bass.

Hartup, W. W. (1983). The peer system. In P. H. Mussen (Series Ed.) & E. M. Hetherington (Vol. Ed.), *Handbook of child psychology: Vol. 4. Socialization, personality, and social development* (4th ed., pp. 103–196). New York: Wiley.

Haugen, E. (1977). Norm and deviation in bilingual communities. In P. Hornby (Ed.), *Bilingualism: Psychological, social, and educational implications* (pp. 91–102). New York: Academic Press.

Hawkins, J. (2005). Review of Boehm Test of Basic Concepts-3. In R. A. Spies & B. S. Plake (Eds.), *The sixteenth mental measurements yearbook* [Electronic version]. Retrieved from http://web5s.silverplatter.com.arugula.cc.columbia.edu:2048/webspirs/start.ws?customer=waldo&databases=YB

Hayes, A., & Batshaw, M. L. (1993). Down syndrome. *Pediatric Clinics of North America*, *40*, 523–535.

Heath, S. B. (1983). *Ways with words: Language, life and work in communities and classrooms*. Cambridge, UK: Cambridge University Press.

Heath, S. B. (1986). Separating "things of the imagination" from life: Learning to read and write. In W. H. Teale & E. Sluzby (Eds.), *Emergent literacy: Writing and reading* (pp. 156–172). Norwood, NJ: Ablex.

Heaton, P., & Wallace, G. H. (2004). Annotation: The savant syndrome. *Journal of Child Psychology and Psychiatry*, *45*(5), 899–911.

Hedrick, D., Prather, E., & Tobin, A. (1975). *Sequenced Inventory of Communication Development*. Seattle: University of Washington Press.

Hedrick, D., Prather, E., & Tobin, A. (1984). *Sequenced Inventory of Communication Development—Revised Edition*. Seattle: University of Washington Press.

Heller, J. H., & Edwards, C. (1993, November). *Facilitating language learning via enhancement of the listening environment*. Paper presented at the second National Head Start Research Conference, Washington, DC.

Heller, K. A., Holtzman, W., & Messick, S. (1982). *Placing children in special education: A strategy for equity*. Washington, DC: National Academy Press.

Hembree-Kigin, T. L., & McNeil, C. B. (1995). *Parent–child interaction therapy*. New York: Plenum Press.

Henderson, S., Byrne, D. G., & Duncan-Jones, P. (1981). *Neurosis and the social environment*. New York: Academic Press.

Henderson, S., Duncan-Jones, P., Byrne, D. G., & Scott, R. (1980). Measuring social relationships: The Interview Schedule for Social Interaction. *Psychological Medicine*, *10*(4), 723–734.

Hernandez, D. J. (1993, November). *Childhood transformed: Family composition and the family economy*. Paper presented at the second National Head Start Research Conference, Washington, DC.

Hess, A. K. (2001). Test review of the *Conners' Rating Scales—Revised* (CRS-R). In B. S. Plake & J. C. Impara (Eds.), *The fourteenth mental measurements yearbook* [Electronic version]. Retrieved from http://web5.silverplatter.com/webspirs/start.ws?customer=waldo&databases=(YB)

Hetherington, E. M., & Kelly, J. (2002). *For better or for worse: Divorce reconsidered*. New York: Norton.

Hiebert, E. H., Hutchinson, T. A., & Raines, P. A. (1991). Alternative assessments of literacy: Teachers' actions and parents' reactions. In J. Zutell & S. McCormick (Eds.), *44th Yearbook of the National Reading Conference* (pp. 97–104). Chicago, IL: National Reading Conference.

High/Scope Educational Research Foundation. (2003). High/Scope Child Observation Record (COR) for ages 2½–6. Ypsilanti, MI: High/Scope Press.

Hill, E. L., & Frith, U. (2003). Understanding autism: Insights from mind and brain. In U. Frith & E. L. Hill (Eds.), *Autism: Mind and brain* (pp. 1–19). New York: Oxford University Press.

Hill, P. M., & McCune-Nicholich, L. (1981). Pretend play and patterns of cognition in Down's syndrome. *Child Development*, *52*, 611–617.

Hill, R. B. (1970). *Family development in three generations.* Cambridge, MA: Schenkman.

Hill, R. B. (1972). *The strengths of African-American families.* New York: Emerson Hall.

Hill, R. B., & Billingsley, A. (1993). *Research on the African American family: A holistic perspective.* Westport, CT: Auburn House.

Hilliard, A., III. (1989). Teachers and cultural styles in a pluralistic society. *NEA Today, 7*(6), 65–69.

Hills, J. R. (1993). Hills' handy hints: Regression effects in educational measurement. *Educational Measurement: Issues and Practice, 12*, 31–34.

Hinshaw, S. P., & Anderson, C. A. (1996). Conduct and oppositional defiant disorders. In E. J. Mash & R. A. Barkley (Eds.), *Child psychopathology* (pp. 113–149). New York: Guilford Press.

Hintze, J. M. (2005). Psychometrics of direct observation. *School Psychology Review, 34*, 507–519.

Hintze, J. M., Christ, T. J., & Methe, S. A. (2006). Curriculum-based assessment. *Psychology in the Schools, 43*, 45–56.

Hintze, J. M., & Shapiro, E. S. (1995). Best practices in the systematic observation of classroom behavior. In A. Thomas & J. Grimes (Eds.), *Best practices in school psychology III* (pp. 651–660). Washington, DC: National Association of School Psychologists.

Hintze, J. M., Volpe, R. J., & Shapiro, E. S. (2002). Best practices in systematic direct observation of student behavior. In A. Thomas & J. Grimes (Eds.), *Best practices in school psychology IV* (Vol. 2, pp. 993–1006). Bethesda, MD: National Association of School Psychologists.

Hirsh-Pasek, K., Kochanoff, A., Newcombe, N. S., & de Villiers, J. (2005). Using scientific knowledge to inform preschool assessment: Making the case for "empirical validity." *Society for Research in Child Development Social Policy Report, 9*(1), 1, 3, 5–11, 13, 15–19.

Hobbs, N. (1966). Helping disturbed children: Psychological and ecological strategies. *American Psychologist, 21*, 1105–1115.

Hobbs, N. (1975). *The classification of children.* San Francisco: Jossey-Bass.

Hobbs, N. (1978). Families, schools, and communities: An ecosystem for children. *Teachers College Record, 79*(4), 756–766.

Hobson, R. P., & Bishop, M. (2004). The pathogenesis of autism: Insights from congenital blindness. In U. Frith & E. L. Hill (Eds.), *Autism: Mind and brain* (pp. 109–126). New York: Oxford University Press.

Hoge, R. D. (1985). The validity of direct observation measures of pupil classroom behavior. *Review of Educational Research, 55*, 469–483.

Holbrook, M. C., & Koenig, A. J. (Eds.). (2000). *Foundations of education: Vol. 2. Instructional strategies for teaching children and youth with visual impairments* (2nd ed.). New York: American Foundation for the Blind Press.

Holland, J., McIntosh, D., & Huffman, L. (2004). The role of phonological awareness, rapid automatized naming, and orthographic processing in word reading. *Journal of Psychoeducational Assessment, 22,* 233–260.

Holman, A. (1983). *Family assessment: Tools for understanding and intervention.* Beverly Hills, CA: Sage.

Holroyd, J. (1974). The Questionnaire on Resources and Stress: An instrument to measure family response to a handicapped member. *Journal of Community Psychology, 2*(1), 92–94.

Holroyd, J. (1987). *Questionnaire on Resources and Stress for families with a chronically ill or handicapped member: Manual.* Brandon, VT: Clinical Psychology.

Holroyd, J., Brown, N., Wikler, L., & Simmons, J. Q. (1975). Stress in families of institutionalized and non-institutionalized autistic children. *Journal of Community Psychology, 3*(1), 26–31.

Holroyd, J., & Guthrie, D. (1979). Stress in families of children with neuromuscular disease. *Journal of Clinical Psychology, 35*(4), 734–739.

Holroyd, J., & McArthur, D. (1976). Mental retardation and stress on the, parents: A contrast between Down's syndrome and childhood autism. *American Journal of Mental Deficiency, 80*(4), 431–436.

Hoover, H. D., Hieronymous, A. N., Frisbie, D. A., & Dunbar, S. B. (1996). *Iowa Tests of Basic Skills (ITBS).* Chicago: Riverside.

Horn, J. L., & Cattell, R. B. (1966). Refinement and test of the theory of fluid and crystallized intelligence. *Journal of Educational Psychology, 57*, 253–276.

Horn, J. L. (1985). Remodeling old models of intelligence: Gf–Gc theory. In B. B. Wollman (Ed.), *Handbook of intelligence* (pp. 253–276). New York: Wiley.

Horn, J. L., & Noll, J. (1997). Human cognitive capabilities: Gf–Gc theory. In D. P. Flanagan, J. L. Genshaft, & P. L. Harrison (Eds.), *Contemporary intellectual assessment* (pp. 53–91). New York: Guilford Press.

Hosp, M. K., & Fuchs, L. S. (2005). Using CBM as an indicator of decoding, word reading, and comprehension: Do the relations change with grade? *School Psychology Review, 34*, 9–26.

Howard, J., Beckwith, L., Rodning, C., & Kropenske, V. (1989). The development of young children of substance abusing parents: Insights from seven years of research. *Zero to Three, 9*, 8–12.

Howell, K. W. (1986). Direct assessment of academic performance. *School Psychology Review, 15*, 324–335.

Howes, C. (1980). Peer play scale as an index of complexity of peer interaction. *Developmental Psychology, 16*, 371–372.

Howes, C. (1987). Social competence with peers in young children: Developmental sequences. *Developmental Review, 7*, 252–272.

Howes, C. (1988). Relations between early child care and schooling. *Developmental Psychology, 24*, 53–57.

Howes, C., & Matheson, C. (1992). Sequences in the development of competent play with peers: Social and social pretend play. *Developmental Psychology, 28*, 961–974.

Howes, C., & Stewart, P. (1987). Child's play with adults, toys, and peers: An examination of family and child-care influences. *Developmental Psychology, 23*(3), 423–430.

Howlin, P. (2000). Outcome in adult life for more able individuals with autism or Asperger syndrome. *Autism, 4*, 63–83.

Howlin, P., & Rutter, M. (1987). *The treatment of autistic children*. Chichester, UK: Wiley.

Howlin, P., Wing, L., & Gould, J. (1995). The recognition of autism in children with Down syndrome: Implications for intervention and some speculations about pathology. *Developmental Medicine and Child Neurology, 37*, 398–414.

Hresko, W. P., Reid, D. K., & Hammill, D. D. (1999). *Test of Early Language Development—Third Edition (TELD-3)*. Austin, TX: PRO-ED.

Huang, A. M., Hunter, L. R., Reinert, H. R., & Wishon, P. H. (1992). Assessment of children with mental retardation and other handicapping conditions. In E. V. Nutall, I. Romero, & J. Kalesink (Eds.), *Assessing and screening preschoolers* (pp. 311–326). Needham Heights, MA: Allyn & Bacon.

Huebner, E. S. (1989). Test review of the Developmental Profile-Second Edition. In J. C. Conoley & J. J. Kramer (Eds.), *The tenth mental measurement yearbook* [Electronic version]. Retrieved from http://web5.silverplatter.com/webspirs/start.ws?customer=waldo&databases=(YB)

Hughes, M., Dote-Kwan, J., & Dolendo, J. (1998). A close look at cognitive play of preschoolers with visual impairments in the home. *Exceptional Children, 64*, 451–462.

Hunt, J. M. (1961). *Intelligence and experience*. New York: Ronald Press.

Huntley, M. (1996). *Griffiths Mental Development Scales from Birth to Two Years: Manual for the 1996 revision*. Oxford, England: Test Agency.

Hurford, D. P. (2003a). Test review of the Comprehensive Test of Phonological Processing. In B. S. Plake, J. C. Impara, & R. A. Spies (Eds.), *The fifteenth mental measurements yearbook* [Electronic version]. Retrieved from http://web5s.silverplatter.com.arugula.cc.columbia.edu:2048/webspirs/start.ws?customer=waldo&databases=YB

Hurford, D. P. (2003b). Test review of the Fluharty Preschool Speech and Language Screening Test—Second Edition (Fluharty-2). In B. S. Plake, J. C. Impara, & R. A. Spies (Eds.), *The fifteenth mental measurements yearbook* [Electronic version]. Retrieved from http://web5s.silverplatter.com/webspirs/start.ws?customer=waldo&databases=YB

Hurford, D. P. (2005). Test review of the Utah Test of Language Development—Fourth Edition (ULTD-4). In R. A. Spies & B. S. Plake (Eds.), *The sixteenth mental measurements yearbook* [Electronic version]. Retrieved from http://web5s.silverplatter.com/webspirs/start.ws?customer=waldo&databases=YB

Huttenlocher, P. (1994). Synaptogenesis, synapse elimination and neural plasticity in human cerebral cortex. In C. A. Nelson (Ed.), *Minnesota Symposia on Child Psychology: Vol. 27. Threats to optimal development: Integrating biological, psychological and social risk factors* (pp. 35–54). Hillsdale, NJ: Erlbaum.

Hyman, S. L., Rodier, P. M., & Davidson, P. (2001). Pervasive developmental disorders in young children. *Journal of the American Medical Association, 285*(24), 3141–3142.

Ilg, F. L., & Ames, L. B. (1972). *School readiness*. New York: Harper & Row.

Ilg, F. L., Ames, L. B., Haines, J., & Gillespie, C. (1978). *School readiness* (rev. ed.). New York: Harper & Row.

Inchaurralde, C. (2005). Test review of the Prereading Inventory of Phonological Awareness (PIPA). From R. A. Spies & B. S. Plake (Eds.), *The sixteenth mental measurements yearbook* [Electronic version]. Retrieved from http://web5s.silverplatter.com.arugula.cc.columbia.edu:2048/webspirs/start.ws?customer=waldo&databases=YB

Individuals with Disabilities Education Act (IDEA) of 1990, Pub. L. No. 101-476, 104 Stat. 1141 (1991).

Individuals with Disabilities Education Act (IDEA) Amendments of 1997, Pub. L. 105-17, 111 Stat. 37 (1997).

Individuals with Disabilities Education Improvement Act (IDEA) of 2004, Pub. L. No. 108-446, 118 Stat. 2647 (2004).

Ingram, D. (1981). *Procedures for the phonological analysis of children's language*. Baltimore: University Park Press.

Ireton, H. I. (1992). *Child Development Inventory*. Minneapolis, MN: Behavior Science Systems.

Irwin, D. M., & Bushnell, M. M. (1980). *Observational strategies for child study*. New York: Holt, Rinehart & Winston.

Iverson, A. M. (1992). Test review of the Family Day Care Rating Scale. In J. J. Kramer & J. C. Conoley (Eds.), *The eleventh mental measurements yearbook* [Electronic version]. Retrieved from http://web5.silverplatter.com/webspirs/start.ws?customer=waldo&databases=(YB)

Ives, M., & Munro, N. (2002). *Caring for a child with autism: A practical guide for parents*. London: Kingsley.

Izard, C. E. (2002). Translating emotion theory and research into preventative interventions. *Psychological Bulletin*, *128*(5), 796–824.

Izard, C. E., Fantazzo, C. A., Castle, J. M., Haynes, O. M., Rayias, M. F., & Putnam, P. H. (1995). The ontogeny and significance of infants' facial expressions in the first 9 months of life. *Developmental Psychology*, *31*(6), 997–1013.

Jacobson, J. W., & Mulick, J. A. (1996). *Manual of diagnosis and professional practice in mental retardation*. Washington, DC: American Psychological Association.

Jaffe, P. G., Baker, L. L., & Cunningham, A. J. (Eds.). (2004). *Protecting children from domestic violence: Strategies for community intervention*. New York: Guilford Press.

Jansky, J., & de Hirsch, K. (1972). *Preventing reading failure: Prediction, diagnosis, intervention*. New York: Harper & Row.

Jarrold, C., Boucher, J., & Smith, P. (1993). Symbolic play in autism: A review. *Journal of Autism and Developmental Disorders*, *23*, 281–308.

Jaudes, P. K., & Shapiro, L. D. (1999). Child abuse and developmental disabilities. In J. A. Silver, B. J. Amster, & T. Haecker (Eds.), *Young children and foster care* (pp. 21–34). Baltimore: Brookes.

Jedrysek, E., Klapper, Z., Pope, L., & Wortis, J. (1972). *Psychoeducational evaluation of the preschool child*. New York: Grune & Stratton.

Jensen, V. K., Larrieu, J. A., & Mack, K. K. (1997). Differential diagnosis between attention deficit/hyperactivity disorder and pervasive developmental disorder—not otherwise specified. *Clinical Pediatrics*, *36*(10), 555–561.

Jitendra, A. K., & Rohena-Diaz, E. (1996). Language assessment of students who are linguistically diverse: Why a discrete approach is not the answer. *School Psychology Review*, *25*, 40–56.

Joe, J. R., & Malach, R. S. (2004). Families with American Indian roots. In E. W. Lynch & M. J. Hanson (Eds.), *Developing cross-cultural competence: A guide for working with children and their families* (3rd ed., pp. 109–134). Baltimore: Brookes.

Johnson, D. L., Howie, V. M., Owen, M., Baldwin, C. D., & Luttman, D. (1993). Assessment of three-year-olds with the Stanford–Binet Intelligence Scale—Fourth Edition. *Psychological Reports*, *73*, 51–57.

Johnson, J. A. (2003). Test review: Stanford–Binet Intelligence Scales—Fifth Edition. In R. A. Spies & B. S. Plake (Eds.), *The sixteenth mental measurements yearbook*. [Electronic version].

Johnson, J. E., Ershler, J., & Bell, C. (1980). Play behavior in a discovery-based and a formal education preschool program. *Child Development*, *51*, 271–274.

Johnston, C., & Murray, C. (2003). Incremental validity in the psychological assessment of children and adolescents. *Psychological Assessment*, *15*(4), 496–507.

Johnston, J. R. (2005). Test review of the Utah Test of Language Development-Fourth Edition (ULTD-4). From R. A. Spies & B. S. Plake (Eds.), *The sixteenth mental measurements yearbook* [Electronic version]. Retrieved from http://web5s.silverplatter.com/webspirs/start.ws?customer=waldo&databases=YB

Johnston, P. H., & Allington, R. L. (1991). Remediation. In R. Barr, M. L. Kamil, P. B. Mosenthal, & P. D. Pearson (Eds.), *Handbook of reading research* (Vol. 2, pp. 984–1012). New York: Longman.

Joseph, G. E., & Strain, P. S. (2004). Comprehensive evidence-based social–emotional curricula for young children. *Topics in Early Childhood Special Education*, *23*(2), 65–76.

Juel, C., & Leavell, J. A. (1988). Retention and nonretention of at-risk readers in first grade and their subsequent achievement. *Journal of Learning Disabilities*, *21*, 571–580.

Kaderavek, J. N., & Sulzby, E. (2000). Issues in emergent literacy for children with language impairments. In L. R. Watson, E. Crais, & T. L. Layton (Eds.), *Handbook of early language impairment in children: Vol. II. Assessment and treatment* (pp. 199–244). Albany, NY: Delmar Thomson.

Kadesjö, B., & Gillberg, C. (2000). Tourette's disorder: Epidemiology and comorbidity in primary school children. *Journal of the American Academy of Child and Adolescent Psychiatry, 39*, 548–555.

Kagan, J. (1994). On the nature of emotion. In N. A. Fox (Ed.), The Development of Emotion Regulation: Biological and Behavioral Considerations. *Monographs of the Society for Research in Child Development, 59*(2–3, Serial No. 240), 7–24.

Kagan, R., & Schlosberg, S. (1989). *Families in perpetual crisis*. New York: W. W. Norton.

Kagan, S. L. (1990). Readiness 2000: Rethinking rhetoric and responsibility. *Phi Delta Kappan, 72*, 272–279.

Kaminer, R. K., & Cohen, H. J. (1988). How do you say, "Your child is retarded"? *Contemporary Pediatrics, 5*, 36–49.

Kaminer, R. K., Jedrysek, E., & Soles, B. (1984). Behavior problems of young children. In J. M. Berg (Ed.). *Perspectives and Progress in Mental Retardation* (Vol. 2, pp. 289–298). Baltimore: University Park Press.

Kaminer, R. K., & Robinson, C. (1993). Perspective: Developmental therapies in early interververtion. *Infants and Young Children, 3*, 5–8.

Kaminiski, R. A., & Good, R. H. (1996). Toward a technology for assessing basic early literacy skills. *School Psychology Review, 25*(2), 215–227.

Kamo, M. (1995). Test review of the Social Skills Rating System (SSRS). From J. C. Conoley & J. C. Impara (Eds.), *The twelfth mental measurements yearbook* [Electronic version]. Retrieved from http://web5.silverplatter.com/webspirs/start.ws?customer=waldo&databases=(YB)

Kamphaus, R. W. (2001). Test review of the Metropolitan Readiness Tests – Sixth Edition (MRT-6). From J. C. Impara & B. S. Plake (Eds.), *The fourteenth mental measurements yearbook* [Electronic version]. Retrieved from http://web5.silverplatter.com/webspirs/start.ws?customer=waldo&databases=(YB)

Kamphaus, R. W., & Frick, P. J. (2002). *Clinical assessment of child and adolescent personality and behavior* (2nd ed.). Boston: Allyn & Bacon.

Kanner, L. (1943). Autistic disturbance of affective contact. *Nervous Child, 2*, 217–250.

Kaplan, C. (1993). Reliability and validity of test-session behavior observations: Putting the horse before the cart. *Journal of Psychoeducational Assessment, 11*(4), 314–322.

Kaplan, E., Goodglass, H., & Weintraub, S. (2000). *The Boston Naming Test—Second Edition (BNT-2)*. Philadelphia, PA: Lippincott, Williams, & Wilkins.

Karnes, M. B., Johnson, J. L., & Beauchamp, K. D. (1989). Developing problem-solving skills to enhance task persistence of handicapped preschool children. *Journal of Early Intervention, 13*(1), 61–72.

Karpel, M. A., & Strauss, E. S. (1983). *Family evaluation*. New York: Gardner Press.

Kasari, C., & Sigman, M. (1996). Expression and understanding of emotion in atypical development: Autism and Down's syndrome. In M. Lewis & M. W. Sullivan (Eds.), *Emotional development in atypical children* (pp. 109–130). Mahwah, NJ: Erlbaum.

Kaufman, A. S., & Kaufman, N. L. (1983). *Kaufman Assessment Battery for Children*. Circle Pines, MN: American Guidance Service.

Kaufman, A. S., & Kaufman, N. L. (1993). *Kaufman Survey of Early Academic and Language Skills*. Circle Pines, MN: American Guidance Service.

Kaufman, A. S., & Kaufman, N. L. (2004). *Kaufman Assessment Battery for Children, Second Edition (KABC-II)*. Circle Pines, MN: American Guidance Service.

Kaufman, J. C., Kaufman, A. S., Kaufman-Singer, J., & Kaufman, N. L. (2005). The Kaufman Assessment Battery for Children—Second Edition, and the Kaufman Adolescent and Adult Intelligence Test. In D. P. Flanagan & P. L. Harrison (Eds.), *Contemporary intellectual assessment* (2nd ed., pp. 344–370). New York: Guilford Press.

Keenan, K., & Shaw, D. D. (1997). Developmental and social influences on young girls' early problem behavior. *Psychological Bulletin, 121*(1), 95–113.

Keenan, K., Shaw, D. S., Delliquadri, E., Giovannelli, J., & Walsh, B. (1998). Evidence for the continuity of early problem behaviors: Application of a developmental model. *Journal of Abnormal Child Psychology, 26*(6), 441–452.

Keith, T. Z. (1990). Confirmatory and hierarchical analysis of the Differential Ability Scales. *Journal of Psychoeducational Assessment, 8*, 391–405.

Keller, H. (2005). Review of Boehm Test of Basic Concepts-3. In R. A. Spies & B. S. Plake (Eds.), *The sixteenth mental measurements yearbook* [Electronic version]. Retrieved from http://web5s.silverplatter.com.arugula.cc.columbia.edu:2048/webspirs/start.ws?customer=waldo&databases=YB

Kelly, J. F., & Barnard, K. E. (2000). Assessment of parent–child interaction: Implications for early intervention. In J. P. Shonkoff & S. J. Meisels (Eds.), *Handbook of early childhood intervention* (2nd ed., pp. 258–289). New York: Cambridge University Press.

Kent, R. N., & Foster, S. L. (1977). Direct observational procedures: Methodological issues in naturalistic settings. In A. R. Ciminero, K. W. Calhoun, & H. E. Adams (Eds.), Handbook of behavioral assessment (pp. 279–328). New York: Wiley.

Keogh, B. K., & Becker, L. D. (1973). Early detection of learning problems: Questions, cautions, and guidelines. *Exceptional Children, 40*, 5–11.

Keogh, B. K., Coots, J. J., & Bernheimer, L. P. (1995). School placement of children with nonspecific developmental delays. *Journal of Early Intervention, 20*, 65–78.

Kerlinger, F. N. (1973). *Foundations of behavioral research*. New York: Holt, Rinehart & Winston.

Kessler, C. (1984). Language acquisition in bilingual children. In N. Miller (Ed.), *Bilingual and language disability: Assessment and remediation* (pp. 26–54). San Diego, CA: College-Hill Press.

Kieth, P. B. (2001). Test review of the School-Age Care Environment Rating Scale (SACERS). From J. C. Impara & B. S. Plake (Eds.), *The fourteenth mental measurements yearbook* [Electronic version]. Retrieved from http://web5.silverplatter.com/webspirs/start.ws?customer=waldo&databases=(YB)

Kim, U., & Kagan, S. L. (1999). Stepping back and looking forward: Thinking about assessment for young children. *Instructional Leader, 12*, 1–5, 11.

King, B. H., State, M. W., Shah, B., Davanso, P., & Dykens, E. (1997). Mental retardation: A review of the past 10 years: Part I. *Journal of the American Academy of Child and Adolescent Psychiatry, 36*, 1656–1663.

Kirby, J. R., Parrila, R. K, & Pfeiffer, S. L. (2003). Naming speed and phonological awareness as predictors of reading development. *Journal of Educational Psychology, 95*, 453–464.

Kirnan, J. P. (1998). Test review of Child Developmental Inventory (CDI). From J. C. Impara & B. S. Plake (Eds.), *The thirteenth mental measurements yearbook* [Electronic version]. Retrieved from http://web5s.silverplatter.com.arugula.cc.columbia.edu:2048/webspirs/start.ws?customer=waldo&databases=YB

Klecker, B. M. (2001). Test review of the Attention Deficit Disorders Evaluation Scale—Second Edition (ADDES). In B. S. Plake & J. C. Impara (Eds.), *The fourteenth mental measurements yearbook* [Electronic version]. Retrieved from http://web5.silverplatter.com/webspirs/start.ws?customer=waldo&databases=(YB)

Kleinman, S. N., & Prizant, B. M. (2000). Ecologically valid assessment of two- to five-year-olds. In L. R. Watson, E. Crais, & T. L. Layton (Eds.), *Handbook of early language impairment in children: Assessment and treatment* (pp. 39–71). Albany, NY: Delmar Thomson.

Klin, A., Jones, W., Schultz, R., & Volkmar, F. (2004). The enactive mind, or from action to congition: Lessons from autism. In U. Frith & E. L. Hill (Eds.), *Autism: Mind and brain* (pp. 127–159). New York: Oxford University Press.

Klin, A., Lang, J., Cicchetti, D. V., & Volkmar, F. R. (2000). Brief report: Inter-rater reliability of clinical diagnosis and DSM-IV criteria for autistic disorder: Results of the DSM-IV Autism Field Trial. *Journal of Autism and Developmental Disorders, 30*(2), 163–167.

Knoff, H. M. (2001a). Review of the Early Screening Project. In B. S. Plake & J. C. Impara (Eds.), *The fourteenth mental measurements yearbook* [Electronic version]. Retrieved from http://web5s.silverplatter.com.arugula.cc.columbia.edu:2048/webspirs/start.ws?customer=waldo&databases=(YB)

Knoff, H. M. (2001b). *Review of the* Conners' Rating Scales—Revised. In B. S. Plake & J. C. Impara (Eds.), *The fourteenth mental measurements yearbook* [Electronic version]. Retrieved from http://web5s.silverplatter.com.arugula.cc.columbia.edu:2048/webspirs/start.ws?customer=waldo&databases=(YB)

Knutson, J. F. (1995). Psychological characteristics of maltreated children: Putative risk factors and consequences. *Annual Review of Psychology, 46*, 401–431.

Kochanek, T., Kabacoff, R., & Lipsitt, L. (1987). Early detection of handicapping conditions in infancy and early childhood: Toward a multivariate model. *Journal of Applied Developmental Psychology, 8*, 411–420.

Kochanek, T., Kabacoff, R., & Lipsitt, L. (1990). Early identification of developmentally disabled and at-risk preschool children. *Exceptional Children, 56*, 528–538.

Koegel, L. K., Koegel, R. L., & Smith, A. (1997). Variables related to differences in standardized test outcomes for children with sutism, *Journal of Autism and Developmental Disorders, 27*(3), 233–243.

Koenen, K. C., Moffitt, T. E., Caspi, A., Taylor, A., & Purcell, S. (2003). Domestic violence is associated with environmental suppression of IQ in young children. *Development and Psychopathology, 15*(2), 297–311.

Kolata, G. (1992, February 25). Discovery of worsening family ills spurs rush to tap protein bonanza. *The New York Times.*

Konold, T. (2001). Test review of the Kindergarten Language Screening Test—Second Edition (KLST-2). In B. S. Plake & J. C. Impair (Eds.), *The fourteenth mental measurements yearbook* [Electronic version]. Retrieved from the Buros Institute's *Test Reviews Online* website: www.unl.edu/buros

Koppitz, E. M. (1968). *Psychological evaluation of children's human figure drawing.* New York: Grune & Stratton.

Koppitz, E. M. (1975). *The Bender Gestalt Test for Young Children. New York: Grune & Stratton.*

Korbin, J. (1981). *Child abuse and neglect: Cross-cultural perspectives.* Berkeley: University of California Press.

Kozloff, M. A. (1984). A training program for families with autism. In E. Schopler & G. Mesibov (Eds.), *The effects of autism on the family* (pp. 163–186). New York: Plenum Press.

Kozma, C., & Stock, J. S. (1993). What is mental retardation? In R. Smith (Ed.), *Children with mental retardation: A parents' guide* (pp. 1–49). Rockville, MD: Woodbine House.

Kraijer, D. (2000). Review of adaptive behavior studies in mentally retarded persons with autism/pervasive developmental disorder. *Journal of Autism and Developmental Disorders, 30*(1), 39–47.

Krantz, P. J., & Risley, T. R. (1977). Behavior ecology in the classroom. In K. D. O'Leary & S. G. O'Leary (Eds.), *Classroom management: The successful use of behavior modification* (2nd ed., pp. 349–367). New York: Pergamon Press.

Kratochwill, T. R., & Wetzel, R. J. (1977). Observer agreement, credibility, and judgment: Some considerations in presenting observer agreement data. *Journal of Applied Behavior Analysis, 10*, 133–139.

Kretschmer, L., & Kretschmer, R. (2001). Deafness and hearing impairment in young children. In T. Layton, E. Crais, & L. Watson (Eds.), *Handbook of early language impairment in children: Nature* (pp. 541–626). Albany, NY: Delmar Thomson.

Krug, D. A., Arick, J. R., & Almond, P. J. (1993). *Autism Screening Instrument for Educational Planning—Second Edition (ASIEP-2).* Austin, TX: PRO-ED.

LaFreniere, P. J., & Dumas, J. E. (1995). *Social Competence and Behavior Evaluation: Preschool Edition (SCBE).* Los Angeles: Western Psychological Services.

Lahey, M. (1988). *Language disorders and language development.* New York: Macmillan.

Lamb, M. E. (Ed.). (2004). *The role of the father in child development* (4th ed.). Hoboken, NJ: Wiley.

Landy, S., & Menna, R. (2006). *Early intervention with multi-risk families: An integrative approach.* Baltimore: Brookes.

Landy, S., Menna, R., & Clipsham, C. K. (2006). Reaching and engaging hard-to-reach families. In S. Landy & R. Menna (Eds.), *Early intervention with multi-risk: An integrative approach* (pp. 179–197). Baltimore: Brookes.

Last, C. G., Herson, M., Kazdin, A. E., Francis, G., & Grubb, H. J. (1987). Psychiatric illness in the mothers of anxious children. *American Journal of Psychiatry, 144*, 1580–1583.

Laurent, J., Swerdlik, M., & Ryburn, M. (1992). Review of validity research on the Stanford–Binet Intelligence Scale Fourth Edition. *Psychological Assessment, 4*, 102–112.

Lavigne, J. V., Arend, R., Rosenbaum, D., Binns, H. J., Christoffel, K. K., & Gibbons, D. (1998a). Psychiatric disorders with onset in the preschool years: I. Stability of diagnoses. *Journal of the American Academy of Child and Adolescent Psychiatry, 37*(12), 1246–1254.

Lavigne, J. V., Arend, R., Rosenbaum, D., Binns, H. J., Christoffel, K. K., & Gibbons, D. (1998b). Psychiatric disorders with onset in the preschool years: II. Correlates and predictors of stable case status. *Journal of the American Academy of Child and Adolescent Psychiatry, 37*(12), 1255–1261.

Lavigne, J. V., Gibbons, R. D., Christoffel, K. K., Arend, R., Rosenbaum, D., Binns, H., et al. (1996). Prevalence rates and correlates of psychiatric disorders among preschool children. *Journal of the American Academy of Child and Adolescent Psychiatry, 35*(2), 204–214.

Lawry, J., Danko, C. D., & Strain, P. S. (2000). Examining the role of the classroom environment in the prevention of problem behaviors. *Young Exceptional Children*, *32*(2), 11–19.

Lazar, I., & Darlington, R. (1982). Lasting effects of early education: A report from the Consortium for Longitudinal Studies. *Monographs of the Society for Research in Child Development*, *47*(2–3, Serial No. 195), pp. 1–151.

Le-Ager, C., & Shapiro, E. S. (1995). Template matching as a strategy for assessment of and intervention for pre-school students with disabilities. *Topics in Early Childhood Special Education*, *15*(2), 187–218.

LeBuffe, P. A., & Naglieri, J. A. (1999). *Devereux Early Childhood Assessment (DECA)*. Lewisville, NC: Kaplan Press.

LeCouteur, A., Rutter, M., Lord, C., Rios, P., Robertson, S., Holdgrafer, M., et al. (1989). Autism Diagnostic Interview: A standardized investigator-based instrument. *Journal of Autism and Developmental Disorders*, *19*(3), 363–387.

Leff, S. S., & Lakin, R. (2005). Playground-based observational systems: A review and implications for practitioners and researchers. *School Psychology Review*, *34*(4), 475–489.

Leslie, A. M. (1987). Pretense and representation: The origins of "theory of mind." *Psychological Review*, *94*, 412–426.

Leslie, A. M., & Roth, D. (1993). What autism teaches us about meta-representation. In S. Baron-Cohen, H. Tager-Flusberg, & D. J. Cohen (Eds.), *Understanding other minds: Perspectives from autism* (pp. 83–111). Oxford: Oxford University Press.

Lewis, M., & Sullivan, M. W. (1996). The role of situation and child status on emotional interactions. In M. Lewis & M. W. Sullivan (Eds.), *Emotional development in atypical children* (pp. 43–63). Mahwah, NJ: Erlbaum.

Lewis, M. H., & Bodfish, J. W. (1998). Repetitive behavior disorders in autism. *Mental Retardation and Developmental Disabilities Research Reviews*, *4*, 80–89.

Liberman, I. Y., & Shankweiler, D. (1985). Phonology and the problems of learning to read and write. *Remedial and Special Education*, *6*(6), 8–17.

Lichtenstein, R. (1990). Psychometric characteristics and appropriate use of the Gesell School Readiness Screening Test. *Early Childhood Research Quarterly*, *5*, 359–378.

Lichtenstein, R., & Ireton, H. (1984). *Preschool screening: Identifying young children with developmental and educational problems*. Orlando, FL: Grune & Stratton.

Lidz, C. S. (1981). *Improving assessment of schoolchildren*. San Fransicso: Jossey-Bass.

Lidz, C. S. (1983a). Dynamic assessment and the preschool child. *Journal of Psychological Assessment*, *1*, 59–72.

Lidz, C. S. (1983b). Issues in assessing preschool children. In K. D. Paget & B. A. Bracken (Eds.), *The psychoeducational assessment of preschool children* (pp. 17–27). New York: Grune & Stratton.

Lidz, C. S. (1990). The Preschool Learning Assessment Device: An approach to the dynamic assessment of young children. *European Journal of Psychology of Education*, *2*, 167–175.

Lidz, C. S. (1991). *Practitioner's guide to dynamic assessment*. New York: Guilford Press.

Lidz, C. S. (1997). Dynamic assessment approaches. In D. P. Flanagan, J. L. Genshaft, & P. L. Harrison (Eds.), *Contemporary intellectual assessment* (pp. 281–296). New York: Guilford Press.

Lidz, C. S. (2001). Multicultural issues and dynamic assessment. In J. G. Ponterotto & L. A. Suzuki (Eds.), *Handbook of multicultural assessment: Clinical, psychological, and educational applications* (2nd ed., pp. 523–539). San Francisco: Jossey-Bass.

Lidz, C. S. (2003). *Early childhood assessment*. New York: Wiley.

Lidz, C. S. (2005). Dynamic assessment with young children: We've come a long way baby! *Journal of Early Childhood and Infant Psychology*, *1*, 99–112.

Lidz, C. S., Eisenstat, G., Evangelista, N., Robinson, F., Stokes, J., Thies, L., et al. (1999). Flexible assessment: Position paper. *The School Psychologist*, *53*(1), 12–15, 21.

Lidz, C. S., & Pena, E. (1996). Dynamic assessment: The model, its relevance as a nonbiased approach, and its application to Latino American preschool children. *Language, Speech, and Hearing Services in Schools*, *27*, 367–384.

Lidz, C. S., & Thomas, C. (1987). The Preschool Learning Assessment Device: Extension of a static approach. In C. S. Lidz (Ed.), *Dynamic assessment: An interactional approach to evaluating learning potential* (pp. 288–326). New York: Guilford Press.

Lieberman, A. F. (2004). Child–parent psychotherapy. In A. J. Sameroff, S. C. McDonough, & K. L. Rosenblum (Eds.), *Treating parent–infant relationship problems: Strategies for intervention* (pp. 97–122). New York: Guilford Press.

Lieberman, A. F., Weston, D., & Pawl, J. H. (1991). Preventative intervention and outcome in anxiously attached dyads. *Child Development*, *62*, 199–209.

Linares, N. (1981). Rules for calculating mean length of utterance in morphemes for Spanish.

In J. Erickson & D. Omark (Eds.), *Communication assessment of the bilingual bicultural child* (pp. 291–296). Baltimore: University Park Press.

Lindamood, C. H., & Lindamood, P. C. (1991). *Lindamood Auditory Conceptualization Test—Revised.* Austin, TX: PRO-ED.

Lindamood, C. H., & Lindamood, P. C. (2004). *Lindamood Auditory Conceptualization Test* (3rd ed.). Austin, TX: PRO-ED.

Lindeman, D. P., Goodstein, H. A., Sacks, A., & Young, C. C. (1984). An evaluation of the yellow brick road test through a full prediction–performance matrix. *Journal of School Psychology, 22,* 111–117.

Linder, P. E. (1997). Parents in a family literacy program: Their attitudes, beliefs, and behaviors regarding literacy learning. In W. M. Linek & E. G. Sturtevant (Eds.), *Exploring literacy* (pp. 119–131). Commerce, TX: College Reading Association.

Linder, T. W. (1990). *Transdisciplinary play-based assessment: A functional approach to working with young children.* Baltimore: Brookes.

Linder, T. W. (1993). *Transdisciplinary play-based intervention.* Baltimore: Brookes.

Linder, T. W. (1996). *Transdisciplinary play-based assessment: A functional approach to working with young children* (rev. ed.). Baltimore: Brookes.

Linn, M. I., Goodman, J. F., & Lender, W. L. (2000). Played out? Passive behavior by children with Down syndrome during unstructured play. *Journal of Early Intervention, 23,* 264–278.

Linn, R. L. (1994). Criterion-referenced measurement: A valuable perspective clouded by surplus meaning. *Educational Measurement: Issues and Practice, 13*(4), 12–14.

Linver, M. R., Brooks-Gunn, J., & Cabrera, N. (2004). The Home Observation for Measurement of the Environment (HOME) Inventory: The derivation of conceptually derived subscales. *Parenting: Science and Practice, 4,* 99–114.

Lloyd, B. H., & Abidin, R. R. (1985). Revision of the Parenting Stress Index. *Journal of Pediatric Psychology, 10,* 169–177.

Locke, J. L. (1994). Phases in the child's development of language. *American Scientist, 82,* 436–445.

Locke, H. J., & Wallace, K. M. (1959). Short marital-adjustment and prediction tests: Their reliability and validity. *Marriage and Family Living, 21,* 251–255.

Loeber, R., Keenan, K., Lahey, B. B., Green, S., & Thomas, C. (1993). Evidence for developmentally based diagnoses of oppositional defiant disorder and conduct disorder. *Journal of Abnormal Child Psychology, 21*(4), 377–410.

Loesch, D. Z., Bui, Q. M., Butler, E., Huggins, R. M., Grisby, J., Epstein, J., et al. (2003). Effect of the fragile X status categories and the fragile X mental retardation protein levels on executive functioning in males and females with fragile X. *Neuropsychology, 17*(4), 646–657.

Lohman, D. F. (2005). Review of Naglieri and Ford (2003): Does the Naglieri Nonverbal Ability Test identify equal proportions of high-scoring white, black, and Hispanic students? *Gifted Child Quarterly, 49*(1), 19–28.[

Longo, A. (2003). Test review of the Expressive One-Word Picture Vocabulary Test—2000 Edition (EOWPVT). In J. C. Impara, B. S. Plake, & R. A. Spies (Eds.), *The fifteenth mental measurements yearbook* [Electronic version]. Retrieved from http://web5.silverplatter.com/webspirs/start.ws?customer=waldo&databases=(YB)

Lonigan, C. J., Fischel, J. E., Whitehurst, G. J., Arnold, D. S., & Valdez-Menchaca, M. C. (1992). The role of otitis media in the development of expressive language disorder. *Developmental Psychology, 28,* 430–440.

Lopez, E. C. (2002). Best practices in working with school interpreters to deliver psychological services to children and families. In A. Thomas & J. Grimes (Eds.), *Best practices in school psychology IV* (Vol. 2, pp. 1419–1432). Bethesda, MD: National Association of School Psychologists.

Lord, C. (1995). Follow-up of two-year-olds referred for possible autism. *Journal of Child Psychology and Psychiatry, 36,* 1365–1382.

Lord, C., Pickles, A., McLennon, J., Rutter, M., Bregman, J., Folstein, S., et al. (1997). Diagnosing autism: Analysis of data from the Autism Interview. *Journal of Autism and Developmental Disorders, 27*(5), 501–517.

Lord, C., & Risi, S. (1998). Frameworks and methods in diagnosing autism spectrum disorders. *Mental Retardation and Developmental Disabilities Research Review, 4*(2), 90–96.

Lord, C., & Rutter, M. (1994). Autism and pervasive developmental disorders. In M. Rutter, E. Taylor, & L. Hersov (Eds.), *Child and adolescent psychiatry* (pp. 569–593). Oxford: Blackwell.

Lord, C., Rutter, M., DiLavore, P. C., & Risi, S. (2002). *Autism Diagnostic Observation Schedule.* Los Angeles: Western Psychological Services.

Lord, C., Rutter, M., & LeCouteur, A. (1994). Autism Diagnostic Interview—Revised (ADI-R): A revised version of a diagnostic interview for caregivers of individuals with possible pervasive disorders. *Journal of Autism and Developmental Disorders, 24,* 659–685.

Lord, C., & Schopler, E. (1985). Differences in sex ratios in autism as a function of measured intelligence. *Journal Autism and Developmental Disorders, 15,* 185–193.

Lord, C., & Schopler, E. (1989). Stability of assessment results of autistic and non-autistic language-impaired children from preschool years to early school age. *Journal of Child Psychology and Psychiatry, 30,* 575–590.

Lord, C., Storoschuk, S., Rutter, M., & Pickles, A. (1999). Using the ADI-R to diagnose autism in preschool children. *Infant Mental Health Journal, 14,* 234–252.

Los Angeles Unified School District. (1988, Fall). *Guide to psychoeducational assessment* (exp. ed.). Los Angeles: Author.

Loveland, K. A., & Kelly, M. L. (1991). Development of adaptive behavior in preschoolers with autism or Down syndrome. *American Journal on Mental Retardation, 96,* 13–20.

Lowe, M., & Costello, A. J. (1988). *Symbolic Play Test* (2nd ed.). London, England: NFER-Nelson.

Luckasson, R., Borthwick-Duffy, S., Buntinx, W. H. E., Coulter, D. L., Craig, E. M., Reeve, A., et al. (2002). *Mental retardation: Definition, classification and systems of supports* (10th ed.). Washington, DC: American Association on Mental Retardation.

Luckasson, R., Coulter, D. A., Reiss, S., Schalock, R. L., Snell, M. E., Stark, J. A., et al. (1992). *Mental Retardation: Definition, classification, and systems of supports* (9th ed.). Washington, DC: American Association on Mental Retardation.

Lucyshyn, J. M., Dunlap, G., & Albin, R. W. (Eds.). (2002). *Families and positive behavior support: Addressing problem behavior in family contexts.* Baltimore: Brookes.

Lucyshyn, J. M., Horner, R. H., Dunlap, G., Albin, R. W., & Ben, K. R. (2002). Positive behavior support with families. In J. M. Lucyshyn, G. Dunlap, & R. W. Albin (Eds.), *Families and positive behavior support: Addressing problem behavior in family contexts* (pp. 3–43). Baltimore: Brookes.

Luiz, D. M., Foxcroft, C. D., & Stewart, R. (2001). The construct validity of the Griffiths Scales of Mental Development. *Child: Care, Health and Development, 27*(1), 73–83.

Lund, N. J., & Duncan, J. F. (1993). *Assessing children's language in naturalistic contexts* (3rd ed.). Englewood Cliffs, NJ: Prentice-Hall.

Luster, T., & McAdoo, H. (1994). Factors related to the achievement and adjustment of young African-American children. *Child Development, 61,* 311–346.

Luthar, S. S. Burack, J. A., Cicchetti, D., & Weisz, J. R. (Eds.). (1997). *Developmental psychology: Perspectives on adjustment, risk, and disorder.* New York: Cambridge University Press.

Lynch, E. W. (2004a). Conceptual framework: From cultural shock to cultural learning. In E. W. Lynch & M. J. Hanson (Eds.), *Developing cross-cultural competence: A guide for working with children and their families* (3rd ed., pp. 19–39). Baltimore: Brookes.

Lynch, E. W. (2004b). Developing cross-cultural competence. In E. Lynch & M. Hanson (Eds.), *Developing cross-cultural competence: A guide for working with young children and their families* (2nd ed., pp. 41–77). Baltimore: Brookes.

Lynch, E. W., & Hanson, M. J. (Eds.). (2004a). *Developing cross-cultural competence: A guide for working with children and their families* (3rd ed.). Baltimore: Brookes.

Lynch, E. W., & Hanson, M. J. (2004b). Steps in the right direction: Implications for service providers. In E. W. Lynch & M. J. Hanson (Eds.), *Developing cross-cultural competence: A guide for working with children and their families* (3rd ed., pp. 449–466). Baltimore: Brookes.

Lyons-Ruth, K., Wolfe, R., Lyubchik, A., & Steingard, R. (2003). Depressive symptoms in parents of children under age 3: Sociodemographic predictors, current correlates, and associated parenting behaviors. In N. Halfon & K. T. McLearn (Eds.), *Child rearing in America: Challenges facing parents with young children* (pp. 217–259). New York: Cambridge University Press.

Lyytinen, P., Poikkeus, A. M., & Laasko, M. L. (1997). Language and symbolic play in toddlers. *International Journal of Behavioral Development, 21,* 289–302.

MacMillan, D. L., Gresham, F. M., Siperstein, G. N., & Bocian, K. H. (1996). The labyrinth of IDEA: School decisions on referred students with subaverage intelligence. *American Journal on Mental Retardation, 101,* 161–174.

Madle, R. A. (2001a). Test review of the Social Competence and Behavior Evaluation—Preschool Edition (SCBE). In B. S. Plake & J. C. Impara (Eds.), *The fourteenth mental mea-*

surements yearbook [Electronic version]. Retrieved from http://web5.silverplatter.com/webspirs/start.ws?customer=waldo&databases=(YB)

Madle, R. A. (2001b). Test review of the Test of Language Development—Third Edition: Primary (TOLD-P3). In B. S. Plake and J. C. Impara (Eds.), *The fourteenth mental measurements yearbook* [Electronic version]. Retrieved from the Buros Institute's *Test Reviews Online* website: www.unl.edu/buros

Madle, R. A. (2005). Test review of the Preschool and Kindergarten Behavior Scales-2 (PKBS-2). In R. A. Spies & B. S. Plake (Eds.), *The sixteenth mental measurements yearbook* [Electronic version]. Retrieved from http://web5.silverplatter.com.arugula.cc.columbia.edu:2048/webspirs/start.ws?customer=waldo&databases=(YB)

Madsen, K. M., Hviid, A., Vestergaard, M., Schendel, D., Wohlfahrt, J., Thorsen, P., et al. (2002). A population-based study of measles, mumps, and rubella vaccination and autism. *New England Journal of Medicine, 347*(19), 1477–1482.

Mahoney, W. J., Szatmari, P., MacLean, J. E., Bryson, S. E., Bartolucci, G., Walter, S. D., et al. (1998). Reliability and accuracy of differentiating pervasive developmental disorder subtypes. *Journal of the American Academy of Child and Adolescent Psychiatry, 37*(3), 278–285.

Main, M., & Goldwyn, R. (1984). Predicting rejection of her infant from mother's representation of her own experience: Implications for the abused–abusing intergenerational cycle. *Child Abuse and Neglect, 8*(2), 203–217.

Majsterek, D. J., Shorr, D. N., & Erion, V. L. (2000). Promoting early literacy through rhyme detection activities during Head Start circle time. *Child Study Journal, 30*(3), 143–151.

Malatesta, C. Z., Culver, C., Tesman, J. R., & Shepard, B. (1989). The development of emotional expression during the first two years of life. *Monographs of the Society for Research in Child Development, 54*(1–2), 1–104.

Malcolm, T. (2005). Test review of the Boehm Test of Basic Concepts—Third Edition: Preschool Version. In R. A. spies & B. S. Plake (Eds.), *The sixteenth mental measurement yearbook* [Electronic version]. Retrieved from http://web5.silverplatter.com/webspirs/start.ws?customer=waldo&databases=(YB)

Malone, D. M., & Landers, M. A. (2001). Mothers' perception of toy play of preschoolers with intellectual disabilities. *International Journal of Disability, Development, and Education, 48*, 91–102.

Malone, D. M., & Stoneman, Z. (1990). Cognitive play of mentally retarded preschool children: Observations in the home and school. *American Journal on Mental Retardation, 94*, 475–487.

Mancini, J. A. (2001). Test review of the Family Environment Scale—Third Edition (FES). From B. S. Plake & J. C. Impara (Eds.), *The fourteenth mental measurements yearbook* [Electronic version]. Retrieved from http://web5.silverplatter.com/webspirs/start.ws?customer=waldo&databases=(YB)

Manikam, R. (2001). Test review of the Test for Auditory Comprehension of Language—Third Edition (TACL-3). In B. S. Plake & J. C. Impara (Eds.), *The fourteenth mental measurements yearbook* [Electronic version]. Retrieved from the Buros Institute's *Test Reviews Online* website: www.unl.edu/buros

Mann, J., ten Have, T., Plunkett, J. W., & Meisels, S. J. (1991). Time sampling: A methodological critique. *Child Development, 62*, 227–241.

Manning, M., Kamii, C., & Kato, T. (2006). DIBELS: Not justifiable. In K. S. Goodman (Ed.), (2006). *The truth about DIBELS: What it is, what it does* (pp. 71–78). Portsmouth, NH: Heinemann.

Mantzicopoulos, P. Y., & Maller, S. J. (2002). The Brigance K & 1 Screen: Factor composition with a Head Start sample. *Journal of Psychoeducational Assessment, 20*, 164–182.

Mantzicopoulos, P. (2003). Flunking kindergarten after Head Start: An inquiry into the contribution of contextual and individual variables. *Journal of Educational Psychology, 95*(2), 268–278.

Mardell-Czudnowski, C. (1989). Test review of the Sequenced Inventory of Communication Development—Revised Edition. In J. C. Conoley & J. J. Kramer, *The tenth mental measurements yearbook* [Electronic version]. Retrieved from the Buros Institute's *Test Reviews Online* website: www.unl.edu/buros

Mardell-Czudnowski, C., & Goldenberg, D. S. (1998). *Developmental Indicators for the Assessment of Learning—Third Edition (DIAL-3)*. Circle Pines, MN: American Guidance Service.

Marschark, M., Lang, H. G., & Albertini, J. A. (2002). *Educating deaf students: From research to practice*. New York: Oxford University Press.

Marshall, H. H. (2003). Opportunity deferred or

opportunity taken?: An updated look at delaying kindergarten entry. *Young Children, 58*(5), 84–93.

Martin, A. (1988). Screening, early intervention and remediation: Obscuring children's potential. *Harvard Educational Review, 58*, 488—501.

Martin, R. P., & Bridger, R. (1999). *Temperament Assessment Battery for Children—Revised (TABC-R)*. Athens, GA: Authors.

Martuzza, R. (1977). *Applying norm-referenced and criterion-referenced measurement in education*. Boston: Allyn & Bacon.

Mascolo, J. (1998). Acknowledging, understanding, and assessing the impact of children's exposure to community violence. *The School Psychologist, 52*(2), 37, 47, 52, 53, 63, 72.

Mash, E. J., & Terdal, L. G. (Eds.) (1988). *Behavioral assessment of childhood disorders* (2nd ed.). New York: Guilford Press.

Mash, E. J., & Terdal, L. J. (Eds.). (1997). *Assessment of childhood disorders* (3rd ed.). New York: Guilford Press.

Mason, J. M. (1980). When children do begin to read: An exploration of four-year-old children's letter and word reading competencies. *Reading Research Quarterly, 15*, 203–227.

Mason, J. M. (1992). Reading stories to preliterate children: A proposed connection to reading. In P. Gough, L. C. Ehri, & R. Treman (Eds.), *Reading acquisition* (pp. 215–241). Hillsdale, NJ: Erlbaum.

Mason, J. M., & Sinha, S. (1993). Emerging literacy in the early childhood years: Applying a Vygotskian model of learning and development. In B. Spodek (Ed.), *Handbook of research on the education of young children* (pp. 137–150). New York: Macmillan.

Masten, A. S., & Coatsworth, J. D. (1998). The development of competence in favorable and unfavorable environments. *American Psychologist, 53*, 205–220.

Mattes, L. J., & Omark, D. R. (1984). *Speech and language assessment for the bilingual handicapped*. San Diego, CA: College-Hill Press.

Mattson, S. N., Riley, E. P., Gramling, L., Delis, D. C., & Lyons Jones, K. (1998). Neurophysiologic comparison of alcohol-exposed children with or without physical features of fetal alcohol syndrome. *Neuropsychology, 12*(1), 146–153.

May, D. C., & Kundert, D. K. (1992). Kindergarten screenings in New York State: Tests, purposes, and recommendations. *Psychology in the Schools, 29*, 35–41.

May, D. C., & Kundert, D. K. (1993). Prefirst placement: How common and how accurate? *Psychology in the Schools, 30*, 161–167.

May, D. C., Kundert, D. K., Nikoloff, O., Welch, E., Garrett, M., & Brent, D. (1994). School readiness: An obstacle to intervention and inclusion. *Journal of Early Intervention, 18*, 290–301.

May, D. C., & Welch, E. (1986). Screening for school readiness: The influence of birthdate and sex. *Psychology in the Schools, 23*, 100–105.

Mayes, L. C. (1999). Developing brain and *in utero* cocaine exposure: Effects on neural ontogeny. *Development and Psychopathology, 11*, 685–714.

Mayes, S. D., & Calhoun, S. L. (2001). Nonsignificance of early speech delay in children with autism and normal intelligence and implications for DSM-IV Asperger's disorder. *Autism: International Journal of Research and Practice, 3*, 327–354.

McAdoo, H. (1978). Minority families. In J. Stevens & M. Matthews (Eds.), *Mother/child, father/child relationships* (pp. 177–195). Washington, DC: National Association for the Education of Young Children.

McCarney, S., & Bauer, A. M. (1995). *Attention Deficit Disorders Evaluation Scale, Second Edition (ADDES)*. Columbia, MO: Hawthorne Educational Services.

McCarthy, D. (1972). *McCarthy Scales of Children's Abilities*. New York: Psychological Corporation.

McCartney, K. (1984). Effect of quality of day care environment on children's language development. *Developmental Psychology, 20*(2), 244–260.

McCartney, K., Scarr, S., Phillips, D., Grajek, S., & Schwarz, J. C. (1982). Environmental differences among day care centers and their effects on children's development. In E. F. Sigler & E. W. Gordon (Eds.), *Daycare: Scientific and social policy issues* (pp. 126–151). Boston: Auburn House.

McCarty, F., Abbott-Shin, M., & Lambert, R. (2001). The relationships between teacher beliefs and practices, and Head Start classroom quality. *Early Education and Development, 12*(2), 225–238.

McCauley, R. (2003). Test review of the Fluharty Preschool Speech and Language Screening Test—Second Edition (Fluharty-2). From B. S. Plake, J. C. Impara, & R. A. Spies (Eds.), *The fifteenth mental measurements yearbook* [Electronic version]. Retrieved from http://web5s.silverplatter.com/webspirs/start.ws?customer=waldo&databases=YB

McCauley, R. J. (1995). Test review of the Reynell Developmental Language Scales

(RDLS). In J. C. Conoley & J. C. Impara, *The twelfth mental measurements yearbook* [Electronic version]. Retrieved from the Buros Institute's *Test Reviews Online* website: www.unl.edu/buros

McCauley, R. J., & Swisher, L. (1984). Psychometric review of language and articulation tests for preschool children. *Journal of Speech and Hearing Disorders*, *49*, 34–42.

McCloskey, G. (1990). Selecting and using early childhood rating scales. *Topics in Early Childhood Special Education*, *10*(3), 39–64.

McConaughy, S. H. (1993). Evaluating behavioral and emotional disorders with the CBCL, TRF, and YSR cross-informant scales. *Journal of Emotional and Behavioral Disorders*, *1*(1), 40–52.

McConaughy, S. H. (2005). Direct observational assessment during test sessions and child clinical interviews. *School Psychology Review*, *34*(4), 490–506.

McConaughy, S. H., & Achenbach, T. M. (2004). *Manual for the Test Observation Form for ages 2–18*. Burlington, VT: University of Vermont, Research Center for Children, Youth, and Families.

McCormick, L., & Goldman, R. (1984). Designing an optimal learning program. In L. McCormick & R. Schiefelbusch (Eds.), *Early language intervention: An introduction* (pp. 201–242). Columbus, OH: Merrill.

McCune-Nicholich, L. (1981). Toward symbolic functioning: Structure of early pretend games and potential parallels with language. *Child Development*, *52*, 785–797.

McGill-Franzen, A. (1994). Compensatory and special education: Is there accountability for learning and belief in children's potential? In E. H. Hiebert & B. M. Taylor (Eds.), *Getting reading right from the start* (pp. 13–35). Boston: Allyn & Bacon.

McGill-Franzen, A., & Allington, R. L. (1991). *The School Psychologist*, *53*(3), 92–96.

McGill-Franzen, A., Lanford, C., & Adams, E. (2002). Learning to be literate: A comparison of five urban early childhood programs. *Journal of Educational Psychology*, *94*, 443–464.

McGoldrick, M., Gerson, R., & Shellenberger, S. (1999). *Genograms: Assessment and intervention* (2nd ed.). New York: Norton.

McGrew, K. S. (1997). Analysis of the major intelligence batteries according to the proposed comprehensive Gf–Gc framework. In D. P. Flanagan, J. L. Genshaft, & P. L. Harrison (Eds.), *Contemporary intellectual assessment* (pp. 151–174). New York: Guilford Press.

McKnight, T. (2005). Test review of the Bracken School Readiness Assessment. In R. A. Spies & B. S. Plake (Eds.), *The sixteenth mental measurement yearbook* [Electronic version]. Retrieved from http://web5s.silverplatter.com.arugula.cc.columbia.edu:2048/webspirs/start.ws?cu stomer=waldo&databases=YB

McLean, L. K. S. (1990). Communication development in the first two years of life: A transactional process. *Zero to Three*, *11*(1), 13–19.

McLoyd, V. C. (1998). Socioeconomic disadvantage and child development. *American Psychologist*, *53*, 185–204.

McMahon, R. J., & Forehand, R. L. (2003). *Helping the noncompliant child: Family-based treatment for oppositional behavior* (2nd ed.). New York: Guilford Press.

McNeill, D. (1966). A study of word association. *Journal of Verbal Learning and Verbal Behavior*, *5*(6), 548–557.

McNeill, D. (1970). The development of language. In P. H. Mussen (Ed.), *Carmichael's manual of child psychology* (3rd ed., pp. 1061–1161). New York: Wiley.

McWilliam, R. A., & Bailey, D. B. (1995). Effects of classroom social structure and disability on engagement. *Topics in Early Childhood Special Education*, *15*(2), 123–147.

McWilliam, R. A., & Dunst, C. J. (1985a). *Needs Evaluation for Educators of Developmentally Delayed Students*. Unpublished manuscript, Family, Infant, and Preschool Program, Western Carolina Center, Morganton, NC.

McWilliam, R. A., & Dunst, C. J. (1985b). *Preschool Assessment of the Classroom Environment*. Unpublished manuscript, Family, Infant, and Preschool Program, Western Carolina Center, Morganton, NC.

McWilliam, R. A., Galant, K., & Dunst, C. J. (1984). *Daily Engagement Rating Scale*. Unpublished manuscript, Family, Infant, and Preschool Program, Western Carolina Center, Morganton, NC.

Mecham, M. J. (1989). *Utah Test of Language Development—3*. Austin, TX: PRO-ED.

Mecham, M. J. (2003). *Utah Test of Language Development—Fourth Edition (UTLD-4)*. Austin, TX: PRO-ED.

Meier, R. P. (1991). Language acquisition in deaf children. *American Scientist*, *79*, 60–70.

Meier, R. P., & Newport, E. L. (1990). Out of the hands of babes: On a possible sign advantage in language acquisition. *Language*, *66*, 1–23.

Meisels, S. J. (1985). The efficacy of early intervention: Why are we still asking this question? *Topics in Early Childhood Special Education*, *5*(2), 1–11.

Meisels, S. J. (1987). Uses and abuse of developmental screening and school readiness testing. *Young Children*, *42*(4–6), 68–73.

Meisels, S. J. (1989a). *Developmental screening in early childhood: A guide* (3rd ed.). Washington, DC: National Association for the Education of Young Children.

Meisels, S. J. (1989b). High-stakes testing in kindergarten. *Educational Leadership*, *46*(7), 16–22.

Meisels, S. J. (1991). Dimensions of early identification. *Journal of Early Intervention*, *15*(1), 26–35.

Meisels, S. J. (1992). Doing harm by doing good: Latrogenic effects of early childhood enrollment and promotion policies. *Early Childhood Research Quarterly, 7,* 155–174.

Meisels, S. J. (1999). Assessing readiness. In R. C. Pianta & M. J. Cox (Eds.), *The transition to kindergarten* (pp. 39–66). Baltimore: Brookes.

Meisels, S. J., & Atkins-Burnett, S. (1994). *Developmental screening in early childhood: A guide* (4th ed.). Washington, DC: National Association for the Education of Young Children.

Meisels, S. J., & Atkins-Burnett, S. (2000). The elements of early childhood assessment. In J. P. Shonkoff & S. J. Meisels (Eds.), *Handbook of early childhood intervention* (pp. 231–257). New York: Cambridge University Press.

Meisels, S. J., & Atkins-Burnett, S. (2004). The Head Start national reporting system: A critique. *Public Policy Viewpoint: National Association for the Education of Young Children.* Retrieved from www.naeyc.org/resources/journal

Meisels, S. J., & Atkins-Burnett, S. (2005). *Developmental screening in early childhood: A guide* (5th ed.). Washington, DC: National Association for the Education of Young Children.

Meisels, S. J., Dorfman, A., & Steele, D. (1995). Equity and excellence in group-administered and performance-based assessments. In M. T. Nettles & A. L. Nettles (Eds.), *Equity and excellence in educational testing and assessment* (pp. 243–261). Boston: Kluwer Academic.

Meisels, S. J., Jablon, J. R., Marsden, D. B., Dichtelmiller, M. L., & Dorfman, A. B. (2001). *The Work Sampling System, Fourth Edition.* Ann Arbor, MI: Rebus.

Meisels, S. J., Liaw, F., Dorfman, A. B., & Nelson, F. R. (1995). The Work Sampling System: Reliability and validity of a performance assessment for young children. *Early Childhood Research Quarterly*, *10*, 277–296.

Meisels, S. J., Marsden, D. B., Wiske, M. S., & Henderson, L. W. (1997). *Early Screening Inventory—Revised.* Ann Arbor, MI: Rebus.

Meisels, S. J., & Provance, S. (1989). *Screening and assessment: Guidelines for identifying young disabled and developmentally vulnerable children and their families.* Washington, DC: National Center for Clinical Infant Programs.

Meisels, S. J., Steele, D. M., & Quinn-Leering, K. (1993). Testing, tracking, and retraining young child: An analysis of research and social policy. In B. Spodek (Ed.), *Handbook of research on the education of young children* (pp. 279–292). New York: Macmillan.

Menyuk, P. (1972). Relationships among components of the grammar in language disorder. *Journal of Speech and Hearing Research, 15,* 395–406.

Mercer, C. D., Algozzine, B., & Trifiletti, J. (1979a). Early identification: An analysis of research. *Learning Disabilities Quarterly*, *2*, 12–24.

Mercer, C. D., Algozzine, B., & Trifiletti, J. J. (1979b). Early identification: Issues and considerations. *Exceptional Children*, *21*(2), 52–54.

Mercer, J., & Lewis, J. (1982). *Adaptive Behavior Inventory for Children.* New York: Psychological Corporation.

Merrell, K. W. (2002). *Preschool and Kindergarten Behavior Scales—Second Edition (PKBS-2).* Austin, TX: PRO-ED.

Merrell, K. W., & Holland, W. L. (1997). Social-emotional behavior of preschool-age children with and without developmental delays. *Research in Developmental Disabilities*, *18*, 393–405.

Messick, S. (1984). Assessment in context: Appraising student performance in relation to instructional quality. *Educational Researcher, 13*(3), 3–8.

Messick, S. (1989). Validity. In R. L. Linn (Ed.), *Educational measurement* (pp. 13–103). New York: Macmillan.

Messick, S. (1995). Standards of validity and the validity of standards in performance assessment. *Educational Measurement: Issues and Practice*, *14*(40), 5–8.

Messinger, D., Bauer, C., Das, A., Seifer, R., Lester, B., Lagasse, L., et al. (2004). The maternal lifestyle study: Cognitive, motor, and behavioral outcomes of cocaine-exposed and opiate-exposed infants through three years of age. *Pediatrics*, *113*, 1677–1685.

Michaels, H. (2001). Test review of the School-Age Care Environment Rating Scale (SACERS). From J. C. Impara & B. S. Plake (Eds.), *The fourteenth mental measurements yearbook* [Electronic version]. Retrieved from http://web5s.silverplatter.com/arugula.cc.columbia.edu:2048/webspirs/start.ws?customer=waldo&databases=YB

Miller, J. (Ed.). (1981). *Assessing language production in children: Experimental procedures*. Baltimore: University Park Press.

Miller, J. F., & Chapman, R. (1981). The relation between age and mean length of utterance in morphemes. *Journal of Speech and Hearing Research*, *24*, 154–161.

Miller, L. J. (1993). *First STEp: Screening Test for Evaluating Preschoolers*. San Antonio, TX: Psychological Corporation.

Miller, L. K. (1999). The savant syndrome: Intellectual impairment and exceptional skill. *Psychological Bulletin*, *125*(1), 31–46.

Minuchin, S. (1974). *Families and family therapy.* Cambridge, MA: Harvard University Press.

Mirenda, P. (1995). Test review of the Psychoeducational Profile—Revised. In J. C. Conoley & J. C. Impara (Eds.), *The twelfth mental measurements yearbook* [Electronic version]. Retrieved from http://web5.silverplatter.com/webspirs/start.ws?customer=waldo&databases=(YB)

Mirenda, P. (2001). Test review of Asperger Syndrome Diagnostic Scale (ASDS). In B. S. Blake, J. C. Impara, & R. A. Spies (Eds.), *The fifteenth mental measurements yearbook* [Electronic version]. Retrieved from http://web5.silverplatter.com/webspirs/start.ws?customer=waldo&databases=(YB)

Mitchell, S. K., & Gray, C. A. (1981). Developmental generalizability of the HOME inventory. *Educational and Psychological Measurement*, *41*(4), 1001–1010.

Molnar, G. E., & Kaminer, R. K. (1985). Growth and development. In G. E. Molnar (Ed.), *Pediatric rehabilitation* (pp. 19–41). Baltimore: Williams & Wilkins.

Montes, F., & Risley, T. R. (1975). Evaluating traditional daycare practices: An empirical approach. *Child Care Quarterly*, *4*, 208–215.

Moore, G. T. (1987). The physical environment and cognitive development in childcare centers. In C. S. Weinstein & T. G. David (Eds.), *Spaces for children: The built environment and child development* (pp. 41–72). New York: Plenum Press.

Moos, R. H. (1976). *The human context: Environmental determinants of behavior.* New York: Wiley.

Moos, R. H. & Moos, B. S. (1994). *Family Environment Scale—Third Edition (FES-3)*. Palo Alto, CA: Consulting Psychologists Press.

Morado, C. (1987, April). *Kindergarten alternatives for the child who is "not ready": Programs and policy issues*. Paper presented at the biennial meeting of the Society for Research in Child Development, Baltimore.

Morreale-Sherwin, P. (2001). Test review of the Test of Early Language Development—Third Edition (TELD-3). From J. C. Impara & B. S. Plake (Eds.), *The fourteenth mental measurements yearbook* [Electronic version]. Retrieved from http://web5.silverplatter.com/webspirs/start.ws?customer=waldo&databases=(YB)

Morrow, L. W. (1992). The impact of a literature-based program on literacy development, use of literature, and attitudes of children from minority backgrounds. *Reading Research Quarterly*, *27*(2), 250–275.

Mullen, E. M. (1995). *Mullen Scales of Early Learning: AGS Edition*. Circle Pines, MN: American Guidance Service.

Muma, J. R. (1985). "No news is bad news": A response to McCauley and Swisher (1984). *Journal of Speech and Hearing Disorders*, *50*(3), 290–293.

Muma, J. R. (1986). *Language acquisition: A functional perspective*. Austin, TX: PRO-ED.

Muñoz-Sandoval, A. F., Cummins, J., Alvarado, C. G., Ruef, M., & Schrank, F. A. (2005). *Bilingual Verbal Ability Tests Normative Update*. Itasca, IL: Riverside.

Muris, P., Steerneman, P., & Ratering, E. (1997). Brief report: Inter-rater reliability of the Psychoeducational Profile (PEP). *Journal of Autism and Developmental Disorders*, *27*(5), 621–626.

Mutter, V., Hulme, C., & Snowling, M. (1997). *Phonological Abilities Test*. London: Psychological Corporation.

Myers, B. A. (1989). Misleading cues in the diagnosis of mental retardation and infantile autism in the preschool child. *Mental Retardation*, *27*, 85–90.

Myers, S. P. (1988). Teaching individuals with mental handicaps receptive and productive possessive pronouns using a model procedure. *Dissertation Abstracts International*, *48*(10), 3131B.

Myles, B., Bock, S., & Simpson, R. (2001). *Asperger Syndrome Diagnostic Scale (ASDS)*. Austin, TX: PRO-ED.

Nagel, R. J. (2000). Issues in preschool assessment. In B. A. Bracken (Ed.), *The psychoeducational assessment of preschool children* (3rd ed., pp. 19–32). Boston: Allyn & Bacon.

Naglieri, J. A. (1988). *Draw a Person: A quantita-*

tive scoring system. San Antonio, TX: Psychological Corporation.

Naglieri, J. A. (1997). *Naglieri Nonverbal Ability Test*. San Antonio, TX: Psychological Corporation.

Naglieri, J. A. (2003). Addressing underrepresentation of gifted minority children using the Naglieri Nonverbal Ability Test (NNAT). *Gifted Child Quarterly*, *47*(2), 155–160.

Naglieri, J. A. (2005). The Cognitive Assessment System. In D. P. Flanagan & P. L. Harrison (Eds.), *Contemporary intellectual assessment* (2nd ed., pp. 441–460). New York: Guilford Press.

Naglieri, J. A., Booth, A. L., & Winsler, A. (2004). Comparison of Hispanic Children with and without limited English proficiency on the Naglieri Nonverbal Ability Test. *Psychological Assessment*, *16*(1), 81–84.

Naglieri, J. A., Braden, J. P., & Gottling, S. M. (1993). Confirmatory factor analysis of the planning, attention, simultaneous, successive (PASS) cognitive processing model for a kindergarten sample. *Journal of Psychoeducational Assessment*, *11*, 259–269.

Naglieri, J. A., & Das, J. P. (1997). *Das–Naglieri: Cognitive assessment system*. Itasca, IL: Riverside.

Naglieri, J. A., & Das, J. P. (2005). Planning, attention, simultaneous, successive (PASS) theory: A revision of the concept of intelligence. In D. P. Flanagan, & P. L. Harrison (Eds.). *Contemporary intellectual assessment* (2nd ed., pp. 120–135). New York: Guilford Press.

Naglieri, J. A., & Ford, D. Y. (2005). Increasing minority children's participation in gifted classes using the NNAT: A response to Lohman. *Gifted Child Quarterly*, *49*(1), 29–36.

Naglieri, J. A., & Ronning, M. E. (2000). Comparison of white, African American, Hispanic and Asian children on the Naglieri Nonverbal Ability Test. *Psychological Assessment*, *12*(3), 328–335.

National Association for the Education of Young Children (NAEYC). (1984). *Accreditation criteria and procedures—revised*. Washington, DC: Author.

National Association for the Education of Young Children (NAEYC). (1988). Position statement on the standardized testing of young children 3 through 8 years of age. *Young Children*, *43*(3), 42–47.

National Association for the Education of Young Children (NAEYC). (1991). *Accreditation criteria and procedures of the National Academy of Early Childhood Programs*. Washington, DC: Author.

National Association for the Education of Young Children (NAEYC) & International Reading Association (IRA). (1998). *Learning to read and write: Developmentally appropriate practices for young children*. Joint position statement. Washington, DC: Author.

National Association of Education of Young Children (NAEYC) and the National Association of Early Childhood Specialists in State Departments of Education (NAECS/SDE). (2003). *Early Childhood Curriculum, Assessment, and Program Evaluation: Building an effective, accountable system in programs for children birth through age 8*. Washington, DC: Author.

National Association of Early Childhood Specialists in State Departments of Education. (1987). *Unacceptable trends in kindergarten entry and placement: A position statement*. Lincoln, NE: Author.

National Association of School Psychologists (NASP). (2000). *Directory of bilingual school psychologists*. Bethesda, MD: Author.

National Association of School Psychologists (NASP). (2003a, February). Position statement: Advocacy for appropriate educational services for all children. *Communiqué*, insert.

National Association of School Psychologists (NASP). (2003b, February). Position statement: Rights without labels. *Communiqué* insert.

National Association of State Boards of Education. (1988). *Right from the start. Report of the NASBE task force on early childhood education*. Alexandria, VA: Author.

National Center for Children in Poverty. (2005, July). *Fact sheet*. Retrieved from www.nccp.org/fact.html

National Center for Education Statistics (NCES). (1994). *A statistical agenda for early childhood care and education: Addendum to a guide to improving the national education data system*. Washington, DC: U.S. Department of Education.

National Center on Addiction and Substance Abuse (CASA). (1999). *No safe haven: Children of substance abusing parents*. Retrieved from www.ncsacw.samhsa.gov/resources.asp

National Educational Goals Panel. (1991). *The National Educational Goals report*. Washington, DC: Author.

National Household Survey on Drug Abuse. (2003). Children living with substance-abusing or substance-dependent parents. Office of Applied Studies, Substance Abuse and Mental Health Services Administration. Retrieved from www.oas.samhsa.gov/2k3/children/children.htm

National Institute of Child Health and Human Development (NICHD) Early Child Care Research Network. (2000). The relation of child care to cognitive and language development. *Child Development*, *71*, 958–978.

National Institute of Child Health and Human Development (NICHD) (2003, October). Speech and language impairments. *Disability Fact Sheet*, No. 11.

National Institute of Child Health and Human Development (NICHD) Early Child Care Research Network. (2003). The NICHD study of early child care: Contexts of development and developmental outcomes over the first seven years of life. In J. Brooks-Gunn, A. S. Fuligni, & L. J. Berlin (Eds.), *Early child development in the 21st century* (pp. 181–201). New York: Teachers College Press.

National Institute of Child Health and Human Development (NICHD) Early Child Care Research Network. (2005). Duration and developmental timing of poverty and children's cognitive and social development from birth through third grade. *Child Development*, *76*, 795–810.

National Institute for Early Education Research (NIEER) (2003). Survey finds states are failing nation's children: Inadequate preschool programs. Retrieved 7/29/05 http://nieer.org/meduacebter/index.php?PressID=37.

National Reading Panel (2002). *Teaching children to read: An evidence-based assessment of the scientific research literature on reading and its implications for reading instruction.* Washington, DC: U.S. Department of Health and Human Services, National Institute of Child Health and Human Development.

National Research Council. (2001). *Educating children with autism.* Committee on Educational Interventions for children with Autism. Division of Behavioral and Social Sciences and Education. Washington, DC: National Academy Press.

Natriello, G., McDill, E., & Pallas, A. (1990). *Schooling disadvantaged children: Racing against catastrophe.* New York: Teachers College Press.

Nehring, A. D., Nehring, E. F., Bruni, J. R., & Randolph, P. L. (1992). *Learning Accomplishment Profile—Diagnostic.* Lewisville, NC: Kaplan Early Learning.

Neisworth, J. T., & Bagnato, S. J. (1988). Assessment in early childhood special education: A typology of dependent measures. In S. M. Odom & K. B. Karnes (Eds.), *Early intervention for infants and children with handicaps* (pp. 23–49). Baltimore: Brookes.

Neisworth, J. T., & Bagnato, S. J. (1992). The case against intelligence testing in early intervention. *Topics in Early Childhood Special Education*, *12*, 1–20.

Nellis, L. (2001). Test review of the Bracken Basic Concept Scale—Revised (BBCS-R). In B. S. Plake & J. C. Impara (Eds.), *The fourteenth mental measurements yearbook* [Electronic version]. Retrieved from the Buros Institute's *Test Reviews Online* website: www.unl.edu/buros

Nelson, R. O., & Bowles, P. E. (1975). The best of two worlds: Observations with norms. *Journal of School Psychology*, *13*(1), 3–9.

Neuman, S. B., & Dickinson, D. K. (2001). Introduction. In S. B. Neuman & D. K. Dickinson (Eds.), *Handbook of early literacy research* (Vol. 1, pp. 3–10). New York: Guilford Press.

New York State Department of Health. (1999). *Clinical practice guidelines: The guideline technical report. Autism/pervasive developmental disorders assessment and intervention for young children (ages 0–3 years)* (Publication No. 4217). Albany, NY: Author.

Newborg, J. (2004). *Battelle Developmental Inventory, Second Edition (BDI-2).* Itasca, IL: Riverside.

Newborg, J., Stock, J. R., Wnek, L., Guidubaldi, J., & Svinicki, J. (1984). *Battelle Developmental Inventory.* Chicago: Riverside.

Newborn and Infant Hearing Screening and Intervention Act of 1999. H. R. 1193, IH 106th Cong. 1st session, H.R. 1193.

Newcomer, P. L., & Hammill, D. D. (1997), *Test of Language Development—Primary, Third Edition.* Austin, TX: PRO-ED.

Newman, P. W., Creaghead, N. A., & Secord, W. A. (1985). *Assessment and remediation of articulatory and phonological disorders.* Columbus, OH: Merrill.

Newsom, C., & Hovanitz, C. A. (1997). Autistic disorders. In E. J. Mash & L. G. Terdal (Eds.), *Assessment of childhood disorders* (3rd ed., pp. 408–452). New York: Guilford Press.

Nihira, K., Weisner, T. S., & Bernheimer, L. P. (1994). Ecocultural assessment in families of children with developmental delays: Construct and concurrent validities. *American Journal on Mental Retardation*, *98*(5), 551–566.

Nilsson, J. E., Berkel, L. A., Love, K. M., Wendler, A. M., Flores, L, Y., & Mecklenburg, E. C.

(2003). An 11 year review of *Professional Psychology: Research and Practice*: Content and sample analysis with an emphasis on diversity. *Professional Psychology: Research and Practice, 34*(6), 611–616.

No Child Left Behind (NCLB) Act of 2001, Pub. L. No. 107-110, 115 Stat. 1425 (2002).

Nord, C. W., Brimhall, D., & West, U. (1997). *Fathers' involvement in their children's schools*. Washington, DC: U.S. Department of Education. (ERIC Document Reproduction Service No. ED409 125)

Nordin, V., & Gillberg, C. (1996). Autism spectrum disorders in children with physical or mental disability: I. Clinical and epidemiological aspects. *Developmental Medicine and Child Neurology, 38*, 297–313.

Norris, J. A. (1998). Test review of the Clinical Evaluation of Language Fundamentals—Preschool-2 (CELF Preschool-2). In J. C. Impara & B. S. Plake (Eds.), *The thirteenth mental measurements yearbook* [Electronic version]. Retrieved from the Buros Institute's *Test Reviews Online* website: www.unl.edu/buros

Novak, C. (2001). Test review of the Metropolitan Readiness Tests—Sixth Edition (MRT-6). From J. C. Impara & B. S. Plake (Eds.), *The fourteenth mental measurements yearbook* [Electronic version]. Retrieved from http://web5.silverplatter.com/webspirs/start.ws?customer=waldo&databases=(YB)

Novak, C. (2002). Test review of the Test for Auditory Comprehension of Language—Third Edition (TACL-3). In B. S. Plake & J. C. Impara (Eds.), *The fourteenth mental measurements yearbook* [Electronic version]. Retrieved from the Buros Institute's *Test Reviews Online* website: www.unl.edu/buros

Nunnally, J. C. (1978). *Psychometric theory* (2nd ed.). New York: McGraw-Hill.

Nurss, J. R. (1987). *Readiness for kindergarten* (ERIC Clearinghouse on Elementary and Early Childhood Education). Urbana: University of Illinois.

Nurss, J. R. (1992). Child assessment trends, concerns, and issues. In L. R. Williams & D. P. Fromberg (Eds.), *Encyclopedia of early childhood education* (pp. 275–276). New York: Garland Press.

Nurss, J. R., & McGauvran, M. E. (1995). *Metropolitan Readiness Tests—Sixth Edition (MRT-6)*. San Antonio, TX: Psychological Corporation.

Nuttall, E. V., De Leon, B., & Valle, M. (1990). Best practices in considering cultural factors. In A. Thomas & J. Grimes (Eds.), *Best practices in school psychology* (pp. 219–233). Washington, DC: National Association of School Psychologists.

Nuttall, E. V., Romero, I., & Kalesnik, J. (1999). *Assessing and screening preschoolers: Psychological and educational dimensions* (2nd ed.). Austin, TX: PRO-ED.

Oades-Ses, G., & Alfonso, V. C. (2005). *A critical review of the psychometric integrity of preschool language tests*. Manuscript submitted for publication.

O'Connor, S. (1991). *Assessing school-age child care quality*. Unpublished manuscript, Wellesley School-Age Project, Wellesley, MA.

Oehler-Stinnett, J. J. (1998). Test review of the Parenting Stress Index—Third Edition (PSI-3). From J. C. Impara & B. S. Plake (Eds.), *The thirteenth mental measurements yearbook* [Electronic version]. Retrieved from http://web5.silverplatter.com/webspirs/start.ws.customer=waldo&databases=(YB)

Ohio Department of Education. (1989). *The early childhood identification process: A manual for screening and assessment*. Columbus: Author.

Ohtake, Y., Santos, R. M., & Fowler, S. A. (2000). It's a three-way conversation: Families, service providers, and interpreters working together. *Young Exceptional Children, 4*(1), 12–18.

Oller, J. W., & Damico, J. S. (1991). Theoretical considerations in the assessment of LEP students. In E. V. Hamayan & J. S. Damicao (Eds.), *Limiting bias in the assessment of bilingual students* (pp. 77–110). Austin, TX: PRO-ED.

Olmi, D. J. (1998). Test review of the Autism Screening Instrument for Educational Planning—Second Edition (ASIEP-2). In J. C. Impara & B. S. Plake (Eds.), *The thirteenth mental measurements yearbook* [Electronic version]. Retrieved from http://web5.silverplatter.com/webspirs/start.ws?customer=waldo&databases=(YB)

Olmi, D. J. (2001). Test review of the Test of Word Finding—Second Edition (TWF-2). In B. S. Plake, J. C. Impara, & R. A. Spies, *The fourteenth mental measurements yearbook* [Electronic version]. Retrieved from the Buros Institute's *Test Reviews Online* website: www.unl.edu/buros

Olswang, L. B., & Bain, B. A. (1988). Assessment of language in developmentally disabled infants and preschoolers. In T. D. Wachs & R. Sheehan (Eds.), *Assessment of young developmentally disabled children: Perspectives in developmental psychology* (pp. 285–320). New York: Plenum Press.

Olswang, L. B., & Carpenter, R. L. (1978). Elicitor

effects of the language obtained from young language-impaired children. *Journal of Speech and Hearing Disorders*, *43*(1), 76–88.

Ortiz, S. O. (2002). Best practices in nondiscriminatory assessment. In A. Thomas & J. Grimes (Eds.), *Best practices in school psychology IV* (Vol. 2, pp. 1321–1336). Bethesda, MD: National Association of School Psychologists.

Ortiz, S. O., & Dynda, A. M. (2005). Use of intelligence tests with culturally and linguistically diverse populations. In D. P. Flanagan & P. L. Harrison (Eds.), *Contemporary intellectual assessment* (2nd ed., pp. 545–556). New York: Guilford Press.

Osborne, C., & Berger, L. M. (2006). Parental substance abuse and child health and behavior. Unpublished paper retrieved from http://socwork/wisc.edu/unberger/OB_subabuse.pdf

Osofsky, J. D. (1995). The effects of exposure to violence on young children. *American Psychologist*, *50*, 782–788.

Osofsky, J. D., & Jackson, B. R. (1993–1994). Parenting in violent environments. *Zero to Three*, *14*(3), 8–11.

Osofsky, J. D., & Thompson, M. D. (2000). Adaptive and maladaptive parenting: Perspectives on risk and protective factors. In J. P. Shonkoff & S. J. Meisels (Eds.), *Handbook of early childhood intervention* (pp. 54–75). New York: Cambridge University Press.

Ostrov, J. M. (2005). *Early Childhood Play Project (ECPP): Observational coding manual.* Department of Psychology, University of Buffalo, NY.

Oswald, D. P. (1998a). Test review of the Autism Screening Instrument for Educational Planning—Second Edition (ASIEP-2). From J. C. Impara & B. S. Plake (Eds.), *The thirteenth mental measurements yearbook* [Electronic version]. Retrieved from http://web5.silverplatter.com/webspirs/start.ws?customer=waldo&databases=(YB)

Oswald, D. P. (1998b). Test review of the Gilliam Autism Rating Scale (GARS). In J. C. Impara & B. S. Plake (Eds.), *The thirteenth mental measurements yearbook* [Electronic version]. Retrieved from http://web5.silverplatter.com/webspirs/start.ws?customer=waldo&databases=(YB)

Otis, A., & Lennon, R. (1977-1996). *Otis--Lennon School Ability Test, Seventh Edition.* San Antonio, TX: Psychological Corporation.

Ovando, C. J. (2003). Bilingual education in the United States: Historical development and current issues. *Bilingual Research Journal*, *27*(1), 1–24.

Ovando, C. J., & Collier, V. P. (1998). *Bilingual and ESL classrooms: Teaching in multicultural contexts* (2nd ed.). Boston: McGraw-Hill.

Overton, T. (1992). Review of Transdisciplinary Play-Based Assessment. In J.C. Impara and B. S. Blake (Eds.). *The thirteenth mental measurements yearbook*. Lincoln NE: University of Nebraska Press.

Owens, R. E. (1995). *Language disorders: A functional approach to assessment and intervention* (2nd ed.). Boston: Allyn & Bacon.

Owens, R. E. (2004). *Language disorders: A functional approach to assessment and intervention* (4th ed.). Boston: Allyn & Bacon.

Oyserman, D., Mowbray, C. T., Meares, P. A., & Firminger, K. B. (2003). Parenting among mothers with a serious mental illness. In M. E. Hertzig & E. A. Farber (Eds.), *Annual progress in child psychiatry and child development: 2000–2001* (pp. 177–216). New York: Brunner-Routledge.

Page, T. J., & Iwata, B. A. (1986). Interobserver agreement: History, theory, and current methods. In A. Poling & R. Fuga (Eds.), *Research methods in applied behavior analysis* (pp. 99–126). New York: Plenum Press.

Paget, K. D. (1985). Preschool services in the schools: Issues and implications. *Special Services in the Schools*, *2*, 3–25.

Paget, K. D. (1990). Best practices in the assessment of competence in preschool age children. In A. Thomas & J. Grimes (Eds.), *Best practices in school psychology II* (pp. 107–119). Washington, DC: National Association of School Psychologists.

Paget, K. D. (1991). The individual assessment situation: Basic considerations for preschool-age children. In B. A. Bracken (Ed.), *The psychoeducational assessment of preschool children* (2nd ed., pp. 32–52). Boston: Allyn & Bacon.

Paget, K. D. (2001). Review of the Early Screening Inventory—Revised. In B. S. Plake & J. C. Impara (Eds.), *The fourteenth mental measurements yearbook* [Electronic version]. Retrieved from http://web5s.silverplatter.com.arugula.cc.columbia.edu:2048/webspirs/start/ws?customer=waldo&databases=YB

Paget, K. D., & Barnett, D. W. (1990). Assessment of infants, toddlers, preschool children, and their families: Emergent trends. In T. B. Gutkin & C. R. Reynolds (Eds.), *The handbook of school psychology* (2nd ed., pp. 458–486). New York: Wiley.

Paget, K. D., & Nagle, R. (1986). A conceptual model of preschool assessment. *School Psychology Review*, *15*, 154–165.

Paget, K. D. (2001). Test review of the Early Childhood Environment Rating Scale—Revised Edition (ECERS-R). From J. C. Impara & B. S. Plake (Eds.), *The fourteenth mental measurements yearbook* [Electronic version]. Retrieved from http://web5.silverplatter.com/webspirs/start.ws?customer=waldo&databases=(YB)

Palsha, S. A., & Wesley, P. W. (1998). Improving quality in early childhood environments through on-site consultation. *Topics in Early Childhood Special Education*, *18*(4), 243–253.

Paolito, A. W. (1995). Review of the Symbolic Play Test—Second Edition. In J. C. Conoley & J. C. Impara (Eds.), *The twelfth measurements yearbook* (pp. 1024–1026). Lincoln, NE: Buros Institute of Mental Measurements.

Paradis, J., Crago, M. B., Genesee, F., & Rice, M. (2003). Bilingual children with specific language impairment: How do they compare with their monolingual peers? *Journal of Speech, Language, and Hearing Research*, *46*, 1–15.

Paredes Scribner, J. (2002). Best assessment and intervention practices with second language learners. In A. Thomas & J. Grimes (Eds.), *Best practices in school psychology IV* (pp. 1485–1499). Bethesda, MD: National Association of School Psychologists.

Paris, S. G. (2005). Reinterpreting the development of reading skills. *Reading Research Quarterly, 40*(2), 184–202.

Parker, R. (1996). Incorporating speech–language therapy into an applied behavior analysis program. In C. Maurice, G. Green, & S. C. Luce (Eds.), *Behavioral intervention for young children with autism: A manual for parents and professionals* (pp. 303–305). Austin, TX: PRO-ED.

Parker, R. (2005, January 30). Plan would require students pass yearly tests. *Naples [Florida] Daily News*, p. 15AC.

Parten, M. (1932). Social participation among preschool children. *Journal of Abnormal and Social Psychology*, *27*, 243–269.

Patterson, G. R., Reid, J. B., & Dishion, T. J. (1992). *Antisocial boys*. Eugene, OR: Castalia.

Paul, P. V. (2001). *Language and deafness* (3rd ed.). San Diego, CA: Singular.

Paul, R. (2001). *Language disorders from infancy through adolescence: Assessment & intervention* (2nd ed.). St. Louis: Mosby.

Pavelski, R. (2001). Test review of the Caregiver-Teacher Report Form (C-TRF). From B. S. Plake & J. C. Impara (Eds.), *The fourteenth mental measurements yearbook* [Electronic version]. Retrieved from http://web5.silverplatter.com/webspirs/start.ws?customer=waldo&databases=(YB)

Pearson, B. (1998). Assessing lexical development in bilingual babies and toddlers. *International Journal of Bilingualism*, *2*(3), 347–372.

Pearson, D. P. (2006). Foreword, In K. S. Goodman (Ed.), *The truth about DIBELS: What it is, what is does* (pp. 60–65). Portsmouth, NH: Heinemann.

Pearson, M. E. (1989). Test review of the Sequenced Inventory of Communication Development—Revised Edition. In J. C. Conoley & J. J. Kramer, *The tenth mental measurements yearbook* [Electronic version]. Retrieved from the Buros Institute's *Test Reviews Online* website: www.unl.edu/buros

Pecukonis, M. T. (1993). Daily living. In R. Smith (Ed.), *Children with mental retardation: A parents' guide* (pp. 209–257). Rockville, MD: Woodbine House.

Peisner, E. S., Bryant, D. M., & Clifford, R. M. (1988). *Checklist of kindergarten activities.* Unpublished manuscript.

Peisner-Feinberg, E., & Burchinal, M. (1997). Relations between pre-school children's childcare experiences and concurrent development: The Cost, Quality, and Outcomes Study. *Merrill–Palmer Quarterly*, *43*(3), 451–477.

Peisner-Feinberg, E., Burchinal, M., Clifford, R. M., Culkin, M. L., Howes, C., Kagan, S. L., et al. (1999). *The children of the Cost, Quality, and Outcomes Study go to school.* Chapel Hill: University of North Carolina at Chapel Hill, Frank Porter Graham Child Development Center.

Pellegrini, A. D. (1991). A longitudinal study of popular and rejected children's rough-and-tumble play. *Early Education and Development*, *2*(3), 205–213.

Pellegrini, A. D. (1998). Play and the assessment of young children. In O. N. Saracho and B. Spodek (Eds.), *Multiple perspectives on play in early childhood education* (pp. 220–239). Albany: State University of New York Press.

Pena, E., Quinn, R., & Iglesias, A. (1992). The application of dynamic methods in language assessment: A nonbiased procedure. *Journal of Speical Education*, *26*, 269–280.

Penfield, D. (1995). Review of the Revised Brigance Diagnostic Inventory of Early Development. In J. Conoley & J. Impara (Eds.), *The twelfth mental measurements yearbook* (pp. 852–853). Lincoln, NE: Buros Institute of Mental Measurements.

Pepper, S., & Stewart, B. (1985). *Informal family daycare: A study of caregivers*. Toronto: Ontario Mental Health Foundation.

Perfetti, C. A., Beck, I., Bell, L. D., & Hughes, C. (1988). Phonemic knowledge and learning to read are reciprocal: A longitudinal study of first-grade children. In K. E. Stanovich (Ed.), *Children's reading and the development of phonological awareness* (pp. 39–75). Detroit: Wayne State University Press.

Perlman, M., Zellman, G. L., & Le, V. (2004). Examining the psychometric properties of the Early Childhood Environment Rating Scale—Revised (ECERS-R). *Early Childhood Research Quarterly, 19*(3), 398–412.

Perry, A., & Factor, P. (1989). Psychometric validity and clinical usefulness of the Vineland Adaptive Behavior Scales and the AAMD Adaptive Behavior Scale for an autistic sample. *Journal of Autism and Developmental Disorders, 19*, 41–56.

Perry, B. D. (1997). Incubated in terror: Neurodevelopmental factors in the "cycle of violence." In J. D. Osofsky (Ed.), *Children in a violent society* (pp. 124–149). New York: Guilford Press.

Perry, B. D., & Pate, J. E. (1994). Neurodevelopment and the psychobiological roots of post-traumatic stress disorders. In L. F. Koziol & C. E. Stout (Eds.), *The neuropsychology of mental illness: A practical guide* (pp. 120–147). Springfield, IL: Charles C. Thomas.

Perry, B. D., Pollard, R., Blakley, T., Baker, W., & Vigilante, D. (1995). Childhood trauma, the neurobiology of adaption, and the "use-dependent" development of the brain: How "states" become "traits." *Infant Mental Health Journal, 16*, 271–291.

Perry, M. J., & Schachter, J. P. (2003). Migration of native and foreign born: 1995–2000: Census 2000 Special Reports. Retrieved from www.census.gov/prod/2003pubs/censr-11.pdf

Peterson, C. A., Wall, S., Raikes, H. A., Kisker, E. E., Swanson, M. E., Jerald, J., et al. (2004). Early Head Start: Identifying and serving children with disabilities. *Topics in Early Childhood Special Education, 24*(2), 76–88.

Peverly, S. T., & Kitzen, K. R. (1998). Curriculum-based assessment of reading skills: Considerations and caveats for school psychologists. *Psychology in the Schools, 35*(1), 29–47.

Phelps, L., & Grabowski, J. (1991). Autism, differential diagnosis, and behavioral assessment update. *Journal of Psychopathology and Behavioral Assessment, 13*(2), 107–125.

Piaget, J. (1929). *The child's conception of the world*. New York: Harcourt, Brace.

Piaget, J. (1951). *Play, dreams and imitation in childhood*. New York: Norton.

Piaget, J. (1969). *Collected psychological works*. Moscow: Prosveshchenie.

Pianta, R. C., La Paro, K. M., & Hamré, B. R. (2007). *Classroom Assessment Scoring System Manual*—preschool (pre-K) version. Baltimore: Brookes.

Pianta, R. C., & Walsh, D. J. (1996). *High-risk children in schools: Creating sustaining relationships*. New York: Routledge.

Pickles, A., Bolton, P., MacDonald, H., et al. (1995). Latent-class analysis of recurrence risks for complex phenotypes with selection and measurement error: A twin and family history study of autism. *American Journal of Human Genetics, 57*, 717–726.

Pilowsky, T., Yirmiya, N., Shulman, C., & Dover, R. (1998). The Autism Diagnostic Interview—Revised and the Childhood Autism Rating Scale: Differences between diagnostic systems and comparison between genders. *Journal of Autism and Developmental Disorders, 28*(2), 143–151.

Pineda, D., Ardila, A., Rosselli, M., Arias, B. E., Henao, G. C., Gomez, L. F., et al. (1999). Prevalence of attention-deficit/hyperactivity disorder symptoms in 4 to 17-year-old children in the general population. *Journal of Abnormal Child Psychology, 27*, 455–460.

Plata, M. (1993). Using Spanish-speaking interpreters in special education. *Remedial and Special Education, 14*(5), 19–24.

Plomin, R., & Spinath, F. M. (2004). Intelligence: Genetics, genes, and genomics. *Journal of Personality and Social Psychology, 86*(1), 112–129.

Polk, C. (1994). Therapeutic work with African-American families: Using knowledge of the culture. *Zero to Three, 15*(2), 9–11.

Poole, E. (1934). Genetic development of articulation of consonant sounds in speech. *Elementary English Review, 11*, 159–161.

Popham, W. J. (1984). Specifying the domain of content or behaviors. In R. A. Berk (Ed.), *A guide to criterion-referenced test construction* (pp. 29–48). Baltimore: John Hopkins University Press.

Poteat, G. M. (2001). Test review of the Social Competence and Behavior Evaluation—Preschool Edition (SCBE). In B. S. Plake & J. C. Impara (Eds.), *The fourteenth mental measurements yearbook* [Electronic version]. Retrieved from http://web5.silverplatter.com/webspirs/start.ws?customer=waldo&databases=(YB)

Poteat, G. M. (2005). Review of the Ages and Stages Questionnaires, Second Edition. In R. A. Spies & B. S. Plake (Eds.), *The sixteenth mental measurement yearbook* [Electronic version]. Retrieved fromhttp://web5s.silverplatter.com.arugula.cc.columbia.edu:2048/webspirs/start.ws?customer=waldo&databases=YB

Power, T. J., & Radcliffe, J. (1989). The relationship of play behavior to cognitive ability in developmentally disabled preschoolers. *Journal of Autism and Developmental Disorders, 19,* 97–107.

Power, T. J., & Radcliffe, J. (2000). Assessing the cognitive ability of infants and toddlers through play: The Symbolic Play Test. In K. Gitlin-Weiner, A. Sandgrund, & C. Schaefer (Eds.), *Play diagnosis and assessment* (2nd ed., pp. 58–79). New York: Wiley.

Prather, E., Hedrick, D., & Kern, C. (1975). Articulation development in children aged two to four years. *Journal of Speech and Hearing Research, 40,* 179–191.

Pratt, S. (2001). Test review of the Receptive One-Word Picture Vocabulary Test. In B. S. Plake, J. C. Impara, & R. A. Spies (Eds.), *The fifteenth mental measurements yearbook* [Electronic version]. Retrieved from the Buros Institute's *Test Reviews Online* website: www.unl.edu/buros

Prizant, B. M. (1990). Communication disorders and emotional/behavioral disorders in children and adolescents. *Journal of Speech and Hearing Disorders,* *55*(2), 179–192.

Prizant, B. M. (1992). Test review of the Childhood Autism Rating Scale (CARS). In J. J. Kramer & J. C. Conoley (Eds.), *The eleventh mental measurements yearbook* [Electronic version]. Retrieved from http://web5.silverplatter.com/webspirs/start.ws?customer=waldo&databases=(YB)

Prizant, B. M., Audet, L. R., Burke, G. M., Hummel, L. J., Maher, S. R., & Theodore, G. (1990). Communication disorders and emotional/behavioral disorders in children and adolescents. *Journal of Speech and Hearing Disorders,* *55*(2), 179–192.

Prizant, B. M., & Wetherby, A. M. (1990). Assessing the communication of infants and toddlers: Integrating a socioemotional perspective. *Zero to Three,* *11*(1) 1–12.

Prizant, B. M., & Wetherby, A. M. (1992). Facilitating language and communication development in autism: Assessment and intervention guidelines. In D. E. Berkell (Ed.), *Autism: Identification, education, and treatment* (pp. 107–134). Hillsdale, NJ: Erlbaum.

Prizant, B. M., & Wetherby, A. M. (1993). Communication in preschool autistic children. In E. Schopler, M. E. Van Bourgondien, & M. M. Bristol (Eds.), *Preschool issues in autism* (pp. 95–128). New York: Plenum Press.

Prizant, B. M., Wetherby, A. M., & Roberts, J. E. (1993). Communication disorders in infants and toddlers. In C. H. Zeanah (Ed.), *Handbook of infant mental health* (pp. 260–279). New York: Guilford Press.

Prutting, C. A. (1982). Pragmatics and social competence. *Journal of Speech and Hearing Disorders,* *47*(2), 123–134.

Psychological Corporation. (1983). *Basic Achievement Skills Individual Screener (BASIS).* New York: Author.

Quigley, S., & Kretschmer, R. (1982). *The education of deaf children: Issues, theory and practice.* London: Arnold.

Quine, L., & Paul, J. (1986). First diagnosis of severe mental handicap: Characteristics of unsatisfactory encounters between doctors and patients. *Social Science and Medicine, 22,* 52–62.

Quine, L., & Rutter, D. P. (1994). First diagnosis of severe mental and physical disability: A study of doctor–parent communication. *Journal of Child Psychology and Psychiatry, 35,* 1273–1287.

Rabin, I., & Allen, D. A. (1983). Developmental language disorders: Nosological considerations. In U. Kirk (Ed.), *Neuropsychology of language, reading, and spelling* (pp. 155–189). London: Academic Press.

Rabin, I., & Allen, D. A. (1987). Syndromes in developmental dysphasia and adult aphasia. *Research Publications of the Association for Research in Nervous and Mental Disease, 66,* 57–75.

Rabin, I., & Allen, D. A. (1998). The semantic–pragmatic deficit disorder: Classification issues. *International Journal of Language and Communication Disorders,* *33*(1), 82–87.

Rack, J. P., Hulme, C., Snowling, M. J., & Wightman, J. (1994). The role of phonology in young children learning to read words: The direct-mapping hypothesis. *Journal of Experimental Child Psychology, 57,* 42–71.

Rafoth, M. A., Dawson, P., & Carey, K. (1988). Supporting paper on retention. *Communiqué,* 17–19.

Ramchandani, P., Stein, A., Evans, J., O'Conner, T. G., & ALSPAC Study Team. (2005). Paternal depression in the postnatal period and child development: A prospective population study. *Lancet, 365,* 2201–2205.

Ramey, C. T., & Ramey, S. L. (1998). Early intervention and early experience. *American Psychologist, 53,* 109–120.

Ramsey, P. G. (1998). *Teaching and learning in a diverse world: Multicultural education for young children.* New York: Teachers College Press.

Rathvon, N. (2004). *Early reading assessment.* New York: Guilford Press.

Rauh, V. A., Parker, F. L., Garfinkel, R. S., Perry, J., & Andrews, H. F. (2003). Biological, social, and community influences on third-grade reading levels of minority Head Start children: A multilevel approach. *Journal of Community Psychology, 31*(3), 255–278.

Raver, C. C. (2003). Does work pay psychologically as well as economically? The role of employment in predicting depressive symptoms and parenting among low-income families. *Child Development, 74*(6), 1720–1736.

Reid, D. K., Hresko, W. P., & Hammill, D. D. (2001). *Test of Early Reading Ability—Third Edition (TERA-3)*. Circle Pines, MN: American Guidance Service.

Reid, D. K., Hresko, W. P., Hammill, D. D., & Wiltshire, S. (1991). *Test of Early Reading Ability—Deaf or Hard of Hearing (TERA-D/HH)*. Austin, TX: PRO-ED.

Reid, J. B. (1993). Prevention of conduct disorder before and after school entry: Relating interventions to developmental findings. *Development and Psychopathology, 5*(1–2), 243–262.

Reid, S. (1999). The assessment of the child with autism: A family perspective. *Clinical Child Psychology and Psychiatry, 4*(1), 63–78.

Repacholi, B., & Trapolini, T. (2004). Attachment and preschool children's understanding of maternal versus non-maternal psychological states. *British Journal of Developmental Psychology, 22*, 395–415.

Reschly, D. J. (1988). Minority MMR overrepresentation and special education reform. *Exceptional Children, 54*, 316–323.

Rescorla, L., & Goossens, M. (1992). Symbolic development in toddlers with expressive language impairment (SLI-e). *Journal of Speech and Hearing Research, 35*, 1209–1302.

Rescorla, L., & Lee, E. (2001). Language impairment in young children. In T. Layton, E. Crais, & L. Watson (Eds.), *Handbook of early language impairment in children: Nature* (pp. 1–55). Albany, NY: Delmar Thomson.

Reynell, J. K. (1999). *Reynell Developmental Language Scales—Third Edition*. Wood Dale, IL: Stoelting.

Reynell, J. K., & Gruber, C. P. (1990). *Reynell Developmental Language Scales [U.S. Scales] (RDLS)*. Los Angeles: Western Psychological Services.

Reynolds, A. J. (1991). Early schooling of children at risk. *American Education Research Journal, 28*, 392–422.

Reynolds, A. J., Ou, S., & Topitzes, J. W. (2004). Paths of effects of early childhood intervention on educational attainment and delinquency: A confirmatory analysis of the Chicago child–parent centers. *Child Development, 75*, 1299–1328.

Reynolds, C. R., Gutkin, T., Elliot, S., & Witt, J. (1984). *School psychology: Essentials of theory and Practice*. New York: Wiley.

Reynolds, C. R., & Kamphaus, R. W. (2004). *Behavior Assessment Scale for Children—Second Edition (BASC-2)*. Circle Pines, MN: American Guidance Service.

Reynolds, W. M. (1985). Test review of the Token Test for Children. In J. V. Mitchell Jr., *The ninth mental measurements yearbook* [Electronic version]. Retrieved from the Buros Institute's *Test Reviews Online* website: www.unl.edu/buros

Rhodes, R. L., Ochoa, S. H., & Ortiz, S. H. (2005). *Assessing culturally and linguistically diverse students: A practical guide*. New York: Guilford Press.

Riccio, C. A. (1992). The importance of language assessment. *Child Assessment News, 2*(1), 11–12.

Rice, D. M. (1993). When mental retardation isn't the only problem. In R. Smith (Ed.), *Children with mental retardation: A parents' guide* (pp. 343–375). Rockville, MD: Woodbine House.

Richgels, D. J. (2002). Invented spelling phonemic awareness, and reading and writing instruction. In S. B. Neuman & D. K. Dickinson (Eds.), *Handbook of early literacy research* (pp. 142–158).

Rimland, B., & Fein, D. (1988). Special talents of autistic savants. In L. K. Obler & D. Fein (Eds.), *The exceptional brain* (pp. 474–492). New York: Guilford Press.

Ritvo, E. R., Mason-Brothers, A., Freeman, B. J., Pingree, C., Jenson, W. R., McMahon, W. M., et al. (1990). The UCLA–University of Utah Epidemiological Survey of Autism: The etiologic role of rare diseases. *American Journal of Psychiatry, 147*(12), 1614–1621.

Robbins, D. L., Fein, D., Barton, M. L., & Green, J. A. (2001). The Modified Checklist for Autism in Toddlers: An initial study investigating the early detection of autism and pervasive developmental disorders. *Journal of Autism and Developmental Disorders, 31*(2), 131–144.

Roberts, J. E., Bailey, D. B., & Nychka, H. B. (1991). Teachers' use of strategies to facilitate the communication of preschool children with disabilities. *Journal of Early Intervention, 15*(4), 358–376.

Roberts, J. E., & Crais, E. R. (1989). Assessing communication skills. In D. G. Bailey & M. Wolery (Eds.), *Assessing infants and preschoolers with handicaps* (pp. 339–389). Columbus, OH: Merrill.

Robinson, J., Holmberg, J., Corbitt-Price, J., &

Wiener, P. (2002, November). Collaborations with the MacArthur Story Stem Battery: Using narratives to assess risks in young children. Paper presented at "New Directions in Young Children's Socioemotional Measures" workshop sponsored by the NIMH, the NICHD Research Network on Child and Family Well-Being, and the Science and Ecology of Early Development Initiative, Washington, DC.

Robinson, J., Mantz-Simmons, L., MacFie, J., & the MacArthur Narrative Working Group. (1992). *The narrative coding manual.* Unpublished manuscript, University of Colorado.

Rodier, P. M., & Hyman, S. L. (1998). Early environmental factors in autism. *Mental Retardation and Developmental Disabilities Research Reviews, 4,* 121–128.

Rogers, S. J. (1998). Empirically supported comprehensive treatment for young children with autism. *Journal of Clinical Child Psychology, 27,* 168–179.

Rogers-Warren, A. K. (1982). Behavioral ecology in classrooms for young handicapped children. *Topics in Early Childhood Special Education, 2*(1), 21–32.

Rogers-Warren, A., & Wedel, J. W. (1979). The ecology of preschool classrooms for the handicapped. *New Directions for Exceptional Children, 1,* 1–24.

Roggman, L. A., Boyce, L. K., Cook, G. A., Christiansen, K., & Jones, D. (2004). Playing with daddy: Social toy play, Early Head Start, and developmental outcomes. *Fathering, 2,* 83–108.

Rogoff, B. (2003). *The cultural nature of human development.* New York: Oxford University Press.

Rohrbeck, C. A. (2001). Test review of the ADHD Symptom Checklist—Fourth Edition. In B. S. Plake, J. C. Impara, & R. A. Spies (Eds.), *The fifteenth mental measurements yearbook* [Electronic version]. Retrieved from http://web5.silverplatter.com/webspirs/start.ws?customer=waldo&databases=(YB)

Roid, G. H. (2003a). *Stanford–Binet Intelligence Scales, Fifth Edition: Examiner's manual.* Itasca, IL: Riverside.

Roid, G. H. (2003b). *Stanford–Binet Intelligence Scales, Fifth Edition: Technical manual.* Itasca, IL: Riverside.

Roid, G. H. (2005). *Stanford–Binet Intelligence Scales for Early Childhood.* Itasca, IL: Riverside.

Roid, G. H., & Miller, L. J. (1997). *Leiter International Performance Scale—Revised.* Wood Dale, IL: Stoelting.

Roid, G. H., & Sampers, J. A. (2004). *Merrill–Palmer—Revised Scales of Development.* Wood Dale, IL: Stoelting.

Romaine, S. (1995). *Bilingualism* (2nd ed.). Oxford: Blackwell.

Rose, S. A., & Wallace, I. F. (1985). Visual recognition memory: A predictor of later cognitive functioning patterns. *Child Development, 56,* 843–852.

Rosenbaum, J. F., Biederman, J., Hirshfeld, D. R., Bolduc, E. A., & Cahloff, J. (1991). Behavioral inhibition in children: A possible precursor to panic disorder or social phobia. *Journal of Clinical Psychiatry, 52*(Suppl. 11), 5–9.

Rosenthal, P. A., & Rosenthal, S. (1984). Suicidal behavior in preschool children. *American Journal of Psychiatry, 141,* 520–525.

Rosner, J. (1975). *Test of Auditory Analysis Skills (TAAS).* Novato, CA: Academic Therapy.

Rosner, J. (1979). *Helping children overcome learning difficulties: A step-by-step guide for parents and teachers* (2nd ed.). New York: Walker.

Ross, G., & Lawson, K. (1997). Using the Bayley II: Unresolved issues in assessing the development of prematurely born children. *Journal of Developmental and Behavioral Pediatrics, 18,* 109–111.

Rothbart, M. K., & Bates, J. E. (1998). Temperament. In W. Damon (Series Ed.) & N. Eisenberg (Vol. Ed.), *Handbook of child psychology: Vol. 3. Social, emotional, and personality development* (5th ed., pp. 105–176). New York: Wiley.

Rothbart, M. K., Ziaie, H., & O'Boyle, C. G. (1992). Self-regulation and emotion in infancy. In R. A. Fabes & N. Eisenberg (Eds.), *Emotion and its regulation in early development* (pp. 7–23). San Francisco: Jossey-Bass.

Rothbaum, F., Weisz, J., Pott, M., Miyake, K., & Morelli, G. (2000). Attachment and culture: Security in the United States and Japan. *American Psychologist, 55,* 1093–1104.

Rothlinsberg, B. A. (1995). Test review of the Test of Early Reading Ability—Deaf or Hard of Hearing (TERA-D-HH). From J. C. Conoley & J. C. Impara (Eds.), *The twelfth mental measurements yearbook* [Electronic version]. Retrieved from http://web5.silverplatter.com/webspirs/start.ws?customer=waldo&databases=(YB)

RTI International. (n.d.). *NICHD Study of Early Child Care Phase I Instrument Document.* Retrieved from https://secc.rti.org/instdoc.doc

Rubin, K. H. (1993). The Waterloo Longitudinal Project: Correlates and consequences of social withdrawal from childhood to adolescence. In K. H. Rubin & J. Asendorph (Eds.), *Social withdrawal, inhibition, and shyness in childhood* (pp. 291–314). Hillsdale, NJ: Erlbaum.

Ruff, H. A., & Dubiner, K. (1987). Stability of individual differences in infants' manipulation and exploration of objects. *Perceptual and Motor Skills, 64*, 1095–1101.

Rumsey, J. M., & Denckla, M. B. (1987). Neurobiological research priorities in autism. In E. S. Schopler & G. B. Mesibov (Eds.), *Neurobiological issues in autism* (pp. 43–61). New York: Plenum Press.

Ruskin, E. M., Kasari, C., Mundy, P., & Sigman, M. (1994). Attention to people and toys during social and object mastery in children with Down syndrome. *American Journal on Mental Retardation, 99*, 103–111.

Ruskin, E. M., Mundy, P., Kasari, C., & Sigman, M. (1994). Object mastery motivation of children with Down syndrome. *American Journal on Mental Retardation, 98*(4), 499–509.

Russell, C. M. (1999). A meta-analysis of published research on the effects of nonmaternal care on child development. *Dissertation Abstracts International Section A: Humanities & Social Sciences, 59*(9-A), 3362.

Rutherford, M. D., & Rogers, S. J. (2003). Cognitive underpinnings of pretend play in autism. *Journal of Autism and Developmental Disorders, 33*, 289–302.

Rutter, M. (1980). *Changing youth in a changing society.* Cambridge, MA: Harvard University Press.

Rutter, M. (1981). *Maternal deprivation reassessed* (2nd ed.). Harmondsworth, UK: Penguin Books.

Rutter, M. (1987). Stress, coping, and development: Some issues and some questions. *Journal of Child Psychology and Psychiatry, 22*(4), 323–356.

Rutter, M., Bailey, A., & Lord, C. (2003). *Social Communication Questionnaire (SCQ).* Los Angeles: Western Psychological Services.

Rutter, M., Le Couteur, A., & Lord, C. (2003). *Autism Diagnostic Interview—Revised (ADI-R).* Los Angeles: Western Psychological Services.

Rutter, M., & Schopler, E. (1987). Autism and pervasive developmental disorders: Concepts and diagnostic issues. *Journal of Autism and Developmental Disorders, 17*(2), 159–186.

Sacks, O. (1995). *An anthropologist on Mars.* New York: Knopf.

Sakai, L. M., Whitebook, M., Wishard, A., & Howes, C. (2003). Evaluating the Early Childhood Environment Rating Scale (ECERS): assessing differences between the first and revised edition. *Early Childhood Research Quarterly, 18*(4), 427–445.

Salinger, T. (2001). Assessing the literacy of young children: The case for multiple forms of evidence. In S. B. Neuman & D. K. Dickinson (Eds.), *Handbook of early literacy research* (Vol. 1, pp. 390–418). New York: Guilford Press.

Salvia, J. (1985). Test review of the Token Test for Children. In J. V. Mitchell Jr., *The ninth mental measurements yearbook* [Electronic version]. Retrieved from the Buros Institute's *Test Reviews Online* website: www.unl.edu/buros

Salvia, J., & Ysseldyke, J. E. (1988). Using estimated true scores: A response to Sabers, Feldt, and Reschly. *Journal of Special Education, 22*(3), 367–373.

Salvia, J., & Ysseldyke, J. E. (2004). *Assessment in special and inclusive education* (9th ed.). Boston: Houghton Mifflin.

Salzinger, S., Kaplan, S., & Artemyeff, C. (1983). Mothers' personal social networks and child maltreatment. *Journal of Abnormal Psychology, 92*(1), 68–76.

Sameroff, A. J. (1975). Transactional models in early social relations. *Human Development, 18*(1–2), 65–79.

Sameroff, A. J. (1993, November). *Risk and resilience in children: Identifying targets for service to young children.* Paper presented at the Second National Head Start Research Conference, Washington, DC.

Sameroff, A. J. (2004). Ports of entry and the dynamics of mother–infant interventions. In A. J. Sameroff, S. C. McDonough, & K. L. Rosenblum (Eds.), *Treating parent–infant relationship problems: Strategies for intervention* (pp. 3–28). New York: Guilford Press.

Sameroff, A. J., Gutman, L. M., & Peck, S. C. (2003). Adaptation among youth facing multiple risks. In S. S. Luthar (Ed.), *Resilience and vulnerability: Adaptation in the context of childhood adversities* (pp. 364–391). New York: Cambridge University Press.

Sameroff, A. J., & MacKenzie, M. J. (2003). A quarter-century of the transactional model: How have things changed? *Zero to Three, 24*(1), 14–22.

Sameroff, A. J., McDonough, S. C., & Rosenblum, K. L. (Eds.). (2004). *Treating parent–infant relationship problems: Strategies for intervention.* New York: Guilford Press.

Sameroff, A., Seifer, R., Barocas, R., Zax, M., & Greenspan, S. (1987). Intelligence quotient scores of 4-year-old children: Social–environmental risk factors. *Pediatrics*, *79*, 343–350.

Samudra, K., & Cantwell, D. P. (1999). Risk factors for attention deficit/hyperactivity disorder. In H. C. Quay & A. E. Hogan (Eds.), *Handbook of disruptive behavior disorders* (pp. 199–220). New York: Plenum Press.

Sander, E. (1972). When are speech sounds learned? *Journal of Speech and Hearing Disorders*, *37*, 55–63.

Sandoval, J. (2003). Review of the Woodcock–Johnson III. In B. S. Plake, J. C. Impara, & R. A. Spies (Eds.), *The fifteenth mental measurements yearbook* (pp. 1024–1028). Lincoln, NE: Buros Institute of Mental Measurements.

Sattler, J. M. (1988). *Assessment of children* (3rd ed.). San Diego, CA: Author.

Sattler, J. M. (1998). *Clinical and forensic interviewing of children and families: Guidelines for the mental health, education, pediatric, and child maltreatment fields*. San Diego, CA: Author.

Sattler, J. M. (2001). *Assessment of children* (4th ed.): *Cognitive applications*. San Diego, CA: Author.

Sattler, J. M. (2002). *Assessment of children* (4th ed.): *Behavioral and clinical applications*. San Diego, CA: Author.

Sattler, J. M., & Dumont, R. (2004). *Assessment of children: WISC-IV and WPPSI-III supplement*. San Diego, CA: Author.

Scambler, D., Rogers, S. J., & Wehner, E. A. (2001). Can the Checklist for Autism in Toddlers differentiate young children with autism from those with developmental delays? *Journal of the American Academy of Child and Adolescent Psychiatry*, *40*, 1457–1463.

Scarborough, H. S. (1990). Index of Productive Syntax. *Applied Psycholinguistics*, *11*, 1–22.

Scarborough, H. S. (1998). Predicting the future achievement of second graders with reading disabilities: Contributions of phonemic awareness, verbal memory, rapid serial naming, and IQ. *Annals of Dyslexia*, *48*, 115–136.

Scarborough, H. S. (2001). Connecting early language and literacy to later reading disabilities: Evidence, theory, and practice. In S. B. Neuman & D. K. Dickinson (Eds.). *Handbook of early literacy research* (Vol. 1, pp. 97–110). New York: Guilford Press.

Scarborough, H. S., & Dobrich, W. (1990). Development of children with early language delay. *Journal of Speech and Hearing Research*, *33*(1), 70–83.

Schaefer, C., Gitlin, K., & Sandgrund, A. (Eds.). (1991). *Play diagnosis and assessment*. New York: Wiley.

Schatschneider, C., Fletcher, J. M., Francis, D. J., Carlson, C. D., & Foorman, B. R. (2004). Kindergarten prediction of reading skills: A longitudinal comparative analysis. *Journal of Educational Psychology*, *96*, 265–282.

Schemo, D. J. (2004, March 3). Schools, facing tight budgets, leave programs behind. *The New York Times*, pp. 1, 18.

Schiff-Myers, N. B., Djukic, J., McGovern-Lawler, J., & Perez, D. (1993). Assessment considerations in the evaluation of second-language learners: A case study. *Exceptional Children*, *60*(3), 237–258.

Schodorf, J. K., & Edwards, H. T. (1983). Comparative analysis of parent–child interactions with language-disordered and linguistically normal children. *Journal of Communication Disorders*, *16*(2), 71–83.

Schonkoff, J. P., & Meisels, S. (Eds.). (2000). *Handbook of early childhood intervention* (2nd ed.). New York: Cambridge University Press.

Schopler, E. (Ed.). (1995). *Parent survival manual: A guide to crisis resolution in autism and related developmental disorders*. New York: Plenum Press.

Schopler, E., Lansing, M. D., Reichler, R. J., & Marcus, L. M. (2005). *Psychoeducational Profile: TEACCH Individualized Psychoeducational Assessment for Children with Autistic Spectrum Disorders—Third Edition (PEP-3)*. Austin, TX: PRO-ED.

Schopler, E., Lansing, M., & Waters, L. (1983). *Individualized assessment and treatment for autistic and developmentally disabled children: Vol. 3. Teaching activities for autistic children*. Baltimore: University Park Press.

Schopler, E., Reichler, R. J., Bashford, A., Lansing, M. D., & Marcus, L. M. (1990). *Psychoeducational Profile—Revised (PEP-R)*. Austin, TX: PRO-ED.

Schopler, E., Reichler, R. J., & Lansing, M. (1980). *Individualized assessment and treatment for autistic and developmentally disabled children: Vol. 2. Teaching strategies for parents and professionals*. Baltimore: University Park Press.

Schopler, E., Reichler, R. J., & Renner, B. R. (1988). *The Childhood Autism Rating Scale*. Los Angeles: Western Psychological Services.

Schreibman, L. (1988). *Autism*. Newbury Park, CA: Sage.

Schultz, D., Izard, C. E., & Ackerman, B. P. (2000). Children's anger attribution bias: Relations to family environment and social adjustment. *Social Development*, *9*(3), 284–301.

Schwarting, G. (2001). Test review of the Early Childhood Environment Rating Scale—Revised Edition (ECERS-R). From J. C. Impara

& B. S. Plake (Eds.), *The fourteenth mental measurements yearbook* [Electronic version]. Retrieved from http://web5.silverplatter.com/webspirs/start.ws?customer=waldo&databases=(YB)

Schwarting, G. (2005). Test review of the Pre-reading Inventory of Phonological Awareness (PIPA). From R. A. Spies & B. S. Plake (Eds.), *The sixteenth mental measurements yearbook* [Electronic version]. Retrieved from http://web4s.silverplatter.com.arugula.cc.columbia.edu:2048/webspirs/start.ws?customer=waldo&databases=YB

Schwartz, C. E., Snidman, N., & Kagan, J. (1999). Adolescent social anxiety as an outcome of inhibited treatment in childhood. *Journal of the American Academy of Child and Adolescent Psychiatry, 38*(8), 1008–1015.

Schweinhart, L. J., Barnes, H., & Weikart, D. (1993). Significant benefits: The High/Scope Perry Preschool Study through age 27. *Monographs of the High/Scope Educational Research Foundation, 10.*

Schweinhart, L. J., & Weikart, D. P. (1998). High/Scope Perry Preschool Program effects at age twenty-seven. In J. Crane (Ed.), *Social programs that work* (pp. 148–162). New York: Russell Sage Foundation.

Scott-Little, C., Kagan, S. L., & Frelow, V. S. (2006). Conceptualization of readiness and the content of early learning standards: The intersection of policy and research? *Early Childhood Research Quarterly, 21,* 153–173.

Seay, S. (2006). How DIBELS failed Alabama: A research report. In K. S. Goodman (Ed.), *The truth about DIBELS: What it is, what it does* (pp 60–65). Portsmouth, NH: Heinemann.

Sekino, Y., & Fantuzzo, J. (2005). Validity of the Child Observation Record: An investigation of the relationship between COR dimensions and social–emotional and cognitive outcomes for Head Start children. *Journal of Psychoeducational Assessment, 3,* 242–261.

Seligman, M., & Darling, R. B. (1997). *Ordinary families, special children: A systems approach to childhood disability* (2nd ed.). New York: Guilford Press.

Semel, E., Wiig, E. H., & Secord, W. A. (2003). *Clinical Evaluation of Language Fundamentals—Fourth Edition.* San Antonio, TX: Psychological Corporation.

Semrud-Clikeman, M., & Hynd, G. W. (1993). Assessment of learning and cognitive dysfunction in young children. In J. L. Culbertson & D. J. Willis (Eds.), *Testing young children: A reference guide for developmental, psychoeducational, and psychosocial assessment* (pp. 167–191). Austin, TX: PRO-ED.

Sexton, D., Burrell, B., & Thompson, B. (1992). Measurement integrity of the Family Needs Survey. *Journal of Early Intervention, 16*(4), 343–352.

Seymour, H. N., Roeper, T. W., & de Villiers, J. (2003a). *Diagnostic Evaluation of Language Variation—Criterion Referenced.* San Antonio, TX: The Psychological Corporation.

Seymour, H. N., Roeper, T. W., & de Villiers, J., (2003b). *Diagnostic Evaluation of Language Variation—Screening Test.* San Antonio, TX: Psychological Corporation.

Shah, A., Holmes, N., & Wing, L. (1982). Prevalence of autism and related conditions in adults in a mental handicap hospital. *Applied Research on Mental Retardation, 3,* 303–317.

Shakel, J. (1987). NASP position statement and supporting paper on early intervention services in the schools. *Communiqué, 16*(3), 4–5.

Shanahan, T. (2005). Test review of the Dynamic Indicators of Basic Literacy Skills, Sixth Edition. In R. A. Spies & B. S. Plake (Eds.), *The sixteenth mental measurement yearbook* [Electronic version]. Retrieved from http://web5.silverplatter.com/webspirs/start.ws?customer=waldo&databases=(YB)

Shapiro, E. S. (1987). *Behavioral assessment in school psychology.* Hillsdale, NJ: Erlbaum.

Shapiro, E. S. (1990). An integrated model for curriculum-based assessment. *School Psychology Review, 19,* 331–349.

Shapiro, E. S. (1996). *Academic skills problems: Direct assessment and intervention* (2nd ed.). New York: Guilford Press.

Shapiro, E. S. (2004a). *Academic skills problems: Direct assessment and intervention* (3rd ed.). New York: Guilford Press.

Shapiro, E. S. (2004b). *Academic skills problems workbook* (rev. ed.). New York: Guilford Press.

Shapiro, E. S., & Lentz, F. E. (1986). Behavioral assessment of academic behavior. In T. R. Kratochwill (Ed.), *Advances in school psychology* (Vol. 5, pp. 87–139). Hillsdale, NJ: Erlbaum.

Shapiro, E. S., & Skinner, C. H. (1990). Best practices in observation and ecological assessment. In A. Thomas & J. Grimes (Eds.), *Best practices in school psychology II* (pp. 507–518). Washington, DC: National Association of School Psychologists.

Shapiro, T., & Hertzig, M. (1991). Social deviance in autism: A central integrative failure as a model for social non-engagement. *Psychiatric Clinics of North America, 14*(1), 19–32.

Shaw, D. S., Keenan, K., Vondra, J. I., Delliquadri, E., & Giovannelli, J. (1997). Antecedents of preschool children's internalizing problems: A longitudinal study of low-income families. *Journal of the American Academcy of Child and Adolescent Psychiatry, 36*, 1760–1767.

Shepard, L. A., & Graue, M. E. (1993). The morass of school readiness screening: Research on test use and test validity. In B. Spodek (Ed.), *Handbook of research on the education of young children* (pp. 293–305). New York: Macmillan.

Shepard, L., Kagan, S. L., & Wurtz, E. (Eds.). (1998). *Principles and recommendations for early childhood assessments.* Washington, DC: National Education Goals Panel, Goal 1 Early Childhood Resource Group.

Shepard, L. A., & Smith, M. L. (1985). *Boulder Valley Kindergarten Study: Retention practices and retention effects.* Boulder, CO: Boulder Valley Public Schools.

Shepard, L. A., & Smith, M. L. (1986). Synthesis of research on school readiness and kindergarten retention. *Educational Leadership, 44*, 78–86.

Shepard, L. A., & Smith, M. L. (1987). Effects of kindergarten retention at the end of first grade. *Psychology in the Schools, 24*, 346–357.

Shepard, L. A. & Smith, M. L. (1989). Academic and emotional effects of Kindergarten retention in one school district. In L. A. Shepard & M. L. Smith (Eds.), *Flunking grades: Research and policies on retention* (pp. 79–107). London: Falmer Press.

Shinn, M. R. (1989). Identifying and defining academic problems: CBM screening and eligibility procedures. In M. R. Shinn (Ed.), *Curriculum-based measurement: Assessing special children* (pp. 90–129). New York: Guilford Press.

Shinn, M. R. (Ed.) (1998). *Advanced applications of curriculum-based measurement.* New York: Guilford Press.

Shinn, M. R., Rosenfield, S., & Knutson, N. (1989). Curriculum-based assessment: A comparison of models. *School Psychology Review, 18*, 299–316.

Shipley, K. C., & McAfee, J. G. (1998). *Assessment in speech–language pathology* (2nd ed.). San Diego, CA: Singular.

Shonkoff, J., & Meisels, S. (1991). Defining eligibility for services under PL 99–457. *Journal of Early Intervention, 15*(1), 21–25.

Short, R., Simeonsson, R., & Huntington, G. (1990). Early intervention: Implication of Public Law 99-457 for professional child psychology. *Professional Psychology: Research and Practice, 21*(2), 88–93.

Shpancer, N. (2006). The effects of daycare: Persistent questions, elusive answers. *Early Childhood Research Quarterly, 21*(2), 227–237.

Sicoly, F. (1992). Estimating the accuracy of decisions based on cutting scores. *Journal of psychoeducational assessment, 10*, 26–36.

Siegel, B. (1991). Toward DSM-IV: A developmental approach to autistic disorder. *Psychiatric Clinics of North America, 14*(1), 53–68.

Siegel, B. (2003). *Helping children with autism learn: Treatment approaches for parents and professionals.* New York: Oxford University Press.

Siegel, B. (2004). *Pervasive Developmental Disorders Screening Test—Second Edition (PDDST-II).* San Antonio, TX: Psychological Corporation.

Siegel, B., Pliner, C., Eschler, J., & Elliott, G. (1988). How children with autism are diagnosed: Difficulties in identification of children with multiple developmental delays. *Journal of Developmental and Behavioral Pediatrics, 9*(4), 199–204.

Siegel, B., Vukicevic, J., & Spitzer, R. (1990). Using signal detection methodology to review DSM-III-R: Reanalysis of DSM-III-R national field trials for autistic disorder. *Journal of Psychiatric Research, 24*, 293–311.

Siegler, R. S. (1988). Individual differences in strategy choices: Good students, not-so-good students, and perfectionists. *Child Development, 59*, 833–851.

Siegler, R. S. (1996). *The emerging mind: The process of change in children's thinking.* New York: Oxford University Press.

Siegler, R. S. (1998). *Children's thinking* (3rd ed.). Upper Saddle River, NJ: Prentice Hall.

Sigman, M., & Ungerer, J. A. (1984). Cognitive and language skills in autistic, mentally retarded, and normal children. *Developmental Psychology, 20*, 293–302.

Silvern, S. B. (1988). Continuity and discontinuity between home and early childhood education environments. *Elementary School Journal, 89*, 147–159.

Simeonsson, R. (1991). Early intervention eligibility: A prevention perspective. *Infants and Young Children, 3*(4), 48–55.

Simner, M. (1983). The warning signs of school failure: An updated profile of at-risk kindergarten children. *Topics in Early Childhood Special Education, 3*(3), 17–28.

Slavin, R. E., Madden, N. A., Dolan, L. J., Wasik, B. A., Ross, S. M., & Smith, L. J. (1994). Whenever and wherever we choose: The replication of Success for All. *Phi Delta Kappa, 75*(8), 639–647.

Slobin, D. (1973). Cognitive prerequisites for the development of grammar. In C. Ferguson & D. Slobin (Eds.), *Studies of child language development* (pp. 175–208). New York: Holt, Rinehart & Winston.

Slone, M., Durrheim, K., Lachman, P., & Kaminer, D. (1998). Association between the diagnosis of mental retardation and socioeconomic factors. *American Journal on Mental Retardation, 102*, 535–546.

Smith, B. J., & Shakel, J. A. (1986). Noncategorical identification of preschool handicapped children: Policy issues and options. *Journal of the Division of Early Childhood, 11*, 78–86.

Smith, L. F. (2001). Test review of the Test of Early Reading Ability, Third Edition (TERA-3). From J. C. Impara, B. S. Plake, & R. A. Spies (Eds.), *The fifteenth mental measurements yearbook* [Electronic version]. Retrieved from http://web5.silverplatter.com/webspirs/start.ws?customer=waldo&databases=(YB)

Smith, P. K., & Connolly, K. J. (1980). *The ecology of pre-school behavior.* Cambridge, UK: Cambridge University Press.

Snow, C. (1977). The development of conversation between mothers and babies. *Journal of Child Language, 4*, 1–22.

Snow, C., & Hakuta, K. (1992). The costs of monolingualism. In J. Crawford (Ed.), *Language loyalties* (pp. 384–394). Chicago: University of Chicago Press.

Snow, C. E., Barnes, W. S., Chandler, J., Goodman, I. F., & Hemphill, L. (1991). *Unfulfilled expectations: Home and school influences on literacy.* Cambridge, MA: Harvard University Press.

Snow, C. E., Burns, S., & Griffin, P. (Eds.). (1998). *Preventing reading difficulties in young children.* Washington, DC: National Academy Press.

Snow, C. E., & Ninio, A. (1986). The contracts of literacy: What children learn from reading books. In W. H. Teale & E. Sulzby (Eds.), *Emergent literacy: Writing and reading* (pp. 116–138). Norwood, NJ: Ablex.

Snow, M. E., Hertzig, M., & Shapiro, T. (1987). Expression in emotion in young autistic children. *Journal of the American Academy of Child and Adolescent Psychiatry, 26*(6), 836–838.

Snyder, J., Kilgore, K., Schrepferman, L. M., Brooker, M., Suarez, M., & Prichard, J. (1998). *Child–Peer Observation Code.* Unpublished technical manual, Wichita State University, KS.

Snyder, L. S., & Downey, D. M. (1991). The language–reading relationship in normal and reading-disabled children. *Journal of Speech and Hearing Research, 34*(1), 129–140.

Solomon, R. (2001). Test review of the Bracken Basic Concept Scale—Revised (BBCS-R). In B. S. Plake & J. C. Impara (Eds.), *The fourteenth mental measurements yearbook* [Electronic version]. Retrieved from the Buros Institute's *Test Reviews Online* website: www.unl.edu/buros

South, M., Williams, B. J., McMahon, W. M., Owley, T., Filipek, P. A., Shernoff, E., et al. (2002). Utility of the Gilliam Autism Rating Scale in research and clinical populations. *Journal of Autism and Developmental Disorders, 32*(6), 593–599.

Spanier, U. (1976). Measuring dyadic adjustment: New scales for assessing quality of marriage and similar dyads. *Journal of Marriage and the Family, 38*, 15–25.

Sparrow, S. S., Balla, D. A., & Cicchetti, D. V. (1984). *Vineland Adaptive Behavior Scales.* Circle Pines, MN: American Guidance Service.

Sparrow, S. S., Balla, D. A., & Cicchetti, D. V. (1998). *Vineland Social–Emotional Early Childhood.* Circle Pines, MN: American Guidance Service.

Sparrow, S. S., Cicchetti, D. V., & Balla, D. A. (2005). *Vineland Adaptive Behavior Scales, Second Edition (Vineland-II).* Circle Pines, MN: American Guidance Service.

Spencer, P. E. (1996). The association between language and symbolic play at two years: Evidence from deaf toddlers. *Child Development, 67*, 867–876.

Spenciner, L. J. (2005). Test review of the Learning Accomplishment Profile – Diagnostic (LAP-D). From R. A. Spies & B. S. Plake (Eds.), *The sixteenth mental measurement yearbook* [Electronic version]. Retrieved from http://web5s.silverplatter.com.arugula.cc.columbia.edu:2048/webspirs/start.ws?customer=waldo&databases=YB

Sporakowski, M. (2001). Test review of the Family Environment Scale—Third Edition (FES). From B. S. Slake & J. C. Impara (Eds.), *The fourteenth mental measurements yearbook* [Electronic version]. Retrieved from http://web5.silverplatter.com/webspirs/start.ws?customer=waldo&databases=(YB)

Squires, J., Bricker, D., & Twombly, E. (2002). *Ages and Stages Questionnaires, Social-Emotional (ASQ:SE): A parent-completed, child-monitoring system for social-emotional behaviors.* Baltimore: Brookes.

Squires, J., Potter, L., & Bricker, D. (1999). *The ASQ user's guide* (2nd ed.). Baltimore: Brookes.

Sroufe, L. A. (1996). *Emotional development: The organization of emotional life in early years.* New York: Cambridge University Press.

Sroufe, L. A., Egeland, B., Carlson, E. A., & Collins, W. A. (2005). *The development of the person: The Minnesota study of risk and adaptation from birth to adulthood.* New York: Guilford Press.

Sroufe, L. A., Jacobvitz, D., Mangelsdorf, S., DeAngelo, E., & Ward, M. (1985). Generational boundary dissolution between mothers' and their preschool children. *Child Development, 56*, 317–325.

Stainback, G. J. (1992). Review of Transdisciplinary Play-Based Assessment. In J. C. Impara and B. S. Plake (Eds.), *The thirteenth mental measurements yearbook.* Lincoln, NE: University of Nebraska Press.

Stallman, A. C., & Pearson, P. D. (1990). Formal measures of early literacy. In L. M. Morrow & J. K. Smith (Eds.), *Assessment for instruction in early literacy* (pp. 7–44). Upper Saddle River, NJ: Prentice-Hall.

Stanley, S. D., & Greenwood, C. R. (1981). *CISSAR: Code for Instructional Structure and Student Academic Response: Observer's manual.* Kansas City: University of Kansas, Bureau of Child Research, Juniper Gardens Children's Project.

Stanovich, K., Cunningham, A., & Crammer, B. (1984). Assessing phonological awareness in kindergarten children: Issues of task comparability. *Journal of Experimental Child Psychology, 38*, 175–190.

Stavrou, T. E. (1995). Test review of the Test of Early Reading Ability—Deaf or Hard of Hearing (TERA-D-HH). From J. J. Conoley & J. C. Impara (Eds.), *The twelfth mental measurements yearbook* [Electronic version]. Retrieved from http://web5.silverplatter.com/webspirs/start.ws?customer=waldo&databases=(YB)

Stein, S. (1998). Test review of Child Developmental Inventory (CDI). From J. C. Impara & B. S. Plake (Eds.), *The thirteenth mental measurements yearbook* [Electronic version]. Retrieved from http://web5s.silverplatter.com.arugula.cc.columbia.edu:2048/webspirs/start.ws?customer=waldo&databases=YB

Stewart, L. H., & Kaminski, R. (2002). Best practices in developing local norms for academic problem solving. In A. Thomas & J. Grimes (Eds.), *Best practices in school psychology IV* (pp. 737–752). Bethesda, MD: National Association of School Psychologists.

Stiggins, R. J. (1994). *Student-centered classroom assessment.* New York: Merrill.

Stipek, D. (2002). At what age should children enter kindergarten?: A question for policy makers. *Social Policy Report: Giving Child and Youth Development Knowledge Away. Society for Research in Child Development, 16*(2), 3–19.

Stokes, J. (1989). First language Bengali development. In D. Duncan (Ed.), *Working with bilingual language disability* (pp. 60–74). New York: Chapman & Hall.

Stokes, J., & Duncan, P. (1989). Linguistic assessment procedures for bilingual children. In D. Duncan (Ed.), *Working with bilingual language disability* (pp. 113–131). New York: Chapman & Hall.

Stolarski, V., & Boehm, A. E. (2006). *Boehm Test of Basic Concepts—Third Edition for children with visual impairments.* Manuscript in preparation.

Stolarski, V., Boehm, A. E., & Boisvert, K. (2006). *A tactile version of the Boehm Test of Basic Concepts—Third Edition: Preschool.* Manuscript in preparation.

Stone, B. J., Gridley, B. E., & Gyurke, J. S. (1991). Confirmatory factor analysis of the WPPSI-R at the extreme end of the age range. *Journal of Psychoeducational Assessment, 9*, 263–270.

Stone, W. L., Coonrod, E. E., & Ousley, O. Y. (2000). Brief report: Screening Tool for Autism in Two-Year-Olds (STAT): Development and preliminary data. *Journal of Autism and Developmental Disorders, 30*(6), 607–610.

Stone, W. L., Coonrod, E. E., Turner, L. M., & Pozdol, S. L. (2004). Psychometric properties of the STAT for early autism screening. *Journal of Autism and Developmental Disabilities, 34*, 691–701.

Stone, W. L. & Hogan, K. L. (1993a). *Parent Interview for Autism (PIA).* Nashville, TN: Child Development Center at Vanderbilt University.

Stone, W. L., & Hogan, K. L. (1993b). A structured parent interview for identifying young children with autism. *Journal of Autism and Developmental Disorders, 23*(4), 639–652.

Stone, W. L., Lee, E. B., Ashford, L., Brissie, J., Hepburn, S. L., Coonrod, E. E., et al. (1999). Can autism be diagnosed accurately in children under three years? *Journal of Child Psychology and Psychiatry, 40*, 219–226.

Straus, M. A. (1979). Measuring intrafamily conflict and violence: The Conflict Tactics Scales. *Journal of Marriage and the Family, 41*, 75–88.

Straus, M. A., & Field, C. J. (2003). Psychological aggression by American parents: National data on prevalence, chronicity, and severity. *Journal of Marriage and Family, 65*, 795–808.

Straus, M. A., & Hamby, S. L. (1997). Measuring

physical and psychological maltreatment of children with the Conflict Tactics Scales. In G. Kaufman Kantor & J. L. Jasinski (Eds.), *Out of the darkness: Contemporary perspectives on family violence* (pp. 119–135). Thousand Oaks, CA: Sage.

Straus, M. A., & Kurz, D. (1997). Domestic violence: Are women as likely as men to initiate physical assaults in partner relationships? In M. R. Walsh (Ed.), *Women, men, and gender: Ongoing debates* (pp. 207–231). New Haven, CT: Yale University Press.

Stuart, R. B. (2004). Twelve practical suggestions for achieving multicultural competence. *Professional Psychology: Research and Practice, 35*(1), 3–9.

Stutman, G. (2001). Test review of the Test of Language Development—Third Edition: Primary (TOLD-P:3). In B. S. Plake & J. S. Impaira (Eds.), *The fourteenth mental measurements yearbook* [Electronic version]. Retrieved from the Buros Institute's *Test Reviews Online* website: www.unl.edu/buros

Suen, H. K., Ary, D., & Ary, R. (1986). A note on the relationship among eight indices of interobserver agreement. *Behavioral Assessment, 8*, 301–303.

Suen, H. K. (2001). Test review of the Test of Early Language Development—Third Edition (TELD-3). From J. C. Impara & B. S. Plake (Eds.), *The fourteenth mental measurements yearbook* [Electronic version]. Retrieved from http://web5.silverplatter.com/webspirs/start.ws?customer=waldo&databases=(YB)

Sullivan, P. M., Brookhouser, P. E., Scanlan, J. M., Knutson, J. F., & Schulte, L. E. (1991). Patterns of physical and sexual abuse of communicatively handicapped children. *Journal of Otology, Rhinology, and Laryngology, 100*, 188–194.

Sulzby, E. (1985). Children's emergent reading of favorite storybooks: A developmental study. *Reading Research Quarterly, 20*, 458–481.

Sulzby, E. (1986). Writing and reading: Signs of oral and written language organization in the young child. In W. H. Teale & E. Sulzby (Eds.), *Emergent literacy: Writing and reading* (pp. 50–89). Norwood, NJ: Ablex.

Sweeting, P. (1981, April). *Language assessment of the preschool child*. Paper presented at Observing and Assessing the Preschool Child Workshop, Teachers College, Columbia University, New York.

Switzky, H. (1995). Review of the Symbolic Play Tests, Second Edition. In R. A. Spires & B. S. Blake (Eds.), *The twelfth mental measurements yearbook* [Electronic version]. Retrieved from http://web5s.silverplatter.com.arugula.cc.columbia.edu:2048/webspirs/start/ws?customer=wa;dp&databases=YB.

Sylva, K., Siraj-Blatchford, I., & Taggart, B. (2003). *Assessing quality in the early years: Early Childhood Rating Scale—Extension (ECERS-E): Four curricular subscales*. Stoke-on-Trent: Trentham Books.

Sylva, K., Siraj-Blatchford, I., Taggart, B., Sammons, P., Melhuish, E., Elliot, K., & Totsika, V. (2006). Capturing quality in early childhood through environmental rating scales. *Early Childhood Research Quarterly, 21*(1), 76–92.

Symons, D. K., & Clark, S. E. (2000). A longitudinal study of mother–child relationships and theory of mind in the preschool period. *Social Development, 9*(1), 3–23.

Szatmari, P., Jones, M. B., Zwaigenbaum, L., & MacLean, J. E. (1998). Genetics of autism: Overview and new directions. *Journal of Autism and Developmental Disorders, 28*(5), 351–368.

Tabors, P. O., Roach, K. A., & Snow, C. E. (2002). Home language and literacy environment. In D. K Dickinson & P. O. Tabors (Eds.), *Beginning literacy with language: Young children learning at home and learning at school* (pp. 111–138). Baltimore: Brookes.

Taeschner, T. (1983). *The sun is feminine: A study of language acquisition in bilingual children*. Berlin: Springer-Verlag.

Task Force on Research Diagnostic Criteria: Infancy and Preschool. (2003). Research diagnostic criteria for infants and preschool children: The process and empirical support. *Journal of the American Academy of Child and Adolescent Psychiatry, 42*(12), 1504–1512.

Taylor, M. J., Crowley, S. L., & White, K. R. (1993, April). *Measuring family support and resources: Psychometric investigation of the FSS and the FRS*. Paper presented at the annual meeting of the National Council on Measurement in Education, Atlanta, GA.

Taylor, O. (1986). A cultural and communicative approach to teaching standard English as a second dialect. In O. L. Taylor (Ed.), *Treatment of communication disorders in culturally and linguistically diverse populations* (pp. 153–178). Austin, TX: PRO-ED.

Taylor, R. L. (1989). *Assessment of exceptional students* (2nd ed.). Englewood Cliffs, NJ: Prentice-Hall.

Taylor, R. L. (2005). *Assessment of exceptional children: Educational and psychological procedures* (7th ed.). Upper Saddle River, NJ: Prentice Hall.

Teale, W. H. (1990). Issues in early childhood assessment. In P. Afflerbach (Ed.), *Issues in statewide reading assessment* (pp. 35–53). Washington, DC: ERIC/American Institutes for Research.

Teale, W. H., & Sulzby, E. (1986). Emergent literacy as a perspective for examining how young children become writers and readers. In W. H. Teale & E. Sulzby (Eds.), *Emergent literacy: Writing and reading* (pp. vii–xxv). Norwood, NJ: Ablex.

Telzrow, C. (1995). Test review of *AGS Early Screening Profiles* (AGS). From J. C. Conoley & J. C. Impara (Eds.), *The twelfth mental measurements yearbook* [Electronic version]. Retrieved from http://web5s.silverplatter.com.arugula.cc.columbia.edu:2048/webspirs/start.ws?customer=waldo&databases=YB

Templin, M. (1957). *Certain language skills in children.* Minneapolis: University of Minnesota Press.

Thomas, A., & Chess, S. (1977). *Temperament and development.* New York: Brunner/Mazel.

Thomas, W. P., & Collier, V. P. (1997). *School effectiveness for language minority students.* Washington, DC: National Clearinghouse for Bilingual Education.

Thomas, W. P., & Collier, V. P. (2002). *A national study of school effectiveness for language minority students' long-term academic achievement.* Retrieved from www.crede.uscu.edu/research/llaal.html

Thompson, N. (1998). Test review of the Clinical Evaluation of Language Fundamentals—Preschool-2 (CELF Preschool-2). In J. C. Impara & B. S. Plake (Eds.), *The thirteenth mental measurements yearbook* [Electronic version]. Retrieved from the Buros Institute's *Test Reviews Online* website: www.unl.edu/buros

Thompson, R. A. (1994). Emotion regulation: A theme in search of a definition. In N. A. Fox (Ed.), The development of emotion regulation: Biological and behavioral considerations. *Monographs of the Society for Research in Child Development, 59*(2–3, Serial No. 240), 25–52, 250–283.

Thompson, R. A. (1999). Early attachment and later development. In J. Cassidy & P. R. Shaver (Eds.), *Handbook of attachment: Theory, research, and clinical applications* (pp. 265–286). New York: Guilford Press.

Thorndike, R. L., & Hagen, E. (1955). *Measurement and evaluation in psychology and education.* New York: Wiley.

Thorndike, R. L., Hagen, E. P., & Sattler, J. M. (1986a). *The Stanford–Binet Intelligence Scale: Fourth Edition.* Chicago: Riverside.

Thorndike, R. L., Hagen, E. P., & Sattler, J. M. (1986b). *The Stanford–Binet Intelligence Scale: Fourth Edition. Technical manual.* Chicago: Riverside.

Thorndike, R. M. (1990). Would the real factors of the Stanford–Binet Fourth Edition please come forward? *Journal of Psychoeducational Assessment, 8,* 412–435.

Thurlow, M. L., O'Sullivan, P. J., & Ysseldyke, J. E. (1986). Early screening for special education: How accurate? *Educational Leadership, 44,* 93–95.

Thurlow, M. L., Ysseldyke, J. E., & Wotruba, J. W. (1988). *Student and instructional outcomes under varying student teacher ratios in special education* (Research Report No. 12). Minneapolis: University of Minnesota Alternatives Project.

Thurman, K. S., & Widerstrom, A. H. (1985). *Young children with special needs: A developmental and ecological approach.* Boston: Allyn & Bacon.

Thurman, K. S., & Widerstrom, A. H. (1990). *Infants and young children with special needs: A developmental and ecological approach* (2nd ed.). Baltimore: Brookes.

Tindal, G. (1995). Test review of the Psychoeducational Profile—Revised. In J. C. Conoley & J. C. Impara (Eds.), *The twelfth mental measurements yearbook* [Electronic version]. Retrieved from http://web5.silverplatter.com/webspirs/start.ws?customer=waldo&databases=(YB)

Torgesen, J. K. (2002). The prevention of reading difficulties. *Journal of School Psychology, 40,* 7–26.

Torgesen, J. K., & Bryant, B. R. (1994). *Test of Phonological Awareness (TOPA).* Austin, TX: PRO-ED.

Torgesen, J. K., & Burgess, S. R. (1998). Consistency of reading-related phonological processes throughout early childhood: Evidence from longitudinal–correlational and instruction studies. In J. L. Metsala & L. C. Ehri (Eds.), *Word recognition in beginning literacy* (pp. 161–188). Mahwah, NJ: Erlbaum.

Torgesen, J. K., & Wagner, R. K. (1998). Alternative diagnostic approaches for specific developmental reading disabilities. *Learning Disabilities Research and Practice, 13,* 200–232.

Torrance, E. P. (2000). Preschool creativity. In B. A. Bracken (Ed.), *The psychoeducational assessment of preschool children* (3rd ed., pp. 349–363). Boston: Allyn & Bacon.

Totsika, V., & Sylva, K. (2004). The Home Observation for Measurement of the Environment revisited. *Child and Adolescent Mental Health*, *9*(1), 25–35.

Towne, R. (1992). Test review of the Bankson Language Test-2. In J. J. Kramer & J. C. Conoley (Eds.), *The eleventh mental measurements yearbook* [Electronic version]. Retrieved from the Buros Institute *Test Reviews Online* website: www.unl.edu/Buros

Towne, R. (2001). Test review of the Illinois Test of Psycholinguistic Abilities—Third Edition (ITPA-3). In B. S. Plake, J. C. Impara, & R. A. Spies (Eds.), *The fifteenth mental measurements yearbook* [Electronic version]. Retrieved from the Buros Institute's *Test Reviews Online* website: www.unl.edu/buros

Tramontana, M. G., Hooper, S. R., & Selzer, S. C. (1988). Research on the preschool prediction of later academic achievement: A review. *Developmental Review*, *8*, 78–86.

Travis, L. L., & Sigman, M. (1998). Social deficits and interpersonal relationships in autism. *Mental Retardation and Developmental Disabilities Research Reviews*, *4*, 65–72.

Trivette, C., & Dunst, C. (1988). Inventory of Social Support. In C. Dunst, C. Trivette, & A. Deal (Eds.), *Enabling and empowering families* (pp. 158–163). Cambridge, MA: Brookline Books.

Troster, H., & Brambrig, M. (1994). The play behavior and play materials of blind and sighted infants and preschoolers. *Journal of Visual Impairments and Blindness*, *88*, 421–432.

Tsai, L. Y. (1992). Diagnostic issues in high-functioning autism. In. E. Schopler & G. B. Mesibov (Eds.), *High-functioning individuals with autism* (pp. 11–40). New York: Plenum Press.

Turbiville, V. P., & Marquis, J. G. (2001). Father participation in early education programs. *Topics in Early Childhood Specail Education*, *21*, 223–231.

Turk, K. (1995). Test review of the Kaufman Survey of Early Academic and Language Skills (KSEALS). From J. C. Conoley & J. C. Impara (Eds.), *The twelfth mental measurements yearbook* [Electronic version]. Retrieved from http://web5s.silverplatter.com.arugula.cc.columbia.edu:2048/webspirs/start.ws?customer=waldo&databases=YB

Turner, L. A., & Johnson, B. (2003). A model of mastery motivation for at-risk preschoolers. *Journal of Educational Psychology*, *95*(3), 495–505.

Twombly, M. S., & Fink, G. (2004). *Ages and Stages learning activities*. Baltimore: Brookes.

Tyre, P. (September 11 2006). The new first grade: Too much too soon? *Newsweek, 148*(11), 34–36, 37–40, 41–44.

Ulrey, G. (1982). Influences of preschoolers' behavior on assessment. In G. Ulrey & S. J. Rogers (Eds.), *Psychological assessment of handicapped infants and young children* (pp. 25–34). New York: Thieme-Stratton.

U.S. Census Bureau. (2002). Race and Hispanic or Latino Origin by age and sex for the United States: 2000. Census 2000 Summary File. Retrieved from http://factfinder.census.gov.

U.S. Census Bureau (2003, October). *Current population survey*. Retrieved from http://factfinder.census.gov

U.S. Department of Education (n.d.). The No Child Left Behind Act: A desktop reference. Retrieved from www.ed.gov/admins/lead/account/nclbreference/index.html

U.S. Department for Health and Human Services Administration for Children and Families. (n.d.). Denver Developmental Screening Test-II. Retrieved from www.acf.dhhs.gov/programs/opre/ehs/perf_measures/reports/resources_measuring/res_meas_cdij.html

U.S. Department of Health and Human Services (DHHS). (1999). *Mental health: A report of the Surgeon General*. Rockville, MD: Author.

U.S. Department of Health and Human Services (DHHS). (2001). *Head Start Family and Child Experiences Survey (FACES)*. Rockville, MD: Author.

U.S. General Accounting Office. (1987). *Bilingual education: A new look at the research evidence* (Briefing report to the Chairman, Committee on Education and Labor, House of Representatives). Washington, DC: U.S. Government Printing Office.

Vandell, D. L. (2004). Early child care: The known and the unknown. *Merrill–Palmer Quarterly*, *50*(3), 387–414.

Vandell, D. L., Burchinal, M., Friedman, S., Brownell, C. (2001, April). *Overview of early child care effects at 4.5 years*. Presented as part of a symposium at the meetings of the Society for Research on Child Development, Minneapolis, MN.

Vanderveer, B., & Schweid, E. (1974). Infant assessment: Stability of mental functioning in young retarded children. *American Journal of Mental Deficiency*, *79*, 1–4.

Van Horn, M. L., Bellis, J. M., & Snyder, S. W. (2001). Family Resource Scale—Revised: Psychometrics and validation of a measure of family resources in a sample of low-income families. *Journal of Psychoeducational Assessment*, *19*, 54–68.

Venter, A., Lord, C., & Schopler, E. (1992). A follow-up study of high-functioning autistic children. *Journal of Child Psychology and Psychiatry, 33*(3), 489–507.

Verdugo, M. A., Bermejo, B. G., & Fuertes, J. (1995). The maltreatment of intellectually handicapped children and adolescents. *Child Abuse and Neglect, 19*, 205–215.

Vig, S. (2005). Classification versus labeling. In J. W. Jacobson, J. A. Mulick, & R. Foxx (Eds.), *Dubious and controversial therapies for developmental disabilities* (pp. 85–99). Mahwah, NJ: Erlbaum.

Vig, S. (in press). Young children's object play: A window on development. *Journal of Developmental and Physical Disabilities.*

Vig, S., & Jedrysek, E. (1995). Adaptive behavior of young urban children with developmental disabilities. *Mental Retardation, 33*, 91–98.

Vig, S., & Jedrysek, E. (1996a). Application of the 1992 AAMR definition: Issues for preschool children. *Mental Retardation, 34*, 244–253.

Vig, S., & Jedrysek, E. (1996b). Stanford–Binet Fourth Edition: Useful for young children with language impairment? *Psychology in the Schools, 33*, 124–131.

Vig, S., & Jedrysek, E. (1999). Autistic features in young children with significant cognitive impairment: Autism or mental retardation? *Journal of Autism and Developmental Disorders, 29*, 235–248.

Vig, S., & Kaminer, R. (2002). Maltreatment and developmental disabilities in children. *Journal of Developmental and Physical Disabilities, 14*, 371–386.

Vig, S., & Kaminer, R. (2003). Comprehensive interdisciplinary evaluation as intervention for young children. *Infants and Young Children, 16*, 342–353.

Vig, S., Kaminer, R., & Jedrysek, E. (1987). A later look at borderline and mildly retarded preschoolers. *Journal of Developmental and Behavioral Pediatrics, 8*, 12–17.

Vincent, L., Salisbury, C., Strain, P., McCormick, C., & Tessier, A. (1990). A behavioral–ecological approach to early intervention: Focus on cultural diversity. In J. Shonkoff & S. Meisels (Eds.), *Handbook of early childhood intervention* (pp. 173–195). New York: Cambridge University Press.

Volkmar, F. R., Cichetti, D. V., Dykens, E., Sparrow, S. S., Leckman, J. K., & Cohen, D. J. (1988). An evaluation of the Autism Behavior Checklist. *Journal of Autism and Developmental Disorders, 18*(1), 81–97.

Volkmar, F. R., & Klin, A. (2000). Diagnostic issues in Asperger syndrome. In A. Klin, F. R. Volkmar, & S. S. Sparrow (Eds.), *Asperger syndrome* (pp. 25–71). New York: Guilford Press.

Volkmar, F. R., & Siegel, A. (1979). Young children's responses to discrepant social communications. *Journal of Child Psychology and Psychiatry, 20*(2), 139–149.

Volkmar, F. R., Sparrow, S. S., Goudreau, D., Cicchetti, D. V., Paul, R., & Cohen, D. J. (1987). Social deficits in autism: An operational approach using the Vineland Adaptive Behavior Scales. *Journal of the American Academy of Child and Adolescent Psychiatry, 26*, 156–161.

Volpe, R. J. (2001). Test review of the ADHD Symptom Checklist—Fourth Edition. In B. S. Plake, J. C. Impara, & R. A. Spies (Eds.), *The fifteenth mental measurements yearbook* [Electronic version]. Retrieved from http://web5.silverplatter.com/webspirs/start.ws?customer=waldo&databases=(YB)

Volpe, R. J., DiPerna, J. C., Hintze, J. M., & Shapiro, E. S. (2005). Observing students in classroom settings: A review of seven coding schemes. *School Psychology Review, 34*, 454–473.

Volpe, R. J., & McConaughy, S. H. (2005). Systematic direct observational assessment of student behavior: Its use and interpretation in multiple settings: An introduction to the miniseries. *School Psychology Review, 34*, 451–453.

Vort Corporation (1994). *The Hawaii Early Learning Profile*. Palo Alto, CA: VORT.

Vygotsky, L. S. (1962). *Thought and language*. Cambridge, MA: MIT Press.

Vygotsky, L. S. (1978). *Mind in society: The development of higher psychological processes*. Cambridge, MA: Harvard University Press.

Wagner, R. K., & Torgesen, J. K. (1987). The nature of phonological processing and its causal role in the acquisition of reading skills. *Psychological Bulletin, 101*(2), 192–212.

Wagner, R. K., Torgesen, J. K., & Rashotte, C. A. (1999). *Comprehensive Test of Phonological Processing*. Austin, TX: PRO-ED.

Wahler, R. U. (1980). The insular mother: Her problems in parent–child treatment. *Journal of Applied Behavior Analysis, 13*, 207–219.

Walberg, H. (1984). Improving the productivity of America's schools. *Educational Leadership, 41*, 19–27.

Walden, T., & Knipes, L. (1996). Reading and responding to social signals. In M. Lewis & M. W. Sullivan (Eds.), *Emotional development in atypical children* (pp. 29–42). Mahwah, NJ: Erlbaum.

Walker, H. M., Kavanaugh, K., Stiller, B., Golly, A., Severson, H. H., & Feil, E. (1998). First step to success: An early intervention approach for preventing school antisocial behavior. *Journal of Emotional and Behavior Disorders*, *6*(2), 66–80.

Walker, H. M., & Severson, H. H. (1990). *Systematic Screening for Behavior Disorders (SSBD): User's guide and administration manual*. Longmont, CO: Sopris West.

Walker, H. M., Severson, H. H., & Feil, E. G. (1995). *Early Screening Project: A proven child find process*. Longmont, CO: Sopris West.

Wallace, B. C. (1986). Factors related to academic achievement in low-income minority elementary school children. *Dissertation Abstracts International*, *46*(11), 3300A.

Wallerstein, J. S., & Lewis, J. M. (2004). The unexpected legacy of divorce: Report of a 25-year study. *Psychoanalytic Psychology*, *21*, 353–370.

Walsh, F. (2003). Clinical views of family normality, health, and dysfunction: From deficit to strengths perspective. In F. Walsh (Ed.), *Normal family processes* (3rd ed., pp. 27–57). New York: Guilford Press.

Walsh, K. K. (2002). Thoughts on changing the term mental retardation. *Mental Retardation*, *40*, 70–75.

Walters, E., & Cummings, E. M. (2000). A secure base from which to explore close relationships. *Child Development*, *71*(1), 164–172.

Warner, C., & Nelson, N. W. (2000). Assessment of communication, language, and speech. In B. A. Bracken (Ed.), *The psychoeducational assessment of preschool children* (3rd ed., pp. 145–185). Boston: Allyn & Bacon.

Warren, S. L. (2003). Narrative Emotion Coding System (NEC). In R. N. Emde, D. P. Wolf, & D. Oppenheim (Eds.), *Revealing the inner worlds of young children: The MacArthur Story Stem Battery and parent–child narratives* (pp. 92–105). New York: Oxford University Press.

Warren, S. L., Huston, L., Egeland, B., & Sroufe, L. A. (1997). Child and adolescent anxiety disorders and early attachment. *Journal of the American Academy of Child and Adolescent Psychiatry*, *36*(5), 537–644.

Wasik, B. A., Bond, M. A., & Hindman, A. (2006). The effects of a language and literacy intervention on Head Start children and teachers. *Journal of Educational Psychology*, *98*, 63–74.

Wasyliw, O. (2001a). Test review of the Expressive Vocabulary Test (EVT). In B. S. Plake & J. C. Impara (Eds.), *The fourteen mental measurements yearbook* [Electronic version]. Retrieved from the Buros Institute's *Test Reviews Online* website: www.unl.edu/buros

Wasyliw, O. E. (2001b). Test review of the Peabody Picture Vocabulary Test—III (PPVT-III). From J. C. Impara & B. S. Plake (Eds.), *The fourteenth mental measurements yearbook* [Electronic version]. Retrieved from http://web5.silverplatter.com/webspirs/start.ws?customer-waldo&databases=(YB)

Waterman, B. (1998). Test Review of the Early Language Milestone Scale. In J. C. Impara & B. S. Plake (Eds.), *The thirteenth mental measurements yearbook* [Electronic version]. Retrieved from the Buros Institute *Test Reviews Online* website: www.unl.edu/Buros

Watson, S. T. (1995). Test review of the Brigance K and 1 Screen, Revised. In J. C. Conoley & J. C. Impara (Eds.), *The twelfth mental measurements yearbook* [Electronic version]. Retrieved from http://web5s.silverplatter.com.arugula.cc.columbia.edu:2048/webspirs/start.ws?customer=waldo&databases=YB

Watson, S. T. (2005). Review of the Achenbach System of Empirically Based Assessment (ASEBA). In R. A. Spies & B. S. Plake (Eds.), *The sixteenth mental measurement yearbook* [Electronic version]. Retrieved from http://web5.silverplatter.com.arugula.cc.columbia.edu:2048/webspirs/start.ws?customer=waldo&databases=(YB)

Waxler-Morrison, N., Anderson, J., & Richardson, E. (Eds.). (1990). *Cross-cultural caring: A handbook for health professionals in western Canada*. Vancouver: University of British Columbia Press.

Webster-Stratton, C. (1999). *How to promote children's social and emotional competence*. Thousand Oaks, CA: Sage.

Webster-Stratton, C. (2000). *The Incredible Years training series*. Washington, DC: U.S. Department of Justice, Office of Juvenile Justice and Delinquency Prevention.

Webster-Stratton, C. (2001). *Dina Dinosaur's Classroom-Based Social Skills, Problem-Solving, and Anger Management Curriculum*. Seattle, WA: Incredible Years.

Webster-Stratton, C., & Herbert, M. (1994). *Troubled families—problem children: Working with parents: A collaborative process*. Chichester, UK: Wiley.

Webster-Stratton, C., & Reid, M. J. (2004). Strengthening social and emotional competence in young children: The foundation for early school readiness and success. *Infants and Young Children*, *17*(2), 96–113.

Webster-Stratton, C., Reid, M. J., & Hammond, M. (2004). Treating children with early-onset conduct problems: Intervention outcomes for parent, child and teacher training. *Journal of Clinical Child and Adolescent Psychology*, *33*(1), 105–124.

Wechsler, D. (2004). *WISC-IV Spanish*. San Antonio, TX: Psychological Corporation.

Wechsler, D. (2002). *Wechsler Preschool and Primary Scale of Intelligence—Third Edition*. San Antonio, TX: Psychological Corporation.

Weckerly, J. (2002). Pediatric bipolar disorder. *Journal of Developmental and Behavioral Pediatrics*, *23*(1), 42–56.

Weinstein, C. S. (1979). The physical environment of the school: A review of the research. *Review of Education Research*, *49*(4), 597–610.

Wellman, B., Case, I., Mengurt, I., & Bradbury, D. (1931). Speech sounds in young children. *University of Iowa Studies in Child Welfare*, *5*(2).

Wells, G. (1985). *Language development in the preschool years*. New York: Cambridge University Press.

Welsh, J. S. (1992). Test review of the Childhood Autism Rating Scale (CARS). In J. J. Kramer & J. C. Conoley (Eds.), *The eleventh mental measurements yearbook* [Electronic version]. Retrieved from http://web5.silverplatter.com/webspirs/start.ws?customer=waldo&databases=(YS)

Werner, E., Dawson, G., Munson, J., & Osterling, J. (2005). Variation in early developmental course in autism and its relation with behavioral outcome at 3–4 years of age. *Journal of Autism and Developmental Disorders*, *35*(3), 337–350.

Werner, E., Dawson, G., Osterling, J., & Dinno, N. (2000). Brief report: Recognition of autism spectrum disorder before one year of age: A retrospective study based on home videos. *Journal of Autism and Developmental Disorders*, *30*, 157–162.

Werner, E. E. (1988). Individual differences, universal needs: A 30-year study of resilient high risk infants. *Zero to Three*, *8*(4), 1–5.

Werner, E. E. (2000). Protective factors and individual resilience. In J. P. Shonkoff, & S. J. Meisels (Eds.), *Handbook of early childhood intervention* (pp. 115–132). New York: Cambridge University Press.

Werner, E. E., & Smith, R. (1992). *Overcoming the odds: High risk children from birth to adulthood*. Ithaca, NY: Cornell University Press.

Werner, E. E., & Smith, R. (2001). *Journeys from childhood to midlife: Risk, resilience, and recovery*. Ithaca, NY: Cornell University Press.

Westby, C. E. (1980). Assessment of cognitive and language abilities through play. *Language, Speech, and Hearing Services in Schools*, *11*, 154–168.

Westby, C. E. (1988). *Symbolic Play Scale (SPS)*. Austin, TX: PRO-ED.

Westby, C. E. (1991). A scale for assessing children's pretend play. In C. Schaefer, K. Gitlin, & A. Sandgrund (Eds.), *Play diagnosis and assessment* (pp. 131–161). New York: Wiley.

Westby, C. E. (2000). A scale for assessing development of children's play, In K. Gitlin-Weiner, A. Sandgrund, & C. Schaefer (Eds.), *Play diagnosis and assessment* (2nd ed., pp. 15–57). New York: Wiley.

Wetherby, A. M., & Prizant, B. M. (1992). Profiling young children's communicative competence. In S. F. Warren & J. E. Reichle (Eds.), *Causes and effects in communication and language intervention* (pp. 217–253). Baltimore: Brookes.

Wetherby, A. M., & Prizant, B. M. (1993). Profiling communication and symbolic abilities in young children. *Journal of Childhood Communication Disorders*, *15*(1), 23–32.

White, K. R., & Boyce, G. C. (Eds.). (1993). Comparative evaluation of early intervention alternatives [Special issue]. *Early Education and Development*, *4*.

Whitebrook, M., Howes, C., & Phillips, D. (1990). *Who cares? Childcare teachers and the quality of care in America* (Final report of the National Child Care Staffing Study). Oakland, CA: Child Care Employee Project.

Whitehurst, G. J., & Lonigan, C. J. (1998). Child development and emergent literacy. *Child Development*, *69*, 848–872.

Whitehurst, G. J., & Lonigan, C. J. (2001). Emergent literacy: Development from prereaders to readers. In S. B. Neuman & D. K. Dickinson (Eds.), *Handbook of early literacy research* (Vol. 1, pp. 11–29). New York: Guilford Press.

Whiting, B., & Edwards, C. (1988). *Children of different worlds: The formation of social behavior*. Cambridge, MA: Harvard University Press.

Wieder, S., Poisson, S., Lourie, R. S., & Greenspan, S. I. (1988). Enduring gains: A five-year follow-up report on the clinical infant development program. *Zero to Three*, *8*(4), 6–12.

Wiig, E. H., & Semel, E. M. (1984). *Language assessment and intervention for the Learning disabled* (2nd ed.). Columbus, OH: Merrill.

Wiig, E. H., Secord, W. A., & Semel, E. (2005).

Clinical Evaluation of Language Fundamentals Preschool—Second Edition CELF Preschool-2). San Antonio, TX: Psychological Corporation.

Wilens, T. E., Biederman, J., Brown, S., Tanguay, S., Monuteaux, M. C., Blake, C., et al. (2002). Psychiatric comorbidity and functioning in clinically referred preschool children and school-age youth with ADHD. *Journal of the American Academy of Child and Adolescent Psychiatry, 41*(3), 262–268.

Wilkes, D. (1989). *Administration, classroom program, sponsorship: Are these indices of quality care in day care centers?* Unpublished doctoral dissertation, Georgia State University.

Wilkinson, K. M. (1998). Profiles of language and communication skills in autism. *Mental Retardation and Developmental Disabilities Research Reviews, 4,* 73–79.

Williams, K. (1997). *Expressive Vocabulary Test (EVT).* Bloomington, MN: AGS.

Willig, A. C. (1985). A meta-analysis of selected studies on the effectiveness of bilingual education. *Review of Educational Research, 55,* 269–317.

Willis, W. (2004). Families with African American roots. In E. W. Lynch & M. J. Hanson (Eds.), *Developing cross-cultural competence: A guide for working with children and their families* (3rd ed., pp. 141–177). Baltimore: Brookes.

Wilson, M. S., & Reschly, D. J. (1996). Assessment in school psychology training and practice. *School Psychology Review, 25*(1), 9–23.

Wing, L. (1981a) Asperger's syndrome: A clinical account. *Psychological Medicine, 11,* 115–130.

Wing, L. (1981b). Language, social, and cognitive impairments in autism and severe mental retardation. *Journal of Autism and Developmental Disorders, 11,* 31–44.

Wing, L. (1985). *Autistic children* (2nd ed.). New York: Brunner/Mazel.

Wing, L. (1990). What is autism? In K. Ellis (Ed.), *Autism: Professional perspectives and practice* (pp. 1–24). New York: Chapman & Hall.

Wing, L. (1998). The history of Asperger syndrome. In E. Schopler, G. B. Mesibov, & L. Kunce (Eds.), *Asperger syndrome or high-functioning autism?* (pp. 11–28). New York: Plenum Press.

Wing, L. (2000). Past and future of research on Asperger syndrome. In A. Klin, F. R. Volkmar, & S. S. Sparrow (Eds.), *Asperger syndrome* (pp. 418–432). New York: Guilford Press.

Wing, L., & Gould, J. (1979). Severe impairments of social interaction and associated abnormalities in children: Epidemiology and classification. *Journal of Autism and Developmental Disorders, 9,* 11–30.

Wing, L., & Potter, D. (2002). The epidemiology of autistic spectrum disorders: Is the prevalence rising? *Mental Retardation and Developmental Disabilities Research Reviews, 8,* 151–161.

Wohlwill, J. F., & Heft, H. (1997). The physical environment and the development of the child. In D. Stokols & J. Altman (Eds.), *Handbook of environmental psychology* (pp. 281–328). New York: Wiley.

Wolery, M. (1989). Using direct observation in assessment. In D. B. Bailey & M. Wolery (Eds.), *Assessing infants and preschoolers with handicaps* (pp. 64–96). Columbus, OH: Merrill.

Wolf, R. M. (2001). Test review of the Test of Children's Language (TOCL). In B. S. Plake & J. C. Impara (Eds.), *The fourteenth mental measurements yearbook* [Electronic version]. Retrieved from the Buros Institute's *Test Reviews Online* website: www.unl.edu/buros

Wong, V., Hui, L.-H. S., Lee, W.-C., Leung, L.-S., Ho, P.-K. P., Lau, W.-L. C., et al. (2004). A modified screening tool for autism (Checklist for Autism in Toddlers [CHAT-23]) for Chinese children. *Pediatrics, 114*(2), e166–e176.

Woodcock, R. W., & Johnson, M. B. (1989). *Woodcock—Johnson Psycho-Educational Battery Revised: Tests of Cognitive Ability.* Chicago: Riverside.

Woodcock, R. W., McGrew, K. S., & Mather, N. (2001a). *Woodcock–Johnson III Tests of Achievement, Preschool Cluster.* Itasca, IL: Riverside.

Woodcock, R. W., McGrew, K. S., & Mather, N. (2001b). *Woodcock–Johnson III Tests of Cognitive Abilities.* Itasca, IL: Riverside.

Woodcock, R., Muñoz-Sandoval, A., McGrew, K., Mather, N., & Schrank, F. (2005). *Bateria III Woodcock–Munoz.* Itasca, IL: Riverside.

World Health Organization. (1992). *International classification of diseases* (10th rev.). Geneva: Author.

Wozniak, J., & Biederman, J. (1995). Pre-pubertal mania exists (and co-exists with ADHD). *ADHD Report, 2*(3), 5–6.

Wright, C. (2001). Test review of the Comprehensive Test of Phonological Processing. In B. S. Plake, J. C. Impara & R. A. Spies (Eds.), *The fifteenth mental measurements yearbook* [Electronic Version]. Retrieved from http://web5.silverplatter.com/webspirs/start.ws?customer=waldo&databases=(YB)

Wright, C. R. (2003). Test review of the Comprehensive Test of Phonological Processing. In B. S. Plake, J. C. Impara, & R. A. Spies (Eds.),

The fifteenth mental measurements yearbook [Electronic version]. Retrieved from http://web5s.silverplatter.com.arugula.cc.columbia.edu:2048/webspirs/start/ws?customer=waldo&databases=YB

Wright, L., & Borland, J. H. (1993). Using early childhood developmental portfolios in the identification and education of young, economically disadvantaged, potentially gifted students. *Roeper Review, 15*(4), 205–210.

Wulbert, M., Inglis, S., Kriegsman, E., & Mills, B. (1975). Language delay and associated mother–child interactions. *Developmental Psychology, 2*, 61–70.

Yingling, L. C. (2004). Child and family assessment: Strategies and inventories. In L. Sperry (Ed.), *Assessment of couples and families* (pp. 159–181). New York: Brunner-Routledge.

Yirmiya, N., Sigman, M., & Freeman, B. J. (1994). Comparison between diagnostic instruments for identifying high-functioning children with autism. *Journal of Autism and Developmental Disorders, 24*(3), 281–291.

Yolton, K., & Bolig, R. (1994). Psychosocial, behavioral, and developmental characteristics of toddlers prenatally exposed to cocaine. *Child Study Journal, 24*, 49–68.

Young, J. G., Grasic, J. R., & Leven, L. (1990). Genetic causes of Autism and the pervasive developmental disorders. In S. I. Deutsch, A. Weizman, & R. Weizman (Eds.), *Application of basic neuroscience to child psychiatry* (pp. 183–216). New York: Springer.

Young, J. G., Newcorn, J., & Leven, L. (1989). Pervasive developmental disorders. In H. I. Kaplan & B. J. Sadock (Eds.), *Comprehensive textbook of psychiatry* (5th ed., Vol. 2, pp. 1772–1787). Baltimore: Williams & Wilkins.

Ysseldyke, J. E., & Christenson, S. L. (1987). Evaluating students' instructional environments. *Remedial and Special Education, 8*(3), 17–24.

Ysseldyke, J. E., & Christenson, S. L. (1988). Linking assessment to intervention. In J. L. Graden, J. E. Zins, & M. J. Curtis (Eds.), *Alternative educational delivery systems: Enhancing instructional options for all students* (pp. 91–109). Washington, DC: National Association of School Psychologists.

Ysseldyke, J. E., & Christenson, S. L. (1993–1996). *The Instructional Environment Scale–II (TIES-II)*. Longmont, CO: Sopris West.

Ysseldyke, J. E., & Christenson, S. L. (2002). *Functional Assessment of Academic Behavior: Creating successful learning environments.* Longmon, CO: Sopris West.

Zeanah, C. H., & Boris, N. W. (2000). Disturbances and disorders of attachment in early childhood. In C. H. Zeanah (Ed.), *Handbook of infant mental health* (2nd ed., pp. 353–368). New York: Guilford Press.

Zeitlin, S. (1976). *Kindergarten screening: Early identification of potential high-risk learners.* Springfield, IL: Thomas.

Zentall, S. S. (1983). Learning environments: A review of physical and temporal factors. *Exceptional Education Quarterly, 4*, 90–115.

Zero to Three. (2005). *Diagnostic classification of mental health and developmental disorders of infancy and early childhood: Revised edition (DC:0–3R)*. Washington, DC: Author.

Zhou, Z., & Boehm, A. E. (2004). American and Chinese children's understanding of basic relational concepts in directions. *Psychology in the Schools, 41*, 261–272.

Zigler, E., Balla, D., & Hodapp, R. M. (1986). On the definition and classification of mental retardation. *American Journal of Mental Deficiency, 89*, 215–230.

Zigler, E., & Muenchow, S. (1992). *Head Start: The inside story of America's most successful educational experiment.* New York: Basic Books.

Zimmerman, I. L., Steiner, V. G., & Pond, R. (2002). *Preschool Language Scale—Fourth Edition.* San Antonio, TX: Psychological Corporation.

Zuniga, M. E. (2004). Families with Latino roots. In E. W. Lynch & M. J. Hanson (Eds.), *Developing cross-cultural competence: A guide for working with children and their families* (3rd ed., pp. 179–217). Baltimore: Brookes.

Index

B

C

D

E

F

G

H

Q

R

S

T

U

V

W